CLINICAL MANIFESTATIONS AND ASSESSMENT OF RESPIRATORY DISEASE

FIFTH EDITION

Terry Des Jardins, MEd, RRT

Director
Professor Emeritus
Department of Respiratory Care
Parkland College
Champaign, Illinois

George G. Burton, MD, FACP, FCCP, FAARC

Associate Dean for Medical Affairs
Kettering College of Medical Arts
Kettering, Ohio
Clinical Professor of Medicine and Anesthesiology
Wright State University School of Medicine
Dayton, Ohio

Medical Illustrations By
Timothy H. Phelps, MS, FAMI, CMI

Associate Professor
Johns Hopkins University School of Medicine
Baltimore, Maryland

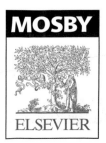

MOSBY

ELSEVIER

MOSBY
ELSEVIER

11830 Westline Industrial Drive
St. Louis, Missouri 63146

CLINICAL MANIFESTATIONS AND ASSESSMENT OF
RESPIRATORY DISEASE, FIFTH EDITION
ISBN 978-0-323-02806-6
ISBN 0-323-02806-3
Copyright © 2006, Mosby Inc.

Previous editions copyrighted 1984, 1990, 1995, 2002

ISBN 978-0-323-02806-6
ISBN 0-323-02806-3

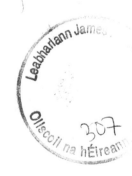

Printed in the United States

Last digit is the print number: 9 8 7 6 5 4 3 2

To
Wenda and Jean

Contributor

Beverly Ervin, MSA, RRT
Kettering College of Medical Arts
Kettering, Ohio

Reviewers

Regina Clark, BS, RRT
Program Director
Respiratory Therapy
Northwest Mississippi Community College
Southaven, Mississippi

Martha DeSilva, MEd, RRT
Program Director
Massasoit Community College
Brockton, Massachusetts

Glenn N. Hojem, MA, RRT
Program Director, Respiratory Care Practitioner
   Program
Program Director, Polysomnography Program
Madison Area Technical College
Madison, Wisconsin

Joe A. Koss, MS
Director of Clinical Education
Respiratory Therapy Program
Indiana University
Indianapolis, Indiana

Robert A. Muller, MA, RRT
Chairman, Allied Health Department
Director, Respiratory Therapy Program
Bergen Community College
Paramus, New Jersey

Debra Waterman, MS
Assistant Professor
Health Services
Mohawk Valley Community College
Utica, New York

"(There is a) manpower shortage of health-care providers who care for the critically ill. This is one of the most pressing issues affecting the future of our aging population and American medicine...it has been generally acknowledged...that the shortages in nursing, respiratory care practitioners, and pharmacists have already reached crisis levels...a severe shortage of (pulmonary/critical care physicians) can be expected by 2007."[1]

"...respiratory therapists are important for patient outcome *and their roles might even be expanded beyond traditional boundaries.* More research is needed to define the ICU multidisciplinary staffing that matches patient needs and optimizes patient outcomes."[2]

1. Irwin RS, Marcus L, Lever A: The Critical Care Professional Societies address the critical care crisis in the United States, *Chest* 125:1512-1513, 2004.
2. Kelly MA, Angus D, Chalfin DB, et al: The critical care crisis in the United States, *Chest* 125: 1514-1517, 2004.

Preface

The use of therapist-driven protocols (TDPs) is increasing and is now an integral part of respiratory health services. TDPs provide much-needed flexibility to respiratory care practitioners and increase the quality of health care because therapy can be modified easily and efficiently according to the needs of the patient.

Central to the success of the TDP is the quality of the respiratory therapist's assessment skills at the bedside and the ability to transfer findings into a treatment plan that follows agreed-upon guidelines. The respiratory care practitioner must be able to recognize when physician- and patient-specific severity indicators have been reached or exceeded and must be able to communicate concerns to the physicians and other health care workers who need to hear them.

This textbook is designed to provide the student with the basic knowledge and understanding essential to assess and treat patients with respiratory diseases. To meet this objective, this text provides the reader with the following:

1. A detailed illustration (both in color and black-and-white) of the major anatomic alterations of the lungs (or related anatomic structures) caused by various respiratory disorders
2. The pathophysiologic mechanisms that are most commonly activated as a result of the anatomic alterations

3. An overview of the cardiopulmonary clinical manifestations caused by the pathophysiologic mechanisms
4. A listing of various treatment modalities used to offset the clinical manifestations caused by the anatomic alterations and pathophysiologic mechanisms

The student is provided with the basic knowledge and helpful tools to gather clinical data systematically, formulate an assessment (i.e., the cause and severity of the clinical data), select an appropriate and cost-effective treatment plan, and document these essential steps clearly and precisely. In addition, students can further test their skills by going through the practice case studies provided in Part XIV. Representative case studies build on the information presented in this book by allowing the student to apply it to an evolving case study built on commonly used TDPs.

Finally, in writing this textbook, we have tried to present a realistic balance between the esoteric language of pathophysiology and the simple, straight-to-the-point approach generally preferred by busy students.

Terry Des Jardins

George G. Burton

Acknowledgments

For the numerous new radiographic images for the fifth edition, our appreciation goes to Joseph Barkmeier, MD, Urbana, Illinois. For the many new graphic illustrations created for this textbook—especially those presented in Chapter 9—a very special thank you goes to Wenda Speers, Marketing and Creative Services, Parkland College, Champaign, Illinois.

For her review and updates for the neonatal and early childhood respiratory disorders, our gratitude goes to Beverly Ervin, RRT, Kettering College of Medical Arts. For the long hours spent in the development and production of this fifth edition, our appreciation also goes to Mindy Hutchinson, Melissa Boyle, and David Stein of Elsevier.

How to Use This Book

Part I, entitled *Assessment of Respiratory Disease,* consists of three sections. **Section I** consists of two chapters. Chapter 1 describes the knowledge and skills involved in the patient interview. Chapter 2 provides the knowledge and skills needed for the physical examination. Chapter 2 also presents a more in-depth discussion of the pathophysiologic basis for the clinical manifestations associated with respiratory diseases.

Section II is composed of Chapters 3 through 8. Collectively these chapters provide the reader with the essential knowledge and understanding base for the assessment of pulmonary function studies, arterial blood gases, oxygenation, the cardiovascular system (including hemodynamic monitoring), important laboratory tests and procedures, and the radiologic examination of the chest.

Section III consists of Chapters 9 and 10. Chapter 9, entitled *The Therapist-Driven Protocol Program and the Role of the Respiratory Care Practitioner,* provides the reader with the essential knowledge base and the step-by-step process needed to assess and implement respiratory care protocols in the clinical setting. The reader is often referred back to this chapter, which is a cornerstone chapter to the textbook. Chapter 10 is entitled *Recording Skills: The Basis for Data Collection, Organization, Assessment Skills, and Treatment Plans.* Chapters 9 and 10 both provide the reader with the fundamentals for collecting and recording assessment data and improving critical thinking skills.

In subsequent chapters on respiratory diseases (**Parts II to XIII**) the student is often referred back to Part I to supplement the discussion of the clinical manifestations commonly associated with each disease. For example, Section II describes many of the known pathophysiologic mechanisms and therefore explains why various clinical manifestations develop in the respiratory disorder under discussion. In addition, the reader is not only shown that acute alveolar hyperventilation and hypoxemia commonly develop during the early stages of pneumonia but also learns why these abnormal arterial blood gases occur.

Again, the reader is frequently referred back to Chapter 9, especially during the overviews that appear in each respiratory disease chapter.

Parts II through **XIII** (Chapters 11 through 45) provide the reader with essential information on common respiratory diseases. Each chapter adheres to the following format: anatomic alterations of the lungs, etiology of the disease process, overview of the cardiopulmonary clinical manifestations associated with the disorder, general management of the disorder, case study, and a brief set of self-assessment questions.

Anatomic Alterations of the Lungs

Each chapter on respiratory disease begins with a detailed illustration showing the anatomic alterations of the lungs caused by the disease. Although a serious effort has been made to illustrate each disorder accurately at the beginning of each chapter, artistic license has been taken to emphasize certain anatomic points and pathologic processes.

The subsequent material in each chapter discusses the disease in terms of (1) the anatomic alterations of the lungs caused by the disease, (2) the pathophysiologic mechanisms activated throughout the respiratory system as a result of the anatomic alterations, (3) the clinical manifestations that develop as a result of the pathophysiologic mechanisms, and (4) the basic respiratory therapy modalities used to improve the anatomic alterations and pathophysiologic mechanisms caused by the disease. When the anatomic alterations and pathophysiologic mechanisms caused by the disorder are improved, the clinical manifestations also should improve.

Etiology

A discussion of the etiology of the disease follows the presentation of anatomic alterations of the lungs. Various causes and predisposing conditions are described.

Overview of the Cardiopulmonary Clinical Manifestations Associated With the Disorder

The overview section represents the central theme of the text. The reader is provided with the clinical manifestations commonly associated with the disease under discussion. In essence the student is given a general "baseline" of the signs and symptoms commonly demonstrated by the patient. By having a working knowledge—and predetermined expectation—of the clinical manifestations associated with a specific respiratory disorder, the practitioner is in a better position to (1) gather clinical data relevant to the patient's respiratory status, (2) formulate an objective and measurable respiratory and severity assessment, and (3) select an effective and safe treatment plan that is based on a valid assessment. If the appropriate data are not gathered and assessed correctly, the ability to treat the patient effectively is lost.

As mentioned earlier, many of the clinical manifestations listed refer the reader back to specific pages in Part I for a broader discussion of the pathophysiologic mechanisms usually responsible for the identified sign or symptom. ◆ When a particular manifestation is unique to the respiratory disorder, however, a discussion of the pathophysiologic mechanisms responsible for the signs and symptoms is presented in the respective chapter.

Because of the dynamic nature of many respiratory disorders, the reader should note the following regarding this section:

- Because the severity of the disease is influenced by a number of factors (e.g., magnitude of the disease, age, general health of the patient), the clinical manifestations may vary remarkably from one patient to another. In fact, they may vary in the same patient from one time to another. Therefore the practitioner should understand that the patient may demonstrate *all* the clinical manifestations presented or just a *few*. In addition, many of the clinical manifestations associated with a respiratory disorder may never appear in some patients (e.g., digital clubbing, cor pulmonale, increased hemoglobin level). As a general rule, however, the patient usually demonstrates most of the manifestations presented during the advanced stages of the disease.
- Some of the clinical manifestations presented in each chapter may not actually be measured (or measurable) in the clinical setting for a variety of practical reasons (e.g., age, mental status, severity of the disorder). They are nevertheless conceptually important and therefore are presented here through extrapolation. For example, the newborn with severe infant respiratory distress syndrome, who obviously has a restrictive lung disorder as a result of the anatomic alterations associated with the disease, cannot actually perform the maneuvers necessary for a pulmonary function study.
- The clinical manifestations presented in each chapter are based only on the one respiratory disorder under discussion. In the clinical setting, the patient often has a combination of respiratory problems (e.g., emphysema compromised by pneumonia) and may have manifestations related to each of the pulmonary disorders.

This section does not attempt to present the "absolute" pathophysiologic bases for the development of a particular clinical manifestation. Because of the dynamic nature of many respiratory diseases, the precise cause of some of the manifestations presented by the patient is not always clear. In most cases, however, the pathophysiologic mechanisms responsible for the various signs and symptoms are known and understood.

General Management or Treatment of the Disease

Each chapter provides a general overview of the more common therapeutic modalities (treatment protocols) used to offset the anatomic alterations and pathophysiologic mechanisms activated by a particular disorder.

Although several respiratory therapy modalities may be safe and effective in treating a respiratory disorder, the respiratory care practitioner must have a clear conception of the following:

1. The way the therapies offset the anatomic alterations of the lungs caused by the disease
2. The way the correction of the anatomic alterations of the lungs offsets the pathophysiologic mechanisms
3. The way the correction of the pathophysiologic mechanisms offsets the clinical manifestations demonstrated by the patient

Without this understanding, the practitioner merely goes through the motions of performing therapeutic tasks with no anticipated or measurable outcomes.

Case Study

The case study provides the reader with a realistic example of (1) the manner in which the patient may arrive in the hospital with the disorder under discussion, (2) the various clinical manifestations commonly associated with the disease, (3) the way the clinical manifestations can be gathered and organized, (4) the way an assessment of the patient's respiratory status is formulated from the clinical manifestations, and (5) the way the treatment plan is developed from the assessment.

The case study provides the reader with an example of the way a respiratory care practitioner would assess and treat a patient with the disorder under discussion. In addition, many of the case studies presented in the text describe a respiratory care practitioner assessing and treating the patient several times—demonstrating the importance of assessment skills and the way therapy is often up-regulated or down-regulated on a moment-to-moment basis in the clinical setting. Finally, it should be noted that Part XIV provides the reader with additional practice case studies (and suggested answers) to further supplement each disease category presented in the textbook (i.e., respiratory disorders discussed in Parts II through XIII).

Self-Assessment Questions

Each disease chapter concludes with a set of self-assessment questions that stress pathophysiologic rather than treatment-based understanding. The student may be asked questions from the disease chapter under discussion or questions arising from Part I, which often provides a broader understanding of the various treatment modalities commonly used to manage the disease under discussion.

Glossary and Appendices

Finally, a glossary and appendices are provided at the end of the text. The appendices include the following:

- A table of symbols and abbreviations commonly used in respiratory physiology
- Medications commonly used in the treatment of cardiopulmonary disorders, including the following:
  - Aerosolized bronchodilators
  - Mucolytic agents
  - Aersolized antiinflammatory agents
  - Xanthine bronchodilators
  - Expectorants
  - Antibiotic agents
  - Positive inotropic agents
  - Diuretics
- The ideal alveolar gas equation
- Physiologic dead space calculation
- Units of measurement
- Poiseuille's law
- $P_{CO_2}/HCO_3^-/pH$ nomogram
- Calculated hemodynamic measurements
- DuBois body surface area chart
- Cardiopulmonary profile
- Answers to the self-assessment questions
- Answers to selected practice case studies

Contents

Introduction

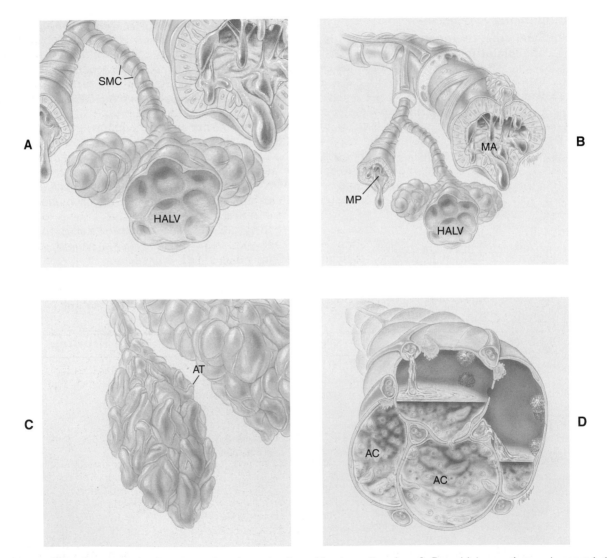

Figure 1 *Common anatomic alterations of the lungs in obstructive lung disorders.* **A,** Bronchial smooth muscle constriction accompanied by air trapping (as seen in asthma). **B,** Tracheobronchial inflammation accompanied by mucus accumulation, partial airway obstruction, and air trapping (as seen in bronchitis). When mucus accumulation causes total airway obstruction, alveolar atelectasis ensues.
Common anatomic alterations of the lungs in restrictive lung disorders. **C,** Alveolar collapse or atelectasis. **D,** Alveolar consolidation (as seen in pneumonia). *SMC,* Smooth muscle constriction; *HALV,* hyperinflated alveoli; *MA,* mucus accumulation; *MP,* mucus plug; *AT,* atelectasis; *AC,* alveolar consolidation.

Introduction

The Assessment Process—An Overview

Assessment is (1) the process of collecting clinical information about the patient's health status, (2) evaluating the data and identifying the specific problems, concerns, and needs of the patient, and (3) the development of a treatment plan that can be managed by the health care provider. The clinical information gathered may consist of subjective and objective data (signs and symptoms) about the patient, the results of diagnostic tests and procedures, the patient's response to therapy, and the patient's general health practices.

The first step in the assessment process is THINKING—even before the actual collection of clinical data begins. In other words, the practitioner must first "think" about why the patient has entered the health care facility and about what clinical data will likely need to be collected. Merely obtaining answers to a specific list of questions does not serve the assessment process well. For example, while en route to evaluate a patient who is said to be having an asthmatic episode, the health care practitioner might mentally consider the following: What are the likely signs and symptoms that can be observed at the bedside during a moderate or severe asthmatic attack? What are the usual emotional responses? What are the anatomical alterations associated with an asthma episode that would be responsible for the signs and symptoms observed? Table 1 presents a broader overview of what the practitioner might think about prior to assessing a patient said to be having an asthmatic episode.

TABLE 1 Examples of What Might Be Considered Before Evaluating a Patient Having an Asthmatic Episode

Questions and/or Considerations	Likely Responses
What are the likely initial observations?	Shortness of breath, use of accessory muscles to breathe, intercostal retractions, pursed-lip breathing; cyanosis, barrel chest
What might be the patient's emotional response to his asthma?	Anxiety, concerned, frightened
What are the anatomic alterations of the lungs associated with asthma?	Bronchospasm; excessive, thick, white, & tenacious bronchial secretions; air trapping; mucus plugging
What are the known causes of asthma?	Extrinsic factors: pollen, grass, house dust, animal dander Intrinsic factors: infection, cold air, exercise, emotional stress
What are the expected vital signs?	Increased respiratory rate, heart rate, and blood pressure
What are the expected chest assessment findings?	Breath sounds: diminished, wheezing, rhonchi Percussion: hyperresonant
What are the expected pulmonary function study findings?	Decreased PEFR, FEF_T, FEV_T/FVC Increased: RV, FRC
What are the expected acute arterial blood gas findings?	Increased pH, decreased $Paco_2$, decreased HCO_3^-, decreased Pao_2, decreased Sao_2 and Spo_2
What are the expected chest radiograph findings?	Translucent lung fields; hyperinflated alveoli; depressed diaphragm
What are the usual respiratory treatments?	Bronchodilator therapy, bronchial hygiene therapy; oxygen therapy
What complications can occur?	Poor response to oxygen & bronchodilator therapy Acute ventilatory failure Severe hypoxia. Mechanical ventilation

To collect data wisely, health care providers must have well-developed skills in observing and listening. In addition, the practitioner must apply his or her mental skills of translation, reason, intuition, and validation to render the clinical data meaningful. Clinically, the collection of data is more useful when the evaluation process is organized into common problem areas, or categories. As the practitioner gathers information under each problem category, a clustering of related data will be generated about the patient. This framework for collecting clinical information enhances the practitioner's ability to establish priorities of care. Furthermore, any time the health care provider interacts with the patient, for any reason, an assessment of the patient's problems, needs, and concerns should be made. To efficiently and correctly gather data, the health care provider must make decisions about what type of assessment is needed, how to obtain the data, the framework and focus of the assessment, and what additional data may be needed before a complete treatment plan can be developed.

Purpose of Assessment

Relative to the purpose, an assessment may involve asking just two or three specific questions or it may involve an in-depth conversation with the patient. An assessment may involve a comprehensive focus (head-to-toe assessment) or a specific or narrow focus. The purpose of the assessment may include any of the following:

- To obtain a baseline databank about the patient's physical and mental status
- To supplement, verify, or refute any previous data
- To identify actual and potential problems
- To obtain data that will help the practitioner establish an assessment and treatment plan
- To focus on specific problems
- To determine immediate needs and to establish priorities
- To determine the cause (etiology) of the problem
- To determine any related or contributing factors
- To identify patient strengths as a basis for changing behavior
- To identify the risk for complications
- To recognize complications

Types of Assessment

There are four major types of assessment: *initial, focused, emergency,* and *ongoing.*

The **initial assessment** is conducted at the first encounter with the patient. In the hospitalized patient, the initial assessment is typically performed by the admitting nurse and is more comprehensive than subsequent assessments. It starts with the reasons that prompted the patient to seek care, and it entails a holistic overview of the patient's health care needs. The general objective of the initial assessment is to rule out as well as to identify (rule in) specific problems. The initial assessment most commonly occurs when the patient has sought medical services for a specific problem or desires a general health status examination. The goals of the initial assessment include prevention, maintenance, restoration, or rehabilitation. In general, the thoroughness of the initial assessment is directly proportional to the length of expected care.

The **focused assessment** consists of a detailed examination of the specific problem areas, or patient complaints. The focused assessment looks at clinical data in detail, considers possible etiologies, looks at possible contributing factors, and examines the patient's personal characteristics that will help—or hinder—the problem. The focused assessment also occurs when the patient describes or presents with a new problem. Common patient complaints include pain, shortness of breath, dizziness, and fatigue. The practitioner must be prepared to evaluate the severity of such problems, assess the possible cause, and determine the appropriate plan of action.

The **emergency assessment** identifies—or rules out—any life-threatening problems or problems that require immediate interventions. When the patient's medical status is life threatening, or time is of the essence, the emergency assessment will include only key data needed for dealing with the immediate problem. Additional information can be gathered after the patient's condition has stabilized. The emergency assessment always follows the basic "ABCs" of cardiopulmonary resuscitation (i.e., the securing of the patient's airway, breathing, and circulation).

The **ongoing assessment** consists of the data collection that occurs during each contact with the patient throughout the patient's hospital stay. Depending on the patient's condition, ongoing assessments may take place hourly, daily, weekly, or monthly. In fact, for the critically ill patient, assessments often take place continuously via electronic monitoring equipment. Ongoing assessments also take place while a patient is receiving anesthesia, as well as afterwards until the effects of the anesthesia have worn off.

Respiratory therapy practitioners routinely make decisions about the frequency, depth, and breadth of the assessment requirements of the patient. To make these decisions effectively, the practitioner must anticipate the potential for a patient's condition to change, the speed at which it could change, and the clinical data that would justify a change. For example, when a patient experiencing an asthmatic episode inhales the aerosol of a selected bronchodilator, assessment decisions are based on the expected onset of drug action, expected therapeutic effects of the medication, and potential adverse effects that may develop.

Types of Data

Clinical information that is provided by the patient, and that cannot be observed directly, is called **subjective data**. When a patient's subjective data describe characteristics of a particular disorder or dysfunction, they are known as **symptoms**. For example, shortness of breath (dyspnea), pain, dizziness, nausea, and ringing in the ears are called symptoms because they cannot be observed directly. The patient must communicate to the health care provider what symptoms he or she is experiencing. The patient is the only source of information about subjective findings.

Characteristics about the patient that can be observed directly by the practitioner are called **objective data**. When a patient's objective data describe characteristics of a particular disorder or dysfunction, they are known as **signs**. For example, swelling of the legs (pedal edema) is a sign of congestive heart failure. Objective data can be obtained through the practitioner's sense of sight, hearing, taste, touch, and smell. Objective information can be measured (or quantified) and it can be replicated from one practitioner to another—a concept called *inter-rater reliability*. For example, the respiratory practitioner can measure the patient's pulse, respiratory rate, blood pressure, inspiratory effort, or arterial blood gases. Because objective data are factual, they have a high degree of certainty.

Sources of Data

Sources of clinical information may include the patient, the patient's significant others, other members of the health care team, the patient's past history, and results from a variety of clinical tests and procedures. The practitioner must confirm that each data source is appropriate, reliable, and valid for the patient's assessment. *Appropriate* means the source is suitable for the specific purpose, patient, or event. *Reliable* means that the practitioner can trust the data

to be accurate and honestly reported. **Valid** means that the clinical data can be verified or confirmed.

The Assessment Process—The Role of the Respiratory Practitioner

When the lungs are affected by disease or trauma, they are anatomically altered to some degree, depending on the severity of the process. In general, the **anatomic alterations** caused by an injury or disease process can be classified as resulting in an obstructive lung disorder, a restrictive lung disorder, or a combination of both. Common anatomic alterations associated with obstructive and restrictive lung disorders are illustrated in Figure 1. Common respiratory diseases and their general classifications are listed in Table 2.

When the normal anatomy of the lungs is altered, certain **pathophysiologic mechanisms** throughout the cardiopulmonary system are activated. These pathophysiologic mechanisms, in turn, produce a variety of **clinical manifestations** specific to the illness. Such clinical manifestations can be readily— and objectively—identified in the clinical setting (e.g., increased heart rate, depressed diaphragm, increased functional residual capacity). Because differing chains of events happen as a result of anatomic alterations of the lungs, treatment selection is most appropriately directed at the basic causes of the clinical manifestations—that is, the anatomic alterations of the lungs. For example, a clinician prescribes a bronchodilator to offset the bronchospasm associated with an asthmatic episode.

The Knowledge Base

A strong knowledge base of the following four factors is essential to good respiratory care assessment and therapy selection skills:

1. Anatomic alterations of the lungs caused by common respiratory disorders
2. Major pathophysiologic mechanisms activated throughout the respiratory system as a result of the anatomic alterations
3. Common clinical manifestations that develop
4. Treatment modalities used to correct the anatomic alterations and pathophysiologic mechanisms caused by the disorder

Specific Components of the Assessment Process

A respiratory care practitioner with good assessment and treatment selection skills must be competent in

TABLE 2   General Classification of Respiratory Diseases

Respiratory Disease	Classification		
	Obstructive	Restrictive	Combination
Chronic bronchitis	X		
Emphysema	X		
Bronchiectasis			X
Asthma	X		
Pneumonia		X	
Lung abscess		X	
Tuberculosis		X	
Fungal disease of the lungs		X	
Pulmonary edema		X	
Flail chest		X	
Pneumothorax		X	
Kyphoscoliosis		X	
Pneumoconiosis			X
Cancer of the lungs		X	
Adult respiratory distress syndrome		X	
Chronic interstitial lung disease		X	
Meconium aspiration syndrome			X
Transient tachypnea of the newborn			X
Idiopathic respiratory distress syndrome		X	
Pulmonary interstitial emphysema			X
Bronchiolitis			X
Bronchopulmonary dysplasia			X
Diaphragmatic hernia		X	
Cystic fibrosis			X
Near drowning	X		

performing the actual assessment process, which has the following components:

1. Quick and systematic collection of the important clinical manifestations demonstrated by the patient
2. Formulation of an accurate assessment of the clinical data—that is, identification of the *cause* and *severity* of the data abnormalities
3. Selection of an optimal treatment modality
4. Quick, clear, and precise documentation of this process

Without this basic knowledge and understanding, the respiratory care practitioner merely goes through the motions of performing assigned therapeutic tasks with no short- or long-term anticipated outcomes that can be measured. In such an environment the practitioner works in an unchallenging task-oriented rather than goal-oriented manner.

That goal-oriented (patient-oriented) respiratory care has become the hallmark of practice was suggested in the early 1990s by analyzing the work performance of other health care disciplines. For example, physical therapists had long been greatly empowered by virtue of the more generic physician's orders under which they work; respiratory therapists, on the other hand, customarily received detailed and specific orders. For example, physical therapists are instructed to "improve back range of motion" or "strengthen quadriceps muscle groups," rather than to "provide warm fomentations to the low back" or "initiate quadriceps setting exercises with 10-pound ankle weights." In addition, physical therapists are permitted to start, up-regulate, down-regulate, or discontinue the therapy on the basis of the patient's current needs and capabilities—not on the basis of a 2-hour-, 2-day-, or 2-week-old physician assessment. Goal achievement, not task completion, is the way the success of physical therapy is routinely measured.

In the current "sicker in, quicker out" cost-conscious environment, a change has come to respiratory care. Under fixed reimbursement programs, shorter lengths of stay have required hospital administrators and medical staff to examine allocation of health care resources. Recent data suggest that fully one third of all hospitalized patients receive respiratory care services; therefore such services have come under close scrutiny. Studies using available peer-reviewed clinical practice guidelines have identified tremendous overuse (and, less frequently, underuse) of therapy modalities, and from this misallocation, the now firmly entrenched "**therapist-driven protocol**" (TDP) approach has emerged as the new "Gold Standard" of respiratory care practice. Observing that the patient (and more accurately, the pulmonary pathophysiology!) should set the pace, some centers have called this "patient-driven protocols," but the appellation of TDP has more strongly caught on. Clinical practice guidelines such as those developed by the American Association of Respiratory Care (AARC) are routinely used as the basis for TDPs in respiratory care.

The American College of Chest Physicians defines respiratory care protocols as follows:

> Patient care plans which are initiated and implemented by credentialed respiratory care workers. These plans are designed and developed with input from physicians, and are approved for use by the medical staff and the governing body of the hospitals in which they are used. They share in common extreme reliance on assessment and evaluation skills. Protocols are by their nature dynamic and flexible, allowing up- or down-regulation of intensity of respiratory services. Protocols allow the respiratory care practitioner authority to evaluate the patient, initiate care, to adjust, discontinue, or restart respiratory care procedures on a shift-by-shift or hour-to-hour basis once the protocol is ordered by the physician. They must contain clear strategies for various therapeutic interventions, while avoiding any misconception that they infringe on the practice of medicine.

Numerous studies have now shown beyond a shadow of a doubt that when respiratory care protocol guidelines are followed appropriately, the outcomes of respiratory care services improve. This improvement is noted in both clinical and economic ways (e.g., shorter ventilator weaning time in post-operative coronary artery bypass graft [CABG] patients). Under this paradigm, respiratory care that is inappropriately ordered is either withheld or modified (whichever is appropriate) and patients who *need* respiratory care services (but are not receiving them) should now be able to receive care. (Chapter 9 discusses the implementation of a good TDP program in detail.) The notion that today's respiratory care practitioner "might" practice in the TDP setting has passed. Respiratory practitioners who find that they are working in an archaic setting where TDPs are not in daily use should critically re-examine their employment options and career goals! To practice in today's health care environment without the cognitive (thinking) skills used in the TDP environment is no longer acceptable.

Experience, however, indicates that at least *some* respiratory care practitioners are not entirely comfortable with the new role and responsibility the TDP paradigm has thrust on them. These workers have difficulty separating the contents of *their* "little black bag" of diagnostic and therapeutic modalities from the one traditionally carried and used by the physician. The choice to be a "protocol safe and ready therapist," however, is no longer elective. The profession of respiratory care has changed and moved on. The Clinical Simulation Examination portion of the National Board for Respiratory Care (NBRC) Advanced Practitioner Examination reflects the actual, no longer just "simulated," bedside practice of respiratory care.

Similar to their physical therapist colleagues, today's respiratory care practitioners are now routinely asked to participate actively in the appropriate allocation of respiratory care services. Modern respiratory care practitioners must process the basic knowledge, skills, and personal attributes to collect and assess clinical data and treat their patients effectively. Under the TDP paradigm, specific indications (clinical manifestations) for a particular respiratory care procedure must first be identified. In other words, a specific treatment plan is only started, up-regulated, down-regulated, or discontinued on the basis of (1) the presence and collection of specific clinical data and (2) an assessment made from the clinical data (i.e., the cause of the clinical data) that justifies the therapy order or change. In addition, after a particular treatment has been administered to the patient, all treatment outcomes must be measured and documented. Clearly, the success or failure of protocol work depends on accurate and timely patient assessment.

In view of the above, it must be stressed that today's respiratory care practitioner must have competent bedside pulmonary assessment skills. Fundamental to this process is the ability to systematically gather clinical data, make an assessment, and develop an appropriate, safe, and effective action plan. Typically, once a treatment regimen has been implemented, the patient's progress is monitored on an ongoing assessment basis. In other words, clinical data are, again, collected, evaluated, and acted on based on the patient's progress toward a predefined goal.

To be fully competent in the assessment of respiratory disorders, the respiratory care practitioner must first have a strong academic foundation in the areas presented in Part I of this textbook. Part I is divided into three sections:

1. Important clinical data obtained at the patient's bedside (patient interview and physical examination)

2. Clinical data obtained from laboratory tests and special procedures (pulmonary function study assessments, arterial blood gas assessments, oxygenation assessments, cardiovascular system assessments, other important laboratory tests and special procedures, and radiologic examination of the chest)
3. Assessment processes for respiratory diseases (using the TDP approach and recording skills essential to that approach)

Part I provides the reader with the essential knowledge base to assess and treat the patient with respiratory disease. The respiratory care practitioner must master this section to work efficiently and safely in a good TDP program. The student will often be referred back to the first part of this textbook (via this symbol ◆) to supplement discussions in the respiratory disease chapters.

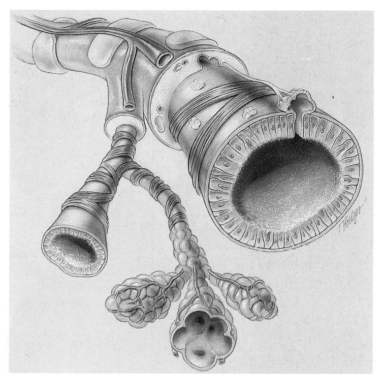

Plate 1 Normal lung (see Fig. 2-49).

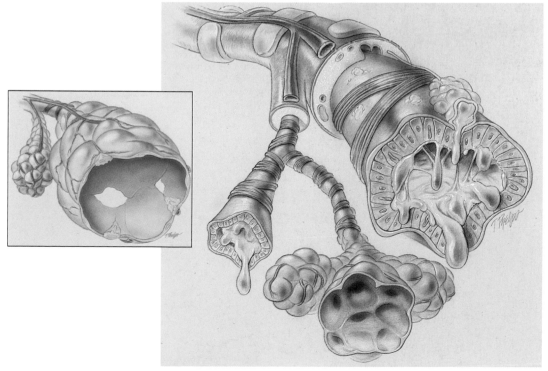

Plate 2 Chronic bronchitis. *Inset,* Weakened distal airways in emphysema, a common secondary anatomic alteration of the lungs (see Fig. 11-1).

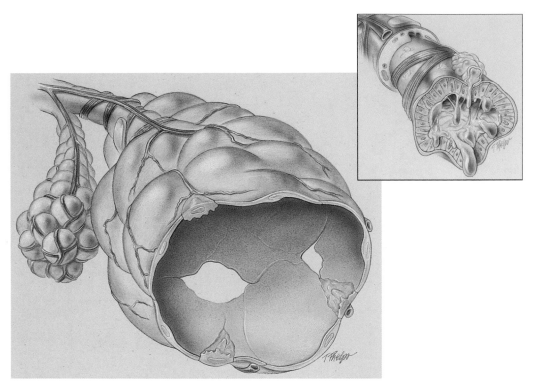

Plate 3 Panlobular emphysema. *Inset,* Excessive bronchial secretions, a common secondary anatomic alteration of the lungs (see Fig. 12-1).

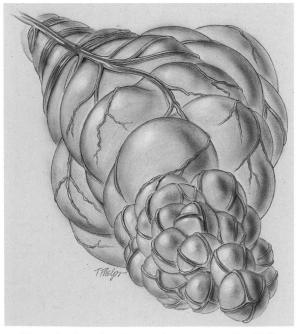

Plate 4 Centrilobular emphysema (see Fig. 12-2).

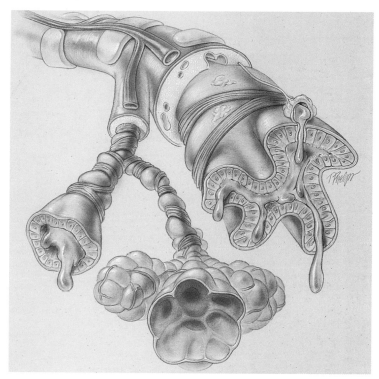

Plate 5 Asthma (see Fig. 13-1).

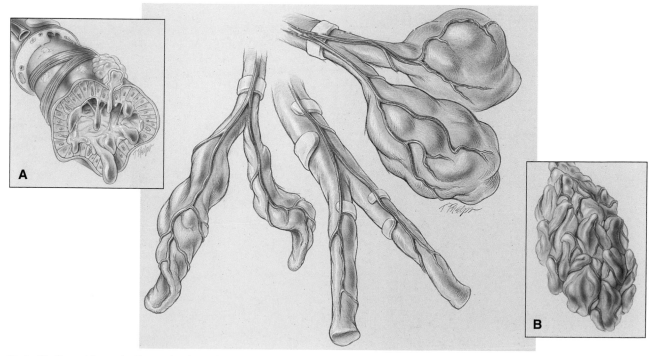

Plate 6 Bronchiectasis. Excessive bronchial secretions **(A)** and atelectasis **(B)** are common secondary anatomic alterations of the lungs (see Fig. 14-1).

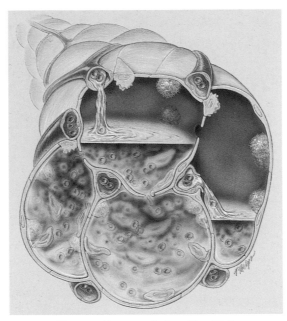

Plate 7 Pneumonia (see Fig. 15-1).

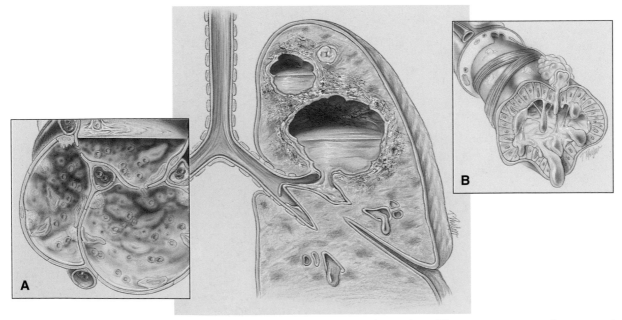

Plate 8 Lung abscess. Alveolar consolidation **(A)** and excessive bronchial secretions **(B)** are common secondary anatomic alterations of the lungs (see Fig. 16-1).

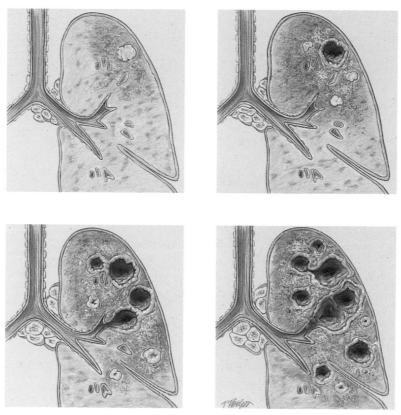

Plate 9 Tuberculosis (see Fig. 17-1).

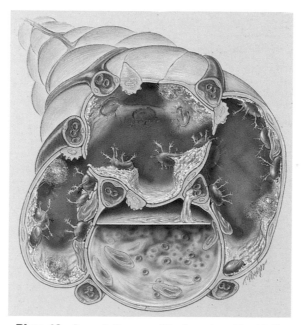

Plate 10 Fungal disease of the lung (see Fig. 18-1).

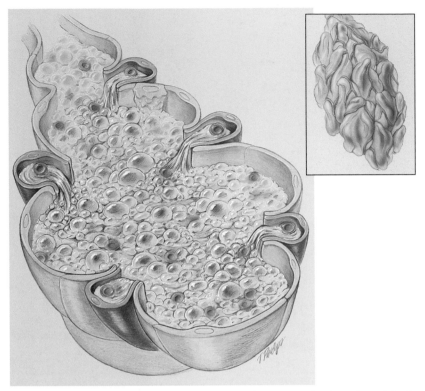

Plate 11 Pulmonary edema. *Inset,* Atelectasis, a common secondary anatomic alteration of the lungs (see Fig. 19-1).

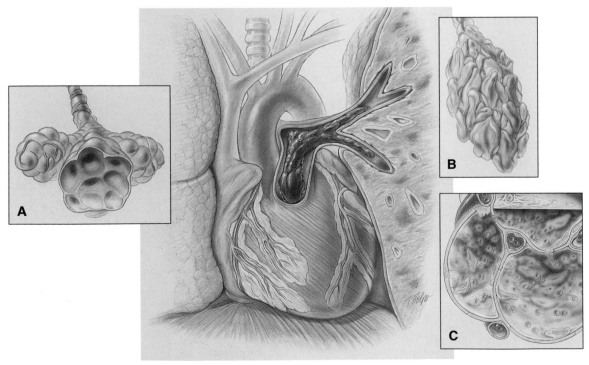

Plate 12 Pulmonary embolism. Bronchospasm **(A)**, atelectasis **(B)**, and alveolar consolidation **(C)** are common secondary anatomic alterations of the lungs (see Fig. 20-1).

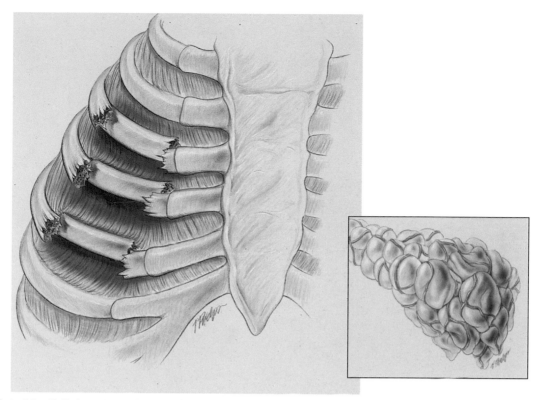

Plate 13 Flail chest. *Inset,* Atelectasis, a common secondary anatomic alteration of the lungs (see Fig. 21-1).

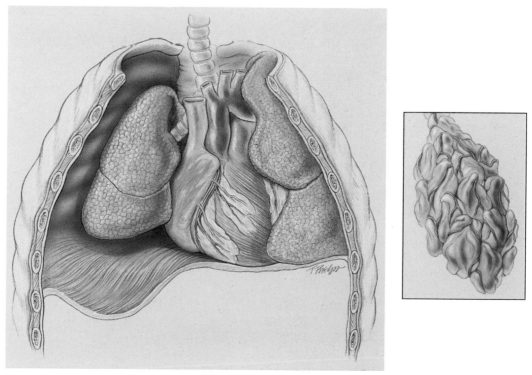

Plate 14 Pneumothorax. *Inset,* Atelectasis, a common secondary anatomic alteration of the lungs (see Fig. 22-1).

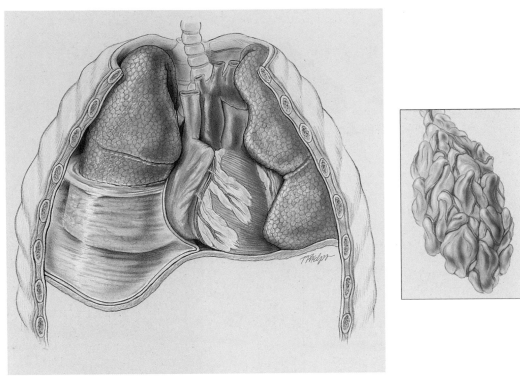

Plate 15 Right-sided pleural effusion. *Inset*, Atelectasis, a common secondary anatomic alteration of the lungs (see Fig. 23-1).

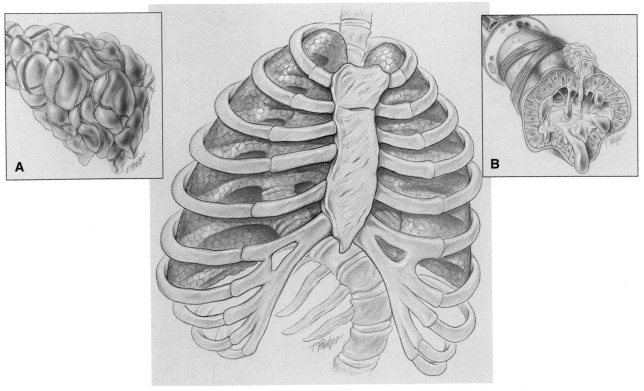

Plate 16 Kyphoscoliosis. Atelectasis **(A)** and excessive bronchial secretions **(B)** are common secondary anatomic alterations of the lungs (see Fig. 24-1).

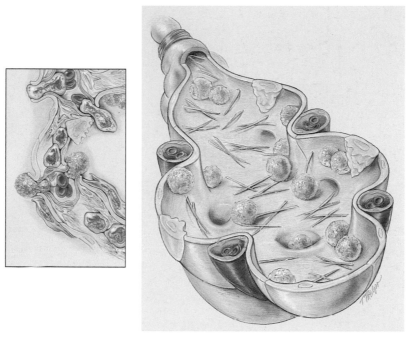

Plate 17 Pneumoconiosis. *Inset*, Fibrotic and thickened cross-section of an alveolus, a common secondary anatomic alteration of the lungs (see Fig. 25-1).

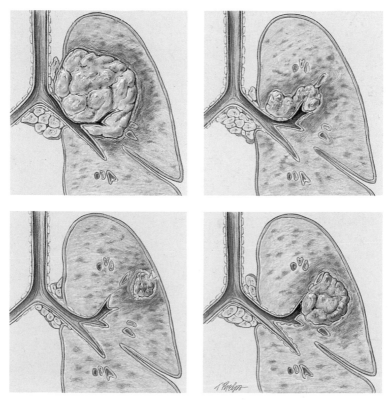

Plate 18 Cancer of the lung (see Fig. 26-1).

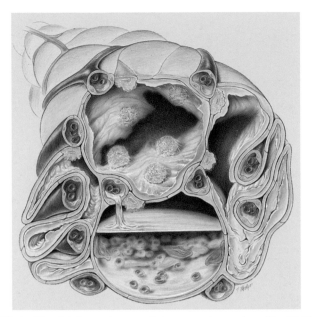

Plate 19 Adult respiratory distress syndrome (see Fig. 27-1).

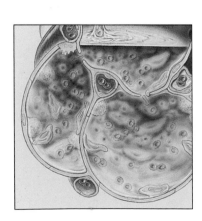

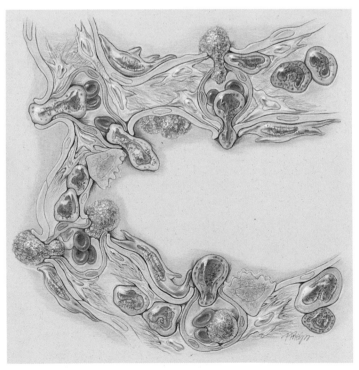

Plate 20 Chronic interstitial lung disease. *Inset*, Alveolar consolidation, a common secondary anatomic alteration of the lungs (see Fig. 28-1).

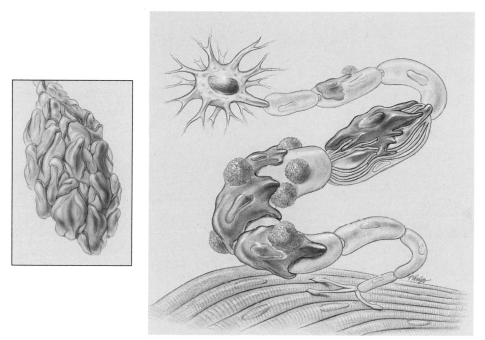

Plate 21   Guillain-Barré syndrome. *Inset*, Atelectasis, a common secondary anatomic alteration of the lungs (see Fig. 29-1).

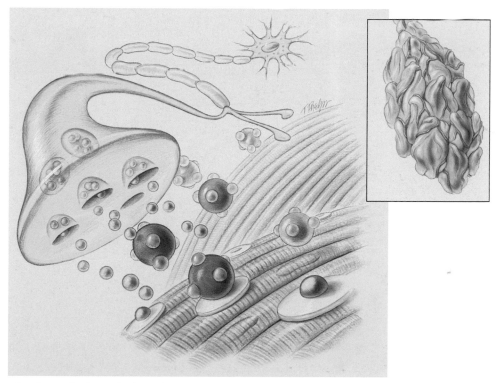

Plate 22   Myasthenia gravis. *Inset*, Atelectasis, a common secondary anatomic alteration of the lungs (see Fig. 30-1).

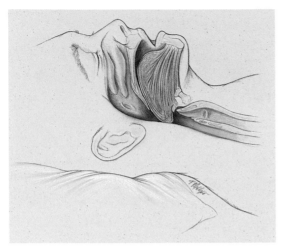

Plate 23 Sleep apnea (see Fig. 31-1).

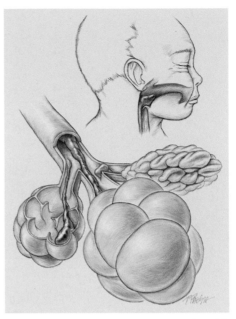

Plate 24 Meconium aspiration syndrome (see Fig. 33-1).

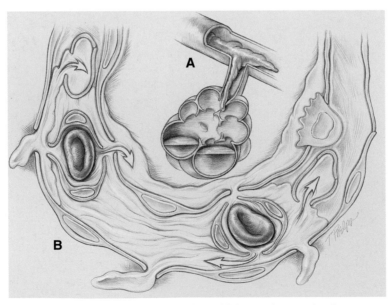

Plate 25 Transient tachypnea of the newborn. **A,** Excessive bronchial secretions and pulmonary capillary congestion. **B,** Cross-section of alveolus with interstitial edema (see Fig. 34-1).

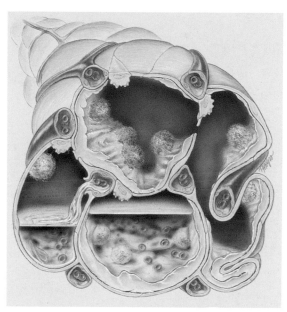

Plate 26   Idiopathic (infant) respiratory distress syndrome (see Fig. 35-1).

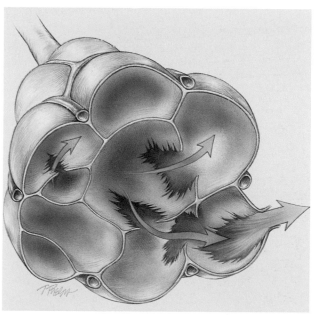

Plate 27   Pulmonary interstitial emphysema (PIE) (see Fig. 36-1).

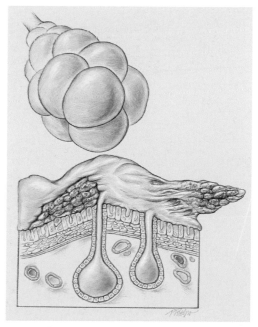

Plate 28   Bronchiolitis caused by respiratory syncytial virus (RSV) (see Fig. 37-1).

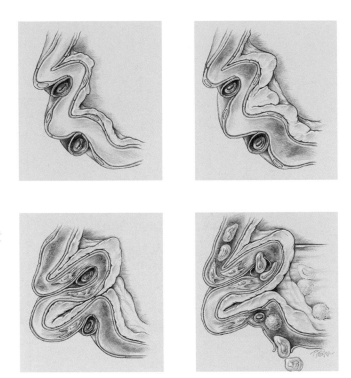

Plate 29   Bronchopulmonary dysplasia (see Fig. 38-1).

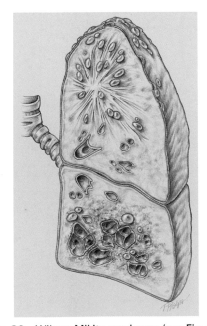

Plate 30   Wilson-Mikity syndrome (see Fig. 38-2).

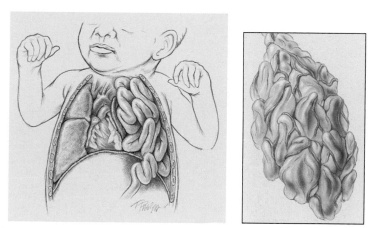

Plate 31 Diaphragmatic hernia. *Inset*, Atelectasis, a common secondary anatomic alteration of the lungs (see Fig. 39-1).

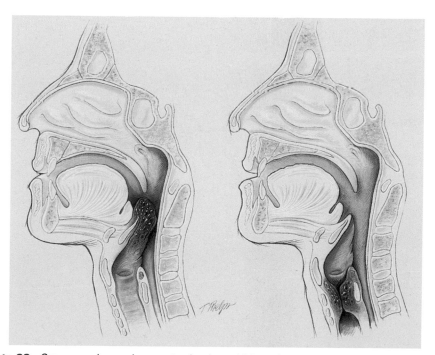

Plate 32 Croup syndrome: laryngotracheobronchitis and acute epiglottitis (see Fig. 40-1).

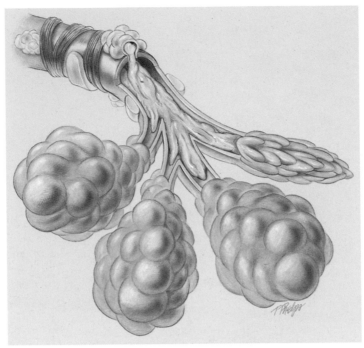

Plate 33 Cystic fibrosis (see Fig. 41-1).

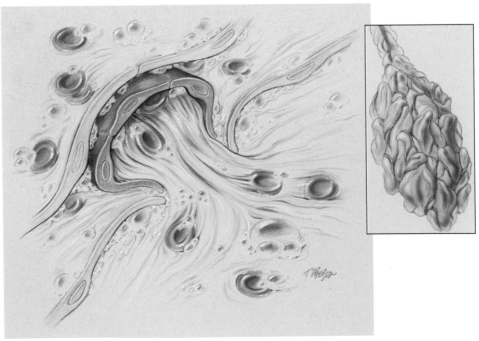

Plate 34 Near wet drowning. *Inset,* Atelectasis, a common secondary anatomic alteration of the lungs (see Fig. 42-1).

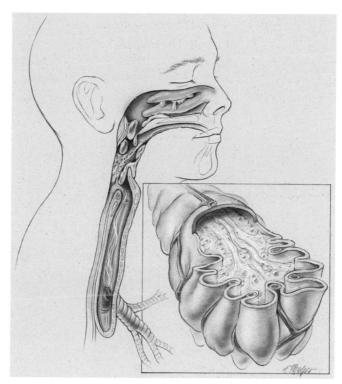

Plate 35 Smoke inhalation and thermal injuries (see Fig. 43-1).

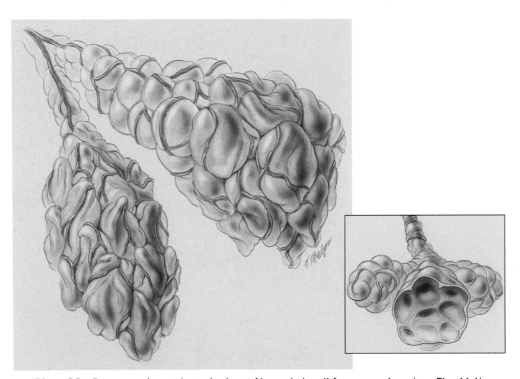

Plate 36 Postoperative atelectasis. *Inset,* Normal alveoli for comparison (see Fig. 44-1).

Assessment of Respiratory Disease

CLINICAL DATA OBTAINED AT THE PATIENT'S BEDSIDE

CHAPTER 1

The Patient Interview

Patient History

A complete patient assessment includes the patient interview. The purpose of the patient history is to gather pertinent subjective and objective data, which in turn can be used to develop a more complete picture of the patient's past and present health. In most clinical settings the patient is asked to fill out a printed history form or checklist. The patient should be allowed ample time to recall important dates, health-related landmarks, and family history. The patient interview is then used to validate what the patient has written and collect additional data on the patient's health status and lifestyle. Although history forms vary, most contain the following:

- Biographical data (age, gender, occupation)
- The patient's chief complaint or reason for seeking care, including the onset, duration, and characteristics of the signs and symptoms
- Present health or history of present illness
- Past health, including childhood illnesses, accidents or injuries, serious or chronic illnesses, hospitalizations, operations, obstetric history, immunizations, last examination date, allergies, current medications, and history of smoking or other habits
- The patient's family history
- Review of each body system, including skin, head, eyes, ears and nose, mouth and throat, respiratory system, cardiovascular system, gastrointestinal system, urinary system, genital system, and endocrine system
- Functional assessment (activities of daily living), including activity and exercise, work performance, sleep and rest, nutrition, interpersonal relationships, and coping and stress management strategies.

Patient Interview

The interview is a meeting between the respiratory care practitioner and the patient. It allows the collection of subjective data about the patient's feelings regarding the condition. During a successful interview, the practitioner performs the following tasks:

1. Gathers complete and accurate data about the patient's impressions about his or her health, including a description and chronology of any symptoms
2. Establishes rapport and trust so the patient feels accepted and comfortable in sharing all relevant information
3. Develops and shows an understanding about the patient's health state, which in turn enhances the patient's participation in identifying problems
4. Builds rapport to secure a continuing working relationship, which facilitates future assessments, evaluations, and treatment plans

Interview skills are an art form that takes time—and experience—to develop. The most important components of a successful interview are communication and understanding. Understanding the various signals of communication is the most difficult part. When understanding (conveying of meaning) breaks down between the practitioner and the patient, no communication can occur. Communication cannot be assumed just because two people have the ability to speak and listen. Communication is about behaviors—conscious and unconscious, verbal and nonverbal. All these behaviors convey meaning. The following paragraphs describe important factors that enhance the sending and receiving of information during communication.

INTERNAL FACTORS

Internal factors encompass what the practitioner brings to the interview—a genuine concern for others, empathy, and the ability to listen. A genuine liking of other people is essential in developing a strong rapport with the patient. It requires a generally optimistic view of people, a positive view of their strengths, and an acceptance of their weaknesses. This affection generates an atmosphere of warmth and caring. The patient must feel accepted unconditionally.

Empathy is the art of viewing the world from the patient's point of view while remaining separate from it. Empathy entails recognition and acceptance of the patient's feelings without criticism. It is sometimes described as feeling *with* the patient rather than feeling *like* the patient. To have empathy the practitioner needs to listen. Listening is not a passive process. Listening is active and demanding. It requires the practitioner's complete attention. If the examiner is preoccupied with personal needs or concerns, he or she will invariably miss something important. Active listening is a cornerstone to understanding. Nearly everything the patient says or does is relevant.

During the interview the examiner should observe the patient's body language and note the patient's facial expressions, eye movement (e.g., avoiding eye contact, looking into space, diverting gaze), pain grimaces, restlessness, and sighing. The examiner should listen to the way things are said. For example, is the tone of the patient's voice normal? Does the patient's voice quiver? Are there pitch breaks in the patient's voice? Does the patient say only a few words and then take a breath?

EXTERNAL FACTORS

A good physical setting enhances the interviewing process. Regardless of the interview's setting (the patient's bedside, an office in the hospital or clinic, or the patient's home), efforts should be made to (1) ensure privacy, (2) prevent interruptions, and (3) secure a comfortable physical environment (e.g., comfortable room temperature, sufficient lighting, absence of noise).

Techniques of Communication

During the interview the patient should be addressed by his or her surname, and the examiner should introduce himself or herself and state the purpose for being there. The following introduction serves as an example: "Good morning, Mr. Jones. I'm Mrs. Smith, and I'm from Respiratory Care. I want to ask you some questions about your breathing so that we can plan your respiratory care here in the hospital."

Verbal skills and techniques used by the examiner to facilitate the interview may include open-ended questions, closed or direct questions, and responses.

OPEN-ENDED QUESTIONS

An open-ended question asks the patient to provide narrative information. The examiner identifies the topic to be discussed but only in general terms. This technique is commonly used (1) to begin the interview, (2) to introduce a new section of questions, or (3) to gather further information whenever the patient introduces a new topic. The following are examples of open-ended questions:

"What brings you to the hospital today?"
"Tell me why you have come to the hospital today."
"How has your breathing been getting along?"
"You said that you have been short of breath. Tell me more about that."

The open-ended question is unbiased; it allows the patient freedom to answer in any way. This type of question encourages the patient to respond at greater length and give a spontaneous account of the condition. As the patient answers, the examiner should stop and listen. Patients often answer in short phrases or sentences and then pause, waiting for some kind of direction from the examiner. What the examiner does next is often the key to the direction of the interview. If the examiner presents new questions on other topics, much of the initial story may be lost. Ideally, the examiner should first respond by saying such things as "Tell me about it" and "Anything else?" The patient will usually add important information to the story.

CLOSED OR DIRECT QUESTIONS

A closed or direct question asks the patient for specific information. This type of question elicits a short one- or two-word answer, a yes or no, or a forced choice. The closed question is commonly used after the patient's narrative to fill in any details the patient may have left out. Closed questions also are used to

BOX 1–1

Comparison of Closed and Open-Ended Questions

Open-Ended	Closed
Used for narrative information	Used for specific information
Call for long answers	Call for short one- or two-word answers
Elicit feelings, options, ideas	Elicit "cold facts"
Build and enhance rapport	Limit rapport and leave interaction neutral

obtain specific facts, such as "Have you ever had this chest pain before?" Closed or direct questions speed up the interview. The use of only open-ended questions is unwieldy and takes an unrealistic amount of time, causing undue stress in the patient. Box 1-1 compares closed and open-ended questions.

RESPONSES—ASSISTING THE NARRATIVE

As the patient answers the open-ended questions, the examiner's role is to encourage free expression but not to let the patient digress. The examiner's responses work to clarify the story. There are nine types of verbal responses. In the first five responses the patient leads; in the last four responses the examiner leads.

The first five responses require the examiner's reactions to the facts or feelings the patient has communicated. The examiner's response focuses on the patient's frame of reference; the examiner's frame of reference is not relevant. For the last four responses the examiner's reaction is not required. The frame of reference shifts from the patient's perspective to the examiner's. These responses include the examiner's thoughts or feelings. The examiner should use these responses only when the situation calls for them. If these responses are used too often, the interview becomes focused more on the examiner than on the patient. The nine responses are described in the following sections.

Facilitation

Facilitation encourages patients to say more, to continue with the story. Examples of facilitating responses include the following: "Mm hmm," "Go on," "Continue," "Uh-huh." This type of response shows patients that the examiner is interested in what they are saying and will listen further. Nonverbal cues, such as maintaining eye contact and shifting

forward in the seat, also encourage the patient to continue talking.

Silence

Silent attentiveness is effective after an open-ended question. It communicates that the patient has time to think and organize what he or she wishes to say without interruption by the examiner.

Reflection

Reflection is used to echo the patient's words. It repeats a part of what the patient has just said to clarify or stimulate further communication. Reflection helps the patient focus on specific areas and continue in his or her own way. The following is a good example:

PATIENT: *"I'm here because of my breathing. It's blocked."*

EXAMINER: *"It's blocked?"*

PATIENT: *"Yes, every time I try to exhale, something blocks my breath and prevents me from getting all my air out."*

Reflection also can be used to express the emotions implicit in the patient's words. The examiner focuses on these emotions and encourages the patient to elaborate:

PATIENT: *"I have three little ones at home. I'm so worried they're not getting the care they need."*

EXAMINER: *"You feel worried and anxious about your children."*

The examiner acts as a mirror reflecting the patient's words and feelings. This technique helps the patient elaborate on the problem.

Empathy

A physical symptom, condition, or disease frequently has accompanying emotions. Patients often have trouble expressing these feelings. An empathic response recognizes these feelings and allows expression of them:

PATIENT: *"This is just great! I used to work out every day, and now I don't have enough breath to walk up the stairs!"*

EXAMINER: *"It must be hard—you used to exercise every day, and now you can't do a fraction of what you used to do."*

The examiner's response does not cut off further communication, which would occur by giving false reassurance (e.g., "Oh, you'll be back on your feet in no time"). Also, it does not deny the patient's feelings, nor does it suggest that the patient's feelings are unjustified. An empathic response recognizes the patient's feelings, accepts them, and allows the patient to express them without embarrassment. It strengthens rapport.

Clarification

Clarification is used when the patient's choice of words is ambiguous or confusing:

> "Tell me what you mean by bad air."

Clarification also is used to summarize and simplify the patient's words. When simplifying the patient's words, the examiner should ask whether the paraphrase is accurate. The examiner is asking for agreement, and this allows the patient to confirm or deny the examiner's understanding.

Confrontation

In using confrontation, the examiner notes a certain action, feeling, or statement made by the patient and focuses the patient's attention on it:

> "You said it doesn't hurt when you cough, but when you cough you grimace."

Alternatively, the examiner may focus on the patient's affect:

> "You look depressed today." "You sound angry."

Interpretation

Interpretation links events and data, makes associations, and implies causes. It provides the basis for inference or conclusion:

> "It seems that every time you have a serious asthma attack, you have had some kind of stress in your life."

The examiner runs the risk of making an incorrect inference. However, even if the patient corrects the inference, the patient's response often serves to prompt further discussion of the topic.

Explanation

Explanation provides the patient with factual and objective information:

> "It is very common for your heart rate to increase a bit after a bronchodilator treatment."

Summary

The summary is the final overview of the examiner's understanding of the patient's statements. It condenses the facts and presents an outline of the way the examiner perceives the patient's respiratory status. It is a type of validation in that the patient can agree or disagree with the examiner's summary. Both the examiner and the patient should participate in the summary. The summary signals that the interview is about to end.

NONPRODUCTIVE VERBAL MESSAGES

In addition to the verbal techniques commonly used to enhance the interview, the examiner must refrain from making nonproductive, defeating verbal messages. These messages restrict the patient's response. They act as barriers to obtaining data and establishing rapport.

Providing Assurance or Reassurance

Providing assurance or reassurance gives the examiner the false sense of having provided comfort. In fact, this type of response probably does more to relieve the examiner's anxiety than that of the patient.

> PATIENT: *"I'm so worried about the mass the doctor found on my chest X-ray. I hope it doesn't turn out to be cancer! What happens to your lung?"*

> EXAMINER: *"Now, don't worry. I'm sure you will be all right. You have a very good doctor."*

The examiner's response trivializes the patient's concern and effectively halts further communication about the topic. Instead, the examiner might have responded in a more empathic way:

> "You are really worried about that mass on your X-ray, aren't you? It must be very hard to wait for the lab results."

This response acknowledges the patient's feelings and concerns and, more important, keeps the door open for further communication.

Giving Advice

A key step in professional growth is to know when to give advice and when to refrain from it. Patients will often seek the examiner's professional advice and opinion on a specific topic:

> "What types of things should I avoid to keep my asthma under control?"

This is a straightforward request for information that the examiner has and the patient needs. The examiner should respond directly, and the answer should be based on knowledge and experience. The examiner should refrain from dispensing advice that is based on a hunch or feeling. For example, consider the patient who has just seen the doctor:

> "Dr. Johnson has just told me I may need an operation to remove the mass they found in my lungs. I just don't know. What would you do?"

If the examiner answers, the accountability for the decision shifts from the patient to the examiner. The examiner is not the patient. The patient must work this problem out. In fact, the patient probably does not really want to know what the examiner would do. In this case, the patient is worried about what he or she might have to do. A better response is reflection:

EXAMINER: *"Have an operation?"*

PATIENT: *"Yes, and I've never been put to sleep before. What do they do if you don't wake up?"*

Now the examiner knows the patient's real concern and can work to help the patient deal with it. For the patient to accept advice, it must be meaningful and appropriate. For example, in planning pulmonary rehabilitation for a male patient with severe emphysema, the respiratory therapist advises him to undertake a moderate walking program. The patient may treat the therapist's advice in one of two ways—either follow it or not. Indeed, the patient may choose to ignore it, feeling that it is not appropriate for him (e.g., he feels he gets plenty of exercise at work anyway).

On the other hand, if the patient follows the therapist's advice, three outcomes are possible: The patient's condition stays the same, improves, or worsens. If the walking strengthens the patient, the condition improves. However, if the patient was not part of the decision-making process to initiate a walking program, the psychologic reward is limited, promoting further dependency. If the walking program does not improve his condition or compromises it, the advice did not work. Because the advice was not the patient's, he can avoid any responsibility for the failure:

> "See, I did what you advised me to do, and it didn't help. In fact, I feel worse! Why did you tell me to do this anyway?"

Although giving advice might be faster, the examiner should take the time to involve the patient in the problem-solving process. A patient who is an active player in the decision-making process is more likely to learn and modify behavior.

Using Authority

The examiner should avoid responses that promote dependency and inferiority:

> "Now, your doctor and therapist know best."

Although the examiner and the patient cannot have equality in terms of professional skills and experience, both are equally worthy human beings and owe each other respect.

Using Avoidance Language

When talking about potentially frightening topics, people often use euphemisms (e.g., "passed on" rather than "died") to avoid reality or hide their true feelings. Although the use of euphemisms may appear to make a topic less frightening, it does not make the topic or the fear go away. In fact, not talking about a frightening subject suppresses the patient's feelings and often makes the patient more fearful. The use of direct and clear language is the best way to deal with potentially uncomfortable topics.

Distancing

Distancing is the use of impersonal conversation that places space between a frightening topic and the speaker. For example, a patient with a lung mass may say, "A friend of mine has a tumor on her lung. She is afraid that she may need an operation" or "There is a tumor in the left lung." By using "the" rather than "my," the patient can deny any association with the tumor. Occasionally, health-care workers also use distancing to soften reality. As a general rule, this technique does not work because it communicates to the patient that the health-care practitioner also is afraid of the topic. The use of frank, specific terms usually helps defuse anxiety rather than causing it.

Professional Jargon

What a health-care worker calls a myocardial infarction, a patient calls a heart attack. The use of professional jargon can sound exclusionary and paternalistic to the patient. Thus health-care practitioners should always try to adjust their vocabulary to the patient's understanding without sounding condescending. Even if patients use medical terms, the examiner cannot assume that they fully understand the meaning. For example, patients often think the term *hypertension* means that they are very tense and therefore take their medication only when they are feeling stressed, not when they feel relaxed.

Asking Leading or Biased Questions

Asking a patient "You don't smoke anymore, do you?" implies that one answer is better than another. The patient is forced either to answer in a way corresponding to the examiner's values or to feel guilty when admitting the other answer. When responding to this type of question, the patient risks the examiner's disapproval and possible alienation, which are undesirable responses from the patient's point of view.

Talking Too Much

Some examiners feel that helpfulness is directly related to verbal productivity. If they have spent the session talking, they leave feeling that they have met the patient's needs. In fact, the opposite is true. The patient needs time to talk. As a general rule, the examiner should listen more than talk.

Interrupting and Anticipating

While patients are speaking, the examiner should refrain from interrupting them, even when the examiner believes that she or he knows what is about to be said. Interruptions do not facilitate the interview. Rather, they communicate to the patient that the examiner is impatient or bored with the interview. Another trap is thinking about the next question while the patient is answering the last one, or anticipating the answer. Examiners who are overly preoccupied with their role as interviewer are not really listening to the patient. As a general rule the examiner should allow for a second or so of silence between the patient's statement and the next question.

Using "Why" Questions

The examiner should be careful in presenting "why" questions. The use of "why" questions often implies blame; it puts the patient on the defensive:

> "Why did you wait so long before calling your doctor?"
> "Why didn't you take your asthma medication with you?"

The only possible answer to a "why" question is "because...," and this places the patient in an uncomfortable position. To avoid this trap, the examiner might say, "I noticed you didn't call your doctor right away when you were having trouble breathing. I'd like to find out what was happening during this time."

NONVERBAL SKILLS

Nonverbal modes of communication include physical appearance, posture, gestures, facial expression, eye contact, voice, and touch. Nonverbal messages are important in establishing rapport and conveying feelings. Nonverbal messages may either support or contradict verbal messages. Therefore an awareness of the nonverbal messages that may be conveyed by either the patient or the examiner during the interview process is important. Box 1-2 provides an overview of nonverbal messages that may occur during an interview.

Physical Appearance

The examiner's general personal appearance, grooming, and choice of clothing send a message to the patient. Professional dress codes vary among hospitals and clinical settings. Depending on the setting, a professional uniform can project a message that ranges from comfortable or casual to formal or distant. Regardless of one's personal choice in clothing and general appearance, the aim should be to convey a competent and professional image.

Posture

An open position is one in which a communicator extends the large muscle groups (i.e., arms and legs are not crossed). An open position shows relaxation, physical comfort, and a willingness to share information. A closed position, with arms and legs crossed, sends a defensive and anxious message.

BOX 1–2

Nonverbal Messages of the Interview

Positive	Negative
Professional appearance	Nonprofessional appearance
Sitting next to patient	Sitting behind a desk
Close proximity to patient	Far away from patient
Turned toward patient	Turned away from patient
Relaxed, open posture	Tense, closed posture
Leaning toward patient	Slouched away from patient
Facilitating gestures	Nonfacilitating gestures
• Nodding of head	• Looking at watch
Positive facial expressions	Negative facial expressions
• Appropriate smiling	• Frowning
• Interest	• Yawning
Good eye contact	Poor eye contact
Moderate tone of voice	Strident, high-pitched voice
Moderate rate of speech	Speech too fast or too slow
Appropriate touch	Overly frequent or inappropriate touch

The examiner should be aware of any posture changes. For example, if the patient suddenly shifts from a relaxed to a tense position, it suggests discomfort with the topic. In addition, the examiner should try to sit comfortably next to the patient during the interview. Sitting too far away or standing over the patient often sends a negative nonverbal message.

Gestures

Gestures send nonverbal messages. For example, pointing a finger may show anger or blame. Nodding of the head or an open hand with the palms turned upward can show acceptance, attention, or agreement. Wringing the hands suggests worry and anxiety. The patient often describes a crushing chest pain by holding a fist in front of the sternum. When a patient has a sharp, localized pain, one finger is commonly used to point to the exact spot.

Facial Expression

An individual's face can convey a wide range of emotions and conditions. For example, facial expressions can reflect alertness, relaxation, anxiety, anger, suspicion, and pain. The examiner should work to convey an attentive, sincere, and interested expression. Patient rapport will deteriorate if the examiner exhibits facial expressions that suggest boredom, distraction, disgust, criticism, and disbelief.

Eye Contact

Lack of eye contact suggests that a person may be insecure, intimidated, shy, withdrawn, confused, bored, apathetic, or depressed. The examiner should work to maintain good eye contact but not stare the patient down with a fixed, penetrating look. Generally, an easy gaze toward the patient's eyes with occasional glances away works well. The examiner, however, should be aware that this approach may not work when interviewing a patient from a culture in which direct eye contact is generally avoided. For example, Asian, Native American, Indochinese, Arab, and some Appalachian people may consider direct eye contact impolite or aggressive, and they may divert their own eyes during the interview.

Voice

Nonverbal messages are reflected through the tone of voice, intensity and rate of speech, pitch, and long pauses. These messages often convey more meaning than the spoken word. For example, a patient's voice may show sarcasm, anxiety, sympathy, or hostility. An anxious patient frequently talks in a loud and fast voice. A soft voice may reflect shyness and fear. A patient with hearing impairment generally speaks in a loud voice. Long pauses may have important meanings. For instance, when a patient pauses for a long time before answering an easy and straightforward question, the honesty of the answer may be questionable. Slow speech with long and frequent pauses, combined with a weak and monotonous voice, suggests depression.

Touch

The meaning of touch is often misinterpreted; it can be influenced by an individual's age, gender, cultural background, past experiences, and the present setting. As a general rule, the examiner should not touch patients during interviews unless he or she knows the patient well and is sure that the gesture will be interpreted correctly. When appropriate, touch (such as a touch of the hand or arm) can be effective in conveying empathy.

To summarize, extensive nonverbal messages, communicated by both the examiner and patient, may occur during the interview. Therefore the examiner must be aware of the patient's various nonverbal messages while working to communicate nonverbal messages that are productive and enhancing to the examiner/patient relationship.

Closing the Interview

The interview should end gracefully. If the session has an abrupt or awkward closing, the patient may be left with a negative impression. This final moment may destroy any rapport gained during the interview. To ease into the closing, the examiner might ask the patient one of the following questions:

"Is there anything else that you would like to talk about?"
"Do you have any questions that you would like to ask me?"
"Are there any other problems that we have not discussed?"

These types of questions give the patient an opportunity for self-expression. The examiner may choose to summarize or repeat what was learned during the interview. This serves as a final statement of the examiner's and the patient's assessment of the situation. Finally, the examiner should thank the patient for the time and cooperation provided during the interview.

SELF-ASSESSMENT QUESTIONS

Matching

Directions: On the line next to the items in Column A, match the items from Column B that best match. Items from Column B may be used once, more than once, or not at all.

Column A

1. Open-ended question
2. Reflection
3. Facilitation
4. Confrontation
5. Closed or direct question

Column B

a. "You are worried about your child."
b. "Tell me more about your shortness of breath."
c. "Mm-hmm, go on."
d. "You sound angry."
e. "Have you had this pain before?"

Essay

6. List five negative nonverbal messages.

   A. _____

   B. _____

   C. _____

   D. _____

   E. _____

Answers appear in Appendix XI.

CHAPTER 2

The Physical Examination and Its Basis in Physiology

◆ Vital Signs

The four major vital signs—*body temperature (T), pulse (P), respiratory rate (R), and blood pressure (BP)*—are excellent bedside clinical indicators of the patient's physiologic and psychologic health. In many patient care settings, the oxygen saturation by **pulse oximetry (Spo$_2$)** measurement is considered to be the fifth vital sign. Table 2-1 shows the normal values that have been established for various age groups. During the initial measurement of a patient's vital signs, the values are compared with these normal values. After several vital signs have been documented, these data are then used as a baseline for subsequent measurements. Isolated vital sign measurements are not as valuable as a *series* of measurements. By evaluating a series of values, the practitioner can identify important vital sign trends for the patient. The identification of vital sign trends that deviate from the patient's normal measurements is much more significant than an isolated measurement.

Although the skills involved in obtaining the vital signs are easy to learn, interpretation and clinical application require knowledge, problem-solving skills, critical thinking, and experience. Even though vital sign measurements are part of routine bedside care, they provide important information and should always be considered as an important part of the assessment process. The frequency with which vital signs should be assessed depends on the individual needs of each patient.

◆ BODY TEMPERATURE

Body temperature is routinely measured to assess for signs of inflammation or infection. Even though the body's skin temperature varies widely in response to environmental conditions and physical activity, the temperature inside the body, the *core temperature,* remains relatively constant—about 37° C (98.6° F), with a daily variation of +/− 0.5° C (1° to 2° F). Under normal circumstances, the body is able to

TABLE 2–1	Average Range for Vital Signs According to Age Group				
				Blood Pressure (mm Hg)	
Age Group	Temperature (F°)	Pulse (bpm)	Respirations (breaths/min)	Systolic	Diastolic
Newborn	96-99.5	100-180	30-60	60-90	20-60
Infant (1 mo.-1 yr)	99.4-99.7	80-160	30-60	75-100	50-70
Toddler (1-3 yrs)	99.4-99.7	80-130	25-40	80-110	55-80
Preschooler (3-6 yrs)	98.6-99	80-120	20-35	80-110	50-80
Child (6-12 yrs)	98.6	65-100	20-30	100-110	60-70
Adolescent (12-18 yrs)	97-99	60-90	12-20	110-120	60-65
Adult	97-99	60-100	12-20	110-140	60-90
Older adult (>70 yrs)	95-99	60-100	12-20	120-140	70-90

maintain this constant temperature through various physiologic compensatory mechanisms, such as the autonomic nervous system and special receptors located in the skin, abdomen, and spinal cord.

In response to temperature changes, the receptors sense and send information through the nervous system to the hypothalamus. The hypothalamus, in turn, processes the information and activates the appropriate response. For example, an increase in body temperature causes the blood vessels near the skin surface to dilate—a process called *vasodilation*. Vasodilation, in turn, allows more warmed blood to flow near the skin surface, thereby enhancing heat loss. In contrast, a decrease in body temperature causes *vasoconstriction*, which works to keep warmed blood closer to the center of the body—thus working to maintain the core temperature.

At normal body temperature, the metabolic functions of all body cells are optimal. When the body temperature increases or decreases significantly from the normal range, the metabolic rate and, therefore, the demands on the cardiopulmonary system also change. For example, during a fever the metabolic rate increases. This action leads to an increase in oxygen consumption and to an increase in carbon dioxide production at the cellular level. According to estimates, for every 1° C increase in body temperature, the patient's oxygen consumption increases about 10%. As the metabolic rate increases, the cardiopulmonary system must work harder to meet the additional cellular demands. Hypothermia reduces the metabolic rate and cardiopulmonary demand.

As shown in Figure 2-1, the normal body temperature is positioned within a relatively narrow range. A patient who has a temperature within the normal range is said to be *afebrile*. A body temperature above the normal range is called *pyrexia*, or *hyperthermia*. When the body temperature rises above the normal range, the patient said to have a *fever*, or to be *febrile*. An exceptionally high temperature, such as 41° C (105.8° F), is called *hyperpyrexia*.

The four common types of fevers are *intermittent*, *remittent*, *relapsing*, and *constant* fevers. An *intermittent fever* is said to exist when the patient's body temperature alternates at regular intervals between periods of fever and periods of normal or below-normal temperatures. In other words, the patient's temperature undergoes peaks and valleys, with the valleys representing normal or below-normal temperatures. During a *remittent fever,* the patient has marked peaks and valleys (more than 2° C or 3.6° F) over a 24-hour period, all of which are above normal— that is, the body temperature does not return to normal between the spikes. A *relapsing fever* is said to exist when short febrile periods of a few days are interspersed with 1 or 2 days of normal temperature. A *continuous fever* is said to exist when the patient's body temperature remains above normal with minimal or no fluctuation.

Hypothermia is a core temperature below normal range. Hypothermia may occur as a result of (1) excessive heat loss, (2) inadequate heat production to counteract heat loss, and (3) impaired hypothalamic thermoregulation. Box 2-1 lists the clinical signs of hypothermia.

Figure 2–1   Range of normal body temperature and alterations in body temperature on the Celsius and Fahrenheit scales. See conversion formulas for Fahrenheit and Celsius scales on left side of figure.

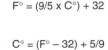

$$F° = (9/5 \times C°) + 32$$

$$C° = (F° - 32) + 5/9$$

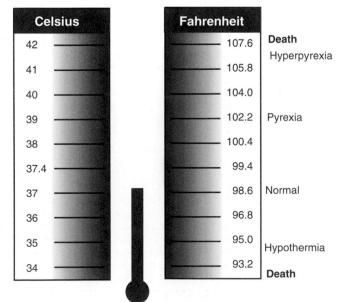

BOX 2–1	BOX 2–2
Clinical Signs of Hypothermia	**Common Therapeutic Interventions for Hypothermia**
• Below normal body temperature • Decreased pulse and respiratory rate • Severe shivering (initially) • Patient indicating coldness or presence of chills • Pale or bluish cool, waxy skin • Hypotension • Decreased urinary output • Lack of muscle coordination • Disorientation • Drowsy or unresponsive • Coma	Remove wet clothing. Provide dry clothing. Place patient in a warm environment (e.g., slowly increase room temperature). Cover patient with warm blankets or electric heating blanket. Apply warming pads (increase temperature slowly). Keep patient's limbs close to body. Cover patient's head with a cap or towel. Supply warm oral or intravenous fluids.

Hypothermia may be caused accidentally or may be induced. *Accidental hypothermia* is commonly seen in the patient who (1) has had an excessive exposure to a cold environment; (2) has been immersed in a cold liquid environment for a prolonged time; or (3) has inadequate clothing, shelter, or heat. A reduced metabolic rate may compound hypothermia in older patients. In addition, older patients often take sedatives, which further depress the metabolic rate. Box 2-2 lists common therapeutic interventions for patients with hypothermia.

Induced hypothermia refers to the intentional lowering of a patient's body temperature to reduce the oxygen demand of the tissue cells. Induced hypothermia may involve only a portion of the body or the whole body. Induced hypothermia is often indicated before certain surgeries, such as heart or brain surgery.

Factors Affecting Body Temperature

Table 2-2 lists several factors that affect body temperature. Knowing these factors can help the practitioner to better assess the significance of expected or normal variations in a patient's body temperature.

TABLE 2–2	**Factors Affecting Body Temperature**
Age	Temperature varies with age. For example, the temperature of the newborn infant is unstable because of immature thermoregulatory mechanisms. However, it is not uncommon for the elderly person to have a body temperature below 36.4° C (97.6° F). The normal temperature decreases with age.
Environment	Normally, variations in environmental temperature do not affect the core temperature. However, exposure to extreme hot or cold temperatures can alter body temperature. If an individual's core temperature falls to 25° C (77° F), death may occur.
Time of day	Body temperature normally varies throughout the day. Typically, an individual's temperature is lowest around 3:00 AM and highest between 5:00 PM and 7:00 PM. Approximately 95% of patients have their highest temperature around 6:00 PM. Body temperature often fluctuates by as much as 2° C (1.8° F) between early morning and late afternoon.
Exercise	Body temperature increases with exercise because exercise increases heat production as the body breaks down carbohydrates and fats to provide energy. During strenuous exercise, the body temperature can increase to as high as 40° C (104° F).
Stress	Physical or emotional stress may increase body temperature because stress can stimulate the sympathetic nervous system, causing the epinephrine and norepinephrine levels to increase. When this occurs, the metabolic rate increases, causing an increased heat production. Stress and anxiety may cause a patient's temperature to increase without underlying disease.
Hormones	Women normally have greater fluctuations in temperature than do men. The female hormone progesterone, which is secreted during ovulation, causes the temperature to increase 0.3° to 0.6° C (0.5° to 1° F). After menopause, women have the same mean temperature norms as men.

Body Temperature Measurement

The measurement of body temperature establishes an essential baseline for clinical comparison as a disease progresses or as therapies are administered. To ensure the reliability of a temperature reading, the practitioner must (1) select the correct measuring equipment, (2) choose the most appropriate site, and (3) use the correct technique or procedure. The four most commonly used sites are the mouth, rectum, ear (tympanic), and axilla. Any of these sites are satisfactory when proper technique is used.

Additional measurement sites include the esophagus and pulmonary artery. Temperatures measured at these sites and in the rectum and tympanic membrane are considered *core temperatures*. The skin, typically that of the forehead or abdomen, may also be used for general temperature purposes. However, practitioners must remember that although skin temperature–sensitive strips or disposable paper thermometers may be satisfactory for general temperature

measurements, the patient's precise temperature should always be confirmed—when indicated—with a glass or tympanic thermometer.

Because body temperature is usually measured orally, the practitioner must be aware of certain external factors that can lead to false oral temperature measurements. For example, drinking hot or cold liquids can cause small changes in oral temperature measurements. The most significant temperature changes have been reported after a patient drinks ice water. Drinking ice water may lower the patient's actual temperature between –0.2° and –1.6° F. Before taking an oral temperature, the practitioner should wait 15 minutes after a patient has ingested ice water. Oral temperature may increase in the patient receiving heated oxygen aerosol therapy and decrease in the patient receiving a cool mist aerosol. Table 2-3 summarizes the body temperature sites, their advantages and disadvantages, and the equipment used.

TABLE 2–3	**Body Temperature Measurements** **Summary of Body Temperature Sites, Advantages and Disadvantages, and** **Equipment Used**		
Site and Temperature	**Advantages and Disadvantages**		**Equipment**
Oral (most common) Average 37° C or 98.6° F	**Advantages:** Convenient. Easy access and patient comfort. **Disadvantages:** Affected by hot or cold liquids. Contraindicated in patients who cannot follow directions to keep mouth closed, who are mouth breathing, or who might bite down and break thermometer. Smoking, drinking, and eating can slightly alter the oral temperature. About 1° F lower than rectal temperature		Glass mercury thermometer, Electronic thermometers
Rectal Average 0.7° C or 0.4° F higher than oral	**Advantages:** Very reliable. Considered most accurate. **Disadvantages:** Contraindicated in patients with diarrhea, patients who have undergone rectal surgery, or patients who have diseases of the rectum. **General Comment:** Used less often now that tympanic thermometers are available.		Glass mercury thermometer
Ear (tympanic) Reflects core temperature. Also calibrated to oral or rectal scales	**Advantages:** Convenient, readily accessible, fast, safe, and noninvasive. Does not require contact with any mucous membrane. Infection control is less of a concern. With the advent of the tympanic membrane thermometer, the ear is now a site where a temperature can be easily and safely measured. Reflects the core body temperature because it measures the tympanic membrane blood supply—the same vascular system that supplies the hypothalamus. Smoking, drinking, and eating do not affect tympanic temperature measurements. Allows rapid temperature measurements in the very young, confused, or unconscious patient. **Disadvantages:** No remarkable disadvantages, assuming site is available.		Tympanic thermometer
Axillary Average 0.6° C or 1° F lower than oral	**Advantages:** Safe and noninvasive. Recommended for infants and children, this is the route of choice in patients whose temperature cannot be measured at other sites. **Disadvantages:** Considered the least accurate and least reliable site because a number of factors can adversely affect the measurement. For example, if the patient has recently been given a bath, the temperature may reflect the temperature of the bath water. Similarly, friction applied to dry the patient's skin may influence the temperature.		Glass mercury thermometer

PULSE

A pulse is generated through the vascular system with each ventricular contraction of the heart (systole). Thus a pulse is a rhythmic arterial blood pressure throb created by the pumping action of the ventricular muscle. Between contractions, the ventricle rests (diastole) and the pulsation disappears. The pulse can be assessed at any location where an artery lies close to the skin surface and can be palpated against a firm underlying structure, such as muscle or bone. Nine common pulse sites are the temporal, carotid, apical, brachial, radial, femoral, popliteal, pedal (dorsalis pedis), and posterior tibial area (Figure 2-2).

In clinical settings, the pulse is usually obtained by palpation. Initially, the practitioner uses the first, second, or third finger and applies light pressure to any one of the pulse sites (e.g., carotid or radial artery) to detect a pulse with a strong pulsation. After locating the pulse, the practitioner may apply a more forceful palpation to count the rate, determine the rhythm, and evaluate the quality of pulsation. The practitioner then counts the number of pulsations for 15, 30, or 60 seconds and then multiplies appropriately to determine the pulse per minute. Shorter time intervals may be used for patients with normal rates or regular cardiac rhythms.

In patients with irregular, abnormally slow, or fast cardiac rhythms, the pulse rates should be counted for 1 minute. To prevent overestimation for any time interval, the practitioner should count the first pulsation as zero and not count pulses at or after the completion of a selected time interval. Counting even one extra pulsation during a 15-second interval leads to an overestimation of the pulse rate by 4. The characteristics of the pulse are described in terms *of rate, rhythm,* and *strength.*

Rate

The normal pulse rate (or heart rate) varies with age. For example, in the newborn the normal pulse rate range is between 100 and 180 beats per minute (bpm). In the toddler the normal range is between 80 and 130 bpm. The normal range for the child is between 65 and 100 bpm, and the normal adult range is between 60 and 100 bpm (see Table 2-1).

A heart rate lower than 60 bpm is called *bradycardia.* Bradycardia may be seen in patients with hypothermia and in physically fit athletes. The pulse may also be lower than expected when the patient is at rest or asleep or as a result of head injury, vomiting, or advanced age. A pulse rate greater than 100 bpm in adults is called *tachycardia.* Tachycardia may occur as a result of hypoxemia, anemia, fever, anxiety, emotional stress, fear, hemorrhage, hypotension, dehydration, shock, and exercise. Tachycardia also is a common side effect in patients receiving certain medications, such as sympathomimetic agents (e.g., adrenaline or dobutamine).

Rhythm

Normally, the ventricular contraction is under the control of the sinus node in the atrium, which generates a normal rate and regular rhythm. Certain conditions and chemical disturbances, such as inadequate blood flow and oxygen supply to the heart or an electrolyte imbalance, can cause the heart to beat irregularly. In children and young adults, it is not uncommon for the heart rate to increase during inspiration and decrease during exhalation. This is called *sinus arrhythmia.*

Strength

The quality of the pulse reflects the strength of left ventricular contraction and the volume of blood flowing to the peripheral tissues. A normal left ventricular contraction combined with an adequate blood volume will generate a strong, throbbing pulse. A weak ventricular contraction combined with an inadequate blood volume will result in a weak, thready pulse wave. An increased heart rate combined with a large blood volume will generate a full, bounding pulse.

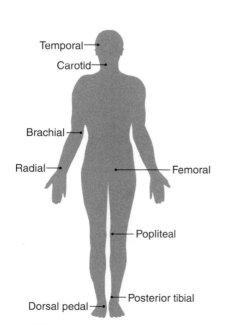

Figure 2–2 The nine common pulse sites.

BOX 2–3

Scale to Rate Pulse Quality

0: Absent or no pulse detected
1+: Weak, thready, easily obliterated with pressure; difficult to feel
2+: Pulse difficult to palpate; may be obliterated by strong pressure
3+: Normal pulse
4+: Bounding, easily palpated and difficult to obliterate

Several conditions may alter the strength of a patient's pulse. For example, heart failure can cause the strength of the pulse to vary every other beat while the rhythm remains regular. This condition is called *pulsus alternans*. The practitioner may detect a pulse that increases markedly in strength during inspiration and decreases back to normal during exhalation, a condition called *pulsus paradoxus* that is common among patients experiencing a severe asthmatic episode. This phenomenon can also be heard when measuring blood pressure.

Finally, the stimulation of the sympathetic nervous system increases the force of ventricular contraction, increasing the volume of blood ejected from the heart and creating a stronger pulse. Stimulation of the parasympathetic nervous system decreases the force of the ventricular contraction, thus leading to a decreased volume of blood ejected from the heart and a weaker pulse. Clinically, the strength of the pulse may be recorded on a scale from 0 to 4+ (Box 2-3).

For peripheral pulses that are difficult to detect by palpation, an ultrasonic Doppler device may also be used. A transmitter attached to the Doppler is placed over the artery to be assessed. The transmitter amplifies and transmits the pulse sounds to an earpiece or to a speaker attached to the Doppler device. The heart rate can also be obtained through auscultation by placing a stethoscope over the apex of the heart.

◆ RESPIRATION

Inspiration is an active process whereby the diaphragm contracts and causes the intrathoracic pressure to decrease. This action, in turn, causes the pressure in the airways to fall below the atmospheric pressure, and air flows in. At the end of inspiration, the diaphragm relaxes and the natural lung elasticity (recoil) causes the pressure in the lung to increase. This action, in turn, causes air to flow out of the lung. Under normal circumstances, expiration is a passive process.

The normal respiratory rate varies with age. For example, in the newborn the normal respiratory rate varies between 30 and 60 breaths per minute. In the toddler, the normal range is between 25 and 40 breaths per minute. The normal range for the preschool child is between 20 and 25 breaths per minute, and the normal adult range is between 12 and 20 breaths per minute (see Table 2-1).

Ideally, the respiratory rate should be counted when the patient is not aware. One good method is to count the respiratory rate immediately after taking the pulse, while leaving the fingers over the patient's artery. As respirations are being counted, the practitioner should observe for variations in the pattern of breathing. For example, an increased breathing rate is called *tachypnea*. Tachypnea is commonly seen in patients with fever, metabolic acidosis, hypoxemia, pain, or anxiety. A respiratory rate below the normal range is called *bradypnea*. Bradypnea may occur with hypothermia, head injuries, and drug overdose. Table 2-4 provides an overview of common abnormal breathing patterns.

TABLE 2–4	**Common Breathing Patterns**	
Pattern	**Graphic Overview**	**Description**
Eupnea	Volume ▲▲▲▲▲ Time (15 seconds)	Normal rate and rhythm; between 12 and 20 breaths per minute in regular rhythm and of moderate depth for an adult

Continued

TABLE 2–4 Common Breathing Patterns—Cont'd

Pattern	Graphic Overview	Description
Bradypnea	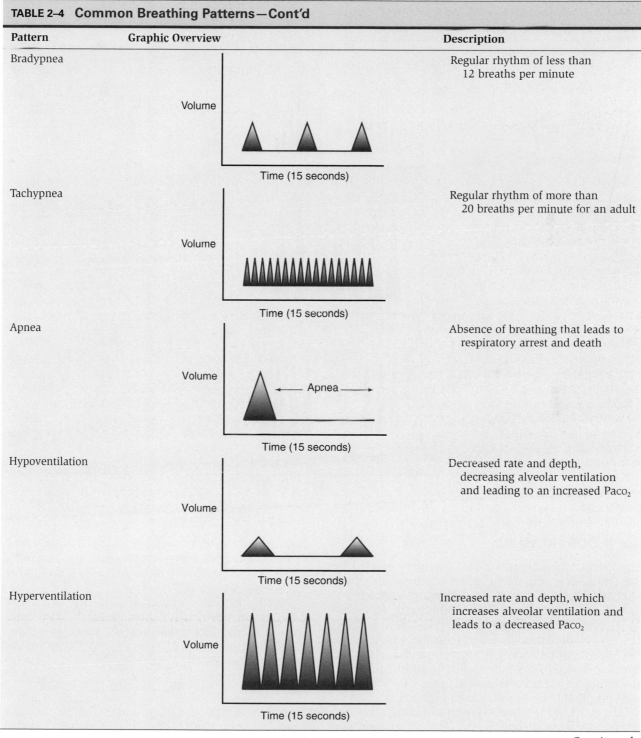	Regular rhythm of less than 12 breaths per minute
Tachypnea		Regular rhythm of more than 20 breaths per minute for an adult
Apnea		Absence of breathing that leads to respiratory arrest and death
Hypoventilation		Decreased rate and depth, decreasing alveolar ventilation and leading to an increased Pa_{CO_2}
Hyperventilation		Increased rate and depth, which increases alveolar ventilation and leads to a decreased Pa_{CO_2}

Continued

TABLE 2–4 Common Breathing Patterns—Cont'd

Pattern	Graphic Overview	Description
Cheyne-Stokes	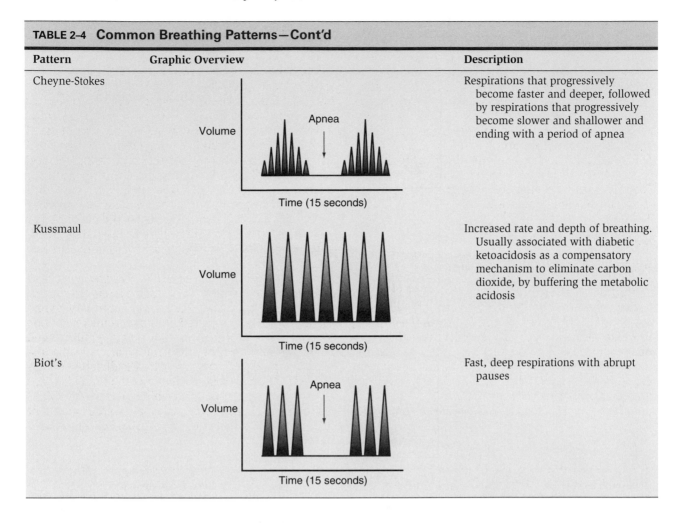	Respirations that progressively become faster and deeper, followed by respirations that progressively become slower and shallower and ending with a period of apnea
Kussmaul		Increased rate and depth of breathing. Usually associated with diabetic ketoacidosis as a compensatory mechanism to eliminate carbon dioxide, by buffering the metabolic acidosis
Biot's		Fast, deep respirations with abrupt pauses

◆ BLOOD PRESSURE

The arterial blood pressure is the force exerted by the circulating volume of blood on the walls of the arteries. The pressure peaks when the ventricles of the heart contract and eject blood into the aorta and pulmonary arteries. The blood pressure measured during ventricular contraction (cardiac systole) is the *systolic blood pressure*. During ventricular relaxation (cardiac diastole), blood pressure is generated by the elastic recoil of the arteries and arterioles. This pressure is called the *diastolic blood pressure*.

The normal blood pressure in the aorta and large arteries varies with age. For example, in the newborn the normal blood pressure range is between 60 and 180 mm Hg. In the toddler the normal range is between 80 and 110 mm Hg. The normal range for the child is between 100 and 110 mm Hg, and the normal adult range is between 110 and 140 mm Hg (see Table 2-1). The numeric difference between the systolic and diastolic blood pressure is the *pulse pressure*. For example, a systolic pressure of 120 mm Hg and a diastolic pressure of 80 mm Hg equal a pulse pressure of 40 mm Hg.

Blood pressure is a function of (1) the blood flow generated by ventricular contraction and (2) the resistance to blood flow caused by the vascular system. Thus blood pressure (BP) equals flow ($\dot{V}$) multiplied by resistance: ($BP = \dot{V} \times R$).

Blood Flow

Blood flow is equal to cardiac output. Cardiac output is equal to product of (1) the volume of blood ejected from the ventricles during each heartbeat (stroke volume) multiplied by (2) the heart rate. Thus a stroke volume (SV) of 75 ml and a heart rate (HR) of 70 beats per minute produce a cardiac output (CO) of 5250 ml/minute, or 5.25 L/min ($CO = SV \times HR$). The average cardiac output in the resting adult is about 5 L/min.

A number of conditions can alter stroke volume and therefore blood flow. For instance, a decreased stroke volume may develop as a result of poor cardiac pumping (e.g., after ventricular failure) or as a result of a decreased blood volume (e.g., after severe hemorrhage). Bradycardia may also reduce cardiac output and blood flow. Conversely, an increased heart rate or blood volume will likely increase cardiac output and blood flow. In addition, an increased heart rate in response to a decreased blood volume (or stroke volume) may also occur as a compensatory mechanism to maintain a normal cardiac output and blood flow.

Resistance

The friction between the components of the blood ejected from the ventricles and the walls of the arteries results in a natural resistance to blood flow. Friction between the blood components and the vessel walls is inversely related to the dimensions of the vessel lumen (size). Thus as the vessel lumen narrows (or constricts), resistance increases. As the vessel lumen widens (or relaxes), the resistance decreases. The autonomic nervous system monitors and regulates the vascular tone.

Table 2-5 presents factors that affect the blood pressure.

Abnormalities

Hypertension

Hypertension is the condition in which an individual's blood pressure is chronically above normal range. Whereas blood pressure normally increases with aging, hypertension is considered a dangerous disease and is associated with an increased risk of morbidity and mortality. According to the Joint National Committee on Detection, Evaluation, and Treatment of High Blood Pressure, the physician may make the diagnosis of hypertension in the adult when an average of two or more diastolic readings, on at least two different visits, is 90 mm Hg or higher or when the average of two or more systolic readings, on at least two visits, is consistently greater than 140 mm Hg.

An elevated blood pressure of unknown cause is called *primary hypertension*. An elevated blood pressure of a known cause is called *secondary hypertension*. Factors associated with hypertension include arterial disease, obesity, a high serum sodium level, pregnancy, obstructive sleep apnea, and a family history of high blood pressure. The incidence of hypertension is higher in men than in women and is twice as common in blacks as in whites. People with mild or moderate hypertension may be asymptomatic or may experience suboccipital headaches (especially

TABLE 2–5	Factors Affecting Blood Pressure
Age	Blood pressure gradually increases throughout childhood, and correlates with height, weight, and age. In the adult, the blood pressure tends to gradually increase with age.
Exercise	Vigorous exercise increases cardiac output and thus blood pressure.
Autonomic nervous system	Increased sympathetic nervous system activity causes an increased heart rate, an increased cardiac contractility, changes in vascular smooth muscle tone to enhance blood flow to vital organs and skeletal muscles, and an increased blood volume. Collectively, these actions cause an increased blood pressure.
Stress	Stress stimulates the sympathetic nervous system and thus can increase blood pressure.
Circulating blood volume	A decreased circulating blood volume, either from blood or fluid loss, causes blood pressure to decrease. Common causes of fluid loss include abnormal, unreplaced fluid losses such as in diarrhea or diaphoresis, and overenthusiastic use of diuretics. Inadequate oral fluid intake can also result in a fluid volume deficit. Excess fluid, such as in congestive heart failure, can cause the blood pressure to increase.
Medications	Any medication that affects one or more of the previous conditions may cause blood pressure changes. For example, diuretics reduce blood volume; cardiac pharmaceuticals may increase or decrease heart rate and contractility; pain medications may reduce sympathetic nervous system stimulation; and specific antihypertension agents may exert their effects as well.
Normal fluctuations	Under normal circumstances, blood pressure varies from moment to moment in response to a variety of stimuli. For example, an increased environmental temperature causes blood vessels near the skin surface to dilate, causing blood pressure to decrease. In addition, normal respirations alter blood pressure: Blood pressure increases during expiration and decreases during inspiration. Blood pressure fluctuations caused by inspiration and expiration may be significant during a severe asthmatic episode.
Race	Black males over 35 years of age often have elevated blood pressures.
Obesity	Blood pressure is often higher in overweight and obese individuals.
Daily variations	Blood pressure is usually lowest early in the morning, when the metabolic rate is lowest.

on rising), tinnitus, light-headedness, easy fatigability, and cardiac palpitations. With sustained hypertension, arterial walls become thickened, inelastic, and resistant to blood flow. This process in turn causes the left ventricle to distend and hypertrophy. Left ventricular hypertrophy may lead to congestive heart failure.

Hypotension

Hypotension is said to be present when the patient's blood pressure falls below 90/60 mm Hg. It is an abnormal condition in which the blood pressure is not adequate for normal perfusion and oxygenation of vital organs. Hypotension is associated with peripheral vasodilation, decreased vascular resistance, hypovolemia, and left ventricular failure. Hypotension can also be caused by analgesics such as meperidine hydrochloride (Demerol) and morphine sulfate, severe burns, prolonged diarrhea, and vomiting. Signs and symptoms include pallor, skin mottling, clamminess, blurred vision, confusion, dizziness, syncope, chest pain, increased heart rate, and decreased urine output. Hypotension is life threatening.

Orthostatic hypotension, also called *postural hypotension,* occurs when blood pressure quickly drops as the individual rises to an upright position or stands. Orthostatic hypotension develops when the peripheral blood vessels—especially in central body organs and legs—are unable to constrict or respond appropriately to changes in body positions. Orthostatic hypotension is associated with decreased blood volume, anemia, dehydration, prolonged bed rest, and antihypertensive medications. The assessment of orthostatic hypotension is made by obtaining pulse and blood pressure readings when the patient is in the supine, sitting, and standing positions.

Pulsus Paradoxus

Pulsus paradoxus is defined as a systolic blood pressure that is more than 10 mm Hg lower on inspiration than on expiration. This exaggerated waxing and waning of arterial blood pressure can be detected using a sphygmomanometer or, in severe cases, by palpating the pulse at the wrist or neck. Commonly associated with severe asthmatic episodes, pulsus paradoxus is believed to be caused by the major intrapleural pressure swings that occur during inspiration and expiration. The reason for this phenomenon is described in the following sections.

Decreased Blood Pressure during Inspiration

During inspiration the asthmatic patient frequently relies on accessory muscles of inspiration. The accessory muscles help produce an extremely negative intrapleural pressure, which in turn enhances intrapulmonary gas flow. The increased negative intrapleural pressure, however, also causes blood vessels in the lungs to dilate, creating pooled blood. Consequently, the volume of blood returning to the left ventricle decreases, causing a reduction in cardiac output and arterial blood pressure during inspiration.

Increased Blood Pressure during Expiration

During expiration, the patient often activates the accessory muscles of expiration in an effort to overcome an increased airway resistance (R_{aw}). The increased power produced by these muscles generates a greater positive intrapleural pressure. Although increased positive intrapleural pressure helps offset R_{aw}, it also works to narrow or squeeze the blood vessels of the lung. This increased pressure on the pulmonary blood vessels enhances left ventricular filling and results in an increased cardiac output and arterial blood pressure during expiration.

◆ OXYGEN SATURATION

Oxygen saturation, often considered the fifth vital sign, is used to establish an immediate baseline Spo_2 value. It is an excellent monitor by which to assess the patient's response to respiratory care interventions. In the adult the normal Spo_2 values range between 95% and 99%. Spo_2 values between 91% and 94% indicate mild hypoxemia. Mild hypoxemia warrants additional evaluation by the respiratory practitioner but does not usually require supplemental oxygen. Spo_2 readings between 86% and 90% indicate moderate hypoxemia. These patients often require supplemental oxygen. Spo_2 values below 85% indicate severe hypoxemia and warrant immediate medical intervention, including the administration of 100% oxygen, ventilatory support, or both. Table 2-6 presents the relationship of the Spo_2 to the Pao_2 for the adult and newborn. Table 2-7 provides an overview of the signs and symptoms of inadequate oxygenation.

TABLE 2–6	Spo_2 and Pao_2 Relationship for the Adult and Newborn			
	Adult		**Newborn**	
Oxygen Status	Spo_2	Pao_2	Spo_2	Pao_2
Normal	95-99%	75-100	91-96%	60-80
Mild hypoxemia	90-95%	60-75	88-90 %	55-60
Moderate hypoxemia	85-90%	50-60	85-89%	50-58
Severe hypoxemia	<85%	<50	<85%	<50

Note: The Spo_2 will be lower than predicted when the following are present: low pH, high $Paco_2$, and high temperature.

TABLE 2–7	Signs and Symptoms of Inadequate Oxygenation	
Central Nervous System		
Apprehension	Early	
Restlessness or irritability	Early	
Confusion or lethargy	Early or late	
Combativeness	Late	
Coma	Late	
Respiratory		
Tachypnea	Early	
Dyspnea on exertion	Early	
Dyspnea at rest	Late	
Use of accessory muscles	Late	
Intercostal retractions	Late	
Takes a breath between each word or sentence	Late	
Cardiovascular		
Tachycardia	Early	
Mild hypertension	Early	
Arrhythmias	Early or late	
Hypotension	Late	
Cyanosis	Late	
Skin is cool or clammy	Late	
Other		
Diaphoresis	Early or late	
Decreased urinary output	Early or late	
General fatigue	Early or late	

◆ Systematic Examination of the Chest and Lungs

The physical examination of the chest and lungs should be performed in a systematic and orderly fashion. The most common sequence is as follows:

- Inspection
- Palpation
- Percussion
- Auscultation

Before the practitioner can adequately inspect, palpate, percuss, and auscultate the chest and lungs, however, he or she must first have a good working knowledge of the topographic landmarks of the lung and chest. Various anatomic landmarks and imaginary vertical lines drawn on the chest are used to identify and document the location of specific abnormalities.

LUNG AND CHEST TOPOGRAPHY

Thoracic Cage Landmarks

Anteriorly, the first rib is attached to the manubrium just beneath the clavicle. After the first rib is identified, the rest of the ribs can easily be located and numbered. The sixth rib and its cartilage are attached to the sternum just above the xiphoid process (Figure 2-3).

Posteriorly, the spinous processes of the vertebrae are useful landmarks. For example, when the patient's head is extended forward and down, two prominent spinous processes can usually be seen at the base of the neck. The top one is the spinous process of the seventh cervical vertebra (C-7); the bottom one is the spinous process of the thoracic vertebra (T-1). When only one spinous process can be seen, it is usually C-7 (see Figure 2-3).

Imaginary Lines

Various imaginary vertical lines are used to locate abnormalities on chest examination (Figure 2-4). The *midsternal line*, which is located in the middle of the sternum, equally divides the anterior chest into left and right hemithoraces. The *midclavicular lines*, which start at the middle of either the right or left clavicle, run parallel to the sternum.

On the lateral portion of the chest, three imaginary vertical lines are used. The *anterior axillary line*

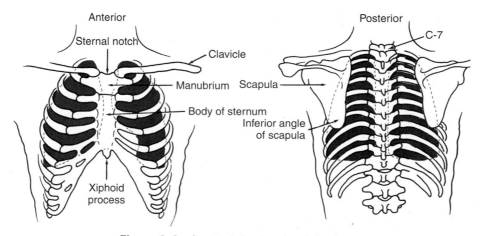

Figure 2–3 Anatomic landmarks of the chest.

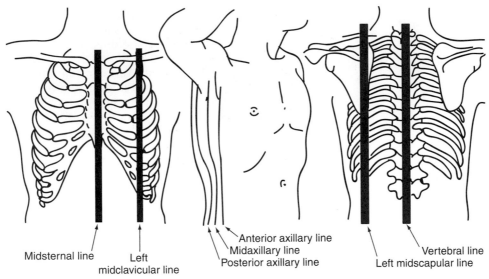

Figure 2–4   Imaginary vertical lines on the chest.

originates at the anterior axillary fold and runs down along the anterolateral aspect of the chest, the *midaxillary line* divides the lateral chest into two equal halves, and the *posterior axillary line* runs parallel to the midaxillary line along the posterolateral wall of the thorax.

Posteriorly, the *vertebral line* (also called the *midspinal line*) runs along the spinous processes of the vertebrae. The *midscapular line* runs through the middle of either the right or the left scapula parallel to the vertebral line.

Lung Borders and Fissures

Anteriorly, the apex of the lung extends about 2 to 4 cm above the medial third of the clavicle. Under normal conditions the lungs extend down to about the level of the sixth rib. Posteriorly, the superior portion of the lung extends to about the level of T-1 and down to about the level of T-10 (Figure 2-5).

The right lung is separated into the upper, middle, and lower lobes by the *horizontal fissure* and the *oblique fissure.* The horizontal fissure runs anteriorly from the fourth rib at the sternal border to the fifth rib at the midaxillary line. The horizontal fissure separates the right anterior upper lobe from the middle lobe. The oblique fissure runs laterally from the sixth or seventh rib and the midclavicular line to the fifth rib at the midaxillary line. From this point the oblique fissure continues to run around the chest posteriorly and upward to about the level of T-3. Anteriorly, the oblique fissure divides the lower lobe from the lower border of the middle lobe. Posteriorly,

the oblique fissure separates the upper lobe from the lower lobe.

The left lung is separated into the upper and lower lobes by the oblique fissure. Anteriorly, the oblique fissure runs laterally from the sixth or seventh rib and the midclavicular line to the fifth rib at the midaxillary line. The fissure continues to run around the chest posteriorly and upward to about the level of T-3.

◆ INSPECTION

The inspection of the patient is an ongoing observational process that begins with the history and continues throughout the patient interview, taking of vital signs, and physical examination. The inspection consists of a series of observations to gather clinical manifestations—signs and symptoms—that are directly or indirectly related to the patient's respiratory status. Although many visual observations are based on the practitioner's professional judgment (subjective information), the information gathered is nevertheless considered important objective clinical data when gathered by a trained respiratory care practitioner.

Common Clinical Manifestations Observed during Inspection

Box 2-4 lists common clinical manifestations observed during the inspection of the patient with a pathologic respiratory condition. For example, during a systematic visual inspection, the respiratory practitioner might note the patient's ventilatory pattern. Is the patient using accessory muscles of inspiration?

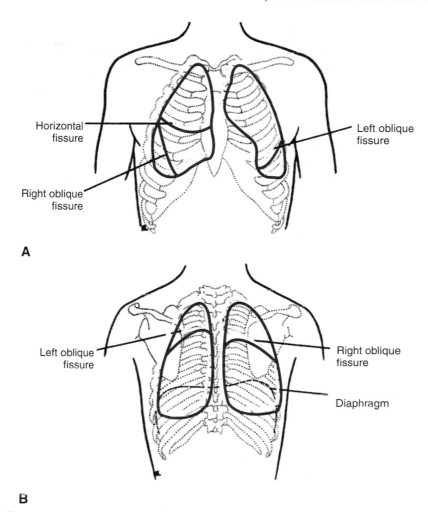

Figure 2–5   Topographic location of lung fissures projected on the anterior chest (**A**) and posterior chest (**B**).

BOX 2–4

Common Clinical Manifestations Observed during Inspection

- Abnormal ventilatory pattern findings
- Use of accessory muscles of inspiration
- Use of accessory muscles of expiration
- Pursed-lip breathing
- Substernal or intercostal retractions
- Nasal flaring
- Splinting due to chest pain or decreased chest expansion
- Abnormal chest shape and configuration
- Abnormal extremity findings:
  - Altered skin color
  - Digital clubbing
  - Pedal edema
  - Distended neck veins
- Cough (note characteristics)

Is the patient engaging in pursed-lip breathing? Are substernal or intercostal retractions occurring during inspiration? Does the patient appear to be splinting or to have decreased chest expansion because of chest pain? Are the shape and configuration of the chest normal? Do the patient's skin, lips, fingers, or toenails appear cyanotic? Does the patient have digital clubbing, pedal edema, or distended neck veins? Is the patient coughing? How strong is the patient's cough? What are the characteristics of the patient's sputum? A more in-depth discussion of the items presented in Box 2-4 can be found in the section on Systematic Examination of the Chest and Lungs (see page 21).

◆ **PALPATION**

Palpation is the process of touching the patient's chest to evaluate the symmetry of chest expansion, the position of the trachea, skin temperature, muscle tone, areas of tenderness, lumps, depressions, and

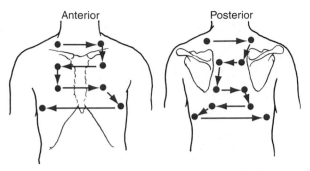

Anterior   Posterior

Figure 2–6 Path of palpation for vocal or tactile fremitus.

tactile and vocal fremitus. When palpating the chest, the clinician may use the heel or ulnar side of the hand, the palms, or the fingertips. As shown in Figure 2-6, both the anterior and posterior chest should be palpated from side to side in an orderly fashion, from the apices of the chest down.

To evaluate the position of the trachea, the examiner places an index finger over the sternal notch and gently moves it from side to side. The trachea should be in the midline directly above the sternal notch. A number of abnormal pulmonary conditions can cause the trachea to deviate from its normal position. For example, a tension pneumothorax, pleural effusion, or tumor mass may push the trachea to the unaffected side, whereas atelectasis and pulmonary fibrosis pull the trachea to the affected side.

Chest Excursion

The symmetry of chest expansion is evaluated by lightly placing each hand over the patient's posterolateral chest so that the thumbs meet at the midline at about the T-8 to T-10 level. The patient is instructed to exhale slowly and completely and then to inhale deeply. As the patient is inhaling, the examiner evaluates the distance that each thumb moves from the midline. Normally, each thumb tip moves equally about 3 to 5 cm from the midline (Figure 2-7).

The examiner next faces the patient and lightly places each hand on the patient's anterolateral chest so that the thumbs meet at the midline along the costal margins near the xiphoid process. The patient is again instructed to exhale slowly and completely and then to inhale deeply. As the patient is inhaling, the examiner observes the distance each thumb moves from the midline.

A number of pulmonary disorders can alter the patient's chest excursion. For example, a bilaterally decreased chest expansion may be caused by both obstructive and restrictive lung disorders. An unequal chest expansion may be caused by alveolar consolidation (e.g., pneumonia), lobar atelectasis, tension

pneumothorax, large pleural effusions, and chest trauma (e.g., fractured ribs).

Tactile and Vocal Fremitus

Vibrations that can be perceived by palpation over the chest are called *tactile fremitus.* This condition is commonly caused by gas flowing through thick secretions that are partially obstructing the large airways. Vibrations that can be perceived by palpation or auscultation over the chest during phonation are called *vocal fremitus.* Sounds produced by the vocal cords are transmitted down the tracheobronchial tree and through the lung parenchyma to the chest wall where the examiner can feel the vibration. Vocal fremitus can often be elicited by having the patient repeat the phrase "ninety-nine" or "blue moon." These are resonant phrases that produce strong vibrations. Normally, fremitus is most prominent between the scapulae and around the sternum, sites where the large bronchi are closest to the chest wall.

Tactile and vocal fremitus decrease when anything obstructs the transmission of vibration. Such conditions include chronic obstructive pulmonary disease, tumors or thickening of the pleural cavity, pleural effusion, pneumothorax, and a muscular or obese chest wall. Tactile and vocal fremitus increase in patients with alveolar consolidation, alveolar collapse, pulmonary edema, lung tumors, pulmonary fibrosis, and thin chest walls.

Crepitus (also called *subcutaneous emphysema*) is a coarse, crackling sensation that may be palpable over the skin surface. It occurs when air escapes from the thorax and enters the subcutaneous tissue. It may occur after a tracheostomy and mechanical ventilation, open thoracic injury, or thoracic surgery.

◆ PERCUSSION

Percussion over the chest wall is performed to determine the size, borders, and consistency of air, liquid, or solid material in the underlying lung. When percussing the chest, the examiner firmly places the distal portion of the middle finger of the nondominant hand between the ribs over the surface of the chest area to be examined. No other portion of the hand should touch the patient's chest. With the end of the middle finger of the dominant hand, the examiner quickly strikes the distal joint of the finger positioned on the chest wall and then quickly withdraws the tapping finger (Figure 2-8). The examiner should perform the chest percussion in an orderly fashion from top to bottom, comparing the sounds generated on both sides of the chest, both anteriorly and posteriorly (Figure 2-9).

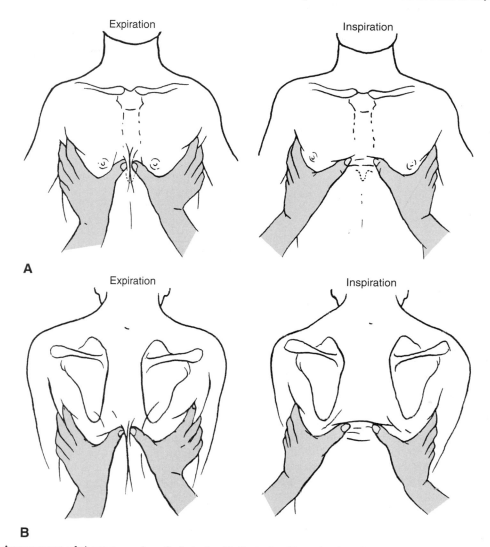

Figure 2-7 Assessment of chest excursion. **A**, Anterior. **B**, Posterior. Note the thumbs move apart on inspiration as the volume of the thorax increases.

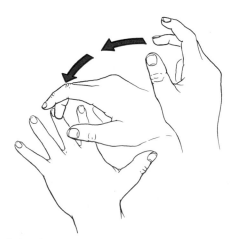

Figure 2-8 Chest percussion technique to include all important areas.

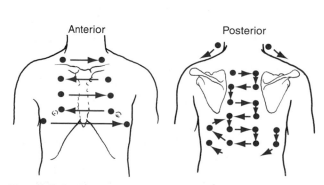

Figure 2–9 Path of systematic percussion to include all important areas.

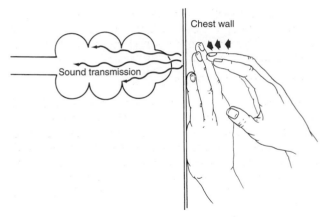

Figure 2–10   Chest percussion of a normal lung.

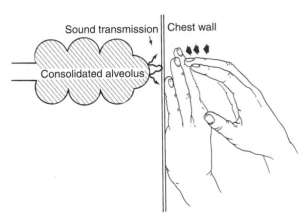

Figure 2–11   A short, dull, or flat percussion note is typically produced over areas of alveolar consolidation.

In the normal lung the sound created by percussion is transmitted throughout the air-filled lung and is typically described as loud, low in pitch, and long in duration. The sounds elicited by the examiner vibrate freely throughout the large surface area of the lungs and create a sound similar to that elicited by knocking on a watermelon (Figure 2-10).

Resonance may be muffled somewhat in the individual with a heavily muscular chest wall and in the obese person. When percussing the anterior chest, the examiner should take care not to confuse the normal borders of cardiac dullness with pulmonary pathology. In addition, the upper border of liver dullness is normally located in the right fifth intercostal space and midclavicular line. Over the left chest, tympany is produced over the gastric space. When percussing the posterior chest, the examiner should avoid the damping effect of the scapulae.

Abnormal Percussion Notes

A *dull percussion note* is heard when the chest is percussed over areas of pleural thickening, pleural effusion, atelectasis, and consolidation. When these conditions exist, the sounds produced by the examiner do not freely vibrate throughout the lungs. A dull percussion note is described as flat or soft, high in pitch, and short in duration, similar to the sound produced by knocking on a full barrel (Figure 2-11).

When the chest is percussed over areas of trapped gas, a *hyperresonant note* is heard. These sounds are described as very loud, low in pitch, and long in duration, similar to the sound produced by knocking on an empty barrel (Figure 2-12). A hyperresonant note is commonly elicited in the patient suffering

from chronic obstructive pulmonary disease or pneumothorax.

Diaphragmatic Excursion

The relative position and range of motion of the diaphragms also can be determined by percussion. Clinically, this evaluation is called the determination of diaphragmatic excursion. To assess the patient's diaphragmatic excursion, the examiner first maps out the lower lung borders by percussing the posterior chest from the apex down, and identifying the point at which the percussion note definitely changes from a resonant to flat sound. This procedure is performed at maximal inspiration and again at maximal expiration. Under normal conditions the diaphragmatic

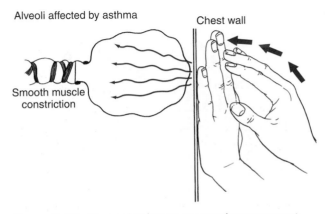

Figure 2–12   Percussion becomes more hyperresonant with alveolar hyperinflation.

excursion should be equal bilaterally and measure about 4 to 8 cm in the adult.

When severe alveolar hyperinflation is present (e.g., severe emphysema, asthma), the diaphragm is low and flat in position and has minimal excursion. Lobar collapse of one lung may pull the diaphragm up on the affected side and reduce excursion. The diaphragms may be elevated and immobile in neuromuscular diseases that affect them.

◆ AUSCULTATION

Auscultation of the chest provides information about the heart, blood vessels, and air flowing in and out of the tracheobronchial tree and alveoli. A stethoscope is used to evaluate the frequency, intensity, duration, and quality of the sounds. During auscultation the patient should ideally be in the upright position and instructed to breathe slowly and deeply through the mouth. The anterior and posterior chest should be auscultated in an orderly fashion from the apex to base while comparing the right side of the chest with the left (Figure 2-13). When examining the posterior chest, the examiner should ask the patient to rotate the shoulders forward so that a greater surface area of the lungs can be auscultated.

Normal Breath Sounds

Three different breath sounds can be auscultated over the normal chest. They are called *bronchial*, *bronchovesicular*, and *vesicular* breath sounds.

Bronchial Breath Sounds

Bronchial breath sounds have a harsh, hollow, or tubular quality. They are loud, high in pitch, and about equal in duration in length of inspiration and expiration. A slight pause occurs between these two components. Bronchial breath sounds are normally auscultated directly over the trachea and are caused by the turbulent flow of gas through the upper airway. Clinically, these sounds are also called *tracheal, tracheobronchial,* and *tubular breath sounds.*

Bronchovesicular Breath Sounds

Bronchovesicular breath sounds are auscultated directly over the mainstem bronchi. They are softer and lower in pitch than bronchial breath sounds and do not have a pause between the inspiratory and expiratory phase. These sounds are reduced in intensity and pitch as a result of the filtering of sound that occurs as gas moves between the large airways and alveoli.

Anteriorly, bronchovesicular breath sounds can be heard directly over the mainstem bronchi between the first and second ribs. Posteriorly, they are heard between the scapulae near the spinal column between the first and sixth ribs, especially on the right side (Figure 2-14, *A*).

Vesicular Breath Sounds

Vesicular breath sounds are the normal sounds of gas rustling or swishing through the small bronchioles and possibly the alveoli. Under normal conditions, vesicular breath sounds are auscultated over most of the lung field, both anteriorly and posteriorly (see Figure 2-14, *B*). Vesicular breath sounds are described as soft and low in pitch and are primarily heard during inspiration. As the gas molecules enter the alveoli, they are able to spread out over a large surface area and, as a result of this

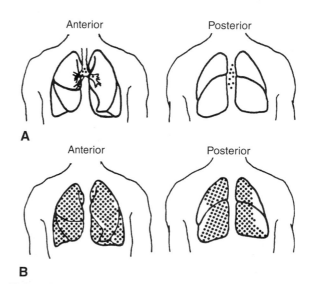

Figure 2-14 The location at which bronchovesicular breath sounds (**A**) and vesicular breath sounds (**B**) are normally auscultated.

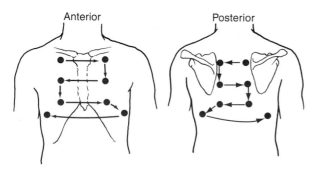

Figure 2-13 Path of systematic auscultation to include all important areas. Note the exact similarity of this pathway to Figure 2-6.

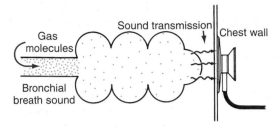

Figure 2–15 Auscultation of vesicular breath sounds over a normal lung unit.

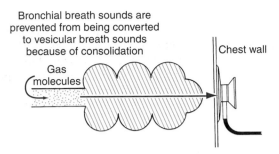

Figure 2–16 Auscultation of bronchial breath sounds over a consolidated lung unit.

action, create less gas turbulence. As gas turbulence decreases, the breath sounds become softer and lower in pitch, similar to the sound of the wind in the trees. Vesicular breath sounds also are heard during the initial third of exhalation as gas leaves the alveoli and bronchioles and moves into the large airways (Figure 2-15).

Adventitious (Abnormal) Breath Sounds

Adventitious breath sounds are additional or different sounds that are not normally heard over a particular area of the thorax. Bronchial breath sounds heard over an area of the chest that normally demonstrates vesicular breath sounds are one example. Several different types of adventitious breath sounds exist, each indicating a particular pulmonary abnormality.

Bronchial Breath Sounds

If gas molecules are not permitted to dissipate throughout the parenchymal areas (because of alveolar consolidation or atelectasis, for example) the gas molecules have no opportunity to spread out over a larger surface area and therefore become less turbulent. Consequently, the sounds produced in this area are louder because the gas sounds are coming mainly from the tracheobronchial tree and not the lung parenchyma. These sounds are called *bronchial breath sounds.*

It is commonly believed that breath sounds in patients with alveolar consolidation should be diminished because the consolidation acts as a sound barrier. Although alveolar collapse or consolidation does act as a sound barrier and reduces bronchial breath sounds, the reduction is not as great as it would be if the gas molecules were allowed to dissipate throughout normal lung parenchyma. In addition, liquid and solid materials transmit sounds more readily than air-filled spaces and therefore may further contribute to the bronchial quality of the breath sound. Therefore when disease causes alveolar collapse or consolidation, harsher, bronchial-type sounds are heard

over the affected areas rather than the normal vesicular sounds (Figure 2-16).

Diminished Breath Sounds

Breath sounds are diminished or distant in respiratory disorders that lead to alveolar hypoventilation, regardless of the cause. For example, patients with chronic obstructive pulmonary disease often have diminished breath sounds. These patients hypoventilate because of air trapping and increased functional residual capacity. In addition, when the functional residual capacity is increased, the gas that enters the enlarged alveoli during each breath spreads out over a greater-than-normal surface area, resulting in less gas turbulence and a softer sound (Figure 2-17). Heart sounds also may be diminished in patients with air trapping.

Diminished breath sounds also are found in respiratory disorders that cause hypoventilation by compressing the lung. Such disorders include flail chest, pleural effusion, and pneumothorax. Diminished breath sounds also are characteristic of neuromuscular diseases that cause hypoventilation. Such disorders include Guillain-Barré syndrome and myasthenia gravis.

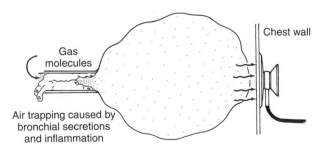

Figure 2–17 As air trapping and alveolar hyperinflation develop in obstructive lung diseases, breath sounds progressively diminish.

Crackles and Rhonchi

Adjectives used in the older literature to describe crackles and rhonchi (moist, wet, dry, crackling, sibilant, coarse, fine, crepitant) depend largely on the auditory acuity and experience of the examiner. Descriptions have little value because only the presence or absence of crackles or rhonchi is important. When fluid accumulation is present in a respiratory disorder, some crackles or rhonchi are almost always present (i.e., "bubbly" or "slurpy" sounds accompanying the breath sounds).

Crackles (rales) are usually fine or medium crackling wet sounds that are typically heard during inspiration. They are formed in the small and medium-sized airways and may or may not change in nature after a strong, vigorous cough.

Rhonchi, on the other hand, usually have a coarse, "bubbly" quality and are typically heard during expiration. They are formed in the larger airways and often change in nature or disappear after a strong, vigorous cough.

Wheezing

Wheezing is the characteristic sound produced by airway obstruction. Found in all bronchospastic disorders, it is one of the cardinal findings in bronchial asthma. The sounds are high-pitched and whistling and generally last throughout the expiratory phase. The mechanism of a wheeze is similar to the vibrating reed of a woodwind instrument. The reed, which partially occludes the mouthpiece of the instrument, vibrates and produces a sound when air is forced through it (Figure 2-18). The softest, higher pitched wheezes occur in the tightest airway obstruction.

Pleural Friction Rubs

If pleuritis accompanies a respiratory disorder, the inflamed pleural membranes resist movement during breathing and create a peculiar and characteristic sound known as a pleural friction rub. The sound is reminiscent of that made by a creaking shoe and is usually heard in the area where the patient complains of pain.

Stridor

Stridor is an abnormal audible high-pitched musical sound caused by an obstruction in the trachea or larynx. It is generally heard during inspiration. Stridor indicates a neoplastic or inflammatory condition, including glottic edema, asthma, diphtheria, laryngospasm, and papilloma (a benign epithelial neoplasm of the larynx). Stridor is usually loud enough to hear without a stethoscope, as in infantile croup.

Whispering Pectoriloquy

Whispering pectoriloquy is the term used to describe the unusually clear transmission of the whispered voice of a patient as heard through the stethoscope. When the patient whispers "one, two, three," the sounds produced by the vocal cords are transmitted not only toward the mouth and nose but throughout the lungs as well. As the whispered sounds travel down the tracheobronchial tree, they remain relatively unchanged, but as the sound disperses throughout the large surface area of the alveoli, it diminishes sharply. Consequently, when the examiner listens with a stethoscope over a normal lung while a patient whispers "one, two, three," the sounds are diminished, distant, muffled, and unintelligible (Figure 2-19).

When a patient who has atelectasis or consolidated lung areas whispers "one, two, three," the sounds produced are prevented from spreading out over a large alveolar surface area. Even though the consolidated area may act as a sound barrier and diminish the sounds somewhat, the reduction in sound is not as great as it would be if the sounds were allowed to dissipate throughout a normal lung. Consequently, the whispered sounds are much louder and more intelligible over the affected lung areas (Figure 2-20).

Table 2-8 provides an overview of the common assessment abnormalities found during inspection, palpation, percussion, and auscultation.

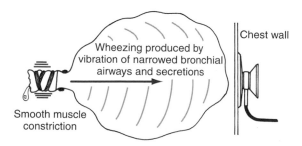

Figure 2–18 Wheezing and rhonchi often develop during an asthmatic episode because of smooth muscle constriction, wall edema, and mucus accumulation.

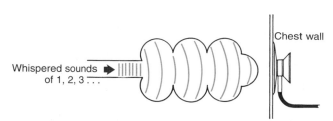

Figure 2–19 Whispered voice sounds auscultated over a normal lung are usually faint and unintelligible.

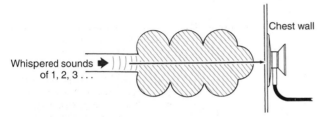

Figure 2–20   Whispering pectoriloquy. Whispered voice sounds heard over a consolidated lung are often louder and more intelligible compared with those of a normal lung.

In-Depth Discussion of Common Clinical Manifestations Observed during Inspection

NORMAL VENTILATORY PATTERN

An individual's breathing pattern is composed of a tidal volume (V_T), a ventilatory rate, and an inspiratory-to-expiratory ratio (I:E ratio). In normal adults the V_T is about 500 ml (7 to 9 ml/kg), the ventilatory rate is about 15 (with a range of 12 to 18) breaths per

---

TABLE 2–8   Common Assessment Abnormalities

Finding	Description	Possible Etiology and Significance
Inspection		
Pursed-lip breathing	Exhalation through mouth with lips pursed together to slow exhalation.	COPD, asthma. Suggests ↑ breathlessness. Strategy taught to slow expiration, ↓ dyspnea.
Tripod position; inability to lie flat	Leaning forward with arms and elbows supported on overbed table.	COPD, asthma in exacerbation, pulmonary edema. Indicates moderate to severe respiratory distress.
Accessory muscle use; intercostal retractions	Neck and shoulder muscles used to assist breathing. Muscles between ribs pull in during inspiration.	COPD, asthma in excerbation, secretion retention. Indicates severe respiratory distress, hypoxemia.
Splinting	Voluntary ↓ in tidal volume to ↓ pain on chest expansion.	Thoracic or abdominal incision. Chest trauma, pleurisy.
↑ AP diameter	AP chest diameter equal to lateral. Slope of ribs more horizontal (90 degrees) to spine.	COPD, asthma, cystic fibrosis. Lung hyperinflation. Advanced age.
Tachypnea	Rate >20 breaths/min; >25 breaths/min in elderly.	Fever, anxiety, hypoxemia, restrictive lung disease. Magnitude of ↑ above normal rate reflects increased work of breathing.
Kussmaul's respirations	Regular, rapid, and deep respirations.	Metabolic acidosis; ↑ in rate aids body in ↑ CO_2 excretion.
Cyanosis	Bluish color of skin best seen in earlobes, under the eyelids, or in nail beds.	↓ Oxygen transfer in lungs, ↓ cardiac output. Nonspecific, unreliable indicator.
Clubbing of fingers	↑ Depth, bulk, sponginess of distal digit of finger.	Chronic hypoxemia. Cystic fibrosis, lung cancer, bronchiectasis.
Abdominal paradox	Inward (rather than normal outward) movement of abdomen during inspiration.	Inefficient and ineffective breathing pattern. Nonspecific indicator of severe respiratory distress.
Palpation		
Tracheal deviation	Leftward or rightward movement of trachea from normal midline position.	Nonspecific indicator of change in position of mediastinal structures. Medical emergency if caused by tension pneumothorax.
Altered tactile fremitus	Increase or decrease in vibrations.	↑ In pneumonia, pulmonary edema; ↓ in pleural effusion, lung hyperinflation; absent in pneumothorax, atelectasis.
Altered chest movement	Unequal or equal but diminished movement of two sides of chest with inspiration.	Unequal movement caused by atelectasis, pneumothorax, pleural effusion, splinting; equal but diminished movement caused by barrel chest, restrictive disease, neuromuscular disease.

Continued

TABLE 2–8 Common Assessment Abnormalities—Cont'd

Finding	Description	Possible Etiology and Significance
Percussion		
Hyperresonance	Loud, lower-pitched sound over areas that normally produce a resonant sound.	Lung hyperinflation (COPD), lung collapse (pneumothorax), air trapping (asthma).
Dullness	Medium-pitched sound over areas that normally produce a resonant sound.	↑ Density (pneumonia, large atelectasis), ↑ fluid pleural space (pleural effusion).
Auscultation		
Fine crackles	Series of short, explosive, high-pitched sounds heard just before the end of inspiration; result of rapid equalization of gas pressure when collapsed alveoli or terminal bronchioles suddenly snap open; similar sound to that made by rolling hair between fingers just behind ear.	Interstitial fibrosis (asbestosis), interstitial edema (early pulmonary edema), alveolar filling (pneumonia), loss of lung volume (atelectasis), early phase of congestive heart failure.
Coarse crackles	Series of short, low-pitched sounds caused by air passing through airway intermittently occluded by mucus, unstable bronchial wall, or fold of mucosa; evident on inspiration and, at times, expiration; similar sound to blowing through straw under water; increase in bubbling quality with more fluid.	Congestive heart failure, pulmonary edema, pneumonia with severe congestion, COPD.
Rhonchi	Continuous rumbling, snoring, or rattling sounds from obstruction of large airways with secretions; most prominent on expiration; change often evident after coughing or suctioning.	COPD, cystic fibrosis, pneumonia, bronchiectasis.
Wheezes	Continuous high-pitched squeaking sound caused by rapid vibration of bronchial walls; first evident on expiration but possibly evident on inspiration as obstruction of airway increases; possibly audible without stethoscope.	Bronchospasm (caused by asthma), airway obstruction (caused by foreign body, tumor), COPD.
Stridor	Continuous musical sound of constant pitch; result of partial obstruction of larynx or trachea.	Croup, epiglottitis, vocal cord edema after extubation, foreign body.
Absent breath sounds	No sound evident over entire lung or area of lung.	Pleural effusion, mainstem bronchi obstruction, large atelectasis, pneumonectomy, lobectomy.
Pleural friction rub	Creaking or grating sound from roughened, inflamed surfaces of the pleura rubbing together; evident during inspiration, expiration, or both and no change with coughing; usually uncomfortable, especially on deep inspiration.	Pleurisy, pneumonia, pulmonary infarct.
Bronchophony, whispered pectoriloquy	Spoken or whispered syllable more distinct than normal on auscultation.	Pneumonia.
Egophony	Spoken "e" similar to "a" on auscultation because of altered transmission of voice sounds.	Pneumonia, pleural effusion.

Modified from Lewis S, Heitkemper MM, Dirksen SR: *Medical-surgical nursing: Assessment and management of clinical problems*, ed 6, vol. 1, St. Louis, 2004, Mosby.

minute, and the I:E ratio is about 1:2. In patients with respiratory disorders, however, an abnormal ventilatory pattern is often present (see Table 2-4 for common abnormal ventilatory patterns).

◆ ABNORMAL VENTILATORY PATTERNS

Although the precise etiology may not always be known, *the cause of an abnormal ventilatory pattern is frequently related to (1) the anatomic alterations*

of the lungs associated with a specific disorder and (2) the pathophysiologic mechanisms that develop because of the anatomic alterations. Therefore to evaluate and assess the various abnormal ventilatory patterns (rate and volume relationships) seen in the clinical setting, the following pathophysiologic mechanisms that can alter the ventilatory pattern must first be understood:

- Lung compliance
- Airway resistance

- Peripheral chemoreceptors
- Central chemoreceptors
- Pulmonary reflexes:

  - Hering-Breuer reflex
  - Deflation reflex
  - Irritant reflex
  - Juxtapulmonary-capillary receptors (J receptors) reflex
  - Reflexes from the aortic and carotid sinus baroreceptors
  - Pain, anxiety, and fever

COMMON PATHOPHYSIOLOGIC MECHANISMS THAT AFFECT THE VENTILATORY PATTERN

Lung Compliance and Its Effect on the Ventilatory Pattern

The ease with which the elastic forces of the lungs accept a volume of inspired air is known as *lung compliance (C_L)*. C_L is measured in terms of unit volume change per unit pressure change. Mathematically, it is written as liters per centimeter of water pressure. In other words, compliance determines how much air in liters the lungs will accommodate for each centimeter of water pressure change in distending pressure.

For example, when the normal individual generates a negative intrapleural pressure change of 2 cm H_2O during inspiration, the lungs accept a new volume of about 0.2 L gas. Therefore the C_L of the lungs is 0.1 L/cm H_2O:

$$C_L = \frac{\Delta V (L)}{\Delta P \text{ (cm } H_2O)}$$

$$= \frac{0.2 \text{ L gas}}{2 \text{ cm } H_2O}$$

$$= 0.1 \text{ L/cm } H_2O$$

The normal compliance of the lungs is graphically illustrated by the volume-pressure curve (Figure 2-21). When C_L increases, the lungs accept a greater volume of gas per unit pressure change. When C_L decreases, the lungs accept a smaller volume of gas per unit pressure change (Figure 2-22).

Although the precise mechanism is not clear, the fact that certain ventilatory patterns occur when lung compliance is altered is well-documented. For example, when C_L decreases, the patient's breathing rate generally increases while the tidal volume simultaneously decreases (Figure 2-23). This type of breathing pattern is commonly seen in restrictive lung disorders such as pneumonia, pulmonary edema,

and adult respiratory distress syndrome. This breathing pattern also is commonly seen during the early stages of an acute asthmatic attack when the alveoli are hyperinflated; C_L progressively decreases as the alveolar volume increases (see Figure 2-21) at high lung volumes.

Airway Resistance and Its Effect on the Ventilatory Pattern

Airway resistance (R_{aw}) is defined as the pressure difference between the mouth and the alveoli (transairway pressure) divided by the flow rate. Therefore the rate at which a certain volume of gas flows through the airways is a function of the pressure gradient and the resistance created by the airways to the flow of gas. Mathematically, R_{aw} is calculated as follows:

$$R_{aw} = \frac{\Delta P \text{ (cm } H_2O)}{\dot{V} \text{ (L/sec)}}$$

For example, if a patient produces a flow rate of 6 L/sec during inspiration by generating a transairway pressure difference of 12 cm H_2O, R_{aw} would be 2 cm H_2O/L/sec:

$$R_{aw} = \frac{\Delta P}{\dot{V}}$$

$$= \frac{12 \text{ cm } H_2O}{6 \text{ L/sec}}$$

$$= 2 \text{ cm } H_2O/L/sec$$

Under normal conditions the R_{aw} in the tracheobronchial tree is about 1.0 to 2.0 cm H_2O/L/sec. However, in large airway obstructive pulmonary diseases (e.g., bronchitis, asthma), the R_{aw} may be extremely high. An increased R_{aw} has a profound effect on the patient's ventilatory pattern.

When airway resistance increases significantly, the patient's ventilatory rate usually decreases while the tidal volume simultaneously increases (see Figure 2-23). This type of breathing pattern is commonly seen in large airway obstructive lung diseases (e.g., chronic bronchitis, bronchiectasis, asthma, cystic fibrosis) during the advanced stages.

The ventilatory pattern adopted by the patient in either a restrictive or an obstructive lung disorder is thought to be based on minimum work requirements rather than gas exchange efficiency. In physics, work is defined as the force multiplied by the distance moved (work = force × distance). In respiratory physiology the change in pulmonary pressure (force)

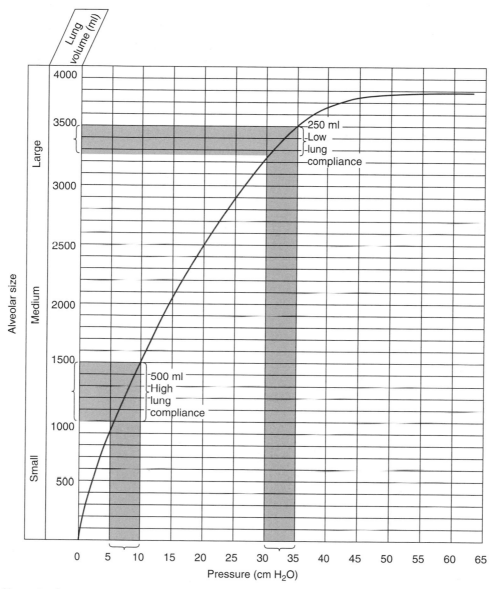

Figure 2–21 Normal volume-pressure curve. The curve shows that lung compliance progressively decreases as the lungs expand in response to more volume. For example, note the greater volume change between 5 and 10 cm H_2O (small and medium alveoli) than between 30 and 35 cm H_2O (large alveoli). (Modified from Des Jardins T: *Cardiopulmonary anatomy and physiology: Essentials for respiratory care,* ed 4, Albany, NY, 2002, Delmar Publishers.)

multiplied by the change in lung volume (distance) may be used to quantify the amount of work required to breathe (work = pressure × volume).

The patient's usual adopted ventilatory pattern may not be seen in the clinical setting because of secondary heart or lung problems. For example, a patient with chronic bronchitis who has adopted a decreased ventilatory rate and an increased tidal volume because of the increased airway resistance

associated with the disorder demonstrates an increased ventilatory rate and decreased tidal volume in response to a secondary pneumonia (a restrictive lung disorder superimposed on a chronic obstructive lung disorder).

Because the patient may adopt a ventilatory pattern based on the expenditure of energy rather than on the efficiency of ventilation, the examiner cannot assume that the ventilatory pattern acquired by the

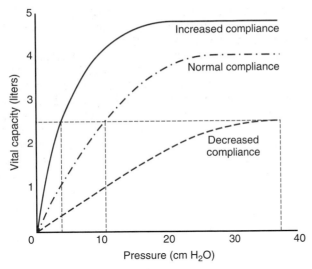

Figure 2–22   The effects of increased and decreased compliance on the volume-pressure curve. As the lung compliance decreases, greater pressure change is required to obtain the same volume of 2.5 L (*dotted lines*).

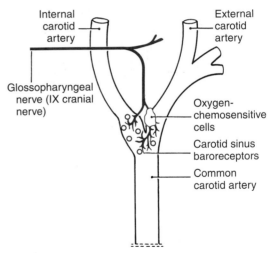

Figure 2–24   Oxygen-chemosensitive cells and the carotid sinus baroreceptors are located on the carotid artery.

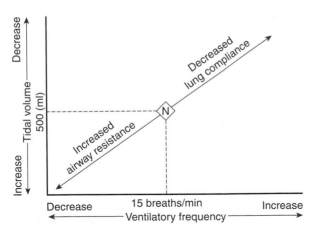

Figure 2–23   The effects of increased airway resistance and decreased lung compliance on ventilatory frequency and tidal volume. *N,* Normal resting tidal volume and ventilatory frequency.

patient in response to a certain respiratory disorder is the most efficient one in terms of physiologic gas exchange.

◆ Peripheral Chemoreceptors and their Effect on the Ventilatory Pattern

The peripheral chemoreceptors (also called *carotid* and *aortic bodies*) are oxygen-sensitive cells that react to a reduction of oxygen in the arterial blood (Pao_2). The peripheral chemoreceptors are located at the

bifurcation of the internal and external carotid arteries (Figure 2-24) and on the aortic arch (Figure 2-25). Although the peripheral chemoreceptors are stimulated whenever the Pao_2 is less than normal, they are generally most active when the Pao_2 falls below 60 mm Hg (Sao_2 of about 90%). Suppression of these chemoreceptors, however, is seen when the Pao_2 falls below 30 mm Hg.

When the peripheral chemoreceptors are activated, an afferent (sensory) signal is sent to the respiratory centers of the medulla by way of the glossopharyngeal nerve (cranial nerve IX) from the carotid bodies and by way of the vagus nerve (cranial nerve X) from the aortic bodies. Efferent (motor) signals are then sent to the respiratory muscles, which results in an increased rate of breathing.

In patients who have a chronically low Pao_2 and a high $Paco_2$ (e.g., during the advanced stages of emphysema), the peripheral chemoreceptors may be totally responsible for the control of ventilation because a chronically high CO_2 concentration in the cerebrospinal fluid (CSF) inactivates the hydrogen ion (H^+) sensitivity of the central chemoreceptors.

Causes of Hypoxemia

In respiratory disease a decreased arterial oxygen level (hypoxemia) is the result of decreased ventilation-perfusion ratios, pulmonary shunting, and venous admixture.

Ventilation-Perfusion Ratios. Ideally, each alveolus should receive the same ratio of ventilation and pulmonary capillary blood flow. In reality, however, this

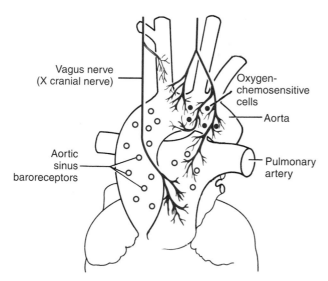

Figure 2–25 Oxygen-chemosensitive cells and the aortic sinus baroreceptors are located on the aortic notch and pulmonary artery.

is not the case. Alveolar ventilation is normally about 4 L/min, and the pulmonary capillary blood flow is about 5 L/min, which makes the overall ratio of ventilation to blood flow 4:5, or 0.8. This relationship is referred to as the *ventilation-perfusion* ($\dot{V}/\dot{Q}$) *ratio* (Figure 2-26).

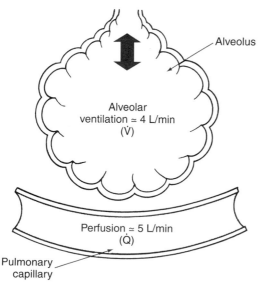

Figure 2–26 The normal overall pulmonary ventilation-perfusion ratio ($\dot{V}/\dot{Q}$) is approximately 0.8. (Modified from Des Jardins T: *Cardiopulmonary anatomy and physiology: Essentials for respiratory care,* ed 4, Albany, NY, 2002, Delmar.)

In a normal individual in the upright position, the alveoli in the upper portions of the lungs (apices) receive moderate amounts of ventilation and little blood flow. Consequently, the $\dot{V}/\dot{Q}$ ratio throughout this region is higher than 0.8. In the lower regions of the lung, alveolar ventilation is moderately increased, and the blood flow is greatly increased because blood flow is gravity dependent. As a result, the $\dot{V}/\dot{Q}$ ratio is lower than 0.8 in this area. The $\dot{V}/\dot{Q}$ ratio progressively decreases from the top to the bottom of the lungs in an individual in the upright position, and the overall average $\dot{V}/\dot{Q}$ ratio is about 0.8. In respiratory disorders the $\dot{V}/\dot{Q}$ ratio is usually altered.

Increased Ventilation-Perfusion Ratio. In some disorders, such as pulmonary embolic disease, the lungs receive less blood flow in relation to ventilation. When this condition develops, the $\dot{V}/\dot{Q}$ ratio increases. A larger portion of the alveolar ventilation therefore will not be physiologically effective and is said to be "wasted" or dead-space ventilation (Figure 2-27).

Decreased Ventilation-Perfusion Ratio. In lung disorders such as asthma or pneumonia the lungs receive less ventilation in relation to blood flow. When this condition develops, the $\dot{V}/\dot{Q}$ ratio decreases. A larger portion of the pulmonary blood flow is not physiologically effective in terms of molecular gas exchange and is said to be "shunted" blood (see the following section on pulmonary shunting). Generally, when the $\dot{V}/\dot{Q}$ ratio decreases, the Pa_{O_2} decreases and the Pa_{CO_2} increases.

Pulmonary Shunting. Pulmonary shunting takes three forms: the anatomic shunt, the capillary shunt, and the shuntlike effect.

Anatomic Shunt. An anatomic right-to-left shunt exists when blood flows from the right side of the heart to the left side without going through the pulmonary capillaries (Figure 2-28). Normally, this is about 2% to 5% of the cardiac output. This normal shunted blood comes from the bronchial, pleural, and thebesian veins, which drain into the left atrium. Shunting may also be caused by congenital heart disease, intrapulmonary arteriovenous fistulas, and pulmonary vascular abnormalities such as hemangiomas.

Capillary Shunt. A capillary shunt is commonly caused by alveolar collapse or atelectasis, alveolar fluid accumulation, and alveolar consolidation (see Figure 2-28, *C*). The sum of the anatomic and capillary shunts is referred to as a *true* or *absolute shunt*. Patients with respiratory disorders causing capillary shunting are refractory to oxygen therapy because the alveoli are unable to provide any O_2/CO_2 exchange function.

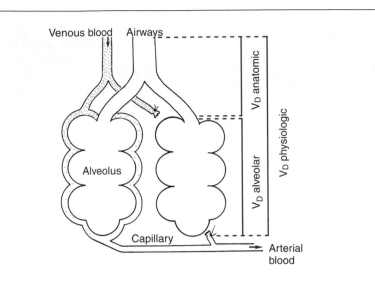

Only the inspired air that reaches the alveoli is physiologically effective. This portion of the inspired gas is referred to as *alveolar ventilation*. The volume of inspired air that does not reach the alveoli is not physiologically effective. This portion of gas is referred to as *dead-space ventilation*. There are three types of dead spaces: anatomic, alveolar, and physiologic.

Anatomic dead space. Anatomic dead space is the volume of gas in the conducting airways: the nose, mouth, pharynx, larynx, and lower portions of the airways down to but not including the respiratory bronchioles. The volume of the anatomic dead space is approximately equal to 1 ml/lb (2.2 ml/kg) of normal body weight.

Alveolar dead space. When an alveolus is ventilated but not perfused with blood, the volume of air in the alveolus is dead space, that is, the air within the alveolus is not physiologically effective in terms of gas exchange. The amount of alveolar dead space is unpredictable.

Physiologic dead space. The physiologic dead space is the sum of the anatomic dead space and the alveolar dead space. Because neither of these two forms of dead space is physiologically effective in terms of gas exchange, the two forms are combined and are referred to as *physiologic dead space*. (See Physiologic Dead Space Calculation, Appendix IV.)

Figure 2–27   Dead-space ventilation (V_D).

Shuntlike Effect. When pulmonary capillary perfusion is in excess of alveolar ventilation, a shuntlike effect can develop. Common causes of this form of shunting are hypoventilation, uneven distribution of ventilation (e.g., bronchospasm, excessive mucus accumulation in the tracheobronchial tree), and alveolar-capillary diffusion defects (although the alveolus may be ventilated in this condition, the blood passing by the alveolus does not have enough time to equilibrate with the alveolar oxygen tension; see Figure 2-28, D). Pulmonary shunting resulting from these conditions can generally be corrected by oxygen therapy.

Table 2-9 lists some respiratory disorders associated with capillary shunting and shuntlike effects.

Venous Admixture. The result of pulmonary shunting is venous admixture, which is the mixing of shunted nonreoxygenated blood with reoxygenated blood distal to the alveoli (i.e., downstream in the pulmonary circulatory system; Figure 2-29). When venous admixture occurs, the shunted nonreoxygenated blood gains oxygen molecules while the reoxygenated blood loses oxygen molecules. The result is a blood mixture that has (1) higher P_{O_2} and C_{aO_2} values than the nonreoxygenated blood and (2) lower P_{O_2} and C_{aO_2} values than the reoxygenated blood—in other words, a blood mixture with P_{aO_2} and C_{aO_2} values somewhere between the original values of the reoxygenated and nonreoxygenated blood. Clinically, this mixed blood is sampled downstream (e.g., from the radial artery) to assess the patient's arterial blood gases.

The peripheral chemoreceptors are frequently stimulated in respiratory disease because they respond to hypoxemia caused by decreased $\dot{V}/\dot{Q}$ ratios, capillary shunting (or a shuntlike effect), and venous admixture. The decreased arterial oxygen tension

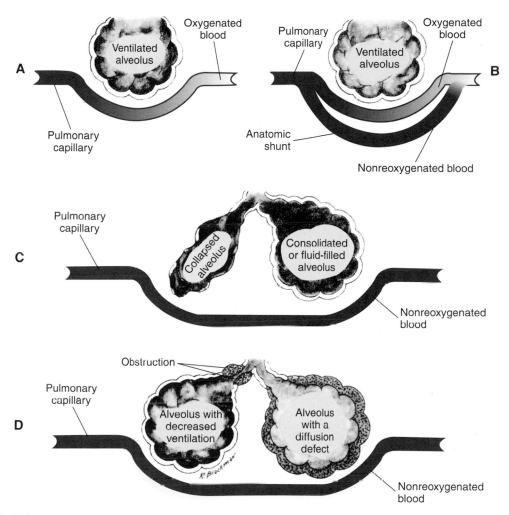

Figure 2–28 Pulmonary shunting. **A**, Normal alveolar-capillary unit. **B**, Anatomic shunt. **C**, Types of capillary shunts. **D**, Types of shuntlike effects. (Redrawn from Des Jardins T: *Cardiopulmonary anatomy and physiology: Essentials for respiratory care*, ed 4, Albany, NY, 2002, Delmar Publishers.)

then stimulates the peripheral chemoreceptors to send a signal to the medulla to increase ventilation (Figure 2-30).

Other Factors that Stimulate the Peripheral Chemoreceptors

Although the peripheral chemoreceptors are primarily activated by a decreased arterial oxygen level, they also are stimulated by a decreased pH (increased H^+ concentration). For example, the accumulation of lactic acid (from anaerobic metabolism) or keto-acids (diabetic acidosis) in the blood increases ventilatory rate almost entirely through the peripheral chemoreceptors. The peripheral chemoreceptors also are activated by hypoperfusion, increased

temperature, nicotine, and the direct effect of Pa_{CO_2}. The response of the peripheral chemoreceptors to Pa_{CO_2} stimulation, however, is relatively small compared with the response generated by the central chemoreceptors.

◆ Central Chemoreceptors and their Effect on the Ventilatory Pattern

Although the mechanism is not fully understood, it is now believed that two special respiratory centers in the medulla, the dorsal respiratory group (DRG) and the ventral respiratory group (VRG), are responsible for coordinating respiration (Figure 2-31). Both the DRG and VRG are stimulated by an increased

TABLE 2–9	Type of Pulmonary Shunting Associated with Common Respiratory Diseases		
Respiratory Diseases		**Capillary Shunt**	**Shuntlike Effect**
Chronic bronchitis			X
Emphysema			X
Asthma			X
Croup/epiglottitis			X
Bronchiectasis*		X	X
Cystic fibrosis*		X	X
Pneumoconiosis*		X	X
Pneumonia		X	
Lung abscess		X	
Pulmonary edema		X	
Near-drowning		X	
Adult respiratory distress syndrome		X	
Chronic interstitial lung disease		X	
Flail chest		X	
Pneumothorax		X	
Pleural diseases		X	
Kyphoscoliosis		X	
Tuberculosis		X	
Fungal diseases		X	
Idiopathic (infant) respiratory distress syndrome		X	
Smoke inhalation		X	

*Shuntlike effect is most common.

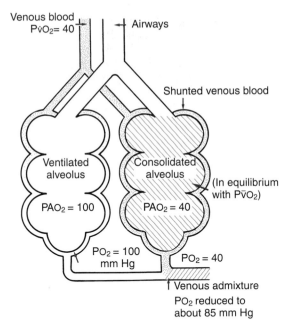

Figure 2–29   Venous admixture occurs when reoxygenated blood mixes with nonreoxygenated blood distal to the alveoli. Technically, the P_{O_2} in the pulmonary capillary system will not equilibrate completely because of the normal $P(A-a)_{O_2}$. The P_{O_2} in the pulmonary capillary system is normally a few mm Hg less than the P_{O_2} in the alveoli.

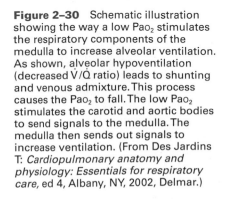

Figure 2–30   Schematic illustration showing the way a low Pa_{O_2} stimulates the respiratory components of the medulla to increase alveolar ventilation. As shown, alveolar hypoventilation (decreased $\dot{V}/\dot{Q}$ ratio) leads to shunting and venous admixture. This process causes the Pa_{O_2} to fall. The low Pa_{O_2} stimulates the carotid and aortic bodies to send signals to the medulla. The medulla then sends out signals to increase ventilation. (From Des Jardins T: *Cardiopulmonary anatomy and physiology: Essentials for respiratory care,* ed 4, Albany, NY, 2002, Delmar.)

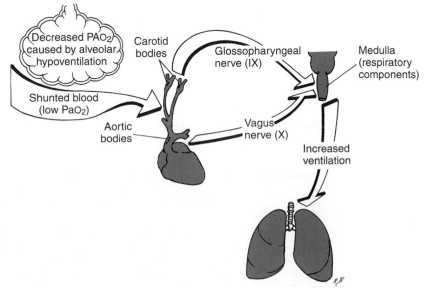

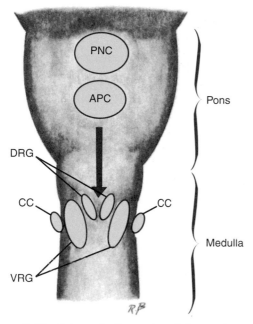

Figure 2–31 Schematic illustration of the respiratory components of the lower brain stem (pons and medulla). *PNC,* Pneumotaxic center; *APC,* apneustic center; *DRG,* dorsal respiratory group; *VRG,* ventral respiratory group; *CC,* central chemoreceptors. (Modified from Des Jardins T: *Cardiopulmonary anatomy and physiology: Essentials for respiratory care,* ed 4, Albany, NY, 2001, Delmar.)

concentration of H^+ in the CSF. The H^+ concentration of the CSF is monitored by the central chemoreceptors, which are located bilaterally and ventrally in the substance of the medulla. A portion of the central chemoreceptor region is actually in direct contact with the CSF. The central chemoreceptors transmit signals to the respiratory neurons by the following mechanism:

1. When the CO_2 level increases in the blood (e.g., during periods of hypoventilation), CO_2

molecules readily diffuse across the blood-brain barrier and enter the CSF. The blood-brain barrier is a semipermeable membrane that separates circulating blood from the CSF. The blood-brain barrier is relatively impermeable to ions such as H^+ and HCO_3^- but is very permeable to CO_2.

2. After CO_2 crosses the blood-brain barrier and enters the CSF, it forms carbonic acid:

$$CO_2 + H_2O \Leftrightarrow H_2CO_3^- \Leftrightarrow H^+ + HCO_3^-$$

3. Because the CSF has an inefficient buffering system, the H^+ produced from the previous reaction rapidly increases and causes the pH of the CSF to decrease.

4. The central chemoreceptors react to the liberated H^+ by sending signals to the respiratory components of the medulla, which in turn increases the ventilatory rate.

5. The increased ventilatory rate causes the Pa_{CO_2} and subsequently the P_{CO_2} in the CSF to decrease. Therefore the CO_2 level in the blood regulates ventilation by its indirect effect on the pH of the CSF (Figure 2-32).

◆ Pulmonary Reflexes and Their Effect on the Ventilatory Pattern

Several reflexes may be activated in certain respiratory diseases and influence the patient's ventilatory rate.

Deflation Reflex

When the lungs are compressed or deflated (e.g., atelectasis), an increased rate of breathing is seen. The precise mechanism responsible for this reflex is not known. Some investigators suggest that the increased rate of breathing may simply result from reduced stimulation of the receptors (the *Hering-Breuer reflex*) rather than the stimulation of specific deflation receptors. Receptors for the Hering-Breuer

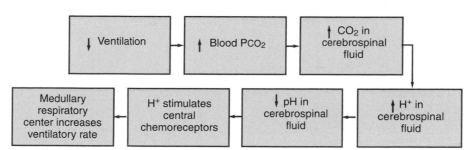

Figure 2–32 Sequence of events in alveolar hypoventilation. The central chemoreceptors are stimulated by hydrogen ions (H^+), which increase in concentration as CO_2 moves into the CSF.

reflex are located in the walls of the bronchi and bronchioles. When these receptors are stretched (e.g., during a deep inspiration), a reflex response is triggered to decrease the ventilatory rate. Other investigators, however, feel that the deflation reflex does not result from the absence of receptor stimulation of the Hering-Breuer reflex because the deflation reflex is still seen when the bronchi and bronchioles are below a temperature of 8° C. The Hering-Breuer reflex does not occur when the bronchi and bronchioles are below this temperature.

Irritant Reflex

When the lungs are compressed, deflated, or exposed to noxious gases, the irritant receptors are stimulated. The irritant receptors are subepithelial mechanoreceptors located in the trachea, bronchi, and bronchioles. When the receptors are activated, a reflex causes the ventilatory rate to increase. Stimulation of the irritant reflex also may produce a cough and bronchoconstriction.

Juxtapulmonary Capillary Receptors

The juxtapulmonary capillary receptors, or J receptors, are located in the interstitial tissues between the pulmonary capillaries and the alveoli. Their precise mechanism of action is not known. When the J receptors are stimulated, a reflex triggers rapid, shallow breathing. The J receptors may be activated by the following:

- Pulmonary capillary congestion
- Capillary hypertension
- Edema of the alveolar walls
- Humoral agents (e.g., serotonin)
- Lung deflation
- Emboli in the microcirculation

Reflexes from the Aortic and Carotid Sinus Baroreceptors

The normal function of the aortic and carotid sinus baroreceptors, located near the aortic and carotid peripheral chemoreceptors, is to activate reflexes that cause (1) decreased heart rate and ventilatory rate in response to increased systemic blood pressure and (2) increased heart rate and ventilatory rate in response to decreased systemic blood pressure.

◆ Pain, Anxiety, and Fever

An increased respiratory rate may result from the chest pain or fear and anxiety associated with the patient's inability to breathe. Chest pain and fear occur in a number of cardiopulmonary pathologies, such as pleurisy, rib fractures, pulmonary hypertension, and angina. An increased respiratory rate also may be caused by fever. Fever is commonly associated with infectious lung disorders such as pneumonia, lung abscess, tuberculosis, and fungal disease.

◆ USE OF THE ACCESSORY MUSCLES OF INSPIRATION

During the advanced stages of chronic obstructive pulmonary disease, the accessory muscles of inspiration are activated when the diaphragm becomes significantly depressed by the increased residual volume and functional residual capacity. The accessory muscles assist or largely replace the diaphragm in creating subatmospheric pressure in the pleural space during inspiration. The major accessory muscles of inspiration are as follows:

- Scalene
- Sternocleidomastoid
- Pectoralis major
- Trapezius

Scalenes

The anterior, medial, and posterior scalene muscles are separate muscles that function as a unit. They originate on the transverse processes of the second to sixth cervical vertebrae and insert into the first and second ribs (Figure 2-33). These muscles normally elevate the first and second ribs and flex the neck. When they are used as accessory muscles of inspiration, their primary role is to elevate the first and second ribs.

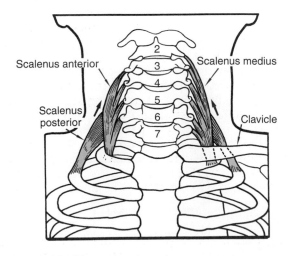

Figure 2–33 The scalene muscles.

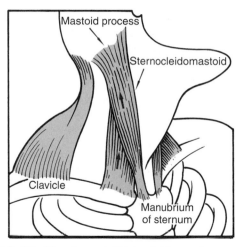

Figure 2–34 The sternocleidomastoid muscle.

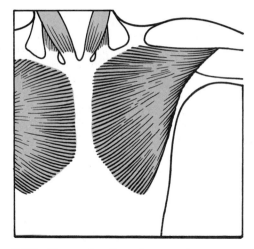

Figure 2–35 The pectoralis major muscles.

Sternocleidomastoids

The sternocleidomastoid muscles are located on each side of the neck (Figure 2-34), where they rotate and support the head. They originate from the sternum and clavicle and insert into the mastoid process and occipital bone of the skull.

Normally, the sternocleidomastoid pulls from its sternoclavicular origin, rotates the head to the opposite side, and turns it upward. When the sternocleidomastoid muscle functions as an accessory muscle of inspiration, the head and neck are fixed by other muscles, and the sternocleidomastoid pulls from its insertion on the skull and elevates the sternum. This action increases the anteroposterior diameter of the chest.

Pectoralis Majors

The pectoralis majors are powerful, fan-shaped muscles that originate from the clavicle and sternum and insert into the upper part of the humerus. The primary function of the pectoralis muscles is to pull the upper part of the arm to the body in a hugging motion (Figure 2-35).

When operating as an accessory muscle of inspiration, the pectoralis pulls from the humeral insertion and elevates the chest, resulting in an increased anteroposterior diameter. Patients with chronic obstructive pulmonary disease usually secure their arms to something stationary and use the pectoralis major muscles to increase the anteroposterior diameter of the chest (Figure 2-36). This braced position is called the *emphysematous habitus*.

Trapezius

The trapezius is a large, flat, triangular muscle that is situated superficially in the upper part of the back

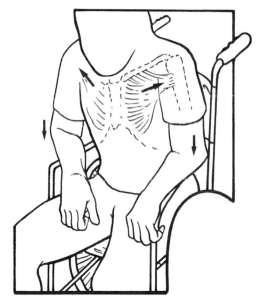

Figure 2–36 The way a patient may appear when using the pectoralis major muscles for inspiration.

and the back of the neck. The muscle originates from the occipital bone, the ligamentum nuchae, the spinous processes of the seventh cervical vertebra, and all the thoracic vertebrae. It inserts into the spine of the scapula, the acromion process, and the lateral third of the clavicle (Figure 2-37). The trapezius muscle rotates the scapula, raises the shoulders, and abducts and flexes the arm. Its action is typified in shrugging the shoulders (Figure 2-38). When used as an accessory muscle of inspiration, the trapezius helps elevate the thoracic cage.

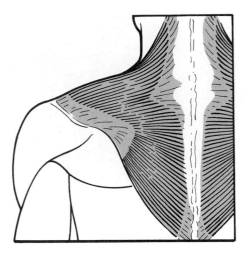

Figure 2–37 The trapezius muscles.

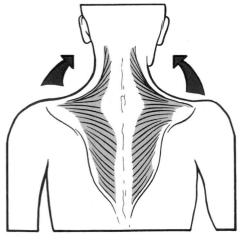

Figure 2–38 The action of the trapezius muscle is typified in shrugging the shoulders.

◆ USE OF THE ACCESSORY MUSCLES OF EXPIRATION

Because of the airway narrowing and collapse associated with chronic obstructive pulmonary disorders, the accessory muscles of exhalation are often recruited when airway resistance becomes significantly elevated. When these muscles actively contract, negative intrapleural pressure increases and offsets the increased airway resistance. The major accessory muscles of exhalation are as follows:

- Rectus abdominis
- External oblique
- Internal oblique
- Transversus abdominis

Rectus Abdominis

A pair of rectus abdominis muscles extends the entire length of the abdomen. Each muscle forms a vertical mass about 4 inches wide, separated by the linea alba. It arises from the iliac crest and pubic symphysis and inserts into the xiphoid process and the fifth, sixth, and seventh ribs. When activated, the muscle assists in compressing the abdominal contents, which in turn push the diaphragm into the thoracic cage (Figure 2-39).

External Obliques

The broad, thin, external oblique muscle is on the anterolateral side of the abdomen. The muscle is the longest and most superficial of all the anterolateral muscles of the abdomen. It arises by eight digitations from the lower eight ribs and the abdominal aponeurosis. It inserts in the iliac crest and into the linea alba. The muscle assists in compressing the abdominal contents. This action also pushes the diaphragm into the thoracic cage during exhalation (see Figure 2-39).

Internal Obliques

The internal oblique muscle is in the lateral and ventral part of the abdominal wall directly under the external oblique muscle. It is smaller and thinner than the external oblique. It arises from the inguinal ligament, the iliac crest, and the lower portion of the lumbar aponeurosis. It inserts into the last four ribs and the linea alba. The muscle assists in compressing the abdominal contents and pushing the diaphragm into the thoracic cage (see Figure 2-39).

Transversus Abdominis

The transversus abdominis muscle is found immediately under each internal oblique muscle. It arises from the inguinal ligament, the iliac crest, the thoracolumbar fascia, and the lower six ribs. It inserts into the linea alba. When activated, it constricts the abdominal contents (see Figure 2-39).

When all four pairs of accessory muscles of exhalation contract, the abdominal pressure increases and drives the diaphragm into the thoracic cage. As the diaphragm moves into the thoracic cage during exhalation, the intrapleural pressure increases and enhances expiratory gas flow (Figure 2-40).

◆ Pursed-Lip Breathing

Pursed-lip breathing occurs in patients during the advanced stages of obstructive pulmonary disease. It is a relatively simple technique that many patients

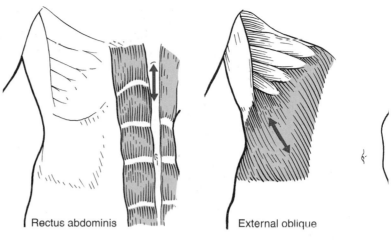

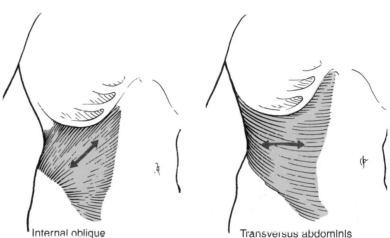

Figure 2–39 Accessory muscles of expiration. *Arrows* indicate the action of these muscles in enlarging the volume of the lungs.

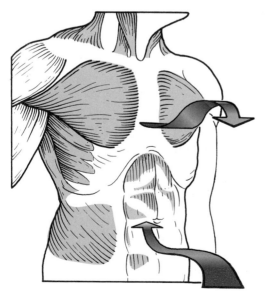

Figure 2–40 When the accessory muscles of expiration contract, intrapleural pressure increases, the chest moves outward, and airflow increases.

learn without formal instruction. During pursed-lip breathing the patient exhales through lips that are held in a position similar to that used for whistling, kissing, or blowing through a flute. The positive pressure created by retarding the airflow through pursed lips provides the airways with some stability and an increased ability to resist surrounding intrapleural pressures. This action offsets early airway collapse and air trapping during exhalation. In addition, pursed-lip breathing has been shown to slow the patient's ventilatory rate and generate a ventilatory pattern that is more effective in gas mixing (Figure 2-41).

◆ Substernal and Intercostal Retractions

Substernal and intercostal retractions may be seen in patients with severe restrictive lung disorders such as pneumonia or adult respiratory distress syndrome. In an effort to overcome the low lung compliance, the patient must generate a greater-than-normal negative intrapleural pressure during inspiration.

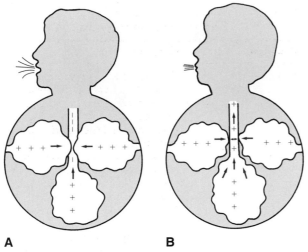

A   **B**

Figure 2–41 **A**, Schematic illustration of alveolar compression of weakened bronchiolar airways during normal expiration in patients with chronic obstructive pulmonary disease (e.g., emphysema). **B**, Effects of pursed-lip breathing. The weakened bronchiolar airways are kept open by the effects of positive pressure created by pursed lips during expiration.

This greater negative intrapleural pressure causes the tissues between the ribs and the substernal area to retract during inspiration (Figure 2-42) . Because the thorax of the newborn is quite flexible (as a result of the large amount of cartilage found in the skeletal structure), substernal and intercostal retractions are seen in infants with idiopathic respiratory distress syndrome (IRDS).

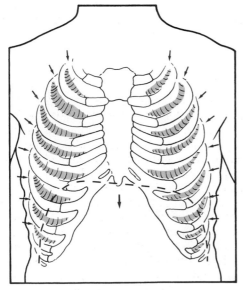

Figure 2–42 Intercostal retraction of soft tissues during forceful inspiration.

◆ NASAL FLARING

Nasal flaring is often seen during inspiration in infants experiencing respiratory distress. It is likely a facial reflex that enhances the movement of gas into the tracheobronchial tree. The dilator naris, which originates from the maxilla and inserts into the ala of the nose, is the muscle responsible for this clinical manifestation. When activated, the dilator naris pulls the alae laterally and widens the nasal aperture, providing a larger orifice for gas to enter the lungs during inspiration (see Chapter 32).

◆ SPLINTING CAUSED BY CHEST PAIN OR DECREASED CHEST EXPANSION

Chest pain is one of the most common complaints among patients with cardiopulmonary problems. It can be divided into two categories: pleuritc and nonpleuritic.

Pleuritic Chest Pain

Pleuritic chest pain is usually described as a sudden, sharp, or stabbing pain. The pain generally intensifies during deep inspiration and coughing and diminishes during breath holding or splinting. The origin of the pain may be the chest wall, muscles, ribs, parietal pleura, diaphragm, mediastinal structures, or intercostal nerves. Because the visceral pleura, which covers the lungs, does not have any sensory nerve supply, pain originating in the parietal region signifies extension of inflammation from the lungs to the contiguous parietal pleura lining the inner surface of the chest wall. This condition is known as *pleurisy* (Figure 2-43). When a patient with pleurisy inhales, the lung expands, irritating the inflamed parietal pleura and causing pain.

Because of the nature of the pleuritc pain, the patient usually prefers to lie on the affected side to allow greater expansion of the uninvolved lung and help splint the chest. Pleuritic chest pain is a characteristic feature of the following respiratory diseases:

- Pneumonia
- Pleural effusion
- Pneumothorax
- Pulmonary infarction
- Lung cancer
- Pneumoconiosis
- Fungal diseases
- Tuberculosis

Nonpleuritic Chest Pain

Nonpleuritic chest pain is usually described as a constant pain that is located centrally. The pain also

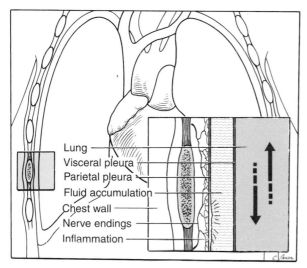

Figure 2–43 When the parietal pleura is irritated, the nerve endings in the parietal pleura send pain signals to the brain.

TABLE 2–10	Common Abnormal Chest Shapes and Configurations
Condition	**Description**
Kyphosis	A "hunchbacked" appearance caused by curvature of the spine
Scoliosis	A lateral curvature of the spine that results in the chest protruding posteriorly and the anterior ribs flattening out
Kyphoscoliosis	The combination of kyphosis and scoliosis (see Figure 25-1)
Pectus carinatum	The forward projection of the xiphoid process and lower sternum (also known as "pigeon breast" deformity)
Pectus excavatum	A funnel-shaped depression over the lower sternum (also called "funnel chest")
Barrel chest	In the normal adult, the anteroposterior diameter of the chest is about half its lateral diameter, or 1:2. When the patient has a barrel chest, the ratio is nearer to 1:1 (Figure 2-44)

may radiate. Nonpleuritic chest pain is associated with the following disorders:

- Myocardial ischemia
- Pericardial inflammation
- Pulmonary hypertension
- Esophagitis
- Local trauma or inflammation of the chest cage, muscles, bones, or cartilage

◆ ABNORMAL CHEST SHAPE AND CONFIGURATION

During inspection the respiratory care practitioner systematically observes the patient's chest for both normal and abnormal findings. Is the spine straight? Are any lesions or surgical scars evident? Are the scapulae symmetric? Common chest deformities are listed in Table 2-10.

◆ ABNORMAL EXTREMITY FINDINGS

The inspection of the patient's extremities should include the following:

- Altered skin color (e.g., cyanotic, pale, with prominent venous distention)
- Presence or absence of digital clubbing
- Presence or absence of peripheral edema
- Presence or absence of distended neck veins

◆ Altered Skin Color

A general observation of the patient's skin color should be routinely performed. For example, does the patient's skin color appear normal—pink, tan, brown, or black? Is the skin cold or clammy? Does the skin appear ashen or pallid? This appearance could be caused by anemia or acute blood loss. Do the patient's eyes, face, trunk, and arms have a yellow, jaundiced appearance (caused by increased bilirubin in the blood and tissue)? Is there redness of the skin, or erythema (often caused by capillary congestion, inflammation, or infection)? Does the patient appear cyanotic?

◆ Cyanosis

Cyanosis is common in severe respiratory disorders. *Cyanosis* is the term used to describe the blue-gray or purplish discoloration of the mucous membranes, fingertips, and toes whenever the blood in these areas contains at least 5 g/dl of reduced hemoglobin. When the normal 14 to 15 g/dl of hemoglobin is fully saturated, the Pa_{O_2} is about 97 to 100 mm Hg, and there is about 20 vol% of oxygen in the blood. In a cyanotic patient with one third (5 g/dl) of the hemoglobin reduced, the Pa_{O_2} is about 30 mm Hg and there is 13 vol% of oxygen in the blood (Figure 2-45).

The detection and interpretation of cyanosis are difficult, and wide individual variations occur among observers. The recognition of cyanosis depends on the acuity of the observer, the light conditions in

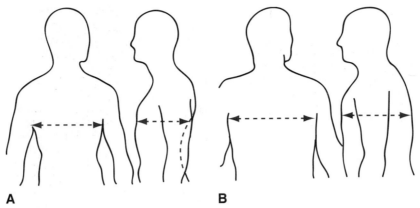

Figure 2–44 **A**, Normally, the anteroposterior diameter is about half the lateral diameter or by a ratio of 1:2. Because of the air trapping and lung hyperinflation in obstructive pulmonary diseases, the natural tendency of the lungs to recoil is decreased and the normal tendency of the chest to move outward prevails. This condition results in an increased anteroposterior diameter and is referred to as the *barrel chest deformity.* The ratio is nearer to 1:1. **B**, The anteroposterior diameter commonly increases with aging. Therefore older individuals may have a slight barrel chest appearance in the absence of any pulmonary disease. Normal infants also usually have an anteroposterior diameter near 1:1.

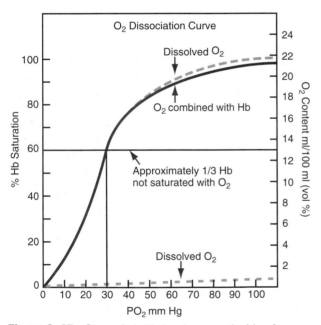

Figure 2–45 Cyanosis is likely whenever the blood contains at least 5 g of reduced hemoglobin. In the normal individual who has about 15 g of hemoglobin per 100 ml of blood, a Po₂ of about 30 mm Hg produces 5 g of reduced hemoglobin. The hemoglobin, however, is still approximately 60% saturated with oxygen.

the examining room, and the pigmentation of the patient. Cyanosis of the nail beds also is influenced by temperature because vasoconstriction induced by cold may slow circulation to the point at which the blood becomes bluish in the surface capillaries even though the arterial blood in the major vessels is not lacking in oxygen.

Central cyanosis, as observed on the mucous membranes of the lips and mouth, is almost always a sign of hypoxemia and therefore has a definite diagnostic value.

In severely anemic patients, cyanosis may never be seen because these patients could not remain alive with 5 g/dl reduced hemoglobin. In the patient with polycythemia, however, cyanosis may be present at a Pao₂ well above 30 mm Hg because the amount of reduced hemoglobin is often greater than 5 g/dl in these patients—even when their total oxygen content is within normal limits. In respiratory disease, cyanosis is the result of (1) a decreased ventilation-perfusion ratio, (2) pulmonary shunting, and/or (3) venous admixture.

◆ Digital Clubbing

Digital clubbing is sometimes noticed in patients with chronic respiratory disorders. Clubbing is characterized by a bulbous swelling of the terminal phalanges of the fingers and toes. The contour of the nail becomes rounded both longitudinally and transversely, which results in an increase in the angle between the surface of the nail and the terminal phalanx (Figure 2-46).

The specific cause of clubbing is unknown. It is a normal hereditary finding in some families without any known history of cardiopulmonary disease. It is believed that the following factors may be causative: (1) circulating vasodilators, such as bradykinin and the prostaglandins, that are released from normal tissues but are not degraded by the lungs because of intrapulmonary shunting; (2) chronic infection; (3) unspecified toxins; (4) capillary stasis from increased venous backpressure; (5) arterial

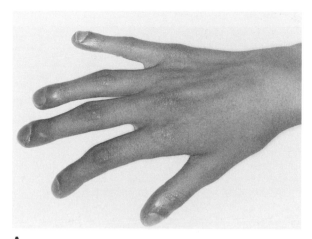

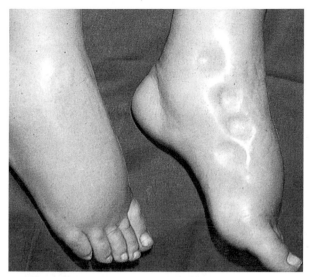

Figure 2–47 Pitting edema. (From Bloom A, Ireland J: *Color atlas of diabetes*, ed2, London, 1992, Mosby-Wolfe.)

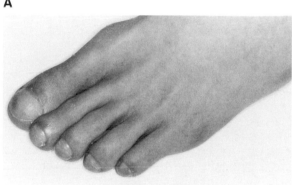

Figure 2–46 Digital clubbing.

hypoxemia; and (6) local hypoxia. Successful treatment of the underlying disease may result in resolution of the clubbing and return of the digits to normal.

◆ Peripheral Edema

Bilateral, dependent, pitting edema is commonly seen in patients with congestive heart failure, cor pulmonale, and hepatic cirrhosis. To assess the presence and severity of pitting edema, the health-care practitioner places a finger or fingers over the tibia or medial malleolus (2 to 4 inches above the foot), firmly depresses the skin for 5 seconds, and then releases. Normally, this procedure leaves no indentation, although a pit may be seen if the person has been standing all day or is pregnant. If pitting is present, it is graded on the following subjective scale: 1+ (mild, slight depression) to 4+ (severe, deep depression) (Figure 2-47).

◆ Distended Neck Veins

In patients with cor pulmonale, severe flail chest, pneumothorax, or pleural effusion, the major veins of the chest that return blood to the right heart may be compressed. When this happens, venous return decreases and central venous pressure (CVP)

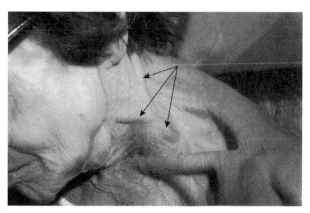

Figure 2–48 Distended neck veins (*arrows*).

increases. This condition is manifested by distended neck veins (also called jugular venous distention; Figure 2-48). The reduced venous return also may cause the patient's cardiac output and systemic blood pressure to decrease. In severe cases, the veins over the entire upper anterior thorax may be dilated.

◆ Sputum Production, Cough, and Hemoptysis

NORMAL HISTOLOGY AND MUCUS PRODUCTION OF THE TRACHEOBRONCHIAL TREE

The wall of the tracheobronchial tree is composed of three major layers: an epithelial lining, the lamina propria, and a cartilaginous layer (Figure 2-49).

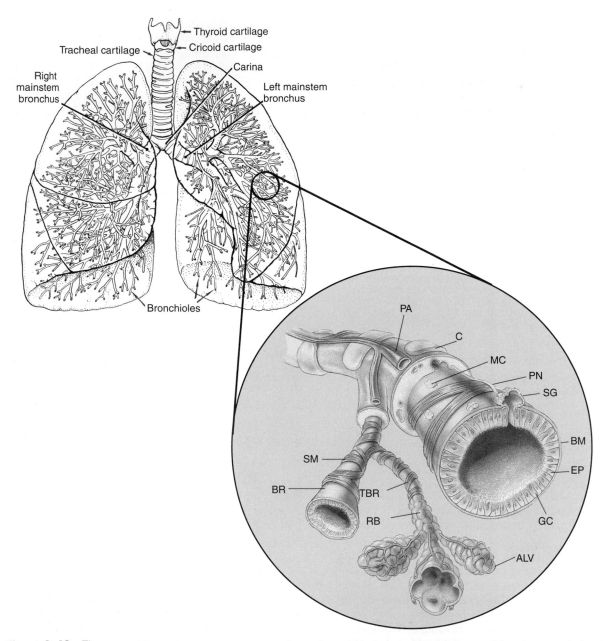

Figure 2–49   The normal lung. *PA,* Pulmonary artery; *C,* cartilage; *PN,* parasympathetic nerve; *SG,* submucosal gland; *SM,* smooth muscle; *MC,* mast cell; *BM,* basement membrane; *EP,* epithelium; *GC,* goblet cell; *BR,* bronchioles; *TBR,* terminal bronchioles; *RB,* respiratory bronchioles; *ALV,* alveoli. (See also Plate 1.)

The *epithelial lining,* which is separated from the lamina propria by a basement membrane, is predominantly composed of pseudostratified, ciliated, columnar epithelium interspersed with numerous mucus- and serum-secreting glands. The ciliated cells extend from the beginning of the trachea to—and sometimes including—the respiratory bronchioles. As the tracheobronchial tree becomes progressively smaller, the columnar structure of the ciliated cells gradually decreases in height. In the terminal bronchioles the epithelium appears more cuboidal than columnar. These cells flatten even more in the respiratory bronchioles (see Figure 2-49).

A mucus layer, commonly referred to as the mucus blanket, covers the epithelial lining of the tracheobronchial tree (Figure 2-50). The viscosity of the

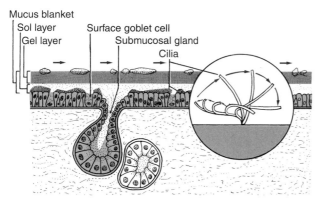

Figure 2–50 The epithelial lining of the tracheobronchial tree.

mucus layer progressively increases from the epithelial lining to the inner luminal surface and has two distinct layers: (1) the sol layer, which is adjacent to the epithelial lining, and (2) the gel layer, which is the more viscous layer adjacent to the inner luminal surface. The mucus blanket is 95% water. The remaining 5% consists of glycoproteins, carbohydrates, lipids, DNA, some cellular debris, and foreign particles.

The mucus blanket is produced by the goblet cells and the submucosal, or bronchial, glands. The goblet cells are located intermittently between the pseudostratified, ciliated columnar cells distal to the terminal bronchioles.

Most of the mucus blanket is produced by the submucosal glands, which extend deeply into the lamina propria and are composed of different cell types: serous cells, mucus cells, collecting duct cells, mast cells, myoepithelial cells, and clear cells, which are probably lymphocytes. The submucosal glands are particularly numerous in the medium-sized bronchi and disappear in the bronchioles. These glands are innervated by parasympathetic (cholinergic) nerve fibers and normally produce about 100 ml of clear, thin bronchial secretions per day.

The mucus blanket is an important cleansing mechanism of the tracheobronchial tree. Inhaled particles stick to the mucus. The distal ends of the cilia continually strike the innermost portion of the gel layer and propel the mucus layer, along with any foreign particles, toward the larynx. At this point, the cough mechanism moves secretions beyond the larynx and into the oropharynx. This mucociliary mechanism is commonly referred to as the *mucociliary transport* or the *mucociliary escalator.* The cilia move the mucus blanket at an estimated average rate of 2 cm/min.

The submucosal layer of the tracheobronchial tree is the *lamina propria.* Within the lamina propria is a loose, fibrous tissue that contains tiny blood vessels, lymphatic vessels, and branches of the vagus nerve.

A circular layer of smooth muscle also is found within the lamina propria. It extends from the trachea down to and including the terminal bronchioles.

The *cartilaginous structures* that surround the tracheobronchial tree progressively diminish in size as the airways extend into the lungs. The cartilaginous layer is completely absent in bronchioles less than 1 mm in diameter (see Figure 2-49).

TYPES OF SPUTUM PRODUCTION

Excessive sputum production is commonly seen in respiratory diseases that cause an acute or chronic inflammation of the tracheobronchial tree (see Figure 11-1 and Plate 2). Depending on the severity and nature of the respiratory disease, sputum production may take several forms. For example, during the early stages of tracheobronchial tree inflammation, the sputum is usually clear, thin, and odorless. As the disease intensifies, the sputum becomes *yellow-green and opaque.* The yellow-green appearance results from an enzyme (myeloperoxidase) that is released during the cellular breakdown of leukocytes. It may also be caused by retained or stagnant secretions or secretions caused by an acute infection.

Thick and tenacious sputum is commonly seen in patients suffering from chronic bronchitis, bronchiectasis, cystic fibrosis, and asthma. Patients with pulmonary edema expectorate a thin, frothy, pinkish sputum. Technically, this fluid is not true sputum. It results from the movement of plasma and red blood cells across the alveolar-capillary membrane into the alveoli. *Hemoptysis* is the coughing up of blood or blood-tinged sputum from the tracheobronchial tree. In true hemoptysis the sputum is usually bright red and interspersed with air bubbles.

Clinically, hemoptysis may be confused with hematemesis, which is blood that originates from the upper gastrointestinal tract and usually has a dark, coffee-ground appearance. Repeated expectoration of blood-streaked sputum is seen in chronic bronchitis, bronchiectasis, cystic fibrosis, pulmonary embolism, lung cancer, necrotizing infections, tuberculosis, and fungal diseases. A small amount of hemoptysis is common after bronchoscopy, particularly when biopsies are taken. *Massive hemoptysis* is defined as coughing up 400 to 600 ml of blood within a 24-hour period. Death from exsanguination resulting from hemoptysis is rare. Table 2-11 provides a general overview and analysis of the types of sputum commonly seen in the clinical setting.

COUGH

A cough is a sudden, audible expulsion of air from the lungs. It is commonly seen in respiratory disease,

TABLE 2-11   Analysis of Sputum Color

Color	Indications and Conditions
Brown/dark	Old blood
Bright red (hemoptysis)	Fresh blood (bleeding tumor, tuberculosis)
Clear and translucent	Normal
Copious	Large amount
Frank hemoptysis	Massive amount of blood
Green	Stagnant sputum or gram-negative bacteria
Green and foul smelling	Pseudomonas or anaerobic infection
Mucoid (white/gray)	Asthma, chronic bronchitis
Pink, frothy	Pulmonary edema
Tenacious	Secretions that are sticky or adhesive or otherwise tend to hold together
Viscous	Thick, viscid, sticky, or glutinous
Yellow or opaque	Presence of white blood cells, bacterial infection

BOX 2-5

Common Factors that Stimulate the Irritant Receptors

- Inflammation
- Infectious agents
- Excessive secretions
- Noxious gases (e.g., cigarette smoke, chemical inhalation)
- Very hot or very cold air
- A mass of any sort compressing the lungs
- Mechanical stimulation (e.g., endotracheal suctioning, compression of the airways)

especially in disorders that cause inflammation of the tracheobronchial tree. In general, a cough is preceded by (1) a deep inspiration, (2) partial closure of the glottis, and (3) forceful contraction of the accessory muscles of expiration to expel air from the lungs. In essence, a cough is a protective mechanism that clears the lungs, bronchi, or trachea of irritants. A cough also prevents the aspiration of foreign material into the lungs. For example, a cough is a common symptom associated with chronic sinusitis and postnasal drip. The effectiveness of a cough depends largely on (1) the depth of the preceding inspiration and (2) the extent of dynamic compression of the airways (see Figure 3-13).

Although a cough may be voluntary, it is usually a reflex response that arises when an irritant stimulates the *irritant receptors* (also called *subepithelial mechanoreceptors*). The irritant receptors are located in the pharynx, larynx, trachea, and large bronchi. When stimulated, the irritant receptors send a signal by way of the glossopharyngeal (cranial nerve IX) and vagus (cranial nerve X) nerves to the cough reflex center located in the medulla. The medulla then causes the glottis to close and the accessory muscles of expiration to contract. Box 2-5 lists common factors that stimulate the irritant receptors.

Clinically, a cough is termed *productive* if sputum is produced and *nonproductive* if no sputum is produced.

Nonproductive Cough

Common causes of a nonproductive cough include (1) irritation of the airway, (2) inflammation of the airways, (3) mucus accumulation, (4) tumors, and (5) irritation of the pleura.

Productive Cough

When the cough is productive, the respiratory practitioner should assess the following:

- Is the cough *strong* or *weak*? In other words, does the patient have a good or poor ability to mobilize bronchial secretions? A good, strong cough may indicate only deep breath and cough therapy, whereas an inadequate cough may indicate chest physical therapy or postural drainage.
- A productive cough should be evaluated in terms of its frequency, pitch, and loudness. A brassy cough may indicate a tumor, whereas a barking or hoarse cough indicates croup.
- Finally, the sputum of a productive cough should be monitored and evaluated continuously in terms of amount (teaspoons, tablespoons, cups), consistency (thin, thick, tenacious), odor, and color (see Table 2-11).

SELF-ASSESSMENT QUESTIONS

Multiple Choice

1. Which of the following pathologic conditions increases vocal fremitus?
   - I. Atelectasis
   - II. Pleural effusion
   - III. Pneumothorax
   - IV. Pneumonia
   - a. III only
   - b. IV only
   - c. II and III only
   - d. I and IV only
   - e. I, III, and IV only

2. A dull or soft percussion note would likely be heard in which of the following pathologic conditions?
   - I. Chronic obstructive pulmonary disease
   - II. Pneumothorax
   - III. Pleural thickening
   - IV. Atelectasis
   - a. I only
   - b. II only
   - c. III only
   - d. II and III only
   - e. III and IV only

3. Bronchial breath sounds are likely to be heard in which of the following pathologic conditions?
   - I. Alveolar consolidation
   - II. Chronic obstructive pulmonary disease
   - III. Atelectasis
   - IV. Fluid accumulation in the tracheobronchial tree
   - a. III only
   - b. IV only
   - c. I and III only
   - d. II and IV only
   - e. I, III, and IV only

4. Wheezing is:
   - I. Produced by bronchospasm
   - II. Generally auscultated during inspiration
   - III. A cardinal finding of bronchial asthma
   - IV. Usually heard as high-pitched sounds
   - a. I only
   - b. I and III only
   - c. II and IV only
   - d. I, III, and IV only
   - e. I, II, III, and IV

5. In which of the following pathologic conditions is transmission of the whispered voice of a patient through a stethoscope unusually clear?
   - I. Chronic obstructive pulmonary disease
   - II. Alveolar consolidation
   - III. Atelectasis
   - IV. Pneumothorax
   - a. I only
   - b. II and III only
   - c. I and IV only
   - d. I, II, and III only
   - e. II, III, and IV only

6. An individual's ventilatory pattern is composed of which of the following?
   - I. Inspiratory and expiratory force
   - II. Ventilatory rate
   - III. Tidal volume
   - IV. Inspiratory and expiratory ratio
   - a. I and III only
   - b. II and III only
   - c. II, III, and IV only
   - d. I, II, and III only
   - e. I, II, III, and IV

7. Which of the following abnormal breathing patterns is commonly associated with diabetic acidosis?
   - a. Orthopnea
   - b. Kussmaul's respiration
   - c. Biot's respiration
   - d. Hypoventilation
   - e. Cheyne-Stokes respiration

8. What is the average compliance of the lungs and chest wall combined?
   - a. 0.05 L/cm H_2O
   - b. 0.1 L/cm H_2O
   - c. 0.2 L/cm H_2O
   - d. 0.3 L/cm H_2O
   - e. 0.4 L/cm H_2O

9. When lung compliance decreases, which of the following is seen?
   - I. Ventilatory rate usually decreases
   - II. Tidal volume usually decreases
   - III. Ventilatory rate usually increases
   - IV. Tidal volume usually increases
   - a. I only
   - b. II only
   - c. III only
   - d. II and III only
   - e. I and IV only

10. What is the normal airway resistance in the tracheobronchial tree?

    a. 0.5 to 1.0 cm H_2O/L/sec
    b. 1.0 to 2.0 cm H_2O/L/sec
    c. 2.0 to 3.0 cm H_2O/L/sec
    d. 3.0 to 4.0 cm H_2O/L/sec
    e. 4.0 to 5.0 cm H_2O/L/sec

11. What is the normal overall ventilation/perfusion ratio ($\dot{V}/\dot{Q}$ ratio)?

    a. 0.2
    b. 0.4
    c. 0.6
    d. 0.8
    e. 1.0

12. When venous admixture occurs, which of the following occur(s)?

    I. The P_{O_2} of the nonreoxygenated blood increases
    II. The C_{aO_2} of the reoxygenated blood decreases
    III. The P_{O_2} of the reoxygenated blood increases
    IV. The C_{aO_2} of the nonreoxygenated blood decreases

    a. I only
    b. IV only
    c. II and III only
    d. III and IV only
    e. I and II only

13. The pathophysiology of some respiratory disorders causes a shuntlike effect, whereas some disorders feature a capillary shunt and others a combination of both. Which of the following respiratory diseases causes a shuntlike effect?

    I. Pneumonia
    II. Asthma
    III. Pulmonary edema
    IV. Adult respiratory distress syndrome

    a. II only
    b. III only
    c. I and III only
    d. II, III, and IV only
    e. I, II, III, and IV

14. What percentage is the normal anatomic shunt?

    a. 2 to 5
    b. 6 to 8
    c. 9 to 10
    d. 11 to 15
    e. 15 to 20

15. When the systemic blood pressure increases, the aortic and carotid sinus baroreceptors initiate reflexes that cause which of the following?

    I. Increased heart rate
    II. Decreased ventilatory rate
    III. Increased ventilatory rate
    IV. Decreased heart rate

    a. I only
    b. II only
    c. III only
    d. II and IV only
    e. I and III only

16. What is the anteroposterior-transverse chest diameter ratio in the normal adult?

    a. 1:0.5
    b. 1:1
    c. 1:2
    d. 1:3
    e. 1:4

17. Which of the following muscles originate from the clavicle?

    I. Scalene muscles
    II. Sternocleidomastoid muscles
    III. Pectoralis major muscles
    IV. Trapezius muscles

    a. I only
    b. II only
    c. IV only
    d. I and IV only
    e. II and III only

18. Which of the following muscles inserts into the xiphoid process and into the fifth, sixth, and seventh ribs?

    a. Rectus abdominis muscle
    b. External oblique muscle
    c. Internal oblique muscle
    d. Transversus abdominis muscle

19. Which of the following is associated with digital clubbing?

    I. Chronic infection
    II. Local hypoxia
    III. Circulating vasodilators
    IV. Arterial hypoxia

    a. II only
    b. IV only
    c. II and IV only
    d. II, III, and IV only
    e. I, II, III, and IV

20. Which of the following is associated with pleuritic chest pain?

    I. Lung cancer
   II. Pneumonia
  III. Myocardial ischemia
  IV. Tuberculosis

a. I only
b. II only
c. III only
d. I and III only
e. I, II, and IV only

Answers appear in Appendix XI.

CLINICAL DATA OBTAINED FROM LABORATORY TESTS AND SPECIAL PROCEDURES

CHAPTER 3

Pulmonary Function Study Assessments

Pulmonary function studies play a major role in the assessment of pulmonary disease. The results from pulmonary function studies are used to (1) evaluate pulmonary causes of dyspnea, (2) differentiate between obstructive and restrictive pulmonary disorders, (3) assess severity of the pathophysiologic impairment, (4) follow the course of a particular disease, (5) evaluate the effectiveness of therapy, and (6) assess the patient's preoperative status.

Normal Lung Volumes and Capacities

As shown in Figure 3-1, gas in the lungs is divided into four separate volumes. The four lung capacities represent different combinations of lung volumes.

LUNG VOLUMES

- *Tidal volume (V_T)*: The volume of gas that normally moves into and out of the lungs in one quiet breath.
- *Inspiratory reserve volume (IRV)*: The volume of air that can be forcefully inspired after a normal tidal volume inhalation.
- *Expiratory reserve volume (ERV)*: The volume of air that can be forcefully exhaled after a normal tidal volume exhalation.
- *Residual volume (RV)*: The amount of air remaining in the lungs after a forced exhalation.

LUNG CAPACITIES

- *Vital capacity (VC)*: $VC = IRV + V_T + ERV$. The volume of air that can be exhaled after a maximal inspiration. There are two major VC measurements: *slow vital capacity (SVC)*, or a VC in which exhalation is performed slowly to offset air trapping, and *forced vital capacity (FVC)*, or a VC in which a maximal effort is made to exhale as rapidly as possible to assess the degree of airflow obstruction.

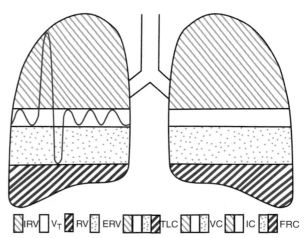

Figure 3–1 Normal lung volumes and capacities. *IRV,* Inspiratory reserve volume; *V_T,* tidal volume; *RV,* residual volume; *ERV,* expiratory reserve volume; *TLC,* total lung capacity; *VC,* vital capacity; *IC,* inspiratory capacity; *FRC,* functional residual capacity.

- *Inspiratory capacity (IC)*: IC = V_T + IRV. The volume of air that can be inhaled after a normal exhalation.
- *Functional residual capacity (FRC)*: FRC = ERV + RV. The lung volume at rest after a normal tidal volume exhalation.
- *Total lung capacity (TLC)*: TLC = IC + FRC. The maximal amount of air that the lungs can accommodate.
- *Residual volume/total lung capacity ratio (RV/TLC × 100)*: The percentage of TLC occupied by the RV.

The amount of air the lungs can accommodate varies with age, weight, height, gender, and, to a much lesser extent, race. Prediction formulas exist that take these variables into account. Table 3-1 lists the normal lung volumes and capacities of the average man and woman aged 20 to 30 years.

Lung volumes and capacities change as a result of pulmonary disorders. These changes are usually classified as either an obstructive lung disorder or a restrictive lung disorder. In **obstructive lung disorders**, the RV, V_T, FRC, and RV/TLC ratio are increased, and the VC, IC, IRV, and ERV are decreased. In **restrictive lung disorders**, the VC, IC, RV, FRC, V_T, and TLC are all decreased. Combined obstructive and restrictive lung disease can exist, as in cystic fibrosis. Figure 3-2 provides a visual comparison of obstructive and restrictive lung disorders.

TABLE 3–1	Lung Volumes and Capacities (in Milliliters) of Normal Recumbent Subjects Between 20 and 30 Years	
Measurement	**Male**	**Female**
Tidal volume (V_T)	500	400 to 500
Inspiratory reserve volume (IRV)	3100	1900 volume
Expiratory reserve volume (ERV)	1200	800 volume
Residual volume (RV)	1200	1000
Vital capacity (VC)	4800	3200
Inspiratory capacity (IC)	3600	2400
Functional residual capacity (FRC)	2400	1800
Total lung capacity (TLC)	6000	4200

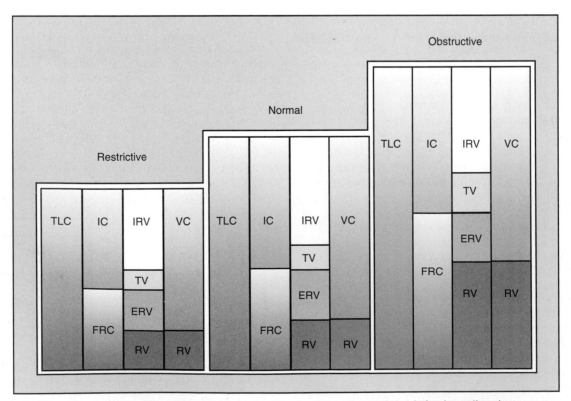

Figure 3–2   Visual comparison of lung volumes and capacities in obstructive and restrictive lung disorders. (From Wilkins RL, Stoller JK, Scanlan CL: *Egan's fundamentals of respiratory care,* ed 8, St. Louis, 2003, Mosby.)

INDIRECT MEASUREMENTS OF THE RESIDUAL VOLUME AND CAPACITIES CONTAINING THE RESIDUAL VOLUME

Because the residual volume (RV) cannot be exhaled, the RV and the lung capacities that contain the RV (FRC and TLC) are measured indirectly in the clinical setting by one of the following methods:

- Closed circuit helium dilution test
- Open circuit nitrogen washout test
- Body plethysmography

Expiratory Flow Rate Measurements

In addition to the volumes and capacities that can be measured by pulmonary function testing, the rate at which gas flows out of the lungs also can be measured. Such measurements provide data on the patency of the airways, the severity of the airway impairment, and the size of the patient's airway.

FORCED VITAL CAPACITY (FVC)

The FVC is the total volume of gas that can be exhaled as forcefully and rapidly as possible after a maximal inspiration. In the healthy individual, the total expiratory time (TET) necessary to perform a FVC is 4 to 6 seconds. In obstructive lung disease (e.g., chronic bronchitis or emphysema), the TET increases because of the increased airway resistance and air trapping associated with the disorder. TETs of more than 10 seconds have been reported in these patients. In the normal individual, the FVC equals the VC. Clinically, the lungs are considered normal if the FVC and the VC are within 200 ml of each other. In the patient with obstructive lung disease, the FVC is lower than the VC because of increased airway resistance and air trapping with maximal effort (Figure 3-3).

A decreased FVC also is a common clinical manifestation in the patient with a restrictive lung disorder (e.g., pneumonia, acute respiratory distress syndrome, atelectasis). This decrease is mainly due to the fact that restrictive lung disorders reduce the patient's ability to fully expand the lungs, thus reducing the vital capacity (VC) necessary to generate a good FVC. However, the TET required to perform a FVC is usually normal or even less than normal because of the high lung elasticity (low lung compliance) associated with restrictive disorders.

A number of pulmonary function tests can be extrapolated from a single FVC maneuver. The most common tests are as follows:

- Forced Expiratory Volume Time (FEV$_T$)
- Forced Expiratory Volume$_1$ $_{sec}$/Forced Vital Capacity Ratio (FEV$_1$/FVC Ratio)
- Forced Expiratory Flow$_{200-1200}$ (FEF$_{200-1200}$)

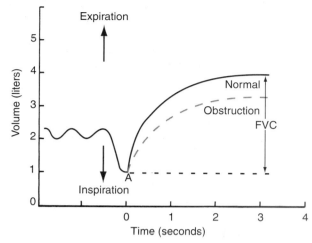

Figure 3-3 Forced vital capacity (FVC). *A* is the point of maximal inspiration and the starting point of an FVC. Note the reduction in FVC in obstructive pulmonary disease, caused by dynamic compression of the airways.

- Forced Expiratory Flow$_{25\%-75\%}$ (FEF$_{25\%-75\%}$)
- Peak Expiratory Flow Rate (PEFR)

FORCED EXPIRATORY VOLUME TIMED (FEV$_T$)

The maximum volume of gas that can be exhaled over a specific period is the FEV$_T$. This measurement is obtained from an FVC measurement. Commonly used time periods are 0.5, 1.0, 2.0, 3.0, 6.0 seconds. The most commonly used time period is 1 second (FEV$_1$). In the normal adult the percentages of the total volume exhaled during these time periods are as follows: FEV$_{0.5}$, 60%; FEV$_1$, 83%; FEV$_2$, 94%; and FEV$_3$, 97%. In obstructive disease, the FEV$_T$ is decreased because the time necessary to exhale a certain volume forcefully is increased (Figure 3-4). Although the FEV$_T$ may be normal in restrictive lung disorders (e.g., pneumonia, acute respiratory distress syndrome, atelectasis), it is commonly decreased because of the decreased VC associated with restrictive disorders (similar to the FVC in restrictive disorders). The FEV$_T$ progressively decreases with age.

FORCED EXPIRATORY VOLUME$_1$ $_{SECOND}$/FORCED VITAL CAPACITY RATIO (FEV$_1$/FVC RATIO OR FEV$_{1\%}$)

The FEV$_1$/FVC ratio compares the amount of air exhaled in 1 second to the total amount exhaled during an FVC maneuver. Because the FEV$_1$/FVC ratio is expressed as a percentage, it is commonly referred to as the forced expiratory volume in 1 second percentage (FEV$_{1\%}$). Simply stated, the FEV$_{1\%}$ provides the percentage of the patient's total volume of air forcefully exhaled (FVC) in 1 second. As already discussed under the FEV$_T$ section, the normal adult

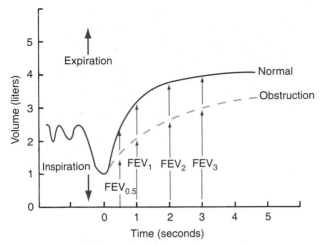

Figure 3–4   FEV$_T$. In obstructive pulmonary disease, more time is needed to exhale a specified volume.

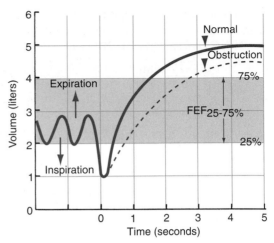

Figure 3–5   FEF$_{25\%-75\%}$. This test measures the average rate of flow between 25% and 75% of an FVC. The flow rate is measured when 25% of the FVC has been exhaled and again when 75% of the FVC has been exhaled. The average rate of flow is derived by dividing the combined flow rates by 2. Note that expiration (in this figure) starts at 1.0 L on the upward axis.

exhales 83 percent or more of the FVC in 1 second (FEV$_1$). Thus the FEV$_{1\%}$ should also be 83% or greater under normal circumstances. The FEV$_{1\%}$ progressively decreases with age.

Clinically, the FVC, FEV$_1$, and FEV$_{1\%}$ are commonly used to (1) assess the severity of a patient's obstructive disorder and (2) determine whether the patient has either an obstructive or restrictive lung disorder. The primary pulmonary function study differences between an obstructive and restrictive lung disorder are as follows: In an *obstructive disorder*, the FEV$_1$ and FEV$_{1\%}$ are both decreased; in a *restrictive disorder*, the FEV$_1$ is decreased and the FEV$_{1\%}$ is normal or increased.

FORCED EXPIRATORY FLOW$_{25\%-75\%}$

The FEF$_{25\%-75\%}$ is the average flow rate generated by the patient during the middle 50% of an FVC measurement (Figure 3-5). This expiratory maneuver is used to evaluate the status of *medium-to-small-sized airways* in obstructive lung disorders. The normal FEF$_{25\%-75\%}$ in the healthy male between 20 and 30 years of age is about 4.5 L/sec (270 L/min). The normal FEF$_{25\%-75\%}$ in the healthy female between 20 and 30 years of age is about 3.5 L/sec (210 L/min). The FEF$_{25\%-75\%}$ is somewhat effort dependent because it depends on the FVC exhaled.

The FEF$_{25\%-75\%}$ progressively decreases in obstructive diseases and with age. The FEF$_{25\%-75\%}$ may also be decreased in moderate or severe restrictive lung disorders. This decrease is believed to be due primarily to the reduced cross-sectional area of the small airways associated with restrictive lung problems. Clinically, the FEF$_{25\%-75\%}$ is often used to further confirm—or rule out—the presence of an obstructive pulmonary disease in the patient with a borderline FEV$_{1\%}$ value.

FORCED EXPIRATORY FLOW$_{200-1200}$

The FEF$_{200-1200}$ measures the average flow rate between 200 and 1200 ml of an FVC (Figure 3-6). The first 200 ml of the FVC is usually exhaled more slowly than at the average flow rate because of (1) the normal inertia involved in the respiratory maneuver and (2) the initial slow response time of the pulmonary function equipment. Because the FEF$_{200-1200}$ measures expiratory flows at high lung volumes (i.e., the initial part of the

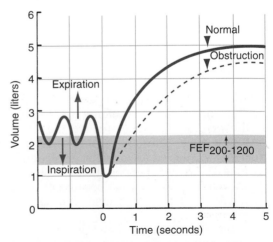

Figure 3–6   FEF$_{200-1200}$. This test measures the average rate of flow between 200 ml and 1200 ml of an FVC. The flow rate is measured when 200 ml have been exhaled and again when 1200 ml have been exhaled. The average rate of flow is derived by dividing the combined flow rates by 2. Note that expiration (in this figure) starts at 1.0 L on the upward axis.

forced vital capacity), it provides a good assessment of the large upper airways. The $FEF_{200-1200}$ is relatively effort-dependent.

The normal $FEF_{200-1200}$ for the average healthy male between 20 and 30 years of age is approximately 8 L/sec (480 L/min). The normal $FEF_{200-1200}$ in the average healthy female between 20 and 30 years of age is approximately 5.5 L/sec (330 L/min). The $FEF_{200-1200}$ decreases in obstructive lung disorders. The $FEF_{200-1200}$ is a good test to determine the patient's response to bronchodilator therapy. In restrictive lung disorders the $FEF_{200-1200}$ is usually normal because it measures the early expiratory flow rates during the first part of a FVC (i.e., when the patient's VC is at its highest level). The $FEF_{200-1200}$ progressively decreases with age.

PEAK EXPIRATORY FLOW RATE (PEFR)

The PEFR (also known as the *peak flow rate*) is the maximum flow rate generated during a FVC maneuver (Figure 3-7). The PEFR provides a good assessment of the large upper airways. It is quite effort-dependent. The normal PEFR in the average healthy male between 20 and 30 years of age is approximately 10 L/sec (600 L/min). The normal PEFR in the average healthy female between 20 and 30 years of age is approximately 7.5 L/sec (450 L/min). The PEFR decreases in obstructive lung diseases. In restrictive lung disorders, the PEFR is usually normal because it measures the early expiratory flow rates during the first part of a FVC (i.e., when the patient's VC is at its highest level). The PEFR progressively decreases with age.

The PEFR also can easily be measured at the patient's bedside with a hand-held peak flowmeter (e.g., Wright peak flowmeter). The hand-held peak flowmeter is used to monitor the degree of airway

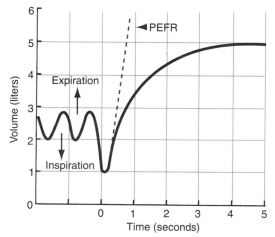

Figure 3-7 PEFR. The steepest slope of the $\Delta\dot{V}/\Delta T$ line is the PEFR ($\dot{V}$).

obstruction on a moment-to-moment basis and is relatively small, inexpensive, accurate, reproducible, and easy for the patient to use. In addition, the mouthpieces are disposable, thus allowing the safe use of the same peak flowmeter from one patient to another. PEFR measurements should routinely be performed at the patient's bedside to assess the degree of bronchospasm, effect of bronchodilators, and day-to-day progress. The PEFR results generated by the patient before and after bronchodilator therapy can serve as excellent objective data by which to assess the effectiveness of therapy.

MAXIMUM VOLUNTARY VENTILATION (MVV)

The MVV is the largest volume of gas that can be breathed voluntarily in and out of the lungs in 1 minute (Figure 3-8). The normal MVV in the average healthy male between 20 and 30 years of age is approximately 170 L/min. The normal MVV in the average healthy female between 20 and 30 years of age is approximately 110 L/min. The MVV progressively decreases in obstructive pulmonary disorders. In restrictive pulmonary disorders, the MVV may be normal or decreased.

FLOW-VOLUME LOOP

Flow-volume loop analysis is helpful in determining the site of airway obstruction. It requires use of a flowmeter (called a pneumotachograph), a spirometer, and a recorder with X-Y graphic capability. As shown in Figure 3-9, the upper half of the flow-volume loop (above the zero flow axis) represents the maximum expiratory flow generated at various lung volumes during an FVC maneuver plotted against volume. This portion of the curve shows the flow generated between the TLC and RV.

The lower half of the flow-volume loop (below the zero flow axis) illustrates the maximum inspiratory flow generated at various lung volumes during a forced inspiration (called a *force inspiratory volume [FIV]*) plotted against the volume inhaled. This portion of the curve shows the flow generated between the RV and TLC. Depending on the sophistication of the equipment, the following information can be obtained from this test:

- FVC
- FEV_T
- $FEF_{25\%-75\%}$
- $FEF_{200-1200}$
- PEFR
- Peak inspiratory flow rate (PIFR)
- $FEF_{50\%}$
- Instantaneous flow at any given lung volume during forced inhalation and exhalation

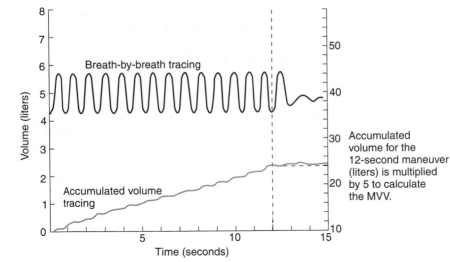

Figure 3–8   Volume/time tracing for an MVV maneuver.

Accumulated volume for the 12-second maneuver (liters) is multiplied by 5 to calculate the MVV.

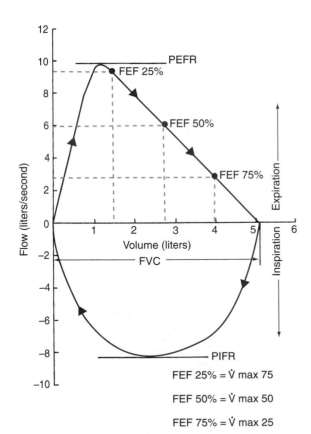

Figure 3–9   Flow-volume loop.

FEF 25% = $\dot{V}$ max 75

FEF 50% = $\dot{V}$ max 50

FEF 75% = $\dot{V}$ max 25

In normal subjects the expiratory flow rate usually decreases linearly with volume after the PEFR has been achieved (this portion of the curve represents approximately the last 70% to 80% of the FVC). In patients with obstructive lung disease, however, flow is frequently decreased at low lung volumes,

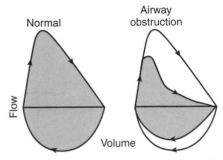

Figure 3–10   Flow-volume loop demonstrating the shape change that results from an obstructive lung disorder. The curve on the right represents intrathoracic airway obstruction.

which causes a perceptible "cuplike" or "scooped-out" appearance in the expiratory flow curve when 50% of the FVC has been exhaled. This portion of the flow curve is referred to as the *forced expiratory flow$_{50\%}$ (FEF$_{50\%}$)*, or $\dot{V}_{max50}$ (Figure 3-10).

FORCED EXPIRATORY TIME (FET)

The growing concern over the appropriate use of high-cost medical technology has led to renewed interest in physical examination methods that are safe, reproducible, inexpensive, and accurate. In the spirit of this trend the forced expiratory time (FET) recently has been reintroduced in the literature. Although controversial in the past, the FET is now presented as a moderately good, simple, and inexpensive bedside test in the screening of obstructive airway disease.

The FET is defined as the time it takes an individual to exhale forcefully through an open mouth from TLC until airflow is no longer audible. The FET is easily measured at the patient's bedside with only a stethoscope and a stopwatch. The patient is asked to inhale deeply (to his/her TLC) and then to exhale as fast and as hard as possible. The cessation of airflow is determined by listening either at the mouth or by stethoscope over the trachea. An FET of 4 seconds or less is normal. An FET of more than 6 seconds suggests airway obstruction.

The auscultated FET, combined with clinical history, physical examination, and X-ray examination, permits the clinician to evaluate the patient's pulmonary function status at the bedside before resorting to more precise (and expensive) pulmonary function studies. The auscultated FET is simple to perform, inexpensive, and fairly reproducible, and it may provide the respiratory care practitioner with useful screening information in the assessment of obstructive airway disease. It also may be used to measure the effectiveness of bronchodilator therapy.

◆ Expiratory Maneuver Findings Characteristic of Restrictive Lung Diseases

In restrictive lung disorders, flow and volume are, in general, reduced equally. Clinically, this phenomenon is referred to as "symmetric" reduction in flows and volumes. The flow-volume loop therefore is a "small version" of normal in restrictive pulmonary disease (Figure 3-11).

◆ Lung Volume and Capacity Findings Characteristic of Restrictive Lung Diseases

The previously described lung volumes and capacity abnormalities develop in response to pathologic conditions that alter the anatomic structures distal to the terminal bronchioles (i.e., the lung parenchyma). Such conditions include the following:

- Lung compression (e.g., secondary to a pneumothorax or pleural effusion)
- Atelectasis (e.g., secondary to a pneumothorax, flail chest, or mucus plugging)
- Consolidation (e.g., pneumonia)
- Calcification (e.g., tuberculosis, asbestosis)
- Fibrosis (e.g., pneumoconiosis, chronic interstitial lung diseases such as sarcoidosis)
- Bronchogenic tumor (e.g., squamous cell carcinoma)
- Cavitations (e.g., tuberculosis, lung abscess)

These conditions cause increased lung rigidity, which decreases lung compliance. Decreased lung compliance in turn causes a reduction in the patient's V_T, RV, FRC, TLC, VC, IRV, and ERV (Figure 3-12). In addition, the patient's ventilatory rate increases and the V_T decreases (see Figure 2-23).

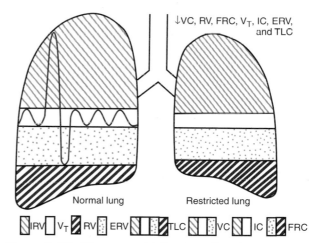

Figure 3–12 The way restrictive lung disorders alter lung volumes and capacities. *IRV,* Inspiratory reserve volume; *V_T,* tidal volume; *RV,* residual volume; *ERV,* expiratory reserve volume; *TLC,* total lung capacity; *VC,* vital capacity; *IC,* inspiratory capacity; *FRC,* functional residual capacity.

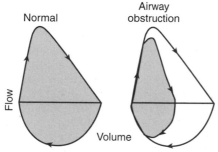

Figure 3–11 Flow-volume loop demonstrating the shape change that results from a restrictive lung disorder. Note the symmetric loss of flow and volume.

◆ Pulmonary Function Study Expiratory Maneuver Findings: RESTRICTIVE LUNG DISEASE

FVC	FEVT	FEF$_{25\%-75\%}$	FEF$_{200-1200}$
↓	N or ↓	N or ↓	N
PEFR	MVV	FEF$_{50\%}$	FEV$_{1\%}$
N	N or ↓	N	N or ↑

◆ Pulmonary Function Study Lung Volume and Capacity Findings: RESTRICTIVE LUNG DISEASE

VT	RV	FRC	TLC
N or ↓	↓	↓	↓
VC	IC	ERV	RV/TLC%
↓	↓	↓	N

◆ Pulmonary Function Study Expiratory Maneuver Findings: OBSTRUCTIVE LUNG DISEASE

FVC	FEVT	$FEF_{25\%-75\%}$	$FEF_{200-1200}$
↓	↓	↓	↓
PEFR	MVV	$FEF_{50\%}$	$FEV_{1\%}$
↓	↓	↓	↓

◆ Expiratory Maneuver Findings Characteristic of Obstructive Lung Diseases

In pulmonary obstructive disease, the expiratory findings develop in response to pathologic conditions that alter the anatomic structures of the tracheobronchial tree. Such pathologic conditions include the following:

- Chronic inflammation and swelling of the peripheral airways (e.g., chronic bronchitis)
- Excessive mucus production and accumulation (e.g., cystic fibrosis)
- A tumor projecting into a bronchus (e.g., bronchogenic cancer)
- Destruction and weakening of the distal airways (e.g., emphysema)
- Bronchial smooth muscle constriction (e.g., asthma)

Because of the decreased expiratory flow rates seen in patients with obstructive pulmonary disease, the $FEF_{50\%}$ portion of the flow-volume loop usually has a "cuplike" or "scooped-out" appearance (see Figure 3-10).

To fully appreciate the way these pathologic conditions cause the expiratory findings seen in obstructive pulmonary disorders, an understanding of the following is essential:

- The manner in which activation of the dynamic airway compression mechanism affects respiratory function in obstructive pulmonary diseases

- Bernoulli's principle and the dynamic compression mechanism in obstructive pulmonary diseases (see next section)
- The way Poiseuille's law relates to respiratory function in obstructive pulmonary diseases (see next section)
- The way the airway resistance equation relates to respiratory function in obstructive pulmonary diseases

DYNAMIC COMPRESSION MECHANISM AND ITS EFFECTS ON RESPIRATORY FUNCTION IN OBSTRUCTIVE PULMONARY DISEASES

Effort-Dependent Portion of a Forced Expiratory Maneuver

Normally, during approximately the first 20% to 30% of an FVC maneuver, the maximum (peak) flow rate depends on the amount of muscular effort exerted by the individual. Therefore the first 20% to 30% of a forced expiratory maneuver is referred to as *effort-dependent*. In other words, the initial maximal flow rate during forced expiration depends on the muscular effort produced by the individual.

Effort-Independent Portion of a Forced Expiratory Maneuver

The flow rate during approximately the last 70% to 80% of an FVC maneuver is effort-independent—that is, after a maximum flow rate has been attained, the flow rate cannot be increased by further muscular effort.

The lung volume at which the patient initiates a forced expiratory maneuver also influences the maximum flow rate. As lung volumes decline, flow also declines. The reduced flow, however, is the maximum flow for that particular volume.

Figure 3-13 illustrates where the effort-dependent and effort-independent portions of a forced expiratory maneuver appear in a normal flow-volume loop.

Dynamic Compression of the Airways

The limitation of the flow rate that occurs during approximately the last 70% to 80% of an FVC maneuver results from dynamic compression of the walls of the airways. As gas flows through the airways during passive expiration, the pressure within the airways diminishes to zero (Figure 3-14, *A*).

During a forced expiratory maneuver, however, as the airway pressure decreases from the alveolus to the atmosphere, a point comes at which the pressure within the lumen of the airways equals the pleural

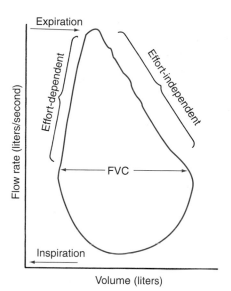

Figure 3–13 The effort-dependent and effort-independent portions of a forced expiratory maneuver in a flow-volume loop measurement. *FVC,* Forced vital capacity.

pressure surrounding the airways. The transpulmonary pressure at this point is zero. This is called the *equal-pressure point.*

Downstream (i.e., toward the mouth) from the equal-pressure point, the lateral pressure within the airway becomes less than the surrounding pleural pressure. Consequently, the airways are compressed.

As muscular effort and pleural pressure increase during a forced expiratory maneuver, the equal-pressure point moves upstream (i.e., toward the alveolus). Ultimately, the equal-pressure point becomes fixed where the individual's flow rate has achieved a maximum (Figure 3-14, *B*). In essence, after dynamic compression occurs during a forced expiratory maneuver, increased muscular effort merely augments airway compression, which in turn increases airway resistance.

As the structural changes associated with obstructive pulmonary diseases intensify, the patient commonly responds by increasing intrapleural pressure during expiration to overcome the increased airway resistance produced by the disease. By increasing intrapleural pressure during expiration, however, the patient activates the dynamic compression mechanism, which in turn further reduces the diameter of the bronchial airways. This results in an even greater increase in airway resistance.

BERNOULLI'S PRINCIPLE AND THE DYNAMIC COMPRESSION MECHANISM IN OBSTRUCTIVE PULMONARY DISEASES

Bernoulli's principle states that when gas flowing through a tube encounters a narrowing or obstruction, the velocity of the gas molecules increases. As a result, the gas molecules collide less frequently with the sides of the tube, and this causes the lateral pressure to drop (Figure 3-15).

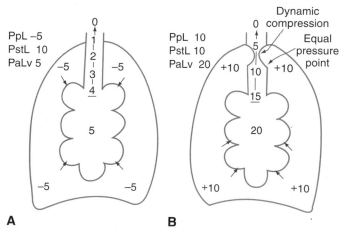

A   **B**

Figure 3–14 The dynamic compression mechanism. **A,** During passive expiration, static elastic recoil pressure *(PstL)* is 10, pleural pressure *(PpL)* at the beginning of expiration is 25, and alveolar pressure *(PaLv)* is 15. For gas to move from the alveolus to the atmosphere during expiration, the pressure must decrease progressively in the airways from +5 to 0. As **A** shows, PpL is always less than the airway pressure. **B,** During forced expiration, PpL becomes positive (+10 in this illustration). When the PpL is added to the PstL of +10, PaLv becomes +20. As the pressure progressively decreases during forced expiration, there is a point at which the pressures inside and outside the airway wall are equal. This point is the equal pressure point. Airway compression occurs downstream (toward the mouth) from this point because the lateral pressure in the lumen is less than the surrounding wall pressure.

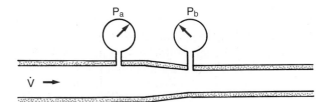

Figure 3-15 Bernouilli's principle (see text). P_a, Upstream pressure; P_b, downstream pressure.

This mechanism may play an insidious role in certain pulmonary disorders. In chronic obstructive pulmonary disease, for example, when the gas flow encounters bronchial narrowing during a forced expiratory maneuver, the decreased lateral pressure that results at the obstructed sites enhances dynamic compression.

POISEUILLE'S LAW AND ITS RELATION TO RESPIRATORY FUNCTION IN OBSTRUCTIVE PULMONARY DISEASES

During a normal inspiration, intrapleural pressure decreases from its normal resting level (about 2 to 3 cm H_2O pressure) and causes the bronchial airways to lengthen and increase in diameter (passive dilation). During expiration, intrapleural pressure increases (or returns to its normal resting state) and causes the bronchial airways to decrease in length and diameter (passive constriction; Figure 3-16). These anatomic changes can affect bronchial gas flow and intrapleural pressure and can be expressed by Poiseuille's law.

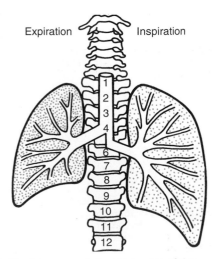

Figure 3-16 The normal change in size of the tracheobronchial tree during inspiration and expiration.

Poiseuille's Law and Its Significance

Although the factors in Poiseuille's law are of little significance during normal, spontaneous breathing, they play a major role in obstructive pulmonary disorders. Poiseuille's law can be expressed for either flow or pressure.

Poiseuille's Law for Flow

Poiseuille's law for flow states that when gas flows through a tube, the following applies

$$\dot{V} = \frac{\Delta P \pi r^4}{8ln}$$

where n is the viscosity of a gas (or fluid), ΔP is the change of pressure from one end of the tube to the other, r is the radius of the tube, l is the length of the tube, and $\dot{V}$ is the gas (or fluid) flow through the tube; π and 8 are constants that will be excluded from the present discussion.

The equation states that flow is directly related to P and r^4 and indirectly related to l and n. Flow decreases in response to a decreased P and tube radius. Flow increases in response to a decreased tube length and viscosity. Conversely, flow increases in response to an increased P and tube radius and decreases in response to an increased tube length and viscosity.

Flow is profoundly affected by the radius of the tube. As Poiseuille's law illustrates, $\dot{V}$ is a function of the fourth power of the radius (r^4). In other words, assuming pressure (ΔP) remains constant, decreasing the radius of a tube by one half reduces the gas flow to $\frac{1}{16}$ of its original flow.

For example, if the radius of a bronchial tube through which gas flows at a rate of 16 ml/sec is reduced to one half its original size because of mucosal swelling, the flow rate through the bronchial tube decreases to 1 ml/sec ($\frac{1}{16}$ the original flow rate; Figure 3-17).

Similarly, decreasing a tube radius by 16% decreases gas flow to one half its original rate. For instance, if the radius of a bronchial tube through which gas flows at a rate of 16 ml/sec is decreased by 16% (because of mucosal swelling, for example), the flow rate through the bronchial tube decreases to 8 ml/sec (half the original flow rate; Figure 3-18).

Poiseuille's Law for Pressure

When it is rearranged for pressure, Poiseuille's law is written as follows:

$$P = \frac{\dot{V}8ln}{\pi r^4}$$

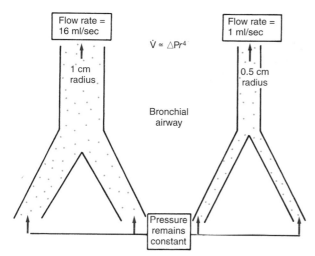

Figure 3–17 Poiseuille's law for flow applied to a bronchial airway with its radius reduced by 50% (see text).

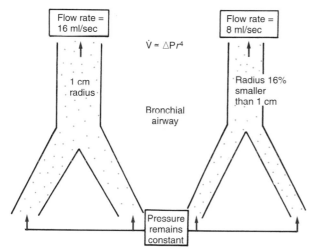

Figure 3–18 Poiseuille's law for flow applied to an airway with its radius reduced by 16% (see text).

For example, if the radius of a bronchus with a driving pressure of 1 cm H_2O is reduced to half its original size because of mucosal swelling, the driving pressure through the bronchus must increase to 16 cm H_2O ($16 \times 1 = 16$) to maintain the same flow rate (Figure 3-19).

Similarly, decreasing the tube radius by 16% increases the pressure to twice its original level. For instance, if the radius of a bronchus with a driving pressure of 10 cm H_2O is decreased by 16% because of mucosal swelling, the driving pressure through the bronchus must increase to 20 cm H_2O (twice its original pressure) to maintain the same flow (Figure 3-20).

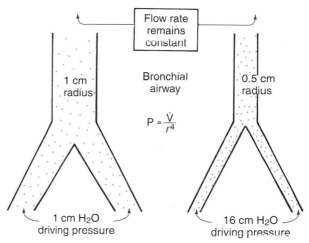

Figure 3–19 Poiseuille's law for pressure applied to an airway with its radius reduced by 50% (see text).

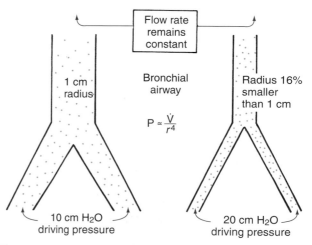

Figure 3–20 Poiseuille's law for pressure applied to an airway with its radius reduced by 16% (see text).

The equation now states that pressure is directly related to $\dot{V}$, l, and n and indirectly related to r^4. Pressure increases in response to a decreased tube radius and decreases in response to decreased flow rate, tube length, or viscosity. The opposite also is true: Pressure decreases in response to an increased tube radius and increases in response to increased flow rate, tube length, or viscosity.

Pressure is a function of the radius to the fourth power; therefore it is profoundly affected by the radius of a tube. In other words, if flow ($\dot{V}$) remains constant, decreasing a tube radius to half its previous size requires an increase in pressure to 16 times its original level.

Poiseuille's Law Rearranged to Simple Proportionalities

When Poiseuille's law is applied to the tracheobronchial tree during spontaneous breathing, the two equations can be rewritten as simple proportionalities:

$$\dot{V} \approx Pr^4$$

$$P \simeq \frac{\dot{V}}{r^4}$$

where P is the intrapleural pressure, $\dot{V}$ is gas flow through the tracheobronchial tree, and r is the radius of the bronchus.

On the basis of the proportionality for flow ($\dot{V}=Pr^4$), it can be stated that because gas flow varies directly with r^4 of the bronchial airway, flow must diminish during exhalation as the radius of the bronchial airways decreases. Stated differently, assuming that the pressure remains constant as the radius (r) of the bronchial airways decreases, the gas flow ($\dot{V}$) also decreases. During normal spontaneous breathing the gas flow reduction during exhalation is negligible.

In terms of the proportionality for pressure ($P \approx \dot{V}/r^4$), if the gas flow is to remain constant during exhalation, the intrapleural pressure must vary indirectly with the fourth power of the radius of the airway. In other words, as the radius of the bronchial airways decreases during exhalation, the driving pressure must increase to maintain a constant gas flow. During normal spontaneous breathing, the need to increase intrapleural pressure during exhalation to maintain a certain gas flow is negligible.

In obstructive pulmonary diseases, however, both gas flow ($\dot{V}$) and intrapleural pressure (ΔP) may change substantially in response to the pathologic processes associated with the disorders.*

AIRWAY RESISTANCE EQUATION AND ITS RELATION TO RESPIRATORY FUNCTION IN OBSTRUCTIVE PULMONARY DISEASES

Changes in driving pressure (ΔP) and gas flow ($\dot{V}$) are used to measure airway resistance (R_{aw}). R_{aw} is measured in centimeters of water per liter per second, according to the following equation:

$$R_{aw} = \Delta P \text{ (cm H}_2\text{O)}/\dot{V} \text{ (L/sec)}$$

Normally, R_{aw} in the tracheobronchial tree is about 1.0 to 2.0 cm H_2O/L/sec. When the R_{aw} equation is applied to a normal ventilatory cycle, R_{aw} is noted to

---

*See a mathematical discussion of Poiseuille's law for flow and pressure in Appendix VI.

be greater during expiration than during inspiration because the radius of the bronchial airways decreases during exhalation and—as Poiseuille's law for flow demonstrates—causes the gas flow ($\dot{V}$) to diminish.

Theoretically, during normal spontaneous breathing gas enters the alveoli during inspiration (when the bronchial airways are dilated) more easily than it leaves the alveoli during expiration (when the caliber of the bronchial airways is smaller). Under normal circumstances, increased R_{aw} during expiration is of no significance. Because of the pathologic processes that develop in obstructive pulmonary diseases, however, R_{aw} may be quite high and may limit expiratory flow.

◆ Lung Volume and Capacity Findings Characteristic of Obstructive Lung Diseases

The changes in lung volumes and capacities listed below develop in response to pathologic conditions of the tracheobronchial tree. Some of the major pathologic conditions that alter the anatomic structures of the tracheobronchial tree are as follows:

- Inflammation and swelling of the peripheral airways
- Excessive mucus production and accumulation
- Bronchial airway obstruction (e.g., from mucus or from a tumor projecting into a bronchus)
- Destruction and weakening of the distal airways
- Smooth muscle constriction of the airways (bronchospasm)

These pathologic conditions cause increased airway resistance (R_{aw}) and airway closure during expiration. When R_{aw} becomes high, the patient's ventilatory rate decreases and the V_T increases. This ventilatory pattern is thought to be an adaptation to reduce the work of breathing (see Figure 2-23).

When bronchial closure develops during expiration, the gas that enters the alveoli during inspiration (when the bronchi are naturally wider) is prevented from leaving the alveoli during expiration. The alveoli then become overdistended with gas, a condition

◆ Pulmonary Function Study Lung Volume and Capacity Findings: OBSTRUCTIVE LUNG DISEASE

VT	RV	FRC	TLC
N or ↑	↑	↑	N or ↑
VC	IC	ERV	RV/TLC ratio
↓	N or ↓	N or ↓	↑

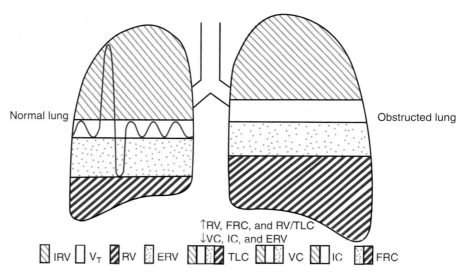

Figure 3–21 The way obstructive lung disorders alter lung volumes and capacities. *IRV,* Inspiratory reserve volume; *V_T,* tidal volume; *RV,* residual volume; *ERV,* expiratory reserve volume; *TLC,* total lung capacity; *VC,* vital capacity; *IC,* inspiratory capacity; *FRC,* functional residual capacity.

Normal lung

Obstructed lung

↑RV, FRC, and RV/TLC
↓VC, IC, and ERV

IRV   V_T   RV   ERV   TLC   VC   IC   FRC

known as *air trapping.* Excluding the V_T, airway closure and air trapping are the major mechanisms responsible for the abnormal lung volume and capacity findings seen in obstructive pulmonary diseases (Figure 3-21).

Pulmonary Diffusion Capacity

Trace gases are used to assess the adequacy of the pulmonary capillary membrane to transfer oxygen and carbon dioxide. Carbon monoxide (CO) is one such trace gas. The pulmonary diffusion capacity of carbon monoxide (D_{LCO}) measures the amount of CO that moves across the alveolar-capillary membrane. CO has an affinity for hemoglobin approximately 210 times greater than that of oxygen. When the patient has a normal hemoglobin concentration, pulmonary capillary blood volume, and ventilatory status, the only limiting factor to the diffusion of CO is the alveolar-capillary membrane (except in carboxyhemoglobinemia, in which the CO already combined with hemoglobin results in a reduced D_{LCO}).

The D_{LCO} decreases in response to lung disorders that affect the alveolar-capillary membrane. For example, the D_{LCO} decreases in emphysema because of the alveolar-capillary destruction associated with the disease. The D_{LCO} also decreases in lung disorders such as the pneumoconioses and other chronic interstitial lung diseases that cause pulmonary fibrosis.

Under normal conditions the average D_{LCO} value for the resting male is 25 ml/min/mm Hg (STPD). A correction for alveolar volume is commonly made (D_{LCO}/V_A). This value is slightly lower in females, presumably because of their smaller normal lung volumes. The carbon monoxide single-breath technique is commonly used for this measurement.

SELF-ASSESSMENT QUESTIONS

Multiple Choice

1. What is the PEFR in the normal healthy female between 20 and 30 years?

   a. 250 L/min
   b. 350 L/min
   c. 450 L/min
   d. 550 L/min
   e. 650 L/min

2. Which of the following can be obtained from a flow-volume loop study?

   I. MEFV
   II. PEFR
   III. FEVT
   IV. $FEF_{25\%-75\%}$

   a. IV only
   b. I and II only
   c. II and III only
   d. I, III, and IV only
   e. I, II, III, and IV

3. Which of the following expiratory maneuver findings are characteristic of restrictive lung disease?

   I. Normal FVC
   II. Decreased $FEF_{25\%-75\%}$
   III. Normal PEFR
   IV. Decreased FEV_T

   a. I and III only
   b. II and IV only
   c. III and IV only
   d. II and III only
   e. I, II, III, and IV

4. The effort-independent portion of an FVC consists of which of the following?

   a. First 20% to 30% of the FVC maneuver
   b. Last 70% to 80% of the FVC maneuver
   c. Middle portion of the FVC maneuver
   d. First 50% of the FVC maneuver
   e. Entire vital capacity maneuver

5. Bernoulli's principle states that when gas flow through a tube encounters a restriction, which of the following occurs?

   I. Velocity of the gas molecules decreases
   II. Lateral gas pressure decreases
   III. Velocity of the gas molecules increases
   IV. Velocity of the gas molecules remains the same

   a. II and V only
   b. II and IV only
   c. I and IV only
   d. II and III only
   e. III and IV only

6. When arranged for flow ($\dot{V}$), Poiseuille's law states that $\dot{V}$ is:

   I. Indirectly related to r^4
   II. Directly related to P
   III. Indirectly related to π
   IV. Directly related to 1

   a. I only
   b. II only
   c. II and III only
   d. III and IV only
   e. II, III, and IV only

7. In an obstructive lung disorder, which of the following occurs?

   I. FRC is decreased
   II. RV is increased
   III. VC is decreased
   IV. IRV is increased

   a. I and III only
   b. II and III only
   c. II and IV only
   d. II, III, and IV only
   e. I, II, and III

8. Under normal conditions, the average D_{LCO} value for the resting male is which of the following?

   a. 10 ml/min/mm Hg
   b. 15 ml/min/mm Hg
   c. 20 ml/min/mm Hg
   d. 25 ml/min/mm Hg
   e. 30 ml/min/mm Hg

9. What is the vital capacity of the normal recumbent male between 20 and 30 years?

   a. 2700 ml
   b. 3200 ml
   c. 4000 ml
   d. 4800 ml
   e. 5400 ml

10. What is the normal percentage of the total volume exhaled during an $FEV_{1.0}$?

    a. 60%
    b. 83%
    c. 94%
    d. 97%
    e. 100%

    Answer appear in Appendix XI.

CHAPTER 4

Arterial Blood Gas Assessments

◆ Blood Gas Findings

As the pathologic processes of a respiratory disorder intensify, the patient's arterial blood gas (ABG) values are usually altered to some degree. Table 4-1 lists normal ABG values.

VENTILATORY ACID-BASE ABNORMALITIES

Ventilatory acid-base abnormalities associated with respiratory diseases are seen in (1) acute alveolar hyperventilation with hypoxemia, (2) acute ventilatory failure with hypoxemia, (3) chronic ventilatory failure with hypoxemia, (4) acute alveolar hyperventilation superimposed on chronic ventilatory failure, and (5) acute ventilatory failure superimposed on chronic ventilatory failure.

◆ Acute Alveolar Hyperventilation with HYPOXEMIA

ABG Changes	Example
pH: increased	7.53
$Paco_2$: decreased	28 mm Hg
HCO_3: decreased	20 mEq/L
Pao_2: decreased	63 mm Hg

Acute Alveolar Hyperventilation With Hypoxemia

When a patient is stimulated to breathe more and has the muscular power and patent airways to do so, alveolar hyperventilation develops (i.e., the $Paco_2$ decreases below the normal value). When a decreased $Paco_2$ is accompanied by alkalemia (a pH above normal), acute alveolar hyperventilation (also called *respiratory alkalosis*) is said to exist. In respiratory disease, acute alveolar hyperventilation is usually accompanied by (and may be caused by) hypoxemia.

The basic pathophysiologic mechanisms that produce the abnormal ABGs in acute alveolar hyperventilation are described in the following sections.

Decreased Pao_2, Decreased $Paco_2$

The decreased Pao_2 seen during acute alveolar hyperventilation usually develops from the decreased $\dot{V}/\dot{Q}$ ratio, capillary shunting (or a shuntlike effect), and venous admixture associated with the pulmonary disorder. The Pao_2 continues to drop as the pathologic effects of the disease intensify. Eventually, the Pao_2 may decline to a point sufficiently low (a Pao_2 of about 60 mm Hg) to stimulate the peripheral chemoreceptors, which in turn causes the ventilatory rate to increase (Figure 4-1). After this increase, the patient's Pao_2 generally remains at a constant level. The increased ventilatory response, however, is often accompanied by a decrease in the $Paco_2$ (Figure 4-2).

The following pathophysiologic mechanisms also may contribute to an increased ventilatory rate and a reduction in the $Paco_2$:

- Decreased lung compliance
- Stimulation of the central chemoreceptors
- Activation of the deflation reflex

TABLE 4–1 Normal Blood Gas Values		
Blood Gas Value*	Arterial	Venous
pH	7.35 to 7.45	7.30 to 7.40
Pco_2	35 to 45 mm Hg	42 to 48 mm Hg
HCO_3^-	22 to 28 mEq/L	24 to 30 mEq/L
Po_2	80 to 100 mm Hg	35 to 45 mm Hg

*Technically, only the oxygen (Po_2) and carbon dioxide (Pco_2) pressure readings are true blood gas values. The pH indicates the balance between the bases and acids in the blood. The bicarbonate (HCO_3^-) reading is an indirect measurement that is calculated from the pH and Pco_2 levels.

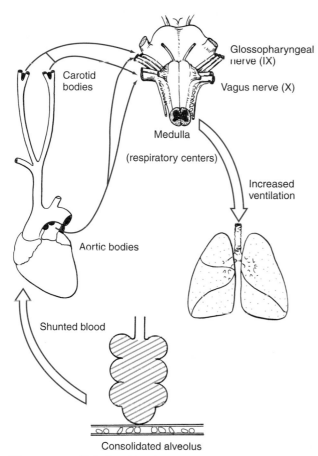

Figure 4–1   Relationship of venous admixture to the stimulation of peripheral chemoreceptors in response to alveolar consolidation.

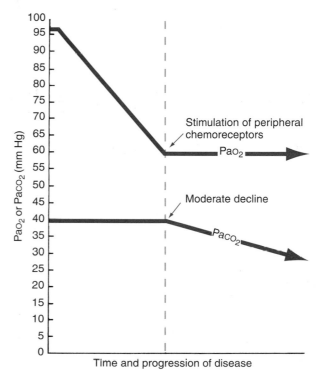

Figure 4–2 Pao_2 and $Paco_2$ trends during acute alveolar hyperventilation.

- Activation of the irritant reflex
- Stimulation of the J receptors
- Pain and anxiety

Decreased HCO_3^-, Increased pH

Sudden changes in the patient's $Paco_2$ level cause an immediate change in the HCO_3^- and pH levels. The reason for this change is the Pco_2/HCO_3^-/pH relationship.

Review of the $Paco_2$/HCO_3^-/pH Relationship

The bulk of the CO_2 is transported from the tissue cells to the lungs as HCO_3^- (Figure 4-3). As the CO_2 level increases, the plasma Pco_2, HCO_3^-, and H_2CO_3 levels increase. The converse also is true: As the level of CO_2 decreases, the plasma Pco_2, HCO_3^-, and H_2CO_3 levels decrease.

Because the blood pH depends on the ratio between the plasma HCO_3^- (base) and H_2CO_3 (acid), acute ventilatory changes immediately alter the pH level.

This relationship is a function of this basic chemical reaction: $CO_2 + H_2O \Leftrightarrow H_2CO_3 \Leftrightarrow HCO_3^- + H^+$. The normal HCO_3^--to-H_2CO_3 ratio is 20:1. Even though plasma HCO_3^- and plasma H_2CO_3 move in the same direction during acute ventilatory changes, acute changes in the H_2CO_3 level play a much more powerful role in altering the pH status than do acute changes in the HCO_3^- level. This difference is due to the 20:1 ratio between HCO_3^- and H_2CO_3.

For every H_2CO_3 molecule increase or decrease, 20 HCO_3^- molecules also must increase or decrease, respectively. If this does not happen, the normal 20:1 ratio between HCO_3^- will change. When the HCO_3^--to-H_2CO_3 ratio is less than 20:1, an *acidosis* exists. When the HCO_3^--to-H_2CO_3 ratio is greater than 20:1, an *alkalosis* exists.

In view of this relationship, during periods of acute alveolar hyperventilation the $PAco_2$ decreases and allows more CO_2 to leave the pulmonary blood. This action necessarily decreases the blood $Paco_2$, H_2CO_3, and HCO_3^- levels (Figure 4-4). Because acute changes in H_2CO_3 levels are more significant than acute changes in HCO_3^- levels, an increased HCO_3^--to-H_2CO_3 ratio develops (a ratio greater than 20:1). This action causes the patient's blood pH to increase, or become more alkaline. The normal buffer line on the Pco_2/HCO_3^-/pH nomogram in Figure 4-5 illustrates the

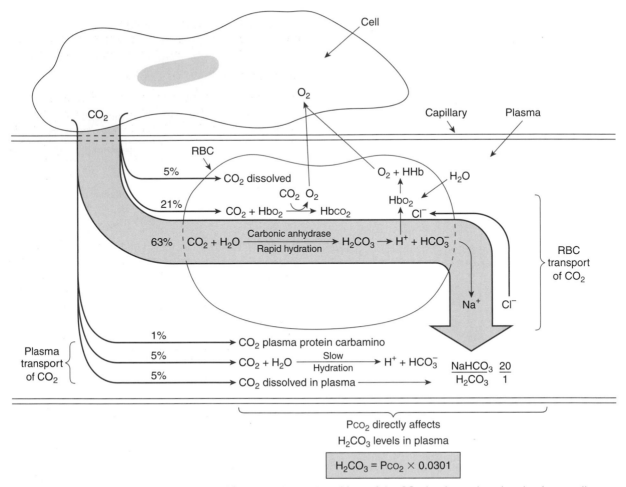

Figure 4–3   The way CO_2 is converted to HCO_3^- at the tissue sites. Most of the CO_2 that is produced at the tissue cells is carried to the lungs in the form of HCO_3^-. *CA,* carbonic anhydrase. (Modified from Des Jardins T: *Cardiopulmonary anatomy and physiology: Essentials for respiratory care,* ed 4, Albany, NY, 2002, Delmar.)

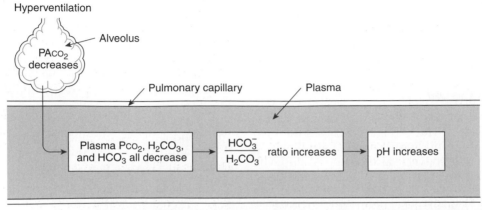

Figure 4–4   Alveolar hyperventilation causes the $P_{A_{CO_2}}$ and the plasma P_{CO_2}, H_2CO_3, and HCO_3^- to decrease. This action increases the HCO_3^-/H_2CO_3 ratio, which in turn increases the blood pH. (Redrawn from Des Jardins T: *Cardiopulmonary anatomy and physiology: Essentials for respiratory care,* ed 4, Albany, NY, 2002, Delmar.)

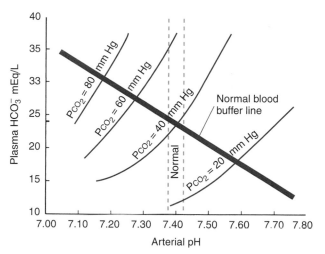

Figure 4–5 $P_{CO_2}/HCO_3^-/pH$ relationship.

expected HCO_3^- and pH changes that develop in response to sudden CO_2 changes.

◆ Acute Ventilatory Failure with HYPOXEMIA

ABG Changes	Example
pH: decreased	7.21
$Paco_2$: increased	79 mm Hg
HCO_3^-: increased (slightly)	28 mM/L
Pao_2: decreased	57 mm Hg

Acute Ventilatory Failure With Hypoxemia

Ventilatory failure is a condition in which the lungs are unable to meet the metabolic demands of the body in terms of CO_2 homeostasis. In other words, the patient is unable to provide the muscular, mechanical work necessary to move gas into and out of the lungs to meet the normal CO_2 metabolic demands of the body. This condition leads to an increased $PAco_2$ and, subsequently, to an increased $Paco_2$ level. Ventilatory failure is not associated with a typical ventilatory pattern. The patient may be apneic or have severe hyperpnea and tachypnea. The bottom line is that ventilatory failure will develop in response to any ventilatory pattern that does not provide adequate alveolar ventilation. When an increased $Paco_2$ is accompanied by acidemia (decreased pH), acute ventilatory failure (also called *respiratory acidosis*) is said to exist. Clinically, this is a medical emergency that requires mechanical ventilation.

The basic pathophysiologic mechanisms that produce the abnormal ABG findings in acute ventilatory failure are discussed in the following sections.

Decreased Pao_2, Increased $Paco_2$

Whenever a respiratory disorder becomes critical over a relatively short period of time, acute ventilatory failure may develop. When this happens, the patient's overall $\dot{V}/\dot{Q}$ ratio decreases. This condition causes the PAo_2 to decrease and the $PAco_2$ to increase. This action in turn causes the Pao_2 to decrease and the $Paco_2$ to increase.

Increased HCO_3^-, Decreased pH

The sudden rise in the $Paco_2$ level causes the H_2CO_3 and HCO_3^- levels to increase (Figure 4-6). Because acute changes in H_2CO_3 are more significant than acute changes in HCO_3^-, a decreased HCO_3^--to-H_2CO_3 ratio develops (a ratio less than 20:1). This action causes a patient's blood pH to decrease, or become less alkaline.

◆ Chronic Ventilatory Failure with HYPOXEMIA

ABG Changes	Example
pH: normal	7.38
$Paco_2$: increased	66 mm Hg
HCO_3^-: increased (significantly)	35 mEq/L
Pao_2: decreased	63 mm Hg

Chronic Ventilatory Failure With Hypoxemia

Chronic ventilatory failure is defined as a greater-than-normal $Paco_2$ level with a normal pH status. Clinically, chronic hypercarbia is most commonly seen in patients with severe chronic obstructive pulmonary disease. Chronic ventilatory failure, however, is seen in other respiratory diseases. Box 4-1 lists some respiratory diseases associated with chronic ventilatory failure during the advanced stages of the disorder.

The basic pathophysiologic mechanisms that produce the abnormal ABG findings in chronic ventilatory failure are described in the following sections.

Decreased Pao_2, Increased $Paco_2$

As a respiratory disorder becomes progressively severe (e.g., chronic bronchitis, emphysema), the work of breathing may become so great and the pulmonary shunting so significant that more oxygen is consumed than is gained. Although the exact mechanism is

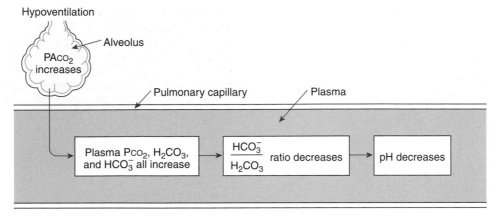

Figure 4–6   Alveolar hypoventilation causes the PA_{CO_2} and the plasma P_{CO_2}, H_2CO_3, and HCO_3^- to increase. This action decreases the HCO_3^-/H_2CO_3 ratio, which in turn decreases the blood pH. (Redrawn from Des Jardins T: *Cardiopulmonary anatomy and physiology: Essentials for respiratory care,* ed 4, Albany, NY, 2002, Delmar.)

BOX 4–1

Respiratory Diseases Associated with Chronic Ventilatory Failure During the Advanced Stages

Chronic Obstructive Pulmonary Diseases (Most Common)

Chronic bronchitis
Emphysema
Bronchiectasis
Cystic fibrosis

Other Respiratory Diseases

Pneumoconiosis
Tuberculosis
Fungal diseases
Kyphoscoliosis

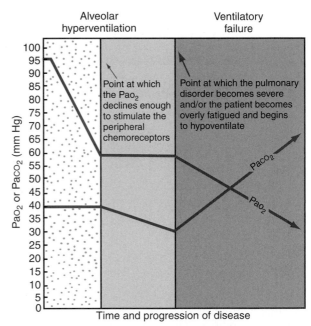

Figure 4–7 Pa_{O_2} and Pa_{CO_2} trends during acute or chronic ventilatory failure.

---

unclear, the patient slowly develops a breathing pattern that uses the least amount of oxygen for the energy expended. In essence, the patient selects a breathing pattern based on *work efficiency* rather than *ventilatory efficiency*.* As a result, the patient's alveolar ventilation slowly decreases, which in turn causes the Pa_{O_2} to decrease and the Pa_{CO_2} to increase further (Figure 4-7).

Increased HCO_3^-, Normal pH

When an individual hypoventilates for a long time, the kidneys try to correct the decreased pH by retaining

HCO_3^- in the blood. Renal compensation in the presence of chronic hypoventilation can be shown when the calculated HCO_3^- and pH readings are higher than expected for a particular P_{CO_2} level. For example, in terms of the absolute $P_{CO_2}/HCO_3^-/pH$ relationship, when the P_{CO_2} level is about 80 mm Hg, the HCO_3^- level should be about 30 mM/L and the pH should be about 7.18, according to the normal blood buffer line (Figure 4-8). If the HCO_3^- and pH levels are greater than these values (i.e., the pH and

---

*See the discussion on altered airway resistance and its effect on the ventilatory patterns, page 32.

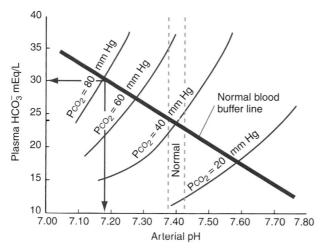

Figure 4–8 Expected pH and HCO_3^- levels when the $Paco_2$ is approximately 80 mm Hg.

HCO_3^- readings cross a Pco_2 isobar* above the normal blood buffer line in the upper left-hand corner of the nomogram), renal retention of HCO_3^- (partial renal compensation) has occurred. When the HCO_3^- level increases enough to return the acidic pH to normal, complete renal compensation is said to have occurred (chronic ventilatory failure).

As a general rule, the kidneys do not overcompensate for an abnormal pH level—that is, should the patient's blood pH level become acidic for a long time as a result of hypoventilation, the kidneys will not retain enough HCO_3^- for the pH value to climb higher than 7.4. The opposite also is true: Should the patient's blood pH become alkalotic for a long time as a result of hyperventilation, the kidneys will not excrete enough HCO_3^- to cause the pH level to fall below 7.4.

In persons who have been hypoventilating over a long period, however, a pH level greater than 7.4 is not uncommon. This higher level is believed to result from water and chloride ion shifts between the intracellular and extracellular spaces that occur while the kidneys are compensating for a decreased blood pH.

The lungs play an important role in maintaining the $Paco_2$, HCO_3^-, and pH levels on a moment-to-moment basis. The kidneys, on the other hand, play an important role in maintaining the HCO_3^- and pH levels during long periods of hyperventilation or hypoventilation. It is a common error to assume that the

---

*The isobars on the $Pco_2/HCO_3^-/pH$ nomogram illustrate the pH changes that develop in the blood as a result of (1) metabolic changes (i.e., HCO_3^- changes) or (2) a combination of metabolic and respiratory (CO_2) changes.

maintenance of HCO_3^- levels in the body is influenced only by the kidneys.

Finally, it should be noted that blood gas analyzers determine HCO_3^- levels on the basis of the patient's in vitro buffer slope. Therefore a nomogram, such as the one shown in Figure 4-5, must be used to determine the expected HCO_3^- and pH values for a particular $Paco_2$ level.

◆ ACUTE VENTILATORY CHANGES SUPERIMPOSED ON CHRONIC VENTILATORY FAILURE

Because acute ventilatory changes frequently are seen in patients already in chronic ventilatory failure, the respiratory care practitioner must be familiar with and be on the alert for (1) acute alveolar hyperventilation superimposed on chronic ventilatory failure and (2) acute ventilatory failure superimposed on chronic ventilatory failure.

Acute Alveolar Hyperventilation Superimposed on CHRONIC VENTILATORY FAILURE

ABG Changes	Example
pH: increased	7.55
$Paco_2$: increased	62 mm Hg
HCO_3^-: increased	38 mEq/L
Pao_2: decreased	51 mm Hg

◆ Acute Alveolar Hyperventilation Superimposed on Chronic Ventilatory Failure

Like any other person (healthy or unhealthy), the patient with chronic ventilatory failure can acquire an acute shunt-producing disease such as pneumonia. Some of these patients have the mechanical reserve to increase their alveolar ventilation significantly in an attempt to maintain their baseline Pao_2. In some of these patients, however, the increased alveolar ventilation is excessive.

When excessive alveolar ventilation occurs, the patient's $PAco_2$ rapidly decreases. This action causes the patient's $Paco_2$ to decrease from its normally high baseline level. As the $Paco_2$ decreases, the arterial pH increases. As this condition intensifies, the patient's baseline ABG values can quickly change from chronic ventilatory failure to acute alveolar hyperventilation superimposed on chronic ventilatory failure (Table 4-2).

If the clinician does not know the past history of the patient with acute alveolar hyperventilation

TABLE 4–2	Examples of Acute Changes in Chronic Ventilatory Failure	
Acute Ventilatory Failure Superimposed on Chronic Ventilatory Failure	Chronic Ventilatory Failure (Baseline Values)	Acute Alveolar Hyperventilation Superimposed on Chronic Ventilatory Failure
7.21 ← – – – – –	pH 7.39	– – – – – → 7.53
110 ← – – – – –	$Paco_2$ 76	– – – – – → 51
43 ← – – – – –	HCO_3^- 41	– – – – – → 37
34 ← – – – – –	Pao_2 61	– – – – – → 46

superimposed on chronic ventilatory failure, he or she might initially interpret the ABG values as partially compensated metabolic alkalosis with severe hypoxemia (see Table 4-3). The clinical manifestation that offsets this interpretation, however, is the presence of marked hypoxemia. This degree of hypoxemia is not commonly seen in patients with metabolic alkalosis. Another tip-off is the presence of a wide alveolar-arterial oxygen tension difference $[P(A-a)o_2]$ in acute alveolar hyperventilation superimposed on chronic ventilatory failure (when measured on room air). A wide $P(A-a)o_2$ is not normally produced in the hypoventilation associated with partially compensated metabolic alkalosis.

Whenever an ABG value appears to reflect partially compensated metabolic alkalosis but is accompanied by significant hypoxemia, the respiratory care practitioner should be alert to the possibility of *acute alveolar hyperventilation superimposed on chronic ventilatory failure.*

Acute Ventilatory Failure Superimposed on CHRONIC VENTILATORY FAILURE

ABG Changes	Example
pH: decreased	7.23
$Paco_2$: increased	107 mm Hg
HCO_3^-: increased	41 mEq/L
Pao_2: decreased	38 mm Hg

◆ Acute Ventilatory Failure Superimposed on Chronic Ventilatory Failure

Some patients who acquire an acute intrapulmonary shunt-producing disease such as pneumonia do not have the mechanical reserve to meet the hypoxemic challenge of the increased shunt. When these patients attempt to maintain their baseline Pao_2 by increasing alveolar ventilation, they begin to consume more oxygen than is gained with the increased alveolar ventilation. When this happens, the patient begins to breathe less. If the alveolar ventilation decreases too much, the patient's $PAco_2$ rapidly increases. This action causes the $Paco_2$ to increase the normally high baseline level. As the $Paco_2$ increases, the arterial pH decreases. As this condition intensifies, the patient's baseline ABG values can quickly change from chronic ventilatory failure to *acute ventilatory failure superimposed on chronic ventilatory failure* (see Table 4-2).

If the respiratory care practitioner judges the severity of the ventilatory failure on the $Paco_2$ alone (in this case, 110 mm Hg), the patient would appear to be in severe ventilatory failure (see Table 4-2). As a general rule, however, when starting at normal baseline ABG values (e.g., a pH of 7.40, a $Paco_2$ of 40 mm Hg, and a HCO_3^- level of 24 mM/L), the pH decreases by 0.05 unit and the HCO_3^- increases by 1 mM/L for every 10 mm Hg increase in $Paco_2$; for every 10 mm Hg decrease in $Paco_2$, the pH will increase by 0.10 unit and the HCO_3^- will decrease by 2 mM/L (Table 4-3).

Because the pH of 7.21 in this example is not as low as expected for a $Paco_2$ level of 110 mm Hg (a pH of 7.05 is expected), the acute ventilatory failure is not as severe as the $Paco_2$ value of 110 mm Hg would lead the respiratory care practitioner to believe

TABLE 4–3	Approximate $Paco_2$/HCO_3^-/pH Relationship	
pH	$Paco_2$ (mm Hg)	HCO_3^- (mM/L)
7.70	10	18
7.60	20	20
7.50	30	22
7.40	40	24
7.35	50	25
7.30	60	26
7.25	70	27
7.20	80	28
7.15	90	29
7.10	100	30
7.05	110	31
7.00	120	32
6.95	130	33

(see Table 4-2). *The severity of acute ventilatory failure depends on the severity of the acidemia.*

Therefore, whenever the $Paco_2$ is high and the pH is not as low as expected, the respiratory care practitioner should be alert to the possibility of *acute ventilatory failure superimposed on chronic ventilatory failure.*

METABOLIC ACID-BASE ABNORMALITIES

◆ METABOLIC ACIDOSIS

ABG Changes	Example
pH: decreased	7.26
$Paco_2$: normal	37 mm Hg
HCO_3^-: decreased	18 mEq/L
Pao_2: normal (or decreased when lactic acidosis is present)	94 mm Hg (or 52 mm Hg when lactic acidosis is present)

Metabolic Acidosis

The presence of other acids not related to an increased $Paco_2$ level or renal compensation can be identified by using the isobars of the $Pco_2/HCO_3^-/pH$ nomogram shown in Figure 4-5. The presence of other acids is verified when the calculated HCO_3^- reading and pH level are both lower than expected for a particular $Paco_2$ level in terms of the absolute $Pco_2/HCO_3^-/pH$ relationship. For example, according to the normal blood buffer line, an HCO_3^- reading of 15 mEq/L and a pH of 7.2 would both be less than expected in a patient who has a Pco_2 of 40 mm Hg. This condition is referred to as *metabolic acidosis.* A number of conditions can cause metabolic acidosis (Box 4-2).

◆ METABOLIC ALKALOSIS

ABG Changes	Example
pH: increased	7.56
$Paco_2$: normal	44 mm Hg
HCO_3^-: increased	27 mEq/L
Pao_2: normal	94 mm Hg

Metabolic Alkalosis

The presence of other bases not related to either a decreased $Paco_2$ level or renal compensation also

---

BOX 4–2

Common Causes of Metabolic Acid-Base Abnormalties

Metabolic Acidosis
Lactic acidosis
Ketoacidosis
Renal failure
Dehydration
Chronic diarrhea

Metabolic Alkalosis
Hypokalemia
Hypochloremia
Gastric suctioning
Vomiting
Use of steroid medications
Excess sodium bicarbonate

---

can be identified by using the $Pco_2/HCO_3^-/pH$ nomogram illustrated in Figure 4-5. The presence of metabolic alkalosis is verified when the calculated HCO_3^- and pH readings are both higher than expected for a particular $Paco_2$ level in terms of the absolute $Pco_2/HCO_3^-/pH$ relationship. For example, according to the normal blood buffer line, an HCO_3^- reading of 35 mEq/L and a pH level of 7.54 would both be higher than expected in a patient who has a $Paco_2$ level of 40 mm Hg (see Figure 4-5). This condition is known as *metabolic alkalosis.* A number of conditions can cause metabolic alkalosis (see Box 4-2).

◆ Assessment of the Hypoxic State

The assessment of the hypoxic state should always accompany the assessment of the patient's ventilatory and acid-base status. In adults, an acceptable therapeutic range for the Pao_2 at sea level is greater than 80 mm Hg.* An acceptable Pao_2 range for newborns is between 40 and 70 mm Hg.

In adults breathing room air, *hypoxemia* is defined as a Pao_2 less than than 80 mm Hg. Clinically, hypoxemia is often classified as *mild, moderate,* or *severe.* Mild hypoxemia may be defined as a Pao_2 less than 80 mm Hg, moderate hypoxemia is generally thought to be present when the Pao_2 is less than 60 mm Hg, and severe hypoxemia is present when the Pao_2 is less than 40 mm Hg.

---

*In adults older than 60 years, subtract 1 mm Hg from 80 mm Hg for each year over 60 years for the normal lower Pao_2 limit at sea level.

The Hazards of Oxygen Therapy in Patients with Chronic Ventilatory Failure with Hypoxemia

In some patients with chronic ventilatory failure and hypoxemia, the administration of moderate to high concentrations of oxygen may suppress ventilation, causing the patient's arterial carbon dioxide (Pa_{CO_2}) to increase and the pH to decrease. This means that when a patient with chronic hypercapnia is given too much oxygen, the patient may develop acute ventilatory failure—superimposed on the already chronic condition. In other words, patients with chronically high CO_2 levels may experience an *acute oxygen-induced hypercapnia*—on top of their already high CO_2 levels—when breathing high concentrations of oxygen. In severe cases, the sudden increase in carbon dioxide and acidemia may depress the patient's central nervous system, cause lethargy, and ultimately lead to coma. Clinically, oxygen-induced hypoventilation is most commonly seen in the relaxed, unstimulated patient with chronic hypercapnia. Patients who are experiencing oxygen-induced hypoventilation are often described as sleepy, lethargic, and hard to arouse, with slow and shallow breathing.

Although the precise mechanism for this phenomenon is not known, one prominent theory suggests that the administration of high concentrations of oxygen may suppress the patient's so-called hypoxic drive to breathe. According to this theory, the sensitivity of the *central chemoreceptors (CO₂ sensors)*, which are located in the medulla, is blunted—or rendered insensitive—when the carbon dioxide level is chronically high. As a result, the patient's primary stimulus to breathe on a moment-to-moment basis falls to the *peripheral chemoreceptors (oxygen sensors)*, which are located near the bifurcation of the common carotid arteries and ascending aorta. Presumably, the excessive administration of oxygen depresses the oxygen peripheral chemoreceptors, which in turn depresses the patient's ventilatory drive. When this occurs, the Pa_{CO_2} increases and the pH decreases.

Other investigators have suggested that the excessive oxygen administration somehow causes the patient's ventilation-perfusion ($\dot{V}/\dot{Q}$) relationships to deteriorate, leading to an acute rise in P_{CO_2} and decrease in pH. Most researchers agree, however, that the oxygen-induced hypercapnia phenomenon most likely is due to a combination of both mechanisms—the (1) oxygen-induced peripheral chemoreceptor depression and (2) the oxygen-induced redistribution of the $\dot{V}/\dot{Q}$ ratio. Regardless of the precise cause of oxygen-induced hypercapnia, the respiratory care practitioner must nevertheless exercise caution when providing oxygen therapy to patients with chronic hypercapnia. Clinically, patients with chronic hypercapnia (e.g., obstructive pulmonary disease) are typically oxygenated with low and precisely controlled concentrations of oxygen. In such patients, oxygen devices that provide a fixed F_{IO_2} regardless of the patient's ventilatory pattern should be used.

SELF-ASSESSMENT QUESTIONS

Multiple Choice

1. During acute alveolar hyperventilation, which of the following occurs?

    I. HCO_3^- decreases
    II. $Paco_2$ increases
    III. H_2CO_3 decreases
    IV. $PAco_2$ increases

    a. I only
    b. II only
    c. III only
    d. I and III only
    e. II and IV only

2. When lactic acidosis is present, which of the following will occur?

    I. pH will likely be lower than expected for a particular $Paco_2$.
    II. HCO_3 will likely be higher than expected for a particular $PAco_2$.
    III. pH will likely be higher than expected for a particular $Paco_2$.
    IV. HCO_3 will likely be lower than expected for a particular $Paco_2$.

    a. I only
    b. II only
    c. III only
    d. II and III only
    e. I and IV only

3. What is the clinical interpretation of the following ABG values (in addition to hypoxemia)?

    pH: 7.17
    $Paco_2$: 77 mm Hg
    HCO_3^-: 27 mEq/L
    Pao_2: 54 mm Hg

    a. Chronic ventilatory failure
    b. Acute alveolar hyperventilation superimposed on chronic ventilatory failure
    c. Acute ventilatory failure
    d. Acute alveolar hyperventilation
    e. Acute ventilatory failure superimposed on chronic ventilatory failure

4. A 74-year-old male with a long history of emphysema and chronic bronchitis enters the emergency room in respiratory distress. His respiratory rate is 34 breaths per minute and labored. His heart rate is 115 beats per minute, and his blood pressure is 170/120. What is the clinical interpretation of the following ABG values (in addition to hypoxemia)?

    pH: 7.57
    $Paco_2$: 68 mm Hg
    HCO_3^-: 37 mEq/L
    Pao_2: 49 mm Hg

    a. Chronic ventilatory failure
    b. Acute alveolar hyperventilation superimposed on chronic ventilatory failure
    c. Acute ventilatory failure
    d. Acute alveolar hyperventilation
    e. Acute ventilatory failure superimposed on chronic ventilatory failure

5. Which of the following is classified as metabolic acidosis?

    a. pH 7.23; $Paco_2$ 63; HCO_3^- 26; Pao_2 52
    b. pH 7.16; $Paco_2$ 38; HCO_3^- 16; Pao_2 86
    c. pH 7.56; $Paco_2$ 27; HCO_3^- 21; Pao_2 101
    d. pH 7.64; $Paco_2$ 49; HCO_3^- 31; Pao_2 91
    e. pH 7.37; $Paco_2$ 66; HCO_3^- 29; Pao_2 73

6. Which of the following cause metabolic acidosis?

    I Hypokalemia
    II. Renal failure
    III. Dehydration
    IV. Hypochloremia

    a. I only
    b. II only
    c. IV only
    d. I and IV only
    e. II and III only

7. According to the $Paco_2/HCO_3^-/pH$ relationship, if the $Paco_2$ suddenly increased to 90 mm Hg in a patient who normally has a pH of 7.4, a $Paco_2$ of 40 mm Hg, and an HCO_3^- of 24 mm/L, the pH will decrease to approximately what level?

    a. 7.15
    b. 7.10
    c. 7.05
    d. 7.00
    e. 6.95

8. What is the lowest acceptable Pa_{O_2} level for an 80-year-old patient?

   a. 55 mm Hg
   b. 60 mm Hg
   c. 65 mm Hg
   d. 70 mm Hg
   e. 80 mm Hg

9. Ketoacidosis can develop from which of the following?

   I. An inadequate oxygen level
   II. Renal failure
   III. An inadequate insulin level
   IV. Anaerobic metabolism
   V. An inadequate glucose level

   a. I only
   b. II and III only
   c. IV and V only
   d. III and V only
   e. II, III, and V only

10. Metabolic alkalosis can develop from which of the following?

    I. Hyperchloremia
    II. Hypokalemia
    III. Hypochloremia
    IV. Hyperkalemia

    a. I only
    b. IV only
    c. I and III only
    d. I and IV only
    e. II and III only

11. During acute alveolar hypoventilation, the blood:

    I. H_2CO_3 increases
    II. pH increases
    III. HCO_3^- increases
    IV. P_{CO_2} increases

    a. II only
    b. IV only
    c. II and III only
    d. I, III, and IV only
    e. I and IV only

12. During acute alveolar hyperventilation, the blood

    I. P_{CO_2} increases
    II. H_2CO_3 decreases
    III. HCO_3^- increases
    IV. pH decreases

    a. II only
    b. IV only
    c. I and III only
    d. II and IV only
    e. II, III, and IV only

13. In chronic hypoventilation, kidney compensation has likely occurred when the

    I. HCO_3^- is higher than expected for a particular Pa_{CO_2}
    II. pH is lower than expected for a particular Pa_{CO_2}
    III. H_2CO_3 is lower than expected for a particular Pa_{CO_2}
    IV. pH is higher than expected for a particular Pa_{CO_2}

    a. I only
    b. II only
    c. I and IV only
    d. III and IV only
    e. I and II only

14. Which of the following represents acute alveolar hyperventilation?

    a. pH 7.56; Pa_{CO_2} 51; HCO_3^- 43
    b. pH 7.45; Pa_{CO_2} 37; HCO_3^- 18
    c. pH 7.53; Pa_{CO_2} 46; HCO_3^- 29
    d. pH 7.54; Pa_{CO_2} 21; HCO_3^- 19
    e. pH 7.47; Pa_{CO_2} 55; HCO_3^- 37

15. Which of the following is compensated metabolic alkalosis?

    a. pH 7.55; Pa_{CO_2} 21; HCO_3^- 17
    b. pH 7.52; Pa_{CO_2} 45; HCO_3^- 29
    c. pH 7.45; Pa_{CO_2} 26; HCO_3^- 19
    d. pH 7.31; Pa_{CO_2} 51; HCO_3^- 31
    e. pH 7.45; Pa_{CO_2} 61; HCO_3^- 41

Answers appear in Appendix XI.

CHAPTER 5

Oxygenation Assessments

Oxygen Transport Review

Oxygen transport between the lungs and the tissue cells is a function of the blood and the heart. Oxygen is carried in the blood in two ways: (1) as dissolved oxygen in the blood plasma, and (2) bound to the hemoglobin (Hb). Most oxygen is carried to the tissue cells bound to the hemoglobin.

Oxygen Dissolved in the Blood Plasma

A small amount of oxygen that diffuses from the alveoli to the pulmonary capillary blood remains in the dissolved form. The term *dissolved* means that the gas molecule (in this case oxygen) maintains its exact molecular structure and freely moves throughout the plasma of the blood in its normal gaseous state. Clinically, it is the dissolved oxygen that is measured to assess the patient's partial pressure of oxygen (Po_2) (Table 4-1).

At normal body temperature, approximately 0.003 ml of oxygen will dissolve in each 100 ml of blood for every 1 mm Hg of Po_2. Therefore in the normal individual with an arterial oxygen partial pressure (Pao_2) of 100 mm Hg, about 0.3 ml of oxygen exists in the dissolved form, in every 100 ml of plasma (0.003×100 mm Hg = 0.3 ml). Clinically, this is written as 0.3 volumes percent (vol%), or as 0.3 vol% oxygen. Relative to the total oxygen transport, only a small amount of oxygen is carried to the tissue cells in the form of dissolved oxygen.

Oxygen Bound to Hemoglobin

In the healthy individual, over 98% of the oxygen that diffuses into the pulmonary capillary blood chemically combines with hemoglobin (Hb). The normal hemoglobin value for the adult male is 14 to 16 g/100 ml of blood. Clinically, the weight measurement of hemoglobin, in reference to 100 ml of blood, is known as the grams percent of hemoglobin (g% Hb). The normal hemoglobin value for the adult female is 12 to 15 g%. The normal infant hemoglobin value is between 14 and 20 g%.

Each gram of Hb (1 g% Hb) is capable of carrying about 1.34 ml of oxygen. Therefore if the hemoglobin level is 12 g%, and the hemoglobin is fully saturated with oxygen (i.e., carrying all the oxygen that is physically possible), about 15.72 vol% will be bound to the hemoglobin:

$$O_2 \text{ bound to Hb} = 1.34 \text{ mL } O_2 \times 12 \text{ g\% Hb}$$
$$= 15.72 \text{ vol\% } O_2 \text{ (15.72 ml}$$
$$\text{of oxygen/100 ml of blood)}$$

Because of normal physiologic shunts (e.g., thebesian venous drainage and bronchial venous drainage), however, the actual normal hemoglobin saturation is only about 97%. Thus the amount of arterial oxygen shown in the above calculation must be adjusted to 97% as follows:

$$15.72 \text{ (vol\% } O_2) \times 0.97 = 15.24 \text{ vol\% } O_2$$

Total Oxygen Content

To calculate the total amount of oxygen in each 100 ml of blood, both the dissolved oxygen and the oxygen bound to the hemoglobin must be added together. The following case example summarizes the mathematics required to determine an individual's total oxygen content.

CASE EXAMPLE

A 44-year-old woman with a long history of asthma arrives in the emergency room in severe respiratory distress. Her vital signs are as follows: respiratory rate 36 breaths/min, heart rate 130 beats/minute, and blood pressure 160/95 mm Hg. Her hemoglobin concentration is 10 g%, and her Pao_2 is 55 mm Hg (Sao_2 85%). On the basis of these data, the patient's total oxygen content is determined as follows:

1. Dissolved O_2

$$\frac{55 \text{ } Pao_2}{\times 0.003 \text{ (dissolved } O_2 \text{ factor)}}$$
$$0.165 \text{ (vol\% } O_2)$$

2. Oxygen bound to hemoglobin

$$\frac{\begin{array}{c} 10\text{ g\% Hb} \\ \times\, 1.34 \text{ (O}_2 \text{ bound to Hb factor)} \end{array}}{13.4 \text{ vol\% O}_2 \text{ (at Sao}_2 \text{ of 100\%)}}$$

$$\frac{\begin{array}{c} 13.4 \text{ vol\% O}_2 \\ \times\, 0.85 \text{ Sao}_2 \end{array}}{11.39 \text{ vol\% O}_2 \text{ (at Sao}_2 \text{ of 85\%)}}$$

3. Total oxygen content

11.39 vol% O_2 (bound to hemoglobin)

+ 0.165 vol% O_2 (dissolved O_2)

11.555 vol% O_2 (total amount of O_2/100 ml of blood)

The total oxygen content can be calculated in the patient's arterial blood (Cao_2), venous blood ($C\bar{v}o_2$), and pulmonary capillary blood, also known as the oxygen content of capillary blood (Cco_2). The mathematics for these calculations are as follows:

Cao_2: Oxygen content of arterial blood
$\quad$ ($Hb \times 1.34 \times Sao_2$) + ($Pao_2 \times 0.003$)
$C\bar{v}o_2$: Oxygen content of mixed venous blood
$\quad$ ($Hb \times 1.34 \times S\bar{v}o_2$) + ($P\bar{v}o_2 \times 0.003$)
Cco_2: Oxygen content of pulmonary capillary blood
$\quad$ ($Hb \times 1.34^*$) + ($PAo_2{}^\dagger \times 0.003$)

As it will be shown later in this chapter, various mathematical manipulations of the Cao_2, $C\bar{v}o_2$, and Cco_2 values are used in several different oxygen transport studies that provide excellent clinical information regarding the patient's ventilatory and cardiac status.

Oxygenation Indices

A number of oxygen transport measurements are available to assess the oxygenation status of the critically ill patient. Results from these studies can provide important information to adjust therapeutic interventions. The oxygen transport studies can be divided into the *oxygen–tension-based indices and the oxygen–saturation- and content-based indices.*[‡]

---

*It is assumed that the hemoglobin saturation with oxygen in the pulmonary capillary blood is 100% of 1.0.

[†]See Ideal Alveolar Gas Equation, Appendix III.

[‡]See Appendix X for a representative example of a cardiopulmonary profile sheet used to monitor the oxygen transport status of the critically ill patient.

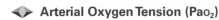

◆ OXYGEN–TENSION-BASED INDICES

◆ Arterial Oxygen Tension (Pao₂)

The Pao_2 has withstood the test of time as a good indicator of the patient's oxygenation status (see the discussion of assessment of the hypoxic state, page 85). In general, an appropriate Pao_2 on an inspired low oxygen concentration almost always indicates good lung oxygenation function. The Pao_2, however, can be misleading in a number of clinical situations. For example, the Pao_2 may give a "false-positive" oxygenation reading when the patient has (1) a low hemoglobin concentration, (2) a decreased cardiac output, (3) peripheral shunting, or (4) hypothermia, or (5) has been exposed to carbon monoxide or cyanide.

◆ Alveolar-Arterial Oxygen Tension Difference [P(A-a)o₂]

The $P(A-a)o_2$ is the oxygen tension difference between the alveoli and arterial blood. The $P(A-a)o_2$ also is known as the *alveolar-arterial oxygen tension gradient.* Clinically, the information required for the $P(A-a)o_2$ is obtained from (1) the patient's calculated alveolar oxygen tension (PAo_2), which is derived from the ideal alveolar gas equation, and (2) the patient's Pao_2 and $Paco_2$, which are obtained from an arterial blood gas analysis.

The ideal alveolar gas equation is written as follows:

$$PAo_2 = (P_B - P_{H_2O})\, F_{IO_2} - Paco_2\ (1.25)$$

where P_B is the barometric pressure, PAo_2 is the partial pressure of oxygen within the alveoli, P_{H_2O} is the partial pressure of water vapor in the alveoli (which is 47 mm Hg), F_{IO_2} is the fractional concentration of inspired oxygen, $Paco_2$ is the partial pressure of arterial carbon dioxide, and the number 1.25 is a factor that adjusts for alterations in oxygen tension resulting from variations in the respiratory exchange ratio, or respiratory quotient (RQ). The RQ is the ratio of carbon dioxide production ($\dot{V}co_2$) divided by oxygen consumption ($\dot{V}o_2$). Under normal circumstances, approximately 250 ml of oxygen per minute are consumed by the tissue cells and approximately 200 ml of carbon dioxide are excreted into the lung. Thus, the RQ is normally about 0.8.

Thus if a patient is receiving an F_{IO_2} of 0.30 on a day when the barometric pressure is 750 mm Hg, and if the patient's $Paco_2$ is 70 mm Hg and Pao_2 is 60 mm Hg, the $P(A-a)o_2$ can be calculated as follows:

$$\begin{aligned} PAo_2 &= (P_B - P_{H_2O})\, F_{IO_2} - Paco_2(1.25) \\ &= (750-47)\,0.30 - 70\,(1.25) \\ &= (703)\,0.30 - 87.5 \\ &= 210.9 - 87.5 \\ &= 123.4 \text{ mm Hg} \end{aligned}$$

Using the Pa_{O_2} obtained from the arterial blood gas, the $P(A-a)_{O_2}$ can now easily be calculated as follows:

$$123.4 \text{ mm Hg } (PA_{O_2})$$
$$- 60.0 \text{ mm Hg } (Pa_{O_2})$$
$$= 63.4 \text{ mm Hg } (P(A-a)_{O_2})$$

The normal $P(A-a)_{O_2}$ on room air at sea level ranges between 7 and 15 mm Hg, and it should not exceed 30 mm Hg. The $P(A-a)_{O_2}$ increases in response to (1) oxygen diffusion disorders (e.g., chronic interstitial lung diseases), (2) decreased ventilation/perfusion ratios disorders (e.g., chronic obstructive pulmonary diseases, atelectasis, consolidation), (3) right-to-left intracardiac shunting (e.g., a patent ventricular septum), and (4) age.

Although the $P(A-a)_{O_2}$ may be useful in patients breathing a low F_{IO_2}, it loses some of its sensitivity in patients breathing a high F_{IO_2}. The $P(A-a)_{O_2}$ increases at high oxygen concentrations. Because of this, the $P(A-a)_{O_2}$ has less value in the critically ill patient who is breathing a high oxygen concentration.

Arterial-Alveolar Oxygen Ratio (Pa_{O_2}/PA_{O_2})

Several variations of the $P(A-a)_{O_2}$ have been introduced over the years. Such oxygenation indices have included the *arterial-alveolar oxygen ratio* (Pa_{O_2}/PA_{O_2}) and the *arterial to inspired oxygen concentration ratio* (Pa_{O_2}/F_{IO_2}). Most experts agree that these studies are not helpful and probably should be abandoned.

OXYGEN–SATURATION- AND CONTENT-BASED INDICES

The oxygen–saturation- and content-based indices can serve as excellent indicators of an individual's cardiac and ventilatory status. These oxygenation studies are derived from the patient's total oxygen content in the arterial blood (Ca_{O_2}), mixed venous blood ($C\bar{v}_{O_2}$), and pulmonary capillary blood (Cc_{O_2}). The Ca_{O_2}, $C\bar{v}_{O_2}$, and Cc_{O_2} are calculated using the following formulas:

$$Ca_{O_2} = (Hb \times 1.34 \times Sa_{O_2}) + (Pa_{O_2} \times 0.003)$$
$$C\bar{v}_{O_2} = (Hb \times 1.34 \times S\bar{v}_{O_2}) + (P\bar{v}_{O_2} \times 0.003)$$
$$Cc_{O_2} = (Hb \times 1.34)* + (PA_{O_2}{}^\dagger \times 0.003)$$

where Hb is grams percent hemoglobin (g% Hb), 1.34 is the approximate amount (ml) of oxygen each g% of Hb is capable of carrying, Sa_{O_2} is the arterial oxygen saturation, Pa_{O_2} is the arterial oxygen tension,

---

*It is assumed that the hemoglobin saturation with oxygen in the pulmonary capillary blood is 100%, or 1.0.
†See Ideal Alveolar Gas Equation, Appendix III.)

0.003 is the dissolved oxygen factor, $S\bar{v}_{O_2}$ is the venous oxygen saturation, $P\bar{v}_{O_2}$ is the venous oxygen tension, and PA_{O_2} is the alveolar oxygen tension.

Clinically, the most common oxygen–saturation- and content-based indices are (1) total oxygen delivery, (2) arterial-venous oxygen content difference, (3) oxygen consumption, (4) oxygen extraction ratio, (5) mixed venous oxygen saturation, and (6) pulmonary shunt.

Total Oxygen Delivery

Total oxygen delivery (D_{O_2}) is the amount of oxygen delivered to the peripheral tissue cells. The D_{O_2} is calculated as follows:

$$D_{O_2} = \dot{Q}_T \times (Ca_{O_2} \times 10)$$

where $\dot{Q}_T$ is total cardiac output (L/min), Ca_{O_2} is oxygen content of arterial blood (ml oxygen/100 ml blood), and the factor 10 is used to convert the Ca_{O_2} to ml O_2/L blood.

Therefore if a patient has a cardiac output of 4 L/min and a Ca_{O_2} of 15 vol%, the D_{O_2} is 600 ml of oxygen per minute:

$$\begin{aligned} D_{O_2} &= \dot{Q}_T \times (Ca_{O_2} \times 10) \\ &= 4 \text{ L/min} \times (15 \text{ vol\%} \times 10) \\ &= 600 \text{ ml } O_2/\text{min} \end{aligned}$$

Normally, the D_{O_2} is approximately 1000 ml of oxygen per minute. Clinically, a patient's D_{O_2} decreases when blood oxygen saturation, hemoglobin concentration, or cardiac output declines. The D_{O_2} increases in response to an increase in blood oxygen saturation, hemoglobin concentration, or cardiac output.

Arterial-Venous Oxygen Content Difference

The arterial-venous oxygen content difference ($C(a-\bar{v})_{O_2}$) is the difference between the Ca_{O_2} and the $C\bar{v}_{O_2}$ ($Ca_{O_2} - C\bar{v}_{O_2}$). Therefore if a patient's Ca_{O_2} is 15 vol% and the $C\bar{v}_{O_2}$ is 8 vol%, the $C(a-\bar{v})_{O_2}$ is 7 vol%:

$$\begin{aligned} C(a-\bar{v})_{O_2} &= Ca_{O_2} - C\bar{v}_{O_2} \\ &= 15 \text{ vol\%} - 8 \text{ vol\%} \\ &= 7 \text{ vol\%} \end{aligned}$$

Normally, the $C(a-\bar{v})_{O_2}$ is about 5 vol%. The $C(a-\bar{v})_{O_2}$ is useful in assessing the patient's cardiopulmonary status because oxygen changes in the mixed venous blood ($C\bar{v}_{O_2}$) often occur earlier than oxygen changes in arterial blood gas. Clinically, the patient's $C(a-\bar{v})_{O_2}$ increases in response to such factors as decreased cardiac output, exercise, seizures, and hyperthermia. It decreases in response to increased cardiac output, skeletal relaxation (e.g., induced by drugs), peripheral shunting (e.g., sepsis), certain poisons (e.g., cyanide), and hypothermia.

Oxygen Consumption

Oxygen consumption ($\dot{V}_{O_2}$), also known as *oxygen uptake,* is the amount of oxygen consumed by the peripheral tissue cells during a 1-minute period. The $\dot{V}_{O_2}$ is calculated as follows:

$$\dot{V}_{O_2} = \dot{Q}_T \, [C(a\text{-}\bar{v})_{O_2} \times 10]$$

where $\dot{V}_T$ is the total cardiac output (L/min), $C(a\text{-}\bar{v})_{O_2}$ is the arterial-venous oxygen content difference, and the factor 10 is used to convert the $C(a\text{-}\bar{v})_{O_2}$ to ml O_2/L.

Therefore if a patient has a cardiac output of 4 L/min and a $C(a\text{-}\bar{v})_{O_2}$ of 6 vol%, the total amount of oxygen consumed by the tissue cells in 1 minute would be 240 ml:

$$\begin{aligned}
\dot{V}_{O_2} &= \dot{Q}_T \, [C(a\text{-}\bar{v})_{O_2} \times 10] \\
&= 4 \text{ L/min} \times 6 \text{ vol\%} \times 10 \\
&= 240 \text{ ml } O_2/\text{min}
\end{aligned}$$

Normally, the $\dot{V}_{O_2}$ is about 250 ml of oxygen per minute. Clinically, the $\dot{V}_{O_2}$ increases in response to seizures, exercise, hyperthermia, and body size. The $\dot{V}_{O_2}$ decreases in response to skeletal muscle relaxation (e.g., induced by drugs), peripheral shunting (e.g., sepsis), certain poisons (e.g., cyanide), and hypothermia. It is often as a function of body weight (i.e., ml/kg or ml/lb).

Oxygen Extraction Ratio

The oxygen extraction ratio (O_2ER), also known as the *oxygen coefficient ratio* or *oxygen utilization ratio,* is the amount of oxygen consumed by the tissue cells divided by the total amount of oxygen delivered. The O_2ER is calculated by dividing the $C(a\text{-}\bar{v})_{O_2}$ by the Ca_{O_2}. Therefore if a patient has a Ca_{O_2} of 15 vol% and a $C\bar{v}_{O_2}$ of 10 vol%, the O_2ER would be 33%:

$$\begin{aligned}
O_2ER &= \frac{Ca_{O_2} - C\bar{v}_{O_2}}{Ca_{O_2}} \\[6pt]
&= \frac{15 \text{ vol\%} - 10 \text{ vol\%}}{15 \text{ vol\%}} \\[6pt]
&= \frac{5 \text{ vol\%}}{15 \text{ vol\%}} \\[6pt]
&= 0.33
\end{aligned}$$

Normally, the O_2ER is about 25%. Clinically, the patient's O_2ER increases in response to (1) a decreased cardiac output, (2) periods of increased oxygen consumption (e.g., exercise, seizures, hyperthermia), (3) anemia, and (4) decreased arterial oxygenation. The O_2ER decreases in response to (1) increased cardiac output, (2) skeletal muscle relaxation (e.g., induced by drugs), (3) peripheral shunting (e.g., sepsis), (4) certain poisons (e.g., cyanide), (5) hypothermia, (6) increased hemoglobin, and (7) increased arterial oxygenation.

Mixed Venous Oxygen Saturation

When a patient has a normal arterial oxygen saturation (Sa_{O_2}) and hemoglobin concentration, the mixed venous oxygen saturation ($S\bar{v}_{O_2}$) is often used as an early indicator of changes in the patient's $C(a\text{-}\bar{v})_{O_2}$, $\dot{V}_{O_2}$, and O_2ER. The $S\bar{v}_{O_2}$ can signal changes in the patient's $C(a\text{-}\bar{v})_{O_2}$, $\dot{V}_{O_2}$, and O_2ER earlier than arterial blood gases because the Pa_{O_2} and Sa_{O_2} levels are often normal during early $C(a\text{-}\bar{v})_{O_2}$, $\dot{V}_{O_2}$, and O_2ER changes.

Normally, the $S\bar{v}_{O_2}$ is approximately 75%. Clinically, the $S\bar{v}_{O_2}$ decreases in response to (1) a decreased cardiac output, (2) exercise, (3) seizures, and (4) hyperthermia. The $S\bar{v}_{O_2}$ increases in response to (1) an increased cardiac output, (2) skeletal muscle relaxation (e.g., induced by drugs), (3) peripheral shunting (e.g., sepsis), (4) certain poisons (e.g., cyanide), and (5) hypothermia.

Over the past several years, there has been a move away from the oxygen–tension-based indices to the oxygen–saturation- and content-based indices when monitoring the oxygenation status of the critically ill patient. Table 5-1 summarizes the way various clinical factors alter the patient's Do_2, $\dot{V}_{O_2}$, $C(a\text{-}\bar{v})_{O_2}$, O_2ER, and $S\bar{v}_{O_2}$.

Pulmonary Shunting

Because pulmonary shunting and venous admixture are frequent complications in respiratory disorders, knowledge of the degree of shunting is desirable in developing patient care plans. The amount of intrapulmonary shunting can be calculated by using the classic shunt equation:

$$\frac{\dot{Q}_S}{\dot{Q}_T} = \frac{Cc_{O_2} - Ca_{O_2}}{Cc_{O_2} - C\bar{v}_{O_2}}$$

where $\dot{Q}_S$ is the cardiac output that is shunted, $\dot{Q}_T$ is the total cardiac output, Cc_{O_2} is the oxygen content of pulmonary capillary blood, Ca_{O_2} is the oxygen content of arterial blood, and $C\bar{v}_{O_2}$ is the oxygen content of venous blood.

To obtain the data necessary to calculate the patient's intrapulmonary shunt, the following information must be gathered:

- BP (barometric pressure)
- Pa_{O_2}
- Pa_{CO_2}

TABLE 5–1 **Clinical Factors Affecting Various Oxygen Transport Study Values**

	Oxygenation Indices and Normal Values				
Clinical Factors	$\dot{D}o_2$ (1000 ml O_2/min)	$\dot{V}o_2$ (250 ml O_2/min)	$C(a\text{-}\bar{v})o_2$ (5 vol%)	O_2ER (25%)	$S\bar{v}o_2$ (75%)
↑ O_2 consumption	~*	↑	↑	↑	↓
↓ O_2 consumption	~	↓	↓	↓	↑
↓ Cardiac output	↓	~	↑	↑	↓
↑ Cardiac output	↑	~	↓	↓	↑
↓ Pao_2	↓	~	~	↑	↓
↑ Pao_2	↑	~	~	↓	↑
↓ Hb	↓	~	~	↑	↓
↑ Hb	↑	~	~	↓	↑
Peripheral shunting	~	↓	↓	↓	↑

*~, Unchanged.

- $P\bar{v}o_2$
- Hb concentration
- PAo_2 (partial pressure of alveolar oxygen)*
- Fio_2 (fractional concentration of inspired oxygen)

A clinical example of the shunt calculation follows:

Shunt Study Calculation in an Automobile Accident Victim

A 22-year-old man is on a volume-cycled mechanical ventilator on a day when the barometric pressure is 755 mm Hg. The patient is receiving an Fio_2 of 0.60. The following clinical data are obtained:

- Hb: 15 g/dl
- Pao_2: 65 mm Hg (Sao_2 = 90%)
- $Paco_2$: 56 mm Hg
- $P\bar{v}o_2$: 35 mm Hg ($S\bar{v}o_2$ = 65%)

With this information the patient's PAo_2, Cco_2, Cao_2, and $C\bar{v}o_2$ can now be calculated. (The clinician should remember that P_{H_2O} represents alveolar water vapor pressure and is always 47 mm Hg.)

1. PAo_2
   $= (PB - P_{H_2O})\, Fio_2 - Paco_2\,(1.25)$
   $= (755 - 47)\, 0.60 - 56\,(1.25)$
   $= (708)\, 0.60 - 70$
   $= 424.8 - 70$
   $= 354.8$

2. Cco_2
   $= (Hb \times 1.34) + (PAo_2 \times 0.003)$
   $= (15 \times 1.34) + (354.8 \times 0.003)$
   $= 20.1 + 1.064$
   $= 21.164$ (vol% O_2)

3. Cao_2
   $= (Hb \times 1.34 \times Sao_2) + (Pao_2 \times 0.003)$
   $= (15 \times 1.34 \times 0.90) + (65 \times 0.003)$
   $= 18.09 + 0.195$
   $= 18.285$ (vol% O_2)

*See Ideal Alveolar Gas Equation, Appendix III.

4. $C\bar{v}o_2$
   $= (Hb \times 1.34 \times S\bar{v}o_2) + (P\bar{v}o_2 \times 0.003)$
   $= (15 \times 1.34 \times 0.65) + (35 \times 0.003)$
   $= 13.065 + 0.105$
   $= 13.17$ (vol% O_2)

With this information the patient's intrapulmonary shunting can now be calculated:

$$\frac{\dot{Q}s}{\dot{Q}\tau} = \frac{Cco_2 - Cao_2}{Cco_2 - C\bar{v}o_2}$$

$$= \frac{21.164 - 18.285}{21.164 - 13.17}$$

$$= \frac{2.879}{7.994}$$

$$= 0.36$$

Therefore 36% of the patient's pulmonary blood flow is perfusing lung tissue that is not being ventilated.

With the proliferation of inexpensive personal computers, much of the shunt equation is now being written in simple programs. What was once a rather esoteric, error-prone procedure is now readily and accurately available to respiratory therapy practitioners.

Table 5-2 shows the clinical significance of pulmonary shunting. Table 5-3 summarizes the way specific respiratory diseases alter various oxygen– saturation- and content-based indices.

Hypoxia

Hypoxia is defined as inadequate oxygenation at the tissue level. It is characterized by tachycardia, increased respiratory rate, hypertension, peripheral

TABLE 5–2 Clinical Significance of Pulmonary Shunting

Degree of Pulmonary Shunting (%)	Clinical Significance
Below 10%	Normal lung status
10% to 20%	Indicates a pulmonary abnormality but is not significant in terms of cardiopulmonary support
20% to 30%	May be life-threatening, possibly requiring cardiopulmonary support
Greater than 30%	Serious life-threatening condition, almost always requiring cardiopulmonary support

TABLE 5–3 Oxygenation Index Changes Commonly Seen in Respiratory Diseases

Pulmonary Disorder	Oxygenation Indices					
	$\dot{Q}s/\dot{Q}T$	Do_2*	Vo_2	$C(a\text{-}\bar{v})o_2$	O_2ER	$S\bar{v}o_2$
Obstructive airway diseases	↑	↓	~†	~	↑	↓
Chronic bronchitis						
Emphysema						
Bronchiectasis						
Asthma						
Cystic fibrosis						
Croup syndrome						
Infectious pulmonary diseases	↑	↓	~	~	↑	↓
Pneumonia						
Lung abscess						
Fungal disorders						
Tuberculosis			~			
Pulmonary edema	↑	↓	~	↑‡	↑	↓
Pulmonary embolism	↑	↓	~	↑‡	↑	↓
Lung collapse	↑	↓		↑‡	↑	↓
Flail chest						
Pneumothorax						
Pleural disease (e.g., hemothorax)						
Kyphoscoliosis	↑	↓	~	~	↑	↓
Pneumoconiosis	↑	↓	~	~	↑	↓
Cancer of the lung	↑	↓	~	~	↑	↓
Adult respiratory distress syndrome	↑	↓	~	~	↑	↓
Idiopathic (infant) respiratory distress syndrome	↑	↓	~	~	↑	↓
Chronic interstitial lung disease	↑	↓	~	~	↑	↓
Sleep apnea	↑	↓	~	~↑‡	↑	↓
Smoke inhalation						
Without surface burns	↑	↓	~	~	↑	↓
With surface burns	↑	↓	↑	↑	↑	↓
Near drowning (wet)	↑	↓	↑	↑	↑	↓

*The Do_2 may be normal in patients with an increased cardiac output, an increased hemoglobin level (polycythemia), or a combination of both. For example, a normal Do_2 is often seen in patients with chronic obstructive pulmonary disease and polycythemia. When the Do_2 is normal, the patient's O_2ER is usually normal.

†~, Unchanged.

‡The increased $C(a\text{-}\bar{v})o_2$ is associated with a decreased cardiac output.

vasoconstriction, dizziness, and mental confusion. Hypoxia can take four forms:

1. Hypoxic hypoxia
2. Anemic hypoxia
3. Circulatory hypoxia
4. Histotoxic hypoxia

When hypoxia is present, alternate anaerobic pathways are activated that result in production of lactic acid. This condition in turn causes the pH to drop and metabolic acidosis to occur.

HYPOXIC HYPOXIA

Hypoxic hypoxia (also known as *hypoxemic hypoxia*) is a condition in which both the Ca_{O_2} and Pa_{O_2} are below normal. Clinically, this type of hypoxia is better known as *hypoxemia* (low oxygen concentration in the blood). Hypoxic hypoxia can develop in any one of the ways discussed in the following paragraphs.

Pulmonary Shunting

Low Alveolar PO_2

When the PA_{O_2} is low, the Pa_{O_2} also will be low. A low PA_{O_2} can develop from (1) alveolar hypoventilation from any cause (e.g., chronic obstructive pulmonary disease, drug overdose, neuromuscular diseases that affect the diaphragm), (2) ascent to high altitudes, and (3) the breathing of gas mixtures that contain less than 21% oxygen (i.e., suffocation).

Diffusion Impairment

When the thickness of the alveolar-capillary membrane is increased, the time necessary for oxygen to move from the alveoli into the blood before it moves into the pulmonary venous circulation may not be adequate. Respiratory disorders associated with diffusion impairment include interstitial fibrosis, alveolar consolidation, atelectasis, and interstitial and alveolar edema.

Ventilation/Perfusion (V̇/Q̇) Ratio Mismatch

When the pulmonary capillary blood flow is greater than alveolar ventilation, a decreased V̇/Q̇ ratio exists. This condition causes a shuntlike effect, which in turn leads to venous admixture and a decreased Pa_{O_2} and Ca_{O_2}.

ANEMIC HYPOXIA

Anemic hypoxia is present when the Pa_{O_2} is normal but the oxygen-carrying ability of the blood is inadequate. Anemic hypoxia is most commonly caused by (1) a low concentration of Hb in the blood or (2) a deficiency in the ability of the Hb to carry oxygen (e.g., carbon monoxide poisoning, methemoglobinemia).

CIRCULATORY HYPOXIA

In circulatory hypoxia, the Pa_{O_2} and Ca_{O_2} may be normal, but the amount of arterial blood flow is not adequate to meet tissue demands. Circulatory hypoxia is most commonly caused by either stagnant hypoxia or arterial-venous shunting. Stagnant hypoxia occurs when peripheral blood flow is decreased or stagnant (pooling). This condition commonly develops in response to a decreased cardiac output, vascular insufficiency, or neurochemical abnormalities. Arterial-venous shunts exist when arterial blood completely bypasses the tissue cells and empties directly into the venous system.

HISTOTOXIC HYPOXIA

Histotoxic hypoxia exists when the ability of the tissue cells to consume oxygen is impaired. Cyanide poisoning causes this type of hypoxia. The Pa_{O_2} and Ca_{O_2} are still normal, but the tissue cells may be extremely hypoxic. Patients with cyanide poisoning have an elevated $P\bar{v}_{O_2}$, $C\bar{v}_{O_2}$, and $S\bar{v}_{O_2}$ as a result of the oxygen not being consumed at the tissue sites.

CHRONIC HYPOXIA

Cor Pulmonale

Cor pulmonale is the term used to denote pulmonary arterial hypertension, right ventricular hypertrophy, increased right ventricular work, and ultimately right ventricular failure. The three major mechanisms involved in producing cor pulmonale in chronic pulmonary disease are (1) the increased viscosity of the blood associated with polycythemia, (2) the increased pulmonary vascular resistance caused by hypoxic vasoconstriction, and (3) the obliteration of the pulmonary capillary bed, particularly in emphysema. Items 1 and 2 are discussed in greater depth in the following paragraphs.

Polycythemia

When pulmonary disorders produce chronic hypoxia, the hormone erythropoietin responds by stimulating the bone marrow to increase red blood cell (RBC) production. RBC production is known as *erythropoiesis*. An increased level of RBCs is called *polycythemia*. The polycythemia that results from hypoxia is an adaptive mechanism that increases the oxygen-carrying capacity of the blood.

Unfortunately, the advantage of the increased oxygen-carrying capacity in polycythemia is at least partially offset by the increased viscosity of the blood when the hematocrit reaches 50% to 60%. Because of the increased viscosity of the blood, a greater driving pressure is needed to maintain a given flow. The work of the right ventricle must increase to generate the pressure needed to overcome the increased viscosity. This can lead to right ventricular hypertrophy, or cor pulmonale.

Hypoxic Vasoconstriction of the Lungs

Hypoxic vasoconstriction of the pulmonary vascular system commonly develops in response to the decreased PA_{O_2} that occurs in chronic respiratory disorders. The decreased PA_{O_2} causes the smooth muscles of the pulmonary arterioles to constrict. The exact mechanism of this phenomenon is unclear. However, PA_{O_2} and not the Pa_{O_2} chiefly controls this response.

The early effect of hypoxic vasoconstriction is to direct blood away from the hypoxic regions of the lungs and thereby offset the shunt effect. However, when the number of hypoxic regions becomes significant— as during the advanced stages of emphysema or chronic bronchitis—a generalized pulmonary vasoconstriction develops, causing the pulmonary vascular resistance to increase substantially. Increased pulmonary vascular resistance leads to pulmonary hypertension, increased work of the right side of the heart, right ventricular hypertrophy, and cor pulmonale.

The cor pulmonale associated with chronic respiratory disorders may develop from the combined effects of polycythemia and pulmonary arterial vasoconstriction. Both of these conditions occur as a result of chronic hypoxia. Clinically, cor pulmonale leads to the accumulation of venous blood in the large veins. This condition causes (1) the neck veins to become distended (see Figure 2-46), (2) the extremities to show signs of peripheral edema and pitting edema (see Figure 2-45), and (3) the liver to become enlarged and tender. A loud pulmonic valve (P_2) closure is commonly heard during auscultation when pulmonary hypertension and cor pulmonale are present. In addition, an electrocardiogram (ECG) often reveals a right-axis deviation when cor pulmonale is present. In lead I, the right-axis deviation is demonstrated as a negative (downward deflection of the QRS complex).

SELF-ASSESSMENT QUESTIONS

Multiple Choice

1. The Pa_{O_2} may give a "false-positive" oxygenation reading when the patient has which of the following?

    I. Hypothermia
    II. Cyanide poisoning
    III. Decreased cardiac output
    IV. Carbon monoxide poisoning
    V. Peripheral shunting

    a. I and II only
    b. II and IV only
    c. III, IV, and V only
    d. II, III, IV, and V only
    e. I, II, III, IV, and V

2. If a hospitalized patient is receiving an FI_{O_2} of 40% on a day when the barometric pressure is 745 mm Hg, and if the patient's Pa_{CO_2} is 65 mm Hg and the Pa_{O_2} is 45 mm Hg, what is the $P(A-a)_{O_2}$?

    a. 153 mm Hg
    b. 198 mm Hg
    c. 230 mm Hg
    d. 267 mm Hg
    e. 343 mm Hg

3. A 46-year-old female with severe asthma arrives in the emergency room with the following clinical data:

    Hb: 11 g%
    Pa_{O_2}: 46 mm Hg
    Sa_{O_2}: 70%

    Based on these clinical data, what is the patient's Ca_{O_2}?

    a. 6.75 vol% O_2
    b. 10.50 vol% O_2
    c. 12.30 vol% O_2
    d. 15.25 vol% O_2
    e. 18.85 vol% O_2

4. If a patient has a cardiac output of 6 L/min and a Ca_{O_2} of 12 vol%, what is the D_{O_2}?

    a. 210 ml/O_2/min
    b. 345 ml/O_2/min
    c. 540 ml/O_2/min
    d. 720 ml/O_2/min
    e. 930 ml/O_2/min

5. If a patient's Ca_{O_2} is 11 vol% and the $C\bar{v}_{O_2}$ is 7 vol%, what is the $C(a-\bar{v})_{O_2}$?

    a. 4 vol%
    b. 7 vol%
    c. 11 vol%
    d. 15 vol%
    e. 18 vol%

6. Clinically, the patient's $C(a-\bar{v})_{O_2}$ increases in response to which of the following?

    I. Hypothermia
    II. Decreased cardiac output
    III. Seizures
    IV. Cyanide poisoning

    a. II only
    b. IV only
    c. II and III only
    d. I and IV only
    e. II, III, and IV only

7. If a patient has a cardiac output of 6 L/min and a $C(a-\bar{v})_{O_2}$ of 4 vol%, what is the $\dot{V}_{O_2}$?

    a. 120 ml O_2/min
    b. 160 ml O_2/min
    c. 180 ml O_2/min
    d. 200 ml O_2/min
    e. 240 ml O_2/min

8. Clinically, the $\dot{V}_{O_2}$ decreases in response to which of the following?

    I. Exercise
    II. Hyperthermia
    III. Body size
    IV. Peripheral shunting

    a. II only
    b. IV only
    c. I and III only
    d. II, III, and IV only
    e. I, II, III, and IV

9. If a patient's Ca_{O_2} is 12 vol% and the $C\bar{v}_{O_2}$ is 7 vol%, what is the O_2ER?

    a. 0.27
    b. 0.33
    c. 0.42
    d. 0.53
    e. 0.75

10. Clinically, the O_2ER increases in response to which of the following?

    I. Decreased cardiac output
    II. Hyperthermia
    III. Anemia
    IV. Exercise

    a. I only
    b. III only
    c. II and IV only
    d. II, III, and IV only
    e. I, II, III, and IV

11. Clinically, the $S\bar{v}o_2$ decreases in response to which of the following?

    I. Increased cardiac output
    II. Peripheral shunting
    III. Hypothermia
    IV. Seizures

    a. I only
    b. IV only
    c. II and III only
    d. I, II, and III only
    e. I, II, III, and IV

12. In the patient with severe emphysema, which of the following oxygenation indices are commonly seen?

    I. Decreased $S\bar{v}o_2$
    II. Increased Vo_2
    III. Decreased $C(a-\bar{v})o_2$
    IV. Increased O_2ER

    a. I only
    b. III only
    c. I and IV only
    d. II and III only
    e. I, II, and III only

13. In the patient with pulmonary edema, which of the following oxygenation indices are commonly seen?

    I. Increased O_2ER
    II. Decreased $S\bar{v}o_2$
    III. Increased $V.o_2$
    IV. Decreased Vo_2

    a. II only
    b. IV only
    c. I and II only
    d. I, II, and III only
    e. I, II, III, and IV

Case Study: Gunshot Victim

A 37-year-old woman is on a volume-cycled mechanical ventilator on a day when the barometric pressure is 745 mm Hg. The patient is receiving an F_{IO_2} of 0.50. The following clinical data are obtained:

Hb: 11 g%
Pao_2: 60 mm Hg (Sao_2 90%)
$P\bar{v}o_2$: 35 mm Hg ($S\bar{v}o_2$ 65)
$Paco_2$: 38 mm Hg
Cardiac output: 6 L/minute

Based on the information above, approximately what is the patient's:

14. Total oxygen delivery:

    a. 430 ml O_2/min
    b. 510 ml O_2/min
    c. 740 ml O_2/min
    d. 806 ml O_2/min
    e. 930 ml O_2/min

15. Arterial-venous oxygen content difference:

    a. 2.45 vol% O_2
    b. 3.76 vol% O_2
    c. 4.20 vol% O_2
    d. 5.40 vol% O_2
    e. 6.10 vol% O_2

16. Intrapulmonary shunting:

    a. 13%
    b. 22%
    c. 26%
    d. 33 %
    e. 37%

17. Oxygen consumption:

    a. 170 ml O_2/min
    b. 200 ml O_2/min
    c. 230 ml O_2/min
    d. 280 ml O_2/min
    e. 320 ml O_2/min

18. Oxygen extraction ratio:

    a. 9.18%
    b. 6.20%
    c. 24%
    d. 26%
    e. 28%

Case Study: Automobile Accident

A 48-year-old woman is on a volume-cycled mechanical ventilator on a day when the barometric pressure is 740 mm Hg. She is receiving intermittent mandatory ventilation of 12 breaths per minute and an F_{IO_2} of 0.60. The following clinical values are obtained:

> Pa_{CO_2}: 37 mm Hg
> Pa_{O_2}: 31 mm Hg (60% saturated)
> $P\bar{v}_{O_2}$: 21 mm Hg (51% saturated)
> Hb: 8 g /dl

Based on the clinical information provided, how much intrapulmonary shunting does the patient have?

19. PA_{O_2} =

20. Cc_{O_2} =

21. Ca_{O_2} =

22. $C\bar{v}_{O_2}$ =

23. $\dot{Q}s/\dot{Q}T$ =

Answers appear in Appendix XI.

CHAPTER 6

Cardiovascular System Assessments

Because the transport of oxygen to the tissue cells and the delivery of carbon dioxide to the lungs is a function of the cardiovascular system, a basic knowledge and understanding of (1) normal heart sounds, (2) normal electrocardiogram (ECG) patterns, (3) common heart arrhythmias, (4) noninvasive hemodynamic monitoring assessments, (5) invasive hemodynamic monitoring assessments, and (6) determinants of cardiac output are essential components of patient assessment.*

◈ Normal Heart Sounds

Although disagreement persists as to their exact origin, it is generally accepted that heart sounds develop in response to sudden changes in blood flow inside the heart that cause the walls of the heart chamber, the valves, and the great vessels to vibrate. The vibration of these structures produces the heart sounds.

When the valves of the heart close, a "lubb-dub" sound is produced. The "lubb" sound is the first heart sound, or S_1. The "dub" sound is the second heart sound, or S_2.

S_1 is associated with the closure of the atrioventricular (AV) valves (i.e., the mitral and tricuspid valves; Figure 6-1). The mitral and tricuspid valves produce separate sounds within S_1; these are referred to as M_1 and T_1. S_1 corresponds to the onset of systole and is louder, longer, and lower pitched than S_2 at the apex. Normally, closure of the mitral valve precedes closure of the tricuspid valve by about 0.02 seconds as the ventricles begin to contract, because the left ventricle is larger and more powerful than the right. However, the mitral valve closes with greater force than the tricuspid valve and therefore is the major source of the S_1 under normal circumstances.

*See Appendix X for an example of a cardiopulmonary profile sheet used to monitor the hemodynamic status of the critically ill patient.

S_2 results from closure of the semilunar valves (i.e., the aortic and pulmonic valves). These valves each generate a separate sound within S_2; they are referred to as A_2 and P_2 (see Figure 6-1). Normally, the A_2 and P_2 sounds are approximately 0.03 seconds apart, with aortic valve closure preceding pulmonary valve closure. A more distinct (wider) split is heard during inspiration as the intrathoracic pressure drops, which allows more blood to return to the right side of the heart. The increased blood volume in the right ventricle causes a delayed pulmonic valve closure. At the same time, the increase in negative intrapleural pressure causes blood vessels in the lungs to dilate and retain blood. This action reduces left ventricular stroke volume and left ventricular systole. As a result, the aortic valve closes earlier. Finally, even though the closure of the aortic valve precedes closure of the pulmonic valve during expiration, the closure sequence is so rapid that A_2 and P_2 are generally heard as a single sound.

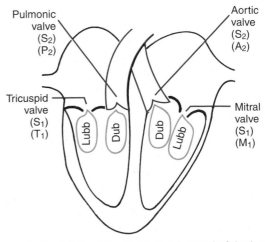

Figure 6-1   Origin of the "lubb-dub" sound of the heart.

◆ Abnormal Heart Sounds

WIDELY SPLIT S₁

Under certain conditions an abnormally wide or split S_1 can be auscultated over the fourth intercostal space to the left of the sternum (patient's left). A widely split S_1 can be produced by electrical or mechanical causes that cause asynchrony of the two ventricles. Some of the electrical causes include right bundle branch block, premature ventricular beats, and ventricular tachycardia.

WIDELY SPLIT S₂

The normal split S_2 (A_2 and P_2) can be accentuated by conditions that cause an abnormal delay in pulmonic valve closure. Such delay may be caused by (1) an increased volume in the right ventricle compared with the left ventricle (e.g., atrial septal defect, ventricle septal defect), (2) chronic right ventricular outflow obstruction (e.g., pulmonic stenosis), (3) acute or chronic dilation of the right ventricle caused by a sudden rise in pulmonary artery pressure (e.g., pulmonary embolism), or (4) electrical delay in activation of the right ventricle (right bundle branch block). The wide split has a duration of 0.04 to 0.05 seconds compared with the normal physiologic split of 0.03 seconds. It can be heard during inspiration and expiration and is best auscultated over the left base of the heart (second intercostal space to the left of the sternum [patient's left]).

PARADOXICALLY SPLIT S₂

A paradoxical split of the S_2 occurs when a reversal of the normal closure sequence occurs with P_2 closure occurring before A_2 closure. The paradoxical split S_2 may be heard when aortic closure is delayed, as in marked volume or pressure loads on the left ventricle (e.g., aortic stenosis) or with conduction defects that delay left ventricular depolarization (e.g., left bundle branch block). The paradoxically split S_2 is best heard during expiration over the left base of the heart (the second intercostal space to the left of the sternum [patient's left]).

FIXED SPLITTING OF THE S₂

Fixed splitting of the S_2 is a split that displays little or no respiratory variation. The fixed splitting of the S_2 occurs when the ventricles are unable to change their volumes with respirations. Such conditions include congestive heart failure, cardiomyopathy, atrial septal defect, or ventricular septal defect (VSD). The fixed split is best heard over the second intercostal space to the left of the sternum (patient's left).

THIRD HEART SOUND (S₃)

The third heart sound, S_3, is a low-frequency sound heard just after S_2. It is also known as an (S_3) gallop or *ventricular gallop*. The S_3 occurs in early diastole during rapid ventricular filling, approximately 0.14 to 0.16 seconds after S_2; it reflects decreased ventricular compliance or an increased ventricular diastolic volume.

The S_3 is normal in children and young adults who have increased diastolic volumes. When normal, it is called a *physiologic third heart sound*. The abnormal S_3 is often heard in patients with coronary artery disease, cardiomyopathies, incompetent valves, left to right shunts, or patent ductus arteriosus. The S_3 may have its origin in either the left or right side of the heart. The S_3 of left ventricular origin is best heard during expiration over the apex (the fifth intercostal space to the left of the sternum at the midclavicular line). The S_3 of right ventricular origin is best heard during inspiration over the left lateral sternal border (the fourth intercostal space to the left of the sternum [patient's left]). Third heart sounds are often associated with sharp outward precordial movements that frequently can be seen or felt.

FOURTH HEART SOUND (S₄)

The fourth heart sound, S_4, is a low-frequency sound heard just before S_1. It is also known as an *atrial gallop*, a *presystolic gallop*, or an S_4 gallop. The S_4 is a diastolic sound that occurs during the late diastolic filling phase at the time when the atria contract. When the ventricles have a decreased compliance or are receiving an increased diastolic volume, they generate a low-frequency vibration—the S_4. The S_4 may be normal in the young but is seldom considered normal in persons older than 20 years. The S_4 may have its origin in either the left or right side of the heart.

The S_4 of left ventricular origin may be auscultated during inspiration or expiration and is best heard at the apex of the heart (the fifth intercostal space in the midclavicular line). Common causes include severe hypertension, aortic stenosis, cardiomyopathies, and left ventricular myocardial infarction.

The S_4 of right ventricular origin is best heard during inspiration over the left lateral sternal border (the fourth intercostal space to the left of the sternum [patient's left]). Common causes include pulmonary valve obstruction, pulmonary stenosis, pulmonary hypertension, and right ventricular myocardial infarction.

EJECTION SOUNDS

Ejection sounds are high-frequency, "clicky" heart sounds that occur just after S_1 with the onset of ventricular ejection. They are caused by the opening of the semilunar valves (aortic or pulmonic) of the heart when one of the valves is diseased or when blood ejection is rapid through a normal heart valve.

Ejection sounds of aortic origin are best heard over the right base of the heart (second intercostal space to the right of the sternum [patient's right]). Aortic ejection sounds are heard in patients with valvular aortic stenosis, aortic insufficiency, coarctation of the aorta, or aneurysm of the ascending aorta. Ejection sounds of pulmonic origin are best heard over the left base of the heart (second intercostal space to the left of the sternum [patient's left]). Pulmonic ejection sounds are heard in pulmonic stenosis, pulmonary hypertension, atrial septal defects, pulmonary embolism, hyperthyroidism, or in conditions that cause enlargement of the pulmonary artery.

MIDSYSTOLIC CLICKS

Midsystolic clicks are high-frequency sounds that occur in early, middle, or late systole. The click occurs at least 0.14 seconds after S_1. The most common cause of a midsystolic click is mitral valve prolapse. Clicks of mitral origin are best heard by stethoscope at the apex or toward the left lateral sternal border.

OPENING SNAP

The opening snap is a short, high-frequency sound that occurs approximately 0.06 to 0.10 seconds after the second heart sound in early diastole. It is best heard between the apex and the left lateral sternal border. The opening snap is commonly caused by audible opening of the mitral valve caused by stiffening (e.g., mitral stenosis) or increased blood flow (e.g., ventricular septal defect or patent ductus arteriosus).

◆ Murmurs

Murmurs are defined as sustained noises (e.g., blowing, harsh, rough, or rumbling sounds) that can be heard during systole, diastole, or both. Murmurs are caused by five major factors: (1) backward regurgitation through a leaking valve, septal defect, or arteriovenous connection; (2) forward blood flow through a narrowed or deformed valve; (3) high rate of blood flow through a normal or abnormal valve; (4) vibration of the loose structures within the heart (e.g., chordae tendineae); or (5) continuous flow through an arteriovenous shunt. Murmurs that occur when the ventricles are contracting are referred to as *systolic murmurs.* Murmurs that occur when the ventricles are relaxing are referred to as *diastolic murmurs.*

SYSTOLIC MURMURS

Systolic murmurs are defined as sustained noises that are audible during systole, or the period between S_1 and S_2. Forward flow across the aortic or pulmonic valves or regurgitant flow from the mitral or tricuspid valve may produce a systolic murmur. Systolic murmurs may be normal and can represent normal blood flow (e.g., thin chest in infants and children or increased blood flow in pregnant women). Systolic murmurs are further classified as *early systolic murmurs, midsystolic murmurs,* and *late systolic murmurs.*

EARLY SYSTOLIC MURMURS

Early systolic murmurs begin with S_1 and peak in the first third of systole. Early murmurs have the greatest intensity in the early part of ventricular contraction. They are commonly caused by a small ventricular septal defect (VSD). The early systolic murmur of a small VSD stops before midsystole because as ejection continues and the ventricular size decreases, the small defect is sealed shut, causing the murmur to soften or cease.

MIDSYSTOLIC MURMURS

A midsystolic murmur begins just after S_1, peaks in the middle of systole, and does not quite extend to S_2. It is a crescendo-decrescendo murmur that builds up and decreases symmetrically. It also is called an *ejection murmur.* This type of murmur is often heard in normal individuals, especially in the young, who usually have increased blood volumes flowing over normal valves. In this setting, it is designated as an *innocent murmur.* A midsystolic murmur may be caused by forward blood flow through a normal, narrow, or irregular valve (i.e., aortic or pulmonic stenosis).

LATE SYSTOLIC MURMUR

A late systolic murmur is heard during the latter half of systole, peaks in the latter third of systole, and extends to S_2. It is a modified regurgitant murmur from backward blood flow through an incompetent valve. It is commonly heard in patients with mitral valve prolapse or tricuspid valve defect.

DIASTOLIC MURMUR

Diastolic murmurs are defined as sustained noises that are audible between S_2 and the next S_1. Unlike systolic murmurs, diastolic murmurs are always considered pathologic. Common causes of diastolic murmurs include aortic regurgitation, pulmonic regurgitation, mitral stenosis, and tricuspid stenosis. Diastolic murmurs are further classified as early diastolic, mid-diastolic, late diastolic, or pandiastolic.

Early Diastolic Murmur

An early diastolic murmur begins with S_2 and peaks in the first third of diastole. An early diastolic murmur is commonly caused by aortic regurgitation, pulmonic regurgitation, or both. The early diastolic murmur of aortic regurgitation has a high-frequency blowing quality and is best heard over the apex of the heart along the left sternal border. The murmur of pulmonic regurgitation occurs after a slight delay after S_2. It has a rough sound and is best heard over the left base of the heart.

Mid-Diastolic Murmur

A mid-diastolic murmur begins after S_2 and peaks in mid-diastole. It is commonly caused by mitral stenosis, tricuspid stenosis, or both. The murmur of mitral stenosis is a low-frequency, crescendo-decrescendo rumble heard at the apex. Mitral stenosis normally causes three distinct abnormal heart sounds: a loud S_1, an opening snap, and a mid-diastolic rumble with a late diastolic accentuation. The diastolic murmur of tricuspid stenosis is similar to that of mitral stenosis, except that it is best heard over the left lateral sternal border.

Late Diastolic Murmur

A late diastolic murmur begins in the latter half of diastole, peaks in the latter third of diastole, and extends to S_1. It is often a component of the murmur of mitral stenosis or tricuspid stenosis. A late diastolic murmur is low in frequency and rumbling in quality.

Pandiastolic Murmur

A pandiastolic murmur begins with S_2 and extends throughout the diastolic period. A pandiastolic murmur can have four major causes: (1) abnormal communication between an artery and vein, (2) abnormal communication between the aorta and the right side of the heart or the left atrium, (3) an abnormal increase in flow or constriction in an artery, and (4) increased or turbulent blood flow through veins. A pandiastolic murmur is commonly heard in infants with patent ductus arteriosus. It is best heard over the left base of the heart (second intercostal space to the left of the sternum [patient's left]).

The ECG

Because the respiratory care practitioner frequently works with critically ill patients who are on cardiac monitors, a basic understanding of normal and

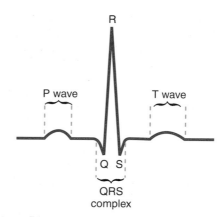

Figure 6–2 ECG pattern of a normal cardiac cycle.

common abnormal ECG patterns is important. An ECG monitors, both visually and on recording paper, the electrical activity of the heart. Figure 6-2 illustrates the ECG pattern of a normal cardiac cycle. The P wave reflects depolarization of the atria. The QRS complex represents the depolarization of the ventricles, and the T wave represents ventricular repolarization.

In normal adults the heart rate is between 60 and 100 beats per minute. In normal infants the heart rate is between 130 and 150 beats per minute. A number of methods can be used to calculate the heart rate. For example, when the rhythm is regular, the heart rate can be determined at a glance by counting the number of large boxes (on the ECG strip) between two QRS complexes and then dividing this number into 300. Therefore if an ECG strip consistently shows four large boxes between each QRS complex, the heart rate is 75 beats per minute ($300 \div 4 = 75$). When the rhythm is irregular, the heart rate can be determined by counting the QRS complexes in a 6-second strip and multiplying by 10. The following heart arrhythmias are commonly seen and should be recognized by the respiratory care practitioner.

Common Heart Arrhythmias

SINUS BRADYCARDIA

In sinus bradycardia the heart rate is less than 60 beats per minute. *Bradycardia* means "slow heart." Sinus bradycardia has a normal P-QRS-T pattern, and the rhythm is regular (Figure 6-3). Athletes often normally demonstrate this finding because of increased cardiac stroke volume and other poorly understood mechanisms. Common pathologic causes of sinus bradycardia include a weakened or damaged sinoatrial (SA) node, severe or chronic hypoxemia, increased intracranial pressure, obstructive sleep

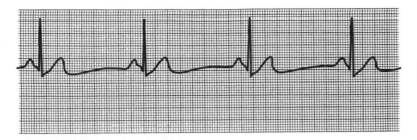

Figure 6–3 Sinus bradycardia. Rate is about 37 beats per minute.

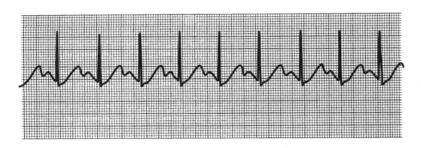

Figure 6–4 Sinus tachycardia. Rate is about 100 beats per minute.

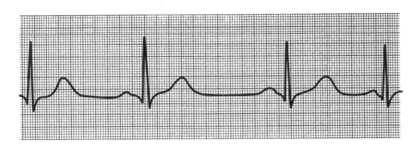

Figure 6–5 Sinus arrhythmia. Note the varying R-R interval.

apnea, and certain drugs (most notably the beta-blockers). Sinus bradycardia may lead to a decreased cardiac output and blood pressure. In severe cases, sinus bradycardia may lead to a decreased vacular perfusion state and tissue hypoxia. The patient may demonstrate a weak or absent pulse, poor capillary refill, cold and clammy skin, and a depressed sensorium.

SINUS TACHYCARDIA

In sinus tachycardia the heart rate is greater than 100 beats per minute. *Tachycardia* means "fast heart." Sinus tachycardia has a normal P-QRS-T pattern, and the rhythm is regular (Figure 6-4). Sinus tachycardia is the normal physiologic response to stress and exercise. Common causes of sinus tachycardia include hypoxemia, severe anemia, hyperthermia, massive hemorrhage, pain, fear, anxiety, hyperthyroidism, and sympathomimetic or parasympatholytic drug administration.

SINUS ARRHYTHMIA

In sinus arrhythmia the heart rate varies by more than 10% from beat to beat. The P-QRS-T pattern is normal (Figure 6-5), but the interval between groups of complexes (i.e., the R-R interval) will vary. A sinus arrhythmia is a normal rhythm in children and young adults. The patient's pulse will often increase during inspiration and decrease during expiration. No treatment is required unless significant alteration occurs in the patient's arterial blood pressure.

ATRIAL FLUTTER

In atrial flutter the normal P wave is absent and replaced by two or more regular sawtooth waves. The QRS complex is normal and the ventricular rate may be regular or irregular, depending on the relationship of the atrial to ventricular beats. Figure 6-6 shows an atrial flutter with a regular rhythm with a 4:1 conduction ratio (i.e., four atrial beats for every ventricular beat). The atrial rate is usually constant,

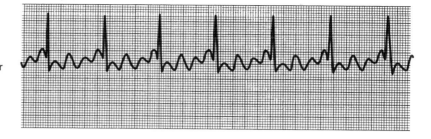

Figure 6–6 Atrial flutter. Atrial rate is greater than 300 beats per minute; ventricular rate is about 60 beats per minute.

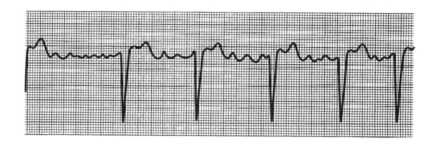

Figure 6–7 Atrial fibrillation.

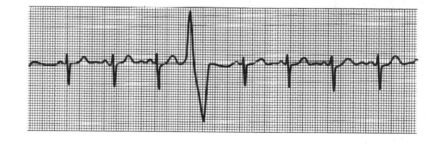

Figure 6–8 Premature ventricular contraction.

between 250 and 350 beats per minute, whereas the ventricular rate is in the normal range. Causes of atrial flutter include hypoxemia, a damaged SA node, and congestive heart failure.

ATRIAL FIBRILLATION

In atrial fibrillation the atrial contractions are disorganized and ineffective, and the normal P wave is absent (Figure 6-7). The atrial rate ranges between 350 and 700 beats per minute. The QRS complex is normal, and the ventricular rate ranges between 100 and 200 beats per minute. Causes of atrial fibrillation include hypoxemia and a damaged SA node. Atrial fibrillation may reduce the cardiac output by 20% because of a loss of atrial filling (the so-called atrial kick).

PREMATURE VENTRICULAR CONTRACTIONS

The premature ventricular contraction (PVC) is not preceded by a P wave. The QRS complex is wide, bizarre, and unlike the normal QRS complex (Figure 6-8). The regular heart rate is altered by the PVC. The heart rhythm may be quite irregular when there are many PVCs. PVCs can occur at any rate. They often occur in pairs, after every normal heartbeat (bigeminal PVCs), and after every two normal heartbeats (trigeminal PVCs). Common causes of PVCs include intrinsic myocardial disease, hypoxemia, acidemia, hypokalemia, and congestive heart failure. PVCs also may be a sign of theophylline or alpha- or beta-agonist toxicity.

VENTRICULAR TACHYCARDIA

In ventricular tachycardia the P wave is generally indiscernible, and the QRS complex is wide and bizarre in appearance (Figure 6-9). The T wave may not be separated from the QRS complex. The ventricular rate ranges between 150 and 250 beats per minute, and the rate is regular or slightly irregular. The patient's blood pressure is often decreased during ventricular tachycardia.

VENTRICULAR FLUTTER

In ventricular flutter the QRS complex has the appearance of a wide sine wave (regular, smooth, rounded ventricular wave; Figure 6-10). The rhythm is regular or slightly irregular. The rate is 250 to 350 beats per minute. There is usually no discernible peripheral pulse associated with ventricular flutter.

VENTRICULAR FIBRILLATION

Ventricular fibrillation is characterized by chaotic electrical activity and cardiac activity. The ventricles literally quiver out of control with no perfusion beat-producing rhythm (Figure 6-11). During ventricular fibrillation, there is no cardiac output or blood pressure, and the patient will die in minutes without treatment.

ASYSTOLE (CARDIAC STANDSTILL)

Asystole is the complete absence of electrical and mechanical activity. As a result, the cardiac output stops and the blood pressure falls to zero. The ECG tracing appears as a flat line and indicates severe damage to the heart's electrical conduction system (see Figure 6-11). Occasionally, periods of disorganized electrical and mechanical activity may be generated during long periods of asystole; this is referred to as an *agonal rhythm* or a *dying heart*.

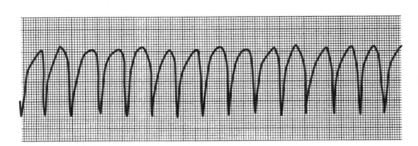

Figure 6–9   Ventricular tachycardia.

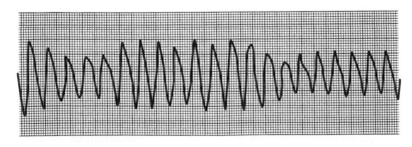

Figure 6–10   Ventricular flutter.

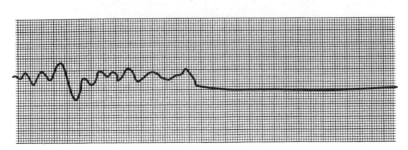

Figure 6–11   Ventricular fibrillation and asystole.

Noninvasive Hemodynamic Monitoring Assessments

Hemodynamics are defined as forces that influence the circulation of blood. The general hemodynamic status of the patient can be monitored noninvasively at the bedside by assessing the heart rate (via an ECG monitor, auscultation, or pulse), blood pressure, and perfusion state. During the acute stages of respiratory disease, the patient frequently demonstrates the hemodynamic changes described in the following paragraphs.

INCREASED HEART RATE (PULSE), CARDIAC OUTPUT, AND BLOOD PRESSURE

Increased heart rate, pulse, and blood pressure develop frequently during the acute stages of pulmonary disease. This can result from the indirect response of the heart to hypoxic stimulation of the peripheral chemoreceptors, primarily the carotid bodies. When the carotid bodies are stimulated, reflex signals are sent to the respiratory muscles, which in turn activate the so-called *pulmonary reflex*, which triggers tachycardia and an increased cardiac output and blood pressure. The increased cardiac output is a compensatory mechanism that at least partially counteracts the hypoxemia produced by the pulmonary shunting in respiratory disorders.

This process is perhaps best understood by assuming that the body's oxygen use remains relatively constant over time. When the cardiac output increases during a period of steady metabolic requirements, oxygen transport increases, and the amount of oxygen extracted from each 100 ml of blood decreases. This results in an increase in the oxygen saturation of the returning venous blood, which in turn reduces the hypoxemia produced by the shunted blood. In other words, venous blood that perfuses underventilated alveoli will have less of a shunt effect if the oxygen content of the systemic venous blood is 13 vol% compared with, say, 10 vol%.

Other causes of increased heart rate, pulse, and blood pressure include severe anemia, high fever, anxiety, massive hemorrhage, certain cardiac arrhythmias, and hyperthyroidism. When the heart rate increases beyond 150 to 175 beats per minute, cardiac output and blood pressure begin to decline (the Starling relationship).

DECREASED PERFUSION STATE

The perfusion state can be evaluated by examining the patient's color, capillary refill, skin, and sensorium. Under normal conditions the patient's nail beds and oral mucosa are pink. If these areas appear cyanotic or mottled, poor perfusion and tissue hypoxia are likely present. When the nail beds are compressed to expel blood, they should normally refill quickly and turn pink when the pressure is released. If the nail beds remain white, perfusion is inadequate. Under normal conditions a patient's skin should be dry and warm. When the skin is diaphoretic (wet), cool, or clammy, local perfusion is inadequate. Finally, when the patient is disoriented as to person, place, and time, a decreased perfusion state and cerebral hypoxia may be present.

Invasive Hemodynamic Monitoring Assessments

Invasive hemodynamic monitoring is used in the assessment and treatment of critically ill patients. Invasive hemodynamic monitors include the measurement of (1) intracardiac pressures and flows via a pulmonary artery catheter, (2) arterial pressure via an arterial catheter, and (3) central venous pressure via a central venous catheter. These monitors provide rapid and precise measurements (assessment data) of the patient's cardiovascular function—which in turn are used to down-regulate or up-regulate the patient's treatment plan in a timely manner.

PULMONARY ARTERY CATHETER

The pulmonary artery catheter (Swan-Ganz) is a balloon-tipped, flow-directed catheter that is inserted at the patient's bedside; the respiratory care professional monitors the pressure waveform as the catheter, with the balloon inflated, is guided by blood flow through the right atrium and right ventricle into the pulmonary artery (Figure 6-12). The pulmonary artery catheter is used directly to measure the right atrial pressure (via the proximal port), pulmonary artery pressure (via the distal port), left atrial pressure (indirectly via the pulmonary capillary wedge pressure), and cardiac output (via the thermodilution technique).

ARTERIAL CATHETER

The arterial catheter (line) is the most commonly used mode of invasive hemodynamic monitoring. It is generally inserted in the radial artery for patient comfort and convenient access reasons. The indwelling arterial catheter allows (1) continuous and precise measurements of systolic, diastolic, and mean blood pressure; (2) accurate information regarding fluctuations in blood pressure; and (3) guidance in the decision to up-regulate or down-regulate therapy for hypotension or hypertension. The arterial catheter also is useful in patients who require frequent or repeated arterial blood gas samples (e.g., the patient

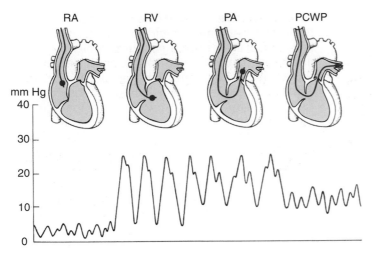

Figure 6-12 Insertion of the pulmonary catheter. The insertion site of the pulmonary catheter may be the basilic, brachial, femoral, subclavian, or internal jugular veins. The latter two are the most common insertion sites. As the catheter advances, pressure readings and waveforms are monitored to determine the catheter's position as it moves through the right atrium *(RA)*, right ventricle *(RV)*, pulmonary artery *(PA)*, and finally into a pulmonary capillary wedge pressure *(PCWP)* position. Immediately after a PCWP reading, the balloon is deflated to allow blood to flow past the tip of the catheter. When the balloon is deflated, the catheter continuously monitors the pulmonary artery pressure. (Redrawn from Des Jardins T: Cardiopulmonary anatomy and physiology: Essentials for respiratory care, ed 4, Albany, NY, 2002, Delmar.)

being mechanically ventilated). The blood samples are readily available, and the patient is not subjected to the pain of repeated arterial punctures.

CENTRAL VENOUS PRESSURE CATHETER

The central venous pressure catheter readily measures the central venous pressure (CVP) and right ventricular filling pressure. It serves as an excellent monitor of right ventricular function. An increased CVP reading is commonly seen in patients who (1) have left ventricular heart failure (e.g., pulmonary edema), (2) are receiving excessively high positive pressure mechanical breaths, (3) have cor pulmonale, or (4) have a severe flail chest, pneumothorax, or pleural effusion.

Table 6-1 summarizes the hemodynamic parameters that can be measured directly. Table 6-2 lists the hemodynamic parameters that can be calculated from results obtained from the direct measurements.*

TABLE 6–1 Hemodynamic Values Measured Directly

Hemodynamic Value	Abbreviation	Normal Range
Central venous pressure	CVP	0-8 mm Hg
Right atrial pressure	RAP	0-8 mm Hg
Mean pulmonary artery pressure	$\overline{PA}$	10-20 mm Hg
Pulmonary capillary wedge pressure (also called *pulmonary artery wedge; pulmonary artery occlusion*)	PCWP PAW PAO	4-12 mm Hg
Cardiac output	CO	4-6 L/min

TABLE 6–2 Hemodynamic Values Calculated from Direct Hemodynamic Measurements

Hemodynamic Value	Abbreviation	Normal Range
Stroke volume	SV	40-80 ml
Stroke volume index	SVI	$40 \pm$ ml/beat/m^2
Cardiac index	CI	3.0 ± 0.5 L/min/m^2
Right ventricular stroke work index	RVSWI	7-12 g/m^2
Left ventricular stroke work index	LVSWI	40-60 g/m^2
Pulmonary vascular resistance	PVR	50-150 dynes $\times$ sec $\times$ cm^{-5}
Systemic vascular resistance	SVR	800-1500 dynes $\times$ sec $\times$ cm^{-5}

*See Appendix VIII for discussion of hemodynamic calculations.

HEMODYNAMIC MONITORING IN RESPIRATORY DISEASES

Because respiratory disorders can have a profound effect on the structure and function of the pulmonary vascular bed, right side of the heart, left side of the heart, or a combination of all three, the results generated by the previously described invasive hemodynamic monitors are commonly used in the assessment and treatment of these patients. For example, respiratory diseases associated with severe or chronic hypoxemia, acidemia, or pulmonary vascular obstruction can increase the pulmonary vascular resistance (PVR) significantly. An increased PVR, in turn, can lead to a variety of secondary hemodynamic changes such as increased CVP, RAP, $\overline{PA}$, RVSWI, and decreased CO, SV, SVI, CI, and LVSWI. Table 6-3 lists common hemodynamic changes seen in pulmonary diseases known to alter the patient's hemodynamic status.

Determinants of Cardiac Output

The cardiac output measured directly by the pulmonary artery catheter is a function of ventricular preload, ventricular afterload, and myocardial contractility.

VENTRICULAR PRELOAD

Ventricular preload refers to the degree the muscle fibers of the ventricle are stretched before contraction (end-diastole). Within normal physiologic limits, the greater the preload, the stronger the ventricular muscle fibers will contract during systole, which in turn leads to a greater force of contraction. This mechanism enables the heart to increase cardiac output in response to an increased venous return.

Because ventricular preload is a function of the pressure generated by the volume of blood returning

TABLE 6–3 Hemodynamic Changes Commonly Seen in Respiratory Diseases

	Hemodynamic Indices											
Disorder	CVP	RAP	$\overline{PA}$	PCWP	CO	SV	SVI	CI	RVSWI	LVSWI	PVR	SVR
COPD Chronic bronchitis Emphysema Cystic fibrosis Bronchiectasis	↑	↑	↑↑	~*	~	~	~	~	↑	~	↑	~
Pulmonary edema (cardiogenic)	~	↑	↑	↑↑	↓	↓	↓	↓	↑	↓	↑	↓
Pulmonary embolism	↑	↑	↑↑	↓	↓	↓	↓	↓	↑	↓	↑	~
Adult respiratory distress syndrome (ARDS)—severe	~↑	~↑	~↑	~	~	~	~	~	~↑	~	~↑	~
Lung collapse Flail chest Pneumothorax Pleural disease (e.g., hemothorax)	↑	↑	↑	↓	↓	↓	↓	↓	↑	↓	↑	↓
Kyphoscoliosis	↑	↑	↑	~	~	~	~	~	↑	~	↑	~
Pneumoconiosis	↑	↑	↑↑	~	~	~	~	~	↑	~	↑	~
Chronic interstitial lung diseases	↑	↑	↑↑	~	~	~	~	~	↑	~	↑	~
Cancer of the lung (tumor mass)	↑	↑	↑	↓	↓	↓	↓	↓	↑	~	↑	~
Hypovolemia	↓↓	↓	↓	↓	↓	↓	↓	↓	↓	↓	~	↑
Hypervolemia (burns)	↑↑	↑	↑	↑	↑	↑	↑	↑	↑	↑	~	~
Right heart failure (cor pulmonale)	↑↑	↑↑	↓	↓	~	~	~	~	~	~	~	~

*~, Unchanged.

to the heart, the ventricular end-diastolic pressure (VEDP), in essence, reflects the ventricular end-diastolic volume (VEDV). Therefore as the VEDP increases or decreases, the VEDV increases or decreases, respectively. The relationship between the VEDP (force) and VEDV (stroke volume) is known as the *Frank-Starling relationship*. Clinically, the patient's ventricular preload is reflected in (1) the degree of neck vein distention, (2) CVP measurements, and (3) pulmonary capillary wedge pressure (PCWP) measurements.

VENTRICULAR AFTERLOAD

Ventricular afterload is defined as the resistance (opposing forces) against which the ventricles must work to eject blood.

The right ventricular afterload is reflected in the PVR. Therefore as the PVR increases or decreases, the right ventricular afterload increases or decreases, respectively. Clinically, conditions that increase PVR include (1) pulmonary vasoconstriction (e.g., alveolar hypoxia), (2) destruction of the pulmonary capillaries (e.g., emphysema), (3) blockage of major pulmonary arteries (e.g., pulmonary emboli), and (4) excessive positive pressure mechanical ventilation.

The left ventricular afterload is reflected in the SVR. Therefore as the SVR increases or decreases, the left ventricular afterload increases or decreases, respectively. The arterial diastolic blood pressure best reflects the left ventricular afterload. For example, as the arterial diastolic pressure increases, the resistance (against which the left side of the heart must work to eject blood) also increases. Clinically, conditions that increase SVR include peripheral vasoconstriction, excessive blood volume, and increased blood viscosity.

MYOCARDIAL CONTRACTILITY

Myocardial contractility refers to the forcefulness of myocardial contraction—independent of preload and afterload. An adequate myocardial contraction is absolutely essential for an adequate cardiac output. For example, when the myocardial contractility is weak or inadequate, the cardiac output is poor, even when the ventricles fill appropriately with blood (preload) and the resistance to outflow is optimal (afterload). An increase in myocardial contractility is called *positive inotropism*. Common positive inotropic drugs include isoproterenol, dopamine, dobutamine, and amrinone. A decrease in myocardial contractility is called *negative inotropism*.

Clinically, no single invasive measurement reflects myocardial contractility. However, the general status of a patient's myocardial contractility can be inferred through various clinical assessments such as pulse, blood pressure, skin temperature, and serial hemodynamic measurements. Myocardial contractility (specifically cardiac ejection fraction) can be measured using a multi-gated acquisition (MUGA) scan, and cardiac wall motion can be assessed with two-dimensional echocardiography. Decreased cardiac contractility is commonly accompanied by increased SVR, ventricular preload, PCWP, and CVP.

SELF-ASSESSMENT QUESTIONS

Multiple Choice

1. In which of the following arrhythmias is there no cardiac output or blood pressure?

a. Ventricular flutter
b. Arial fibrillation
c. Ventricular tachycardia
d. Premature ventricular contractions
e. Ventricular fibrillation

2. The general hemodynamic status of the patient can be monitored noninvasively at the patient's bedside by assessing which of the following?

I. Perfusion state
II. Heart rate
III. Pulse
IV. Blood pressure

a. I only
b. IV only
c. II and III only
d. II, III, and IV only
e. I, II, III, and IV

3. Cardiac output and blood pressure begin to decline when the heart rate increases beyond which of the following?

a. 100 to 125 beats per minute
b. 125 to 150 beats per minute
c. 150 to 175 beats per minute
d. 175 to 200 beats per minute
e. 200 to 250 beats per minute

4. An increased CVP reading is commonly seen in the patient who:

I. Has a severe pneumothorax
II. Is receiving high positive pressure breaths
III. Has cor pulmonale
IV. Is in left heart failure

a. I only
b. III only
c. IV only
d. II, III, and IV only
e. I, II, III, and IV

5. What is the normal range of the mean pulmonary artery pressure?

a. 0 to 5 mm Hg
b. 5 to 10 mm Hg
c. 10 to 20 mm Hg
d. 20 to 30 mm Hg
e. 30 to 40 mm Hg

6. Clinically, a patient's left ventricular afterload increases in response to which of the following?

I. Excessive blood volume
II. Decreased blood viscosity
III. Pulmonary emboli
IV. Pulmonary capillary destruction

a. I only
b. III only
c. II and IV only
d. III and IV only
e. I and II only

7. S_1 is associated with which of the following?

I. "Lubb" sound
II. Closure of atrioventricular valves
III. "Dub" sound
IV. Closure of semilunar valves

a. I only
b. III only
c. I and IV only
d. I and II only
e. II and IV only

8. What is the normal range for the PCWP?

a. 0 to 4 mm Hg
b. 4 to 12 mm Hg
c. 12 to 20 mm Hg
d. 20 to 25 mm Hg
e. 25 to 30 mm Hg

9. The hemodynamic indices in patients with COPD commonly show which of the following?

I. Increased CVP
II. Decreased RAP
III. Increased $\overline{PA}$
IV. Decreased PCWP
V. Increased CO

a. I only
b. III only
c. I and III only
d. II and IV only
e. III, IV, and V only

10. The hemodynamic indices in patients with pulmonary edema commonly show which of the following?
    I. Decreased CVP
    II. Increased RAP
    III. Decreased $\overline{PA}$
    IV. Increased PCWP
    V. Decreased CO

a. I only
b. I and III only
c. II, III, and V only
d. II, IV, and V only
e. I, II, IV, and V

Answers appear in Appendix XI.

CHAPTER 7

Other Important Tests and Procedures

Sputum Examination

A sputum sample can be obtained by expectoration, tracheal suction, or bronchoscopy (discussed below). Sputum samples may be examined for cellular debris, microorganisms, blood, and pus. The amount, color, and constituents of the sputum are important in the assessment and diagnosis of many respiratory disorders, including tuberculosis, pneumonia, cancer of the lungs, and pneumoconiosis.

In addition, a microscopic examination of the sputum can identify such characteristics as color, the presence of blood, odor, and general viscosity. For example, yellow sputum indicates an acute infection. Green sputum is associated with old, retained secretions. Green and foul-smelling secretions are frequently found in patients with anaerobic or Pseudomonas infection. Thick, stringy, and white or mucoid sputum suggests bronchial asthma. Brown sputum suggests the presence of old blood. Red sputum indicates fresh blood.

The microscopic examination of a gram-stained smear of a sputum sample is used to identify the Gram stain reaction—positive or negative—and the shape of the organism causing the infection. Such results,

---

BOX 7–1

Common Organisms Associated With Respiratory Disorders

Gram-Negative Organisms
Klebsiella
Pseudomonas aeruginosa
Haemophilus influenzae
Legionella pneumophila

Gram-Positive Organisms
Streptococcus (80% of all bacterial pneumonias)
Staphylococcus

Viral Organisms
Mycoplasma pneumoniae
Respiratory syncytial virus

---

however, are only presumptive. A positive identification of an organism can be made only by isolating the organism from cultures. Box 7-1 presents common organisms associated with respiratory disorders isolated in the laboratory.

Skin Tests

Skin tests are commonly performed to evaluate allergic reactions or exposure to tuberculous bacilli or fungi. Skin tests entail the intradermal injection of an antigen. A *positive* test result indicates that the patient has been exposed to the antigen. However, it does not mean that the disease is actually present. A *negative* test result indicates that the patient has had no exposure to the antigen. A negative test result also may be seen in patients with a depression of cell-mediated immunity, such as that which develops in HIV infections.

Endoscopic Examinations

BRONCHOSCOPY

The *bronchoscope* is a well-established diagnostic and therapeutic tool used by a number of medical specialists, including those in intensive care units, special procedure rooms, and outpatient settings. With minimal risk to the patient—and without interrupting the patient's ventilation—the flexible fiberoptic bronchoscope allows direct visualization of the upper airways (nose, oral cavity, and pharynx), larynx, vocal cords, subglottic area, trachea, bronchi, lobar bronchi, and segmental bronchi down to the third or fourth generation. Under fluoroscopic control, more peripheral areas can be examined or treated (Figure 7-1). A bronchoscopy may be diagnostic or therapeutic.

A *diagnostic bronchoscopy* is usually performed when an infectious disease is suspected and not otherwise diagnosed or to obtain a lung biopsy when the abnormal lung tissue is located on or near the bronchi.

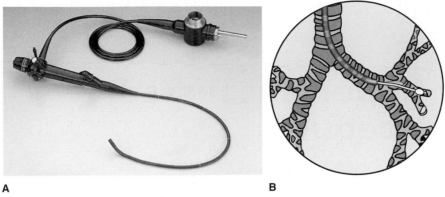

A   **B**

Figure 7–1   Fiberoptic bronchoscope. **A,** The transbronchoscopic balloon-tipped catheter and the flexible fiberoptic bronchoscope. Transbronchoscopic tissue biopsies may be obtained with this device. (From Lewis SM, Heitkemper MM, Dirksen SR: *Medical-surgical nursing: assessment and management of clinical problems,* ed 6, St. Louis, 2004, Mosby.) **B,** The catheter is introduced into a small airway and the balloon inflated with 1.5 to 2 ml air to occlude the airway. Bronchoalveolar lavage is performed by injecting and withdrawing 30-ml aliquots of sterile saline solution, gently aspirating after each instillation. Specimens are sent to the laboratory for analysis. (From Meduri GU et al: Protected bronchoalveolar lavage, *Am Respir Dis* 143:855, 1991.)

A diagnostic bronchoscopy is indicated for a number of clinical conditions, including further inspection and assessment of (1) abnormal radiographic findings (e.g., question of bronchogenic carcinoma or the extent of a bronchial tumor or mass lesion), (2) persistent atelectasis, (3) excessive bronchial secretions, (4) acute smoke inhalation injuries, (5) intubation damage, (6) bronchiectasis, (7) foreign bodies, (8) hemoptysis, (9) lung abscess, (10) major thoracic trauma, (11) stridor or localized wheezing, and (12) unexplained cough. A videotape or colored picture of the procedure may also be obtained to record any abnormalities. When abnormalities are found, additional diagnostic procedures include brushings, biopsies, needle aspirations, and washings. For example, a common diagnostic bronchoscopic technique, termed *bronchoalveolar lavage (BAL),* involves injecting a small amount (30 ml) of sterile saline through the bronchoscope and then withdrawing the fluid for examination of cells. BAL is commonly used to diagnose *Pneumocystis carinii* pneumonia.

Therapeutic bronchoscopy includes (1) suctioning of excessive secretions or mucus plugs—especially when lung atelectasis is forming, (2) the removal of foreign bodies or cancer obstructing the airway, (3) selective lavage (with normal saline or mucolytic agents), and (4) management of life-threatening hemoptysis. Although the virtues of therapeutic bronchoscopy are well established, routine respiratory therapy modalities at the patient's bedside (e.g., chest physical therapy, intermittent percussive ventilation [IPV], postural drainage, deep breathing and coughing techniques, and positive expiratory pressure [PEP] therapy) are considered the first line of defense in the treatment of atelectasis from pooled secretions. Clinically, therapeutic bronchoscopy is commonly used in the management of bronchiectasis, lung abscess,

smoke inhalation and thermal injuries, and lung cancer (see protocol 9-2, page 138).

MEDIASTINOSCOPY

A mediastinoscopy is the insertion of a scope through a small incision in the suprasternal notch; the scope is then advanced into the mediastinum. The test is used to inspect and biopsy lymph nodes in the mediastinal area. This procedure is performed to diagnose carcinoma, granulomatous infections, and sarcoidosis. Mediastinoscopy is done in the operating room while the patient is under general anesthetic.

LUNG BIOPSY

A lung biopsy can be obtained by means of a *transbronchial needle biopsy* or an *open-lung biopsy.* A *transbronchial lung biopsy* entails the passing a forceps or needle through a bronchoscope to obtain a specimen (Figure 7-2). An *open lung biopsy* involves surgery to remove a sample of lung tissue. An incision is made over the area of the lung where the tissue sample is to be collected. In some cases, a large incision may be necessary to reach the suspected problem area. After the procedure a chest tube is inserted for drainage and suction for 7 to 14 days. An open-lung biopsy is usually performed when either a bronchoscopic biopsy or a needle biopsy has been unsuccessful or cannot be performed or when a larger piece of tissue is necessary to establish a diagnosis.

An open biopsy requires a general anesthetic and is more invasive and thus more likely to cause complications. Overall, the risks include pneumothorax, bleeding, bronchospasm, heart arrhythmias, and infection. A needle lung biopsy is contraindicated in patients with lung bullae, cysts, blood coagulation

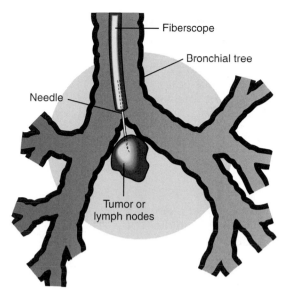

Figure 7-2 Transbronchial needle biopsy. The diagram shows a transbronchial biopsy needle penetrating the bronchial wall and entering a mass of subcarinal lymph nodes or tumor. (Redrawn from DuBois RM, Clarke SW: *Fiberoptic bronchoscopy in diagnosis and management, Orlands, FL*, 1987, Grune and Stratton.

disorders of any type, severe hypoxia, pulmonary hypertension, or cor pulmonale.

A lung biopsy is usually performed to diagnose abnormalities identified on a chest radiograph or computed tomography (CT) scan that are not readily accessible by other diagnostic procedures, such as bronchoscopy. A lung biopsy is especially useful in investigating peripheral lung abnormalities, such as recurrent infiltrates and pleural or subpleural lesions. Additional conditions under which a lung biopsy may be performed include metastatic cancer to the lung and pneumonia with lung abscess.

The tissues from a lung biopsy are sent to a pathology laboratory for examination of malignant cells. Other samples may be sent to a microbiology laboratory to determine the presence of infection. Lung biopsy results are usually available in 2 to 4 days. In some cases, however, it may take several weeks to confirm (by culture) certain infections, such as tuberculosis.

VIDEO-ASSISTED THORACOSCOPY (VATS)

In this newly developed technique, a small incision is made in the chest wall, and a device called a *thoracoscope* is inserted. This device is equipped with a fiberscope that can examine the pleural cavity. The results are displayed on a video monitor (as in bronchoscopy). When pleural lesions are identified, they can be biopsied under video guidance. This procedure is helpful in the diagnosis of tuberculosis, mesothelioma, and metastatic cancer.

Thoracentesis

Thoracentesis (also called *thoracocentesis*) is a procedure in which excess fluid accumulation (pleural effusion) between the chest cavity and lungs (pleural space) is aspirated through a needle inserted through the chest wall (Figure 7-3). A chest radiograph, CT scan, or ultrasound scan may be used to confirm the precise location of the fluid. Once located, a thoracentesis may be performed for *diagnostic* or *therapeutic* purposes.

A *diagnostic thoracentesis* may be performed to identify the etiology of a pleural effusion. The analysis of the pleural fluid may be useful in the diagnosis and staging of a suspected or known malignancy. A pleural biopsy may also be performed during a thoracentesis to collect a tissue sample from the inner lining of the chest wall. A **therapeutic thoracentesis** may be performed to relieve shortness of breath or pain caused by a large pleural effusion, to remove air trapped between the lung and chest wall, or to administer medication directly into the lung cavity to treat the cause of the fluid accumulation or to treat cancer. The fluid in the lung cavity may be classified as either a *transudate* or an *exudate*.

Transudates develop when fluid from the pulmonary capillaries moves into the pleural space. The fluid produced is thin and watery and usually

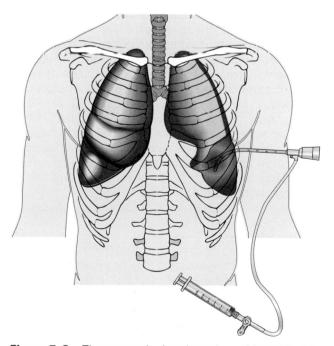

Figure 7-3 Thoracentesis. A catheter is positioned in the pleural space to remove accumulated fluid. Pleural fluid is seen as the dark shadow at the base of the left lung. (From Lewis SM, Heitkemper MM, Dirksen SR: *Medical-surgical nursing: assessment and management of clinical problems*, ed 6, St. Louis, 2004, Mosby.)

has a low white blood count (WBC), a low lactate dehydrogenase (LDH) enzyme level, and a low protein level. The pleural surfaces are not involved in producing the transudate. A transudate may be caused by left ventricular heart failure, cirrhosis, nephritic syndrome, and peritoneal dialysis.

Exudates may be caused by a variety of conditions, including pulmonary infections (e.g., pneumonia, tuberculosis, and fungal diseases), cancer, chest trauma, pancreatitis, autoimmune disease, or a pulmonary embolism. When an infection is present, the fluid usually has a high WBC, a high LDH enzyme level, a high protein level, a large amount of cellular debris, and the presence of bacteria or other infectious organisms. When cancer is present, the fluid usually has a high WBC (often lymphocytes), a high LDH enzyme level, and a high protein level. Abnormal cells also may be found. When a pulmonary embolism is present, a large number of red blood cells are usually present and the WBC and protein levels are both low.

The thoracentesis procedure is generally performed while the patient is in an upright position, leaning forward slightly, typically over a bedside table. Using a local anesthetic, the physician inserts a large-bore thoracentesis needle (16 to 19 gauge), or needle-catheter, between the ribs over the fluid accumulation. The needle or catheter is connected to a small tube with a three-way stopcock, which in turn is attached to either a large syringe or a vacuum and collection bottle. Depending on the purpose of the thoracentesis, up to 1500 ml may be withdrawn. Once the fluid has been collected, the needle or catheter is removed and a bandage is placed over the puncture site. The patient is usually instructed to lie on the puncture site side for about an hour to allow the puncture site to seal.

A thoracentesis is usually a safe procedure. However, a chest radiograph is generally obtained shortly after the procedure to ensure that no complications have developed. Complications may include pneumothorax, pulmonary edema (which sometimes occurs when large amounts of fluid are aspirated), infection, bleeding, and organ damage.

Pleurodesis

On occasion, a thoracentesis may be performed before a procedure called *pleurodesis*. During this procedure a chemical or medication (talc, tetracycline, or bleomycin sulfate) is injected into the chest cavity. The chemical or medication causes an inflammatory reaction over the outer surface of the lung and inside the chest cavity. This procedure is done to cause the surface of the lung to stick to the chest cavity, thus preventing or reducing recurrent fluid accumulation or pneumothorax.

 Hematology, Blood Chemistry, and Electrolyte Findings

Abnormal hematology, blood chemistry, or electrolyte values assist the respiratory care practitioner and physician in the assessment of cardiopulmonary disorders. Knowledge of these laboratory tests provides a greater understanding of the clinical manifestations of a particular cardiopulmonary disorder.

HEMATOLOGY

The most frequent laboratory hematology test is the complete blood count (CBC). The CBC provides important information about the patient's diagnosis, prognosis, response to treatment, and recovery. The CBC includes the red blood cell (RBC) count, hemoglobin, hematocrit, the total WBC, and at least an estimate of the platelet count.

Red Blood Cell Count

The RBCs (erythrocytes) constitute the major portion of the blood cells. The healthy adult male has about 5 million RBCs in each cubic millimeter (mm^3) of blood. The healthy adult female has about 4 million RBCs in each cubic millimeter of blood. Clinically, the total number of RBCs and its indices are useful in assessing the patient's overall oxygen-carrying capacity. The RBC indices are helpful in the identification of specific RBC deficiencies.

Red Blood Cell Indices

Hematocrit (Hct). The Hct is the volume of RBCs in 100 ml of blood and is expressed as a percentage of the total volume. In the healthy adult male the Hct is about 45%; in the healthy adult female the Hct is about 42%. In the healthy newborn the Hct ranges between 45% and 60%. The Hct also is called the *packed cell volume (PCV)*.

Hemoglobin (Hb). Most of the oxygen that diffuses into the pulmonary capillary blood rapidly moves into the RBCs and chemically attaches to the Hb. Each RBC contains approximately 280 million Hb molecules. The Hb value is reported in grams per 100 ml of blood (also referred to as *grams percent of hemoglobin [g% Hb]*). The normal Hb value for the adult male is 14 to 16 g%. The normal adult female Hb value is 12 to 15 g%. Hb constitutes about 33% of the RBC weight.

Mean Cell Volume (MCV). The MCV is the actual size of the RBCs and is used to classify anemias. It is an index that expresses the volume of a single red cell and is measured in cubic microns. The normal MCV is 87 to 103 cubic microns for both men and women.

Mean Corpuscular Hemoglobin Concentration (MCHC). The MCHC is a measure of the concentration or proportion of Hb in an average (mean) RBC. The MCHC is derived by dividing the g% Hb by the Hct. For example, if a patient has 15 g% Hb and a Hct of 45%, the MCHC is 33%. The normal MCHC for men and women ranges between 32% and 36%. The MCHC is most useful in assessing the degree of anemia because the two most accurate hematologic measurements (Hb and Hct—not RBC) are used for the test.

Mean Cell Hemoglobin (MCH). The MCH is a measure of weight of Hb in a single RBC. This value is derived by dividing the total Hb (g% Hb) by the RBC count. The MCH is useful in diagnosing severely anemic patients but not as good as MCHC because the RBC is not always accurate. The normal range for the MCH is 27 to 32 picograms per RBC.

Assessing the RBC count and its indices is useful in the identification of the types of anemias discussed in the following paragraphs.

Normochromic (Normal Hb) and Normocytic (Normal Cell Size) Anemia. Normochromic anemia is most commonly caused by excessive blood loss. The amount of Hb and the number of RBCs are decreased, but the individual size and content remain normal. Clinically, the laboratory report reveals the following:
Hct: below normal
Hb: below normal
MCV: normal
MCHC: normal
MCH: normal

Hypochromic (Decreased Hb) Microcytic (Small Cell Size) Anemia. In hypochromic anemia the size of the RBCs and the Hb content are decreased. This form of anemia is commonly seen in patients with chronic blood loss, iron deficiency, chronic infections, and malignancies. Clinically, the laboratory report reveals the following:
Hct: below normal
Hb: below normal
MCV: below normal
MCHC: below normal
MCH: below normal

Macrocytic (Large Cell Size) Anemia. Macrocytic anemia is commonly caused by folic acid and vitamin B_{12} deficiencies. Patients with macrocytic anemia produce fewer RBCs, but the RBCs that are present are larger than normal. Clinically, the laboratory report reveals the following:
Hct: below normal
Hb: below normal

MCV: above normal (because of the larger RBC size)
MCHC: above normal (because of the larger RBC size)

White Blood Cell Count (WBC)

The major functions of the WBCs (leukocytes) are to (1) fight against infection, (2) defend the body by phagocytosis against foreign organisms, and (3) produce (or at least transport and distribute) antibodies in the immune response. The WBCs are far less numerous than the RBCs, averaging between 5000 and 10,000 cells per cubic millimeter of blood. There are two types of WBCs: granular and nongranular leukocytes. Because the general function of the leukocytes is to combat inflammation and infection, the clinical diagnosis of an injury or infection often entails a differential count, which is the determination of the number of each type of cell in 100 WBCs. Box 7-2 shows a normal differential count. Table 7-1 provides an overview of cell types and common causes for their increase (leukocytosis).

Granular Leukocytes

The granular leukocytes (also called *granulocytes*) are so classified because of the granules present in their cytoplasm. The granulocytes are further divided into

---

BOX 7–2

Normal Differential White Blood Cell Count

Granular Leukocytes
Neutrophils 60% to 70%
Eosinophils 2% to 4%
Basophils 0.5% to 1%

Nongranular Leukocytes
Lymphocytes 20% to 25%
Monocytes 3% to 8%

TABLE 7–1   Common Causes of WBC Increase

Cell Type	Causes of Increase
Neutrophil	Bacterial infection, inflammation
Eosinophil	Allergic reaction, parasitic infection
Basophil	Myeloproliferative disorders
Monocyte	Chronic infections, malignancies
Lymphocyte	Viral infections

the following three types according to the staining properties of the granules: neutrophils, eosinophils, and basophils. Because these cells have distinctive multilobar nuclei, they are often referred to as *polymorphonuclear leukocytes.*

Neutrophils. The neutrophils comprise about 60% to 70% of the total number of WBCs. They have granules that are neutral and therefore do not stain with an acid or a basic dye. The neutrophils are the first WBCs to arrive at the site of inflammation, usually appearing within 90 minutes of the injury. They represent the primary defense against bacterial organisms through the process of phagocytosis. The neutrophils are one of several types of cells called *phagocytes* that ingest and destroy bacterial organisms and particulate matter. The neutrophils also release an enzyme called *lysozyme*, which destroys certain bacteria. An increased neutrophil count is associated with (1) bacterial infection, (2) physical and emotional stress, (3) tumors, (4) inflammatory or traumatic disorders, (5) some leukemias, (6) myocardial infarction, and (7) burns.

Early forms of neutrophils are nonsegmented and are often *band* forms. They almost always signify infection if elevated above 10% of the differential. More mature forms of neutrophils have segmented nuclei. They may increase even in the absence of infection (e.g., with stress [exercise] or the use of corticosteroid medication).

Eosinophils. The cytoplasmic granules of the eosinophils stain red with the acid dye eosin. These leukocytes comprise 2% to 4% of the total number of WBCs. Although the precise function of the eosinophils is unknown, they are thought to play a role in the breakdown of protein material. It is known, however, that the eosinophils are activated by allergies (such as an allergic asthmatic episode) and parasitic infections. Eosinophils are thought to detoxify the agents or chemical mediators associated with allergic reactions. An increased eosinophil count also may be associated with lung cancer, chronic skin infections (e.g., psoriasis, scabies), polycythemia, and tumors.

Basophils. The basophils comprise only about 0.5% to 1% of the total white blood count. The granules of the basophils stain blue with a basic dye. The precise function of the basophils is not clearly understood. Increased basophils are primarily associated with certain myeloproliferative disorders. It is thought that the basophils are involved in allergic and stress responses. They also are considered to be phagocytic and to contain heparin, histamines, and serotonin.

Nongranular Leukocytes

There are two groups of nongranular leukocytes, the monocytes and lymphocytes. The term *mononuclear leukocytes* also is used to describe these cells because they do not contain granules but have spherical nuclei.

Monocytes. The monocytes are the second order of cells to arrive at the inflammation site, usually appearing approximately 5 hours or more after the injury. After 48 hours, however, the monocytes are usually the predominant cell type in the inflamed area. The monocytes are the largest of the WBCs and comprise about 3% to 8% of the total leukocyte count. The monocytes are short-lived, phagocytic WBCs, with a half-life of approximately 1 day. They circulate in the bloodstream from which they move into tissues—at which point they may mature into long-living macrophages (also called *histiocytes*). The macrophages are large wandering cells that engulf larger and greater quantities of foreign material than the neutrophils. When the foreign material cannot be digested by the macrophages, the macrophages may proliferate to form a capsule that surrounds and encloses the foreign material (e.g., fungal spores). Although the monocytes and macrophages do not respond as quickly to an inflammatory process as the neutrophils, they are considered one of the first lines of inflammatory defense. Therefore, an elevated number of monocytes suggests infection and inflammation. The monocytes play an important role in chronic inflammation and also are involved in the immune response and malignancies.

Lymphocytes. Increased lymphocytes are typically seen in viral infections (e.g., infectious mononucleosis). The lymphocytes also are involved in the production of antibodies, which are special proteins that inactivate antigens. For a better understanding of the importance of the lymphocytes and the clinical significance of their destruction or depletion (e.g., *acquired immunodeficiency syndrome [AIDS]*), a brief review of the role and function of the lymphocytes in the immune system is in order.

The lymphocytes can be divided into two categories: B cells and T cells. T and B cells can be identified with an electron microscope according to certain distinguishing surface marks, called *rosettes*: T cells have a smooth surface; B cells have projections. B cells comprise 10% to 30% of the total lymphocytes; T cells comprise 70% to 90% of the total lymphocytes.

The B cells, which are formed in the bone marrow, further divide into either plasma cells or memory cells. The plasma cells secrete antibodies in response to foreign antigens. The memory cells retain the ability to recognize specific antigens long after the initial exposure and therefore contribute to long-term immunity against future exposures to invading pathogens.

The T cells, which are formed in the thymus, are further divided into four functional categories: (1) cytotoxic T cells (also called *killer lymphocytes* or *natural killer cells*), which attack and kill foreign or infected cells; (2) helper T cells, which recognize foreign antigens and help activate cytotoxic T cells and plasma cells (B cells); (3) inducer T cells, which stimulate the production of the different T-cell subsets; and (4) suppressor T cells, which work to suppress the responses of the other cells and help provide feedback information to the system.

The T cells also may be classified according to their surface antigens (i.e., the T cells may display either T4 antigen or T8 antigen). The T4 surface antigen subset, which comprises between 60% and 70% of the circulating T cells, consists mainly of the helper and inducer cells. The T8 surface antigen subset consists mainly of the cytotoxic and suppressor cells.

Sequence of Lymphocyte Responses to Infection

Initially, the macrophages attack and engulf the foreign antigens. This activity in turn stimulates the production of T cells and, ultimately, the antibody-producing B cells (plasma cells). The T4 cells play a pivotal role in the overall modulation of this immune response by (1) secreting a substance called *lymphokine,* which is a potent stimulus to T-cell growth and differentiation; (2) recognizing foreign antigens; (3) causing clonal proliferation of T cells; (4) mediating cytotoxic and suppressor functions; and (5) enabling B cells to secrete specific antibodies.

Because T cells (especially the T4 lymphocytes) have such a central role in this complex immune response, it should not be difficult to imagine the devastating effect that would ultimately follow from the systematic depletion of T lymphocytes. For example, virtually all the infectious complications of AIDS may be explained with reference to the effect that the human immunodeficiency virus (HIV) has on the T cells. A decreased number of T cells increases the patient's susceptibility to a wide range of opportunistic infections and neoplasms. In the healthy, noninfected HIV subject, the T4/T8 ratio is about 2.0. In the HIV-infected patient with AIDS, the T4/T8 ratio is usually 0.5 or less.

Platelet Count

Platelets (also called *thrombocytes*) are the smallest of the formed elements in the blood. They are round or oval, flattened, and disk-shaped in appearance. Platelets are produced in the bone marrow and possibly in the lungs. Platelet activity is essential for blood clotting. The normal platelet count is 150,000 to 350,000/mm^3.

A deficiency of platelets leads to prolonged bleeding time and impaired clot retention. A low platelet count (thrombocytopenia) is associated with (1) massive blood transfusion, (2) pneumonia, (3) cancer chemotherapy, (4) infection, (5) allergic conditions, and (6) toxic effects of certain drugs (e.g., heparin, isoniazid, penicillins, prednisone, streptomycin). A high platelet count (thrombocythemia) is associated with (1) cancer, (2) trauma, (3) asphyxiation, (4) rheumatoid arthritis, (5) iron deficiency, (6) acute infections, (7) heart disease, and (8) tuberculosis.

A platelet count of less than 20,000/mm^3 is associated with spontaneous bleeding, prolonged bleeding time, and poor clot retraction. The precise platelet count necessary for hemostasis is not firmly established. Generally, platelet counts greater than 50,000/mm^3 are not associated with spontaneous bleeding. Therefore various diagnostic or therapeutic procedures, such as bronchoscopy or the insertion of an arterial catheter, are usually safe when the platelet count is greater than 50,000/mm^3.

BLOOD CHEMISTRY

A basic knowledge of the blood chemistry, the normal values, and common health problems that alter these values is an important cornerstone of patient assessment. Table 7-2 lists the blood chemistry tests usually monitored in respiratory care.

ELECTROLYTES

For the cells of the body to function properly, a normal concentration of electrolytes must be maintained. Therefore, the monitoring of the electrolytes is extremely important in the patient whose body fluids are being endogenously or exogenously manipulated (e.g., intravenous therapy, renal disease, diarrhea). Table 7-3 lists electrolytes monitored in respiratory care.

TABLE 7–2   Blood Chemistry Tests Commonly Monitored in Respiratory Care

Chemical	Normal Value	Common Abnormal Findings

Glucose	70 to 110 mg/dl	Hyperglycemia (excess glucose level)
		    Diabetes mellitus
		    Acute infection
		    Myocardial infarction
		    Thiazide and loop diuretics
		Hypoglycemia (low glucose level)
		    Pancreatic tumors or liver disease
		    Pituitary or adrenocortical hyperfunction

Lactic dehydrogenase (LDH)	80 to 120 Wacker units	Increases are associated with the following:
		    Myocardial infarction
		    Chronic hepatitis
		    Pneumonia
		    Pulmonary infarction

Serum glutamic oxaloacetic transaminase (SGOT)	8 to 33 U/ml	Increases are associated with the following:
		    Myocardial infarction
		    Congestive heart failure
		    Pulmonary infarction

Bilirubin	Adult: 0.1 to 1.2 mg/dl
	Newborn: 1 to 12 mg/dl
		Increases are associated with the following;
		    Massive hemolysis
		    Hepatitis

Blood urea nitrogen (BUN)	8 to 18 mg/dl	Increases are associated with acute or chronic renal failure
Serum creatinine	0.6 to 1.2 mg/dl	Increases are associated with renal failure

TABLE 7–3   Electrolytes Commonly Monitored in Respiratory Care

Electrolyte	Normal Value	Common Abnormal Findings	Clinical Manifestations
Sodium (Na$^+$)	136 to 142 mEq/L	Hypernatremia (excess Na$^+$) Dehydration	Desiccated mucous membranes Flushed skin Great thirst Dry tongue

		Hyponatremia (low Na$^+$)
		    Sweating
		    Burns
		    Loss of gastrointestinal secretions
		    Use of some diuretics
		    Excessive water intake
			Abdominal cramps
			Muscle twitching
			Poor perfusion
			Vasomotor collapse
			Confusion
			Seizures

Potassium (K$^+$)	3.8 to 5.0 mEq/L	Hyperkalemia (excess K$^+$)
		    Renal failure
		    Muscle tissue damage
			Irritability
			Nausea
			Diarrhea
			Weakness
			Ventricular fibrillation

		Hypokalemia (low K$^+$)
		    Diuretic therapy
		    Endocrine disorder
		    Diarrhea
		    Reduced intake or loss of K$^+$
		    Chronic stress
			Metabolic alkalosis
			Muscular weakness
			Malaise
			Cardiac arrhythmias
			Hypotension

Continued

TABLE 7–3 **Electrolytes Commonly Monitored in Respiratory Care—cont'd**

Electrolyte	Normal Value	Common Abnormal Findings	Clinical Manifestations

Chloride (Cl^-)	95 to 103 mEq/L	Hyperchloremia (excess Cl^-)
		  Renal tubular acidosis
		Hypochloremia (low Cl^-)
		  Alkalosis
			Deep, rapid breathing
			Weakness
			Disorientation
			Metabolic alkalosis
			Muscle hypertonicity
			Tetany
			Depressed ventilation (respiratory compensation)

Calcium (Ca^{++})	4.5 to 5.4 mEq/L	Hypercalcemia (excess Ca^{++})
		  Malignant tumors
		  Bone fractures
		  Diuretic therapy
		  Excessive use of antacids or milk consumption
		  Vitamin-D intoxication
		  Hyperparathyroidism
			Lethargy, weakness
			Hyporeflexia
			Constipation, anorexia, renal stones
			Mental deterioration

		Hypocalcemia (low Ca^{++})
		  Respiratory alkalosis
		  Pregnancy
		  Vitamin D deficiency
		  Diuretic therapy
		  Hypoparathyroidism
			Paresthesia, cramping of muscles, stridor, convulsions, mental disturbance, Chvostek's sign, Trousseau's sign

SELF-ASSESSMENT QUESTIONS

Multiple Choice

1. In the healthy adult female, what is the Hct?

   a. 31%
   b. 38%
   c. 42%
   d. 45%
   e. 50%

2. Which of the following represent the primary defense against bacterial organisms through phagocytosis?

   a. Eosinophils
   b. Neutrophils
   c. Monocytes
   d. Basophils
   e. Lymphocytes

3. What is the normal Hb value for the adult male?

   a. 10 to 12 g%
   b. 12 to 14 g%
   c. 14 to 16 g%
   d. 16 to 18 g%
   e. 18 to 20 g%

4. What is the normal differential neutrophil count?

   a. 2 to 4%
   b. 20 to 25%
   c. 40 to 50%
   d. 60 to 70%
   e. 75 to 85%

5. In the healthy adult male, what is the RBC count?

   a. $5,000,000/mm^3$
   b. $6,000,000/mm^3$
   c. $7,000,000/mm^3$
   d. $8,000,000/mm^3$
   e. $10,000,000/mm^3$

6. What is the normal WBC count?

   a. 1000 to $5000/mm^3$
   b. 5000 to $10,000/mm^3$
   c. $10,000$ to $15,000/mm^3$
   d. $15,000$ to $20,000/mm^3$
   e. $20,000$ to $25,000/mm^3$

7. Which of the following is activated by allergies (such as an allergic asthmatic episode)?

   a. Eosinophils
   b. Neutrophils
   c. Monocytes
   d. Basophils
   e. Lymphocytes

8. Various clinical procedures such as bronchoscopy or the insertion of an arterial catheter are generally safe when the platelet count is no lower than which of the following?

   a. $150,000/mm^3$
   b. $100,000/mm^3$
   c. $75,000/mm^3$
   d. $50,000/mm^3$
   e. $20,000/mm^3$

9. Which of the following are associated with hyperglycemia?

   I. Diabetes mellitus
   II. Myocardial infarction
   III. Thiazide and loop diuretics
   IV. Acute infection

   a. I and III only
   b. II and IV only
   c. II, III, and IV only
   d. I, II, and III only
   e. I, II, III, and IV

10. Which of the following are clinical manifestations associated with hyponatremia?

    I. Seizures
    II. Confusion
    III. Muscle twitching
    IV. Abdominal cramps

    a. I and III only
    b. II and IV only
    c. II, III, and IV only
    d. I, II, and III only
    e. I, II, III, and IV

Answers appear in Appendix XI.

CHAPTER 8

Radiologic Examination of the Chest

Radiography is the making of a photographic image of the internal structures of the body by passing X-rays through the body to an X-ray film, or radiograph. In patients with respiratory disease, radiography plays an important role in the diagnosis of lung disorders, the assessment of the extent and location of the disease, and the evaluation of the subsequent progress of the disease.

Fundamentals of Radiography

X-rays are created when fast-moving electrons with sufficient energy collide with matter in any form. Clinically, X-rays are produced by an electronic device called an *X-ray tube.*

The X-ray tube is a vacuum-sealed glass tube that contains a cathode and a rotating anode. A tungsten plate approximately ½-inch square is fixed to the end of the rotating anode at the center of the tube. This tungsten block is called the *target.* Tungsten is an effective target metal because of its high melting point, which can withstand the extreme heat to which it is subjected, and because of its high atomic number, which makes it more effective in the production of X-rays.

When the cathode is heated, electrons "boil off." When a high voltage (70 to 150 kV) is applied to the X-ray tube, the electrons are driven to the rotating anode where they strike the tungsten target with tremendous energy. The sudden deceleration of the electrons at the tungsten plate converts energy to X-rays. Although most of the electron energy is converted to heat, a small amount (less than 1%) is transformed to X-rays and allowed to escape from the tube through a set of lead shutters called a *collimator.* From the collimator the X-rays travel through the patient to the X-ray film.

The ability of the X-rays to penetrate matter depends on the density of the matter. For chest radiographs the X-rays may pass through bone, air, soft tissue, and fat. Dense objects such as bone absorb more X-rays (preventing penetration) than objects that are not as dense, such as the air-filled lungs.

After passing through the patient, the X-rays strike the X-ray film. X-rays that pass through low-density objects strike the film at full force and produce a black image on the film. X-rays that are absorbed by high-density objects (such as bone) either do not reach the film at all or strike the film with less force. Relative to the density of the object, these objects appear as light gray to white on the film.

Standard Positions and Techniques of Chest Radiography

Clinically, the standard radiograph of the chest includes two views: a posteroanterior (PA) projection and a lateral projection (either a left or right lateral radiograph) with the patient in the standing position. When the patient is seriously ill or immobilized, an upright radiograph may not be possible. In such cases a supine anteroposterior (AP) radiograph is obtained at the patient's bedside. A lateral radiograph is rarely obtainable under such circumstances.

POSTEROANTERIOR RADIOGRAPH

The standard PA chest radiograph is obtained by having the patient stand (or sit) in the upright position. The anterior aspect of the patient's chest is pressed against a film cassette holder, with the shoulders rotated forward to move the scapulae away from the lung fields. The distance between the X-ray tube and the film is 6 feet. The X-ray beam travels from the X-ray tube, through the patient, and to the X-ray film.

The X-ray is usually taken with the patient's lungs in full inspiration to show the lung fields and related structures to their greatest possible extent. At full inspiration the diaphragm is lowered to approximately the level of the ninth to eleventh ribs posteriorly (Figure 8-1). For certain clinical conditions,

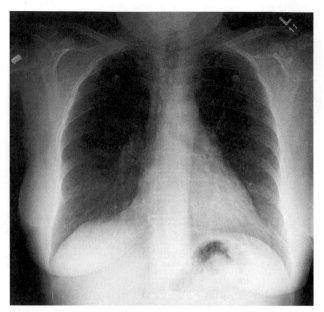

Figure 8–1 Standard PA chest radiograph with the patient's lungs in full inspiration.

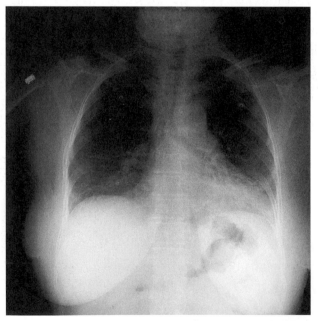

Figure 8–2 A PA chest radiograph of the same patient shown in Figure 8-1 during expiration.

radiographs are sometimes taken at the end of both inspiration and expiration. For example, in patients with obstructive lung disease an expiratory radiograph may be made to evaluate diaphragmatic excursion and the symmetry or asymmetry of such excursion (Figure 8-2).

ANTEROPOSTERIOR RADIOGRAPH

The supine AP radiograph may be taken in patients who are debilitated, immobilized, or too young to tolerate the PA procedure. The AP radiograph is usually taken with a portable X-ray machine at the patient's bedside. The film is placed behind the patient's back, with the X-ray machine positioned in front of the patient approximately 48 inches from the film.

Compared with the PA radiograph, the AP radiograph has a number of disadvantages. For example, the heart and superior portion of the mediastinum are significantly magnified in the AP radiograph. This is because the heart is positioned in front of the thorax as the X-ray beams pass through the chest from the anterior to posterior direction, causing the image of the heart to be enlarged (Figure 8-3).

The AP radiograph also often has less resolution and more distortion. Because the patient is often unable to sustain a maximal inspiration, the lower lung lobes frequently appear hazy, erroneously suggesting pulmonary congestion or pleural effusion. Finally, because the AP radiograph is often taken in the intensive care unit, extraneous shadows, such as those produced by ventilator tubing and indwelling lines, are often present (Figure 8-4).

LATERAL RADIOGRAPH

The lateral radiograph is obtained to complement the PA radiograph. It is taken with the side of the patient's chest compressed against the cassette. The patient's arms are raised, with the forearms resting on the head.

To view the right lung and heart, the patient's right side is placed against the cassette. To view the left lung and heart, the patient's left side is placed against the cassette. Therefore, a right lateral radiograph would be selected to view a density or lesion that is known to be in the right lung. If neither lung is of particular interest, a left lateral radiograph is usually selected to reduce the magnification of the heart. The lateral radiograph provides a view of the structures behind the heart and diaphragmatic dome. It also can be combined with the PA radiograph to give the respiratory care provider a three-dimensional view of the structures or of any abnormal densities (Figure 8-5).

LATERAL DECUBITUS RADIOGRAPH

The lateral decubitus radiograph is obtained by having the patient lie on the left or right side rather than stand or sit in the upright position. The naming of the decubitus radiograph is determined by the

Figure 8–3 Compared with the PA chest radiograph, the heart is significantly magnified in the AP chest radiograph. In the PA radiograph the ratio of the width of the heart to the thorax is normally less than 1:2. The reason the heart appears larger in the AP radiograph is that it is positioned in front of the thorax as the X-ray beams pass through the chest from the anterior to posterior direction. This allows more space for the heart shadow to "fan out" before it reaches the X-ray film.

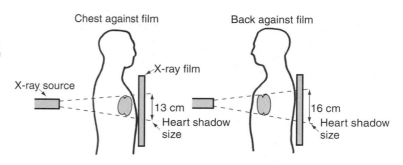

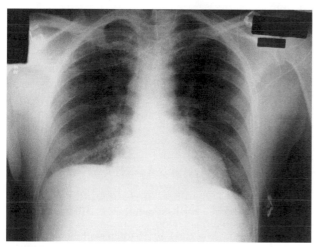

Figure 8–4 AP chest radiograph. The diaphragms are elevated, the lower lung lobes appear hazy, the ratio of the width of the heart to the thorax is greater than 2:1, and extraneous lines are apparent on the patient's left side. X-rays taken with portable machines are frequently performed on patients too ill to be transported to the radiology department. These films, in the best of circumstances, are of poorer quality than erect films taken with standard X-ray apparatus. The films are usually AP projections taken with the X-ray unit in front of and the film plate behind the patient. Overexposure, underexposure, malpositioning, marginal cut-offs, and motion artifact are often present. In this setting, major events such as partial pneumothoraces, pleural effusions, and infiltrates in dependent parts of the lung may go unrecognized. Therefore careful clinical correlation with the patient's pathophysiology and symptomatology is imperative.

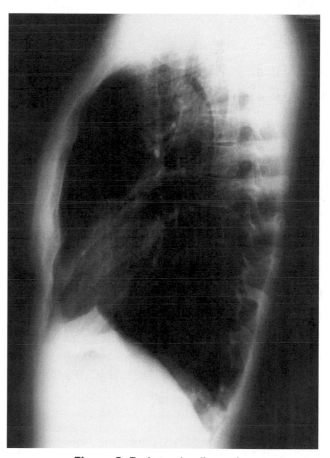

Figure 8–5 Lateral radiograph.

side on which the patient lies; thus a right lateral decubitus radiograph means that the patient's right side is down.

The lateral decubitus radiograph is useful in the diagnosis of a suspected or known fluid accumulation in the pleural space (pleural effusion) that is not easily seen in the PA radiograph. A pleural effusion, which is usually more thinly spread out over the diaphragm in the upright position, collects in the gravity-dependent areas while the patient is in the lateral decubitus position, allowing the fluid to be more readily seen (Figure 8-6).

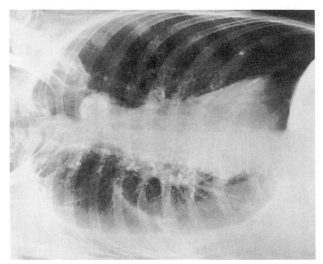

Figure 8-6 Subpulmonic pleural effusion. Right lateral decubitus view. Subdiaphragmatic fluid has run up the lateral chest wall, producing a band of soft tissue density. The medial curvilinear shadow *(arrow)* indicates fluid in the lips of the major fissure.

Inspecting the Chest Radiograph

Before the respiratory care practitioner can effectively identify abnormalities on a chest radiograph, he or she must be able to recognize the normal anatomic structures. Figure 8-7 represents a normal PA chest radiograph with identification of important anatomic landmarks. Figure 8-8 labels the anatomic structures seen on a lateral chest radiograph.

Table 8-1 lists some of the more important radiologic terms used to describe abnormal lung findings.

TECHNICAL QUALITY OF THE RADIOGRAPH

The first step in examining a chest radiograph is to evaluate its technical quality. Was the patient in the correct position when the radiograph was taken? To verify the proper position, check the relationship of the medial ends of the clavicles to the vertebral column. For the PA radiograph the vertebral column should be precisely in the center between the medial ends of the clavicles, and the distance between the right and left costophrenic angles and the spine should be equal. Even a small degree of patient rotation relative to the film can create a false image, erroneously suggesting tracheal deviation, cardiac displacement, or cardiac enlargement.

Second, the exposure quality of the radiograph should be evaluated. Normal exposure is verified by determining whether the spinal processes of the vertebrae are visible to the fifth or sixth thoracic level (T5-T6). X-ray equipment is now available that

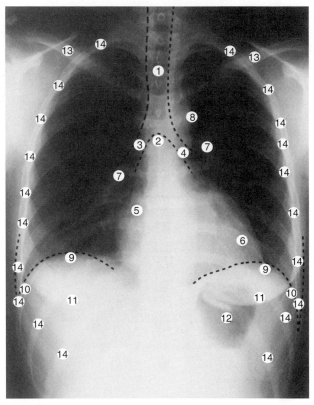

Figure 8-7 Normal PA chest radiograph. *1,* Trachea (note vertebral column in middle of trachea); *2,* carina; *3,* right main stem bronchus; *4,* left main stem bronchus; *5,* right atrium; *6,* left ventricle; *7,* hilar vasculature; *8,* aortic knob; *9,* diaphragm; *10,* costophrenic angles; *11,* breast shadows; *12,* gastric air bubble; *13,* clavicle; *14,* rib.

allows the vertebrae to be seen down to the level of the cardiac shadow. The degree of exposure can be evaluated further by comparing the relative densities of the heart and lungs. For example, because the heart has a greater density than the air-filled lungs, the heart appears whiter than the lung fields. The heart and lungs become more radiolucent (darker) with greater exposure of the radiograph. A radiograph that has been overexposed is said to be "heavily penetrated" or "burned out." Conversely, the heart and lungs on an underexposed radiograph may appear denser and whiter. The lungs may erroneously appear to have infiltrates, and there may be little or no visibility of the thoracic vertebrae.

Third, the level of inspiration at the moment the radiograph was taken should be evaluated. At full inspiration the diaphragmatic domes should be at the level of the ninth to eleventh ribs posteriorly. On radiographs taken during expiration, the lungs appear denser, the diaphragm is elevated, and the heart appears wider and enlarged (see Figure 8-2).

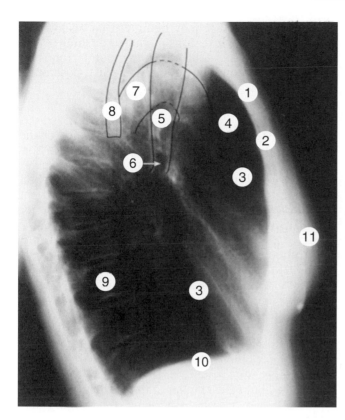

Figure 8–8 Normal lateral chest radiograph. *1,* Manubrium; *2,* sternum; *3,* cardiac shadow; *4,* retrosternal air space in the lung; *5,* trachea; *6,* bronchus, on end; *7,* aortic arch (ascending and descending); *8,* scapulae; *9,* vertebral column; *10,* diaphragm; *11,* breast shadow.

TABLE 8–1 Common Radiologic Terms

Term	Definition
Air cyst	A thin-walled radiolucent area surrounded by normal lung tissue
Bleb	A superficial air cyst protruding into the pleura; also called *bulla*
Bronchogram	An outline of air-containing bronchi beyond the normal point of visibility. An air bronchogram develops as a result of an infiltration or consolidation that surrounds the bronchi, producing a contrasting air column on the radiograph—that is, the bronchi appear as dark tubes surrounded by a white area produced by the infiltration or consolidation
Bulla	A large, thin-walled radiolucent area surrounded by normal lung tissue
Cavity	A radiolucent (dark) area surrounded by dense tissue (white). A cavity is the hallmark of a lung abscess. A fluid level may be seen inside a cavity
Consolidation	The act of becoming solid; commonly used to describe the solidification of the lung caused by a pathologic engorgement of the alveoli, as occurs in acute pneumonia
Homogeneous density	Refers to a uniformly dense lesion (white area); commonly used to describe solid tumors, fluid-containing cavities, or fluid in the pleural space
Honeycombing	A coarse reticular (netlike) density commonly seen in pneumoconiosis
Infiltrate	Any poorly defined radiodensity (white area); commonly used to describe an inflammatory lesion
Interstitial density	A density caused by interstitial thickening
Lesion	Any pathologic or traumatic alteration of tissue or loss of function of a part
Opacity	State of being opaque (white); an opaque area or spot; impervious to light rays, or by extension, X-rays; opposite of translucent or radiolucent
Pleural density	A radiodensity caused by fluid, tumor, inflammation, or scarring
Pulmonary mass	A lesion in the lung that is 6 cm or more in diameter; commonly used to describe a pulmonary tumor
Pulmonary nodule	A lesion in the lung that is less than 6 cm in diameter and composed of dense tissue; also called a *solitary pulmonary nodule* or *"coin" lesion* because of its rounded, coinlike appearance
Radiodensity	Dense areas that appear white on the radiograph; the opposite of radiolucency
Radiolucency	The state of being radiolucent; the property of being partly or wholly permeable to X-rays; commonly used to describe darker areas on a radiograph such as an emphysematous lung or a pneumothorax
Translucent	Permitting the passage of light; commonly used to describe darker areas of the radiograph

SEQUENCE OF EXAMINATION

Although the precise sequence in examining a chest radiograph is not important, the inspection should be done in a systematic fashion. Some practitioners prefer an "inside-out" approach to inspecting the chest radiograph, which entails beginning with the mediastinum and proceeding outward to the extrathoracic soft tissue. Some practitioners prefer the reverse. The following is an "inside-out" method.

Mediastinum

The mediastinum should be inspected for width, contour, and shifts from the midline. The respiratory care practitioner should inspect the anatomy of the mediastinum, including the trachea, carina, cardiac borders, aortic arch, and superior vena cava (see Figure 8-7).

Trachea

On the PA projection the trachea should appear as a translucent column overlying the vertebral column. The diameter of the bronchi progressively tapers a short distance beyond the carina and then disappears (see Figure 8-7). A number of clinical conditions can cause the trachea to shift from its normal position. For example, fluid or gas accumulation in the pleural space causes the trachea to shift away from the affected area. Lung collapse or fibrosis usually causes the trachea to shift *toward* the affected area. The trachea also may be displaced by tumors of the upper lung regions.

Anatomic structures in the chest (e.g., the trachea) move out of their normal position because they are either *pushed* or *pulled* in a given direction. In other words, they may be moved up or down or from side to side by lesions pulling or pushing in that direction. Table 8-2 lists examples of factors that push or pull the trachea out of its normal position in the chest radiograph.

Heart

On the PA projection the ratio of the width of the heart to the thorax (the cardiothoracic ratio) is normally less than 1:2. A small portion of the heart should be seen on the right side of the vertebral column. Two bulges should be seen on the right border of the heart. The upper bulge is the superior vena cava; the lower bulge is the right atrium. Three bulges are normally seen on the left side of the heart. The superior bulge is the aorta, the middle bulge is the main pulmonary artery, and the inferior bulge is the left ventricle (see Figure 8-7). See Table 8-2 for examples of factors that push or pull the heart out of its normal position in the chest radiograph.

Hilar Region

The right and left hilar regions should be evaluated for change in size or position. Normally, the left hilum is about 2 cm higher than the right (see Figure 8-7). An increased density of the hilar region may indicate engorgement of hilar vessels caused by increased pulmonary vascular resistance. Vertical displacement of the hilum suggests volume loss from one or more upper lobes of the lung on the affected side. In infectious lung disorders such as histoplasmosis or tuberculosis the lymph nodes around the hilar region are often enlarged, calcified, or both. Malignant pulmonary lesions, including hilar malignant lymphadenopathy, also may be seen. See Table 8-2

TABLE 8–2 Examples of Factors That Pull or Push Anatomic Structures out of Their Normal Position in the Chest Radiograph

Structure	Examples of Abnormal Position	Lesion

Mediastinum
  Trachea
  Carina
  Heart
  Major vessels
	Leftward shift	Pulled left by upper lobe tuberculosis, atelectasis, or fibrosis
		Pushed left by right upper lobe emphysematous bulla, fluid, gas, or tumor

Left diaphragm	Upward shift	Pulled up by left lower lobe atelectasis or fibrosis Pushed up by distended gastric air bubble
Horizontal fissure	Downward shift	Pulled down by right middle lobe or right lower lobe atelectasis Pushed down by right upper lobe neoplasm
Left lung	Rightward shift	Pulled right by right lung collapse, atelectasis, or fibrosis Pushed right by left-sided tension pneumothorax or hemothorax

for additional factors that push or pull the hilar region out of its normal position in the chest radiograph.

Lung Parenchyma (Tissue)

The lungs should be examined systematically from top to bottom, one lung compared with the other. Normally, tissue markings can be seen throughout the lungs (see Figure 8-7). The absence of tissue markings may suggest a pneumothorax, recent pneumonectomy, or chronic obstructive lung disease (e.g., emphysema) or may be the result of an overexposed radiograph. An excessive amount of tissue markings may indicate fibrosis, interstitial or alveolar edema, lung compression, or an underexposed radiograph. The periphery of the lung fields should be inspected for abnormalities that obscure the lung's interface with the pleural space, mediastinum, or diaphragm. See Table 8-2 for additional examples of factors that push or pull the lung tissue out of its normal position in the chest radiograph.

Pleura

The peripheral borders of the lungs should be examined for pleural thickening, presence of fluid (pleural effusion) or air (pneumothorax) in the pleural space, or mass lesions (see Figure 8-7). The costophrenic angles should be inspected. Blunting of the costophrenic angle suggests the presence of fluid. A lateral decubitus radiograph may be required to confirm the presence of fluid (see Figure 8-6).

Diaphragm

Both the right and left hemidiaphragms should have an upwardly convex, dome-shaped contour. The right and left costophrenic angles should be clear. Normally, the right diaphragm is about 2 cm higher than the left because of the liver below it (see Figure 8-7). Chronic obstructive pulmonary diseases (e.g., emphysema) and diseases that cause gas or fluid to accumulate in the pleural space flatten and depress the normal curvature of the diaphragm. Abnormal elevation of one diaphragm may result from excessive gas in the stomach, collapse of the middle or lower lobe on the affected side, pulmonary infection at the lung bases, phrenic nerve damage, or spinal curvature. See Table 8-2 for additional examples of factors that push or pull the diaphragm out of its normal position in the chest radiograph.

Gastric Air Bubble

The area below the diaphragm should be inspected. A stomach air bubble is commonly seen under the left hemidiaphragm (see Figure 8-7). Free air may appear under either diaphragm after abdominal surgery or in patients with peritoneal abscess.

Bony Thorax

The ribs, vertebrae, clavicles, sternum, and scapulae should be inspected. The intercostal spaces should be symmetric and equal over each lung field (see Figure 8-7). Intercostal spaces that are too close together suggest a loss of muscle tone, commonly seen in patients with paralysis involving one side of the chest. In chronic obstructive pulmonary disease the intercostal spaces are generally far apart because of alveolar hyperinflation. Finally, the ribs should be inspected for deformities or fractures. If a rib fracture is suspected but not seen on the standard chest radiograph, a special rib series (radiographs that focus on the ribs) may be necessary.

Extrathoracic Soft Tissues

The soft tissue external to the bony thorax should be closely inspected. If the patient is a female, the outer boundaries of the breast shadows should be identified (see Figure 8-7). If the patient has undergone a mastectomy, there will be a relative hyperlucency on the side of the mastectomy. Large breasts can create a significant amount of haziness over the lower lung fields, giving the false appearance of pneumonia or pulmonary congestion. Although nipple shadows are easily identified when they are bilaterally symmetric, one may become less visible when the patient is slightly rotated. The other nipple then appears abnormally opaque and may be mistaken for a pulmonary nodule. After a tracheostomy or pneumothorax, subcutaneous air bubbles (called *subcutaneous emphysema*) often form in the soft tissue, especially if the patient is on a positive-pressure ventilator.

Other Radiologic Techniques

COMPUTED TOMOGRAPHY

Computed tomography (CT) scanning provides a series of cross-sectional (transverse) pictures (called *tomograms*) of the structures within the body at numerous levels. The procedure is painless and noninvasive and requires no special preparation. CT uses a narrowly collimated beam of X-rays that rotates in a continuous 360-degree motion around the patient to image the body in cross-sectional slices. Several detectors, positioned at different angles, record the X-rays that pass through the body. A computer uses the different X-ray absorption levels to create a representative cross-sectional image based

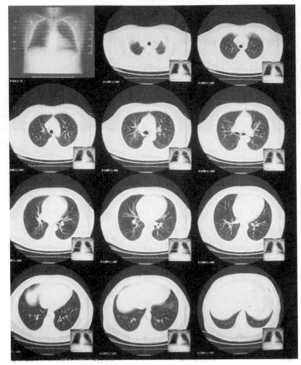

Figure 8–9 Overview of normal lung window CT scan. The apex appears in the two views in the upper right hand corner of this figure; the diaphragm at the base of the lungs appears in the lower right hand view.

on the density of the structures being scanned. This cross-sectional slice is called an *axial view,* or *computerized axial tomogram.* Up to 250 images, approximately 1 mm apart, can be generated on a chest CT scan. These "cuts" are often called a *high resolution CT (HRCT)* scan. In essence, each CT scan provides an image of what a "slice" through the body looks like at specific points—similar to cutting a piece of fruit in half and viewing the cross section of the structures inside the fruit. Dense structures, such as bone, appear white on the tomogram, whereas structures with a relatively low density, such as the lungs, appear dark or black. Therefore a dense tumor in the lungs would appear as a white object surrounded by dark lungs.

The resolution of a CT scan can easily be adjusted to primarily view lung tissue—commonly called a *lung window CT scan*—or bone and mediastinal structures—commonly referred to as a *mediastinal window CT scan.* In a mediastinal window CT scan, the lung tissue is overexposed and appears mostly black; the bones and mediastinal organs appear mostly white. Figure 8-9 provides an overview of a normal lung window CT scan. Figure 8-10 shows a close-up of one "slice" of a normal lung window CT scan. Figure 8-11 provides a close-up view of one slice of a normal mediastinal window CT scan.

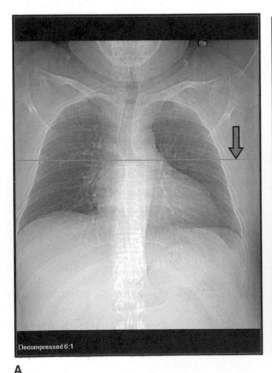

A

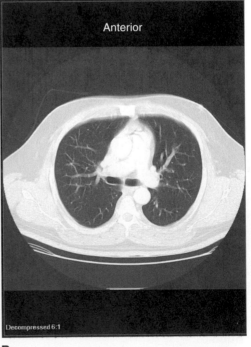

B

Figure 8–10 Close-up of a normal lung window CT scan. **A,** The portion of the chest the CT scan is taken. **B,** The actual cross-sectional slice, or axial view of the chest.

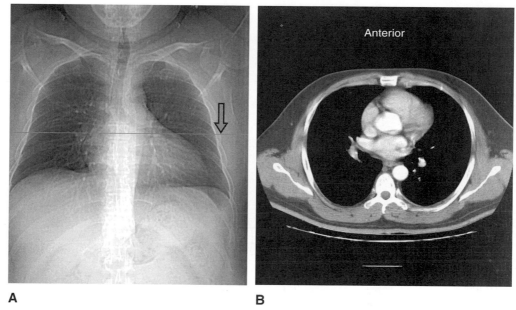

A   **B**

Figure 8–11 Close up of normal CT mediastinal window. **A,** The portion of the chest the CT scan is taken. **B,** The actual cross-sectional slice, or axial view of the chest. Note that the lungs are overexposed and appear mostly black. The bone and mediastinal organs appear mostly white.

Finally, for poorly defined lesions evident on the standard radiograph, the CT scan is a useful supplement in determining the precise location, size, and shape of the lesion. The CT scan is especially helpful in confirming the presence of a mediastinal mass, small pulmonary nodules, small lesions of the bronchi, pulmonary cavities, a small pneumothorax, pleural effusion, and small tumors (as small as 0.3 to 0.5 cm).

POSITRON EMISSION TOMOGRAPHY

The *positron emission tomography (PET)* scan shows both the anatomic structures and the metabolic activity of the tissues and organs scanned. Used in conjunction with a chest X-ray and CT scan for comparison, the PET scan is an excellent diagnostic tool for early detection of cancerous lesions. The unique aspect of the PET scan is its ability to evaluate the metabolic rate of certain tissue cells that may be cancerous. In other words, the PET scan is able to detect cancerous cells in the tissues of the body before changes develop in the anatomic shape of the organ.

Before undergoing the scan, the patient is injected intravenously (IV) with a solution of glucose that has been tagged with a radioactive chemical isotope (generally fluorine 18 deoxyglucose, or F18-FDG compound). Cancer cells metabolize glucose at extremely high rates. The PET scan measures the way

cells burn glucose. When present, the cancer cells rapidly consume the tagged glucose. As the glucose molecules break down, end products are produced that emit *positrons*. The positrons collide with electrons that give off *gamma rays*. The gamma rays are converted to dark spots on the PET scan image. These dark spots are commonly referred to as "hot spots." The presence of a hot spot on a PET scan likely confirms a rapidly growing tumor.

Clinically, a PET scan is an excellent tool to rule out suspicious findings (i.e., a possible cancerous area) that are identified on either the chest radiograph or CT scan. For example, Figure 8-12 shows a chest radiograph that identifies two suspicious findings—one small nodule in the right upper lung lobe and a larger density in the left lower lung lobe, just behind the heart. Figure 8-13 shows two CT scans that also identify the two suspicious findings and their precise location. Figures 8-14 through 8-16 show PET scans that all confirm a hot spot (likely cancer) in the lower left lobe. However, the PET scan shown in Figure 8-17 confirms that the nodule in the right upper lobe is benign (i.e., no hot spot noted).

Although the PET scan is relatively painless (i.e., tantamount to IV insertion), it is lengthy. It may take up to 90 minutes to complete the scan. After the injection, the patient quietly rests in a reclining chair between 30 and 60 minutes before the scan is performed. This allows time for the body to absorb

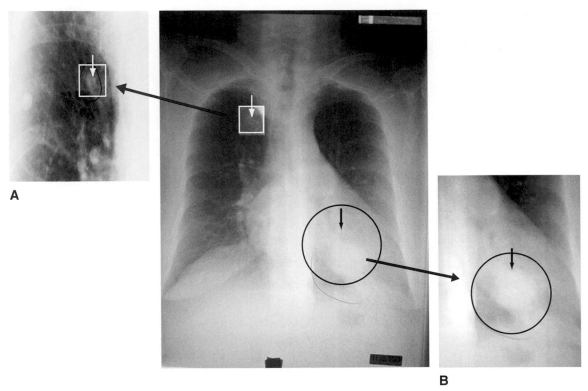

Figure 8–12   Chest radiograph identifying two suspicious findings: in the right upper lobe **(A)** and in the left lower lobe **(B)**, just behind the heart (see *white arrows*).

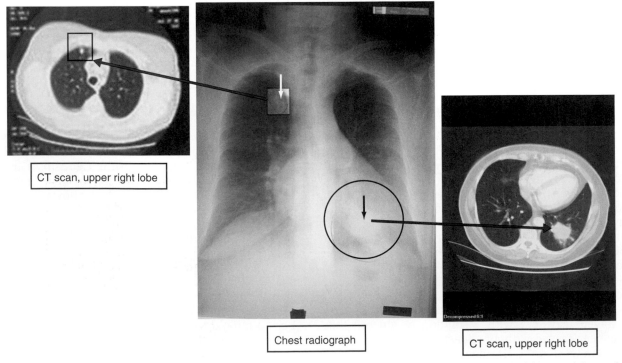

Figure 8–13   Same chest radiograph as shown in Figure 8-12. Note the CT scan also identifies the suspicious nodules and their precise location.

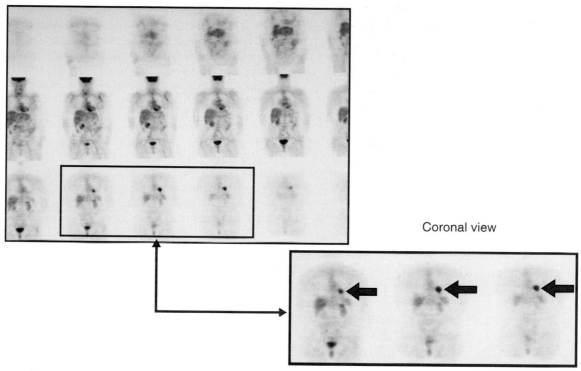

Coronal view

Figure 8–14 PET scan: coronal views. The last three views show a "hot spot" in left lower lung lobe.

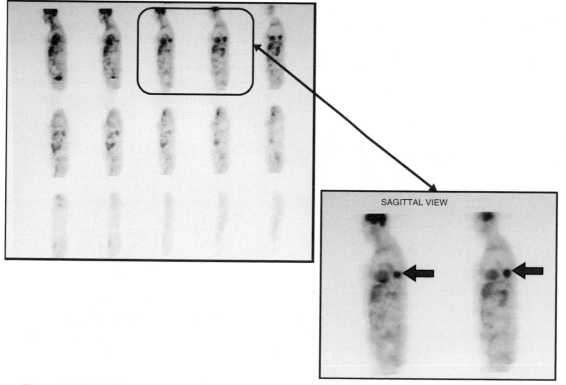

SAGITTAL VIEW

Figure 8–15 PET scan: sagittal views. The encircled images show a "hot spot" in the lower left lobe.

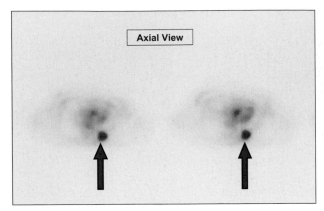

Figure 8–16   PET scan: axial view. A "hot spot" is further confirmed in left lower lung lobe.

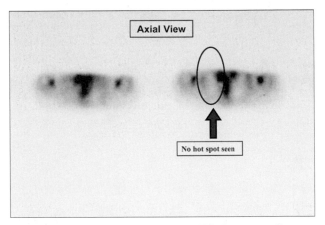

Figure 8–17   PET scan: axial view. This image confirms that the small nodule identified in the upper right lobe in the chest radiograph and CT scan is benign (i.e., no "hot spot" is evident).

the compound. This step may be difficult or impossible for patients who are unable to remain motionless for long periods of time. PET scans are very expensive to perform, compared to CT or MRI studies.

POSITRON EMISSION TOMOGRAPHY AND COMPUTED TOMOGRAPHY SCAN

As described in the preceding sections, PET and CT are both standard imaging tools used by the radiologist to pinpoint the location of cancer or infection within the body before developing a treatment strategy. Individually, however, each scan has its own benefits and limitations. For example, the PET scan detects the metabolic activity of growing cancer cells

in the body, and the CT scan provides a detailed picture of the internal anatomy that shows the precise location, size, and shape of a tumor or mass. On the other hand, because the PET scan and CT scan are done at different times and locations, variations in the patient's body position often make the interpretation of the two images difficult.

Technology has now been developed that allows both the PET scan and the CT scan to be merged together at the same time. The image produced is called a *PET/CT scan* (also known as a *PET/CT fusion*). The PET/CT scan provides an image far superior to that afforded by either technology independently. When combined, the CT scan provides the anatomic detail regarding the precise size, shape, and location of the tumor, and the PET scan provides the metabolic activity of the tumor or mass. The PET/CT image provides excellent image quality and high sensitivity and specificity in detecting malignant lesions in the chest. Figure 8-18 shows a CT/PET scan alongside a CT scan and a PET scan—all the images show the same malignant nodule in the right upper lung lobe.

The benefits of a combined PET/CT scan include earlier diagnosis, accurate staging and localization, and precise treatment and monitoring. With the high quality and accuracy of the PET/CT image, the patient has a better chance at a favorable outcome, without the need for unnecessary procedures. In addition, the PET/CT scan provides early detection of the recurrence or metastasis of cancer, revealing tumors that might otherwise be obscured by scars from surgery and radiation therapy. This is because the combined PET/CT scan provides the radiologist with a more complete overview of what is occurring in the patient's body—both anatomically and metabolically—at the same time.

MAGNETIC RESONANCE IMAGING

Magnetic resonance imaging (MRI) uses magnetic resonance as its source of energy to take cross-sectional (transverse, sagittal, or coronal) images of the body. It uses no ionizing radiation. The patient is placed in the cylindrical-shaped imager, and the body part in question is exposed to a magnetic field and radiowave transmission. The MRI produces a high-contrast image that can detect subtle lesions (Figure 8-19).

The MRI is superior to CT scanning in identifying complex congenital heart disorders, bone marrow diseases, adenopathy, and lesions of the chest wall. The MRI is an excellent supplement to CT scanning for study of the mediastinum and hilar region. For most abnormalities of the chest, however, CT scanning is

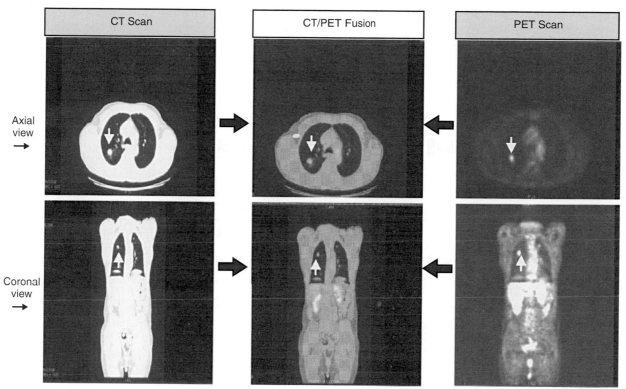

Figure 8–18 CT/PET scan (center). CT scan, CT/PET fusion, and PET scan, all showing the same malignant nodule in right upper lobe (see *white arrow*). Note: The CT/PET fusion is normally presented in color (e.g., red, blue, yellow).

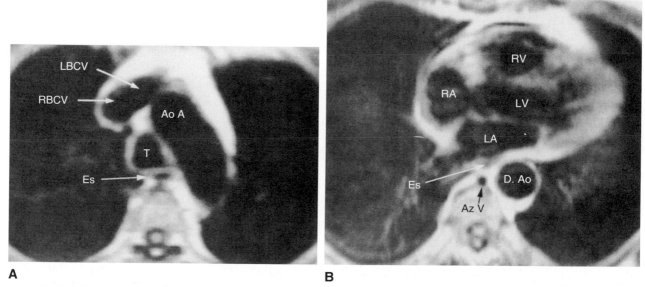

Figure 8–19 Anatomy of mediastinum on MRI. **A,** *LBCV,* Left brachiocephalic vein; *RBCV,* right brachiocephalic vein; *Ao A,* aortic arch; *T,* trachea; *Es,* esophagus. **B,** *RV,* Right ventricle; *LV,* left ventricle; *RA,* right atrium; *LA,* left atrium; *D Ao,* descending aorta; *Es,* esophagus; *Az V,* azygos vein. (From Armstrong P, Wilson AG, Dee P: *Imaging of diseases of the chest,* St. Louis, 1990, Mosby.)

generally better than MRI for motion (patient motion causes loss of resolution), spatial resolution, and cost reasons.

Because the MR imager generates an intense magnetic field, objects made of ferromagnetic material are strongly attracted to it. Therefore patients with ferromagnetic cerebral aneurysm clips or ferromagnetic prosthetic cardiac valves should not undergo MRI because the magnetic force of the MR image can cause these devices to shift and harm the patient. The magnetic force of the MR imager also can interfere with the normal function of cardiac pacemakers and most ventilators.

PULMONARY ANGIOGRAPHY

Pulmonary angiography is useful in identifying pulmonary emboli or arteriovenous malformations. It involves the injection of a radiopaque contrast medium through a catheter that has been passed through the right side of the heart and into the pulmonary artery. The injection of the contrast material into the pulmonary circulation is followed by rapid serial pulmonary angiograms. The pulmonary vessels are filled with radiopaque contrast material and therefore appear white. Figure 8-20 shows an abnormal angiogram in which the major blood vessels appear absent distal to pulmonary emboli in the left lung.

VENTILATION/PERFUSION SCAN

A ventilation/perfusion scan is useful in determining the presence of pulmonary embolism. The perfusion

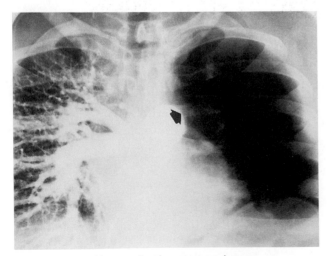

Figure 8–20   Abnormal pulmonary angiogram. Radiopaque material injected into the blood is prevented from flowing into the left lung past the pulmonary embolism *(arrow)*. No vascular structures are seen distal to the obstruction.

scan is obtained by injecting small particles of albumin, called *macroaggregates,* tagged with a radioactive material such as iodine 131 or technetium 99m. After injection the radioactive particles are carried in the blood to the right side of the heart, from which they are distributed throughout the lungs by the blood flow in the pulmonary arteries. The radioactive particles that travel through unobstructed arteries become trapped in the pulmonary capillaries because they are between 20 and 50 µm in diameter and the diameter of the average pulmonary capillary is approximately 8 to 10 µm.

The lungs are then scanned with a gamma camera that produces a picture of the radioactive distribution throughout the pulmonary circulation. The dark areas show good blood flow, and the white or light areas represent decreased or complete absence of blood flow. The macroaggregates eventually break down, pass through the pulmonary circulation, and are excreted by the liver. The injection of these radioactive particles has no significant effect on the patient's hemodynamics because the patent pulmonary capillaries far outnumber those "embolized" by the radioactive particles. In addition to pulmonary emboli, a perfusion scan defect (white or light areas) may be caused by a lung abscess, lung compression, loss of the pulmonary vascular system (e.g., emphysema), atelectasis, or alveolar consolidation.

The perfusion scan is supplemented with a ventilation scan. During the ventilation scan the patient breathes a radioactive gas such as xenon 133 from a closed-circuit spirometer. A gamma camera is used to create a picture of the gas distribution throughout the lungs. A normal ventilation scan shows a uniform distribution of the gas, with the dark areas reflecting the presence of the radioactive gas and therefore good ventilation. White or light areas represent decreased or complete absence of ventilation. See Figure 20-5 for an abnormal perfusion scan and a normal ventilation scan of a patient with a severe pulmonary embolism. An abnormal ventilation scan also may be caused by airway obstruction (e.g., mucus plug or bronchospasm), loss of alveolar elasticity (e.g., emphysema), alveolar consolidation, or pulmonary edema.

FLUOROSCOPY

Fluoroscopy is a technique by which X-ray motion pictures of the chest are taken. Fluoroscopy subjects the patient to a larger dose of X-rays than does standard radiography. Therefore it is used only in selected cases, as in the assessment of abnormal diaphragmatic movement (e.g., unilateral paralysis) or for localization of lesions to be biopsied during fiberoptic bronchoscopy.

BRONCHOGRAPHY

Bronchography entails the instillation of a radiopaque material into the lumen of the tracheobronchial tree. A chest radiograph is then taken, providing a film called a *bronchogram*. The contrast material provides a clear outline of the trachea, carina, right and left main stem bronchi, and segmental bronchi. Bronchography is occasionally used to diagnose bronchogenic carcinoma and determine the presence or extent of bronchiectasis (Figure 8-21). CT of the chest has largely replaced this technique.

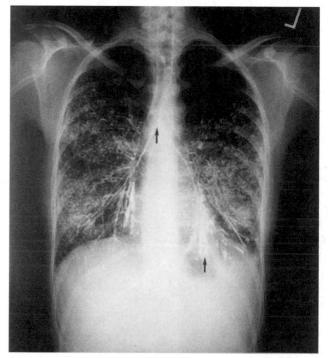

Figure 8–21 Bronchogram obtained using contrast medium in a patient with a history of bronchiectasis. *Arrows* indicate the carina and the bronchi leading to the posterior basilar segment of the left lower lobe. (From Rau JL, Jr, Pearce DJ: *Understanding chest radiographs,* Denver, 1984, Multi-Media Publishing.)

SELF-ASSESSMENT QUESTIONS

Multiple Choice

1. Clinically, the standard radiograph of the chest includes which of the following?

    I. AP radiograph
    II. Lateral decubitus radiograph
    III. Lateral radiograph
    IV. PA radiograph

    a. I only
    b. IV only
    c. III and IV only
    d. I and II only
    e. I, III, and IV only

2. Compared with the PA radiograph, the AP radiograph:

    I. Magnifies the heart
    II. Is usually more distorted
    III. Frequently appears more hazy
    IV. Often has extraneous shadows

    a. I only
    b. II only
    c. III and IV only
    d. I, III, and IV only
    e. I, II, III, and IV

3. To view the right lung and heart in the lateral radiograph, the:

    a. Left side of the patient's chest is placed against the cassette
    b. Anterior portion of the patient's chest is placed against the cassette
    c. Right side of the patient's chest is placed against the cassette
    d. Posterior portion of the patent's chest is placed against the cassette

4. A right lateral decubitus radiograph means that the:

    a. Right side of the chest is down
    b. Posterior side of the chest is up
    c. Left side of the chest is down
    d. Anterior side of the chest is up

5. A leftward shift of the mediastinum is commonly seen on the chest radiograph in response to which of the following?

    I. Left upper lobe atelectasis
    II. Right upper lobe gas
    III. Left upper lobe fibrosis
    IV. Right upper lobe tumor

    a. I and III only
    b. III and IV only
    c. II, III, and IV only
    d. I, II, III, and IV

6. The normal exposure of the radiograph is verified by determining whether the spinal processes of the vertebrae are visible to which level?

    a. C1 to C3
    b. C3 to C5
    c. T2 to T4
    d. T5 to T6
    e. T10 to T12

7. A radiograph that is described as being "heavily penetrated" is which of the following?

    I. Darker in appearance
    II. More translucent
    III. Whiter in appearance
    IV. More opaque in appearance

    a. I only
    b. III only
    c. IV only
    d. III and IV only
    e. I and II only

8. When the radiograph is taken at full inspiration, the diaphragmatic domes should be at the level of the:

    a. First to fourth ribs posteriorly
    b. Fourth to sixth ribs posteriorly
    c. Sixth to ninth ribs posteriorly
    d. Ninth to eleventh ribs posteriorly
    e. Eleventh to twelfth ribs posteriorly

9. Which of the following involves X-ray motion pictures of the chest?

    a. Bronchography
    b. Fluoroscopy
    c. MRI
    d. CT
    e. Pulmonary angiography

10. The MRI is superior to CT scanning for identifying which of the following?

    I. Lesions of the chest
    II. Bone marrow diseases
    III. Congenital heart disorders
    IV. Adenopathy

    a. I and II only
    b. III and IV only
    c. II and III only
    d. II, III, and IV only
    e. I, II, III, and IV

Answers appear in Appendix XI.

CHAPTER 9

The Therapist-Driven Protocol Program and the Role of the Respiratory Care Practitioner

Therapist-driven protocols (TDPs) are an integral part of respiratory care health services. According to the American Association of Respiratory Care (AARC), the purposes of respiratory TDPs are to:

- Deliver individualized diagnostic and therapeutic respiratory care to patients.
- Assist the physician with evaluating patients' respiratory care needs and to optimize the allocation of respiratory care services.
- Determine the indications for respiratory therapy and the appropriate modalities for providing high-quality, cost-effective care that improves patient outcomes and decreases length of stay.
- Empower respiratory care practitioners to allocate care using signs- and symptom-based algorithms for respiratory treatment.

To further support the AARC's purpose statement on TDPs, the American College of Chest Physicians (ACCP) defines respiratory therapy protocols as follows:

> ...Patient care plans which are initiated and implemented by credentialed respiratory care workers. These plans are designed and developed with input from physicians, and are approved for use by the medical staff and the governing body of the hospitals in which they are used. They share in common

extreme reliance on assessment and evaluation skills. Protocols are by their nature dynamic and flexible, allowing up- or down-regulation of intensity of respiratory services. Protocols allow the respiratory care practitioner authority to evaluate the patient, initiate care, to adjust, discontinue, or restart respiratory care procedures on a shift-by-shift or hour-to-hour basis once the protocol is ordered by the physician. They must contain clear strategies for various therapeutic interventions, while avoiding any misconception that they infringe on the practice of medicine.

Respiratory TDPs provide the respiratory care practitioner with a wide-ranging flexibility to both *assess* and *treat* the patient—but only within pre-approved and clearly defined boundaries outlined by the physician and/or the medical staff. In addition, respiratory TDPs give the practitioner specific authority to (1) gather clinical information related to the patient's respiratory status, (2) make an assessment of the clinical data collected, and (3) start, increase, decrease, or discontinue certain respiratory therapies on a moment-to-moment, hour-to-hour, shift-by-shift, or day-to-day basis. The innate beauty of respiratory TDPs is that (1) the physician is always in the "information loop" regarding patient care and (2) therapy can be quickly modified in response to the specific and immediate needs of the patient.

RCP STAFF	HOSPITAL SHIFTS 365 DAYS/YR	THERAPIST-DRIVEN PROTOCOL PROGRAM		
		Clinical Data	Assessment	Tx Selection
TDP SAFE AND READY	Days / Evenings / Nights	Systematic Collection of Clinical Data	Uniform and Accurate Assessment	Uniform and Optimal Tx Selections

Figure 9–1   The promise of a good TDP program.

Numerous clinical research studies have verified these facts: Respiratory TDPs (1) significantly improve respiratory therapy outcomes and (2) appreciably lower therapy costs.

The essential components of a good TDP program, however, do not come easy. This is because a strong TDP program promises that the respiratory care practitioner (RCP), who is identified as "TDP safe and ready" is qualified to (1) systematically collect the appropriate clinical data, (2) formulate a uniform and accurate assessment, and (3) select a uniform and optimal treatment within the limits set by the protocol (Figure 9-1). The converse, however, is also true: When the respiratory care practitioner is not "TDP safe and ready," the collection of clinical data is not done at all or is incomplete. As a result, nonuniform or inaccurate assessments are made, resulting in nonuniform or inaccurate treatment selections (Figure 9-2). This inappropriate and ineffective type of respiratory therapy leads to the misallocation of care, the administration of unneeded care, and—most important—the nonprovision of needed patient care.

The bottom line is poor-quality patient care and unnecessary costs. To be sure, the development and implementation of a strong TDP program require some fundamental knowledge, training, and practice, but the benefits are worth the price. The essential components of a good TDP program are discussed in the following paragraphs.

The "Knowledge Base" Required for a Successful TDP Program

As shown in Figure 9-3, the essential knowledge base for a successful TDP program includes (1) the anatomic alterations of the lungs caused by common respiratory disorders, (2) the major pathophysiologic mechanisms activated throughout the respiratory and cardiac systems as a result of the anatomic alterations, (3) the common clinical manifestations that develop as a result of the activated pathophysiologic mechanisms, and (4) the treatment modalities used to correct them. In other words, the clinical manifestations demonstrated by the patient do not arbitrarily appear but are the result of anatomic lung alterations and pathophysiologic events.

Hence, it is essential that the respiratory practitioner know and understand that certain anatomic alterations of the lung will lead to specific—and often predictable—clinical manifestations. Each respiratory disease chapter presented in this textbook describes these four essential knowledge components necessary for TDP work. In the clinical setting, this knowledge base enhances the assessment process essential to a good TDP program.

RCP STAFF	HOSPITAL SHIFTS 365 DAYS/YR	NO THERAPIST-DRIVEN PROTOCOL PROGRAM		
		Clinical Data	Assessment Nonuniform and Inaccurate	Tx Selection Nonuniform and Nonoptimal
NOT TDP SAFE AND READY	Days / Evenings / Nights	Incomplete or NO Collection of Clinical Data	Assessment / Assessment / Assessment	Tx Selection / Tx Selection / Tx Selection

Figure 9–2   No Assessment Program in Place.

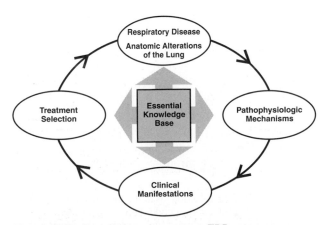

Figure 9–3   Foundations for a strong TDP program. Overview of the essential knowledge base for assessment of respiratory diseases.

The "Assessment Process Skills" Required for a Successful TDP Program

Using the aforementioned knowledge base, the respiratory care practitioner must also be competent in performing the actual assessment process. This means that the practitioner can (1) quickly and systematically gather the clinical information demonstrated by the patient, (2) formulate an accurate assessment of the clinical data (i.e., identify the cause and severity of the problem), (3) select an optimal treatment modality, and (4) document this process quickly, clearly, and precisely. In the clinical setting, the practice—and mastery—of the assessment process is absolutely central and essential to the success of a good TDP program (Figure 9-4). In other words, immediately after the respiratory care practitioner identifies the appropriate *clinical manifestations* (clinical indicators), an *assessment* of the data and *treatment plan* must be formulated. For the most part, the assessment is primarily directed at the anatomic alterations of the lungs that are causing the clinical indicators (e.g., bronchospasm) and the *severity* of the clinical indicators.

For example, an appropriate assessment for the clinical indicator of wheezing might be bronchospasm—the anatomic alteration of the lungs. If the practitioner assesses the cause of the wheezing correctly as bronchospasm, then the correct treatment selection would be a bronchodilator treatment from the Aerosolized Medication Therapy Protocol (see Protocol 9-4, p. 140). If, however, the cause of the wheezing is correctly assessed to be excessive airway secretions,

then the appropriate treatment plan would entail a specific treatment modality under the *Bronchial Hygiene Therapy Protocol,* such as cough and deep breathing or chest physical therapy (see Protocol 9-2, p. 138). Table 9-1 illustrates common clinical manifestations (i.e., clinical indicators), assessments, and treatment selections made by the respiratory care practitioner.

SEVERITY ASSESSMENT

The *frequency* at which a respiratory therapy modality is to be administered is just as important as the correct selection of a respiratory therapy treatment. Often, the frequency of treatment must be up-regulated or down-regulated on a shift-by-shift, hour-to-hour, minute-to-minute, or even (in life-threatening situations) second-to-second basis. Such frequency changes must be made in response to a severity assessment. In a good TDP program, the well-seasoned respiratory care practitioner routinely and systematically documents many severity assessments throughout each working day. For the new practitioner, however, a predesigned *Severity Assessment Rating Form* may be used to enhance this important part of the assessment process. One excellent, semiquantitative method of accomplishing this is illustrated in Table 9-2. The clinical application of this severity assessment is provided in the following case example:

Severity Assessment Case Example

A 67-year-old-male arrived in the emergency room in respiratory distress. The patient was well known to the TDP team; he had been diagnosed with chronic bronchitis several years before this admission (3 points). The patient had no recent surgery history, and he was ambulatory, alert, and cooperative (0 points). He complained of dyspnea and was using his accessory muscles of inspiration (3 points). Auscultation revealed bilateral rhonchi over both lung fields (3 points). His cough was weak and productive of thick gray secretions (3 points). A chest X-ray revealed pneumonia (consolidation) in the left lower lung lobe (3 points). On room air his arterial blood gas values were pH 7.52, $Paco_2$ 54, HCO_3^- 41, and Pao_2 52—acute alveolar hyperventilation on chronic ventilatory failure (3 points).

Using the Severity Assessment Form shown in Table 9-2, the following treatment selection and administration frequency would be appropriate:

Total score: 17

Treatment selection: Chest physical therapy

Frequency of administration: Four times a day; and as needed

Overview of TDP Program

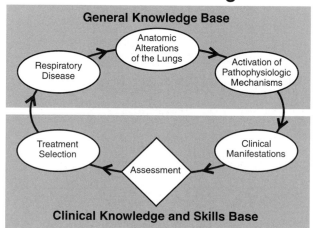

Figure 9–4 The way knowledge, assessment, and a TDP program interface.

TABLE 9–1   Clinical Manifestations, Assessments, and Treatment Selections Commonly Made by the Respiratory Care Practitioner

Clinical Data (indicators)	Assessments	Treatment Selections
Vital Signs		
↑Breathing rate, ↑blood pressure, ↑pulse	Respiratory distress	Treat underlying cause
Airways		
Wheezing	Bronchospasm	Bronchodilator treatment
Inspiratory stridor	Laryngeal edema	Cool mist
Rhonchi	Secretions in large airways	Bronchial hygiene treatment
Crackles	Secretions in distal airways	Treat underlying cause—e.g., congestive heart failure (CHF) Hyperinflation treatment
Cough		
Strong cough	Good ability to mobilize secretions	None
Weak cough	Poor ability to mobilize secretions	Bronchial hygiene treatment
Secretions		
Amount: > 30 ml/24 hrs	Excessive bronchial secretions	Bronchial hygiene treatment
White and translucent sputum	Normal sputum	None
Yellow or opaque sputum	Acute airway infection	Treat underlying cause
Green sputum	Old, retained secretions and infections	Bronchial hygiene treatment
Brown sputum	Old blood	Bronchial hygiene treatment
Red sputum	Fresh blood	Notify physician
Frothy secretions	Pulmonary edema	Treat underlying cause—e.g., congestive heart failure (CHF) Hyperinflation treatment
Alveoli		
Bronchial breath sounds	Atelectasis	Hyperinflation treatment, oxygen treatment
Dull percussion note	Infiltrates or effusion	Treat underlying cause
Opacity on chest X-ray	Fibrosis	No specific treatment
Restrictive pulmonary function test values	Consolidation	No specific, effective respiratory care treatment
Depressed diaphragm on X-ray	Air trapping and hyperinflation	Treat underlying cause
Pleural Space		
Hyperresonant percussion note	Pneumothorax	Evacuate air* and hyperinflation treatment
Dull percussion note	Pleural effusion	Evacuate fluid* and hyperinflation treatment
Thorax		
Paradoxical movement of the chest wall	Flail chest	Mechanical ventilation*
Barrel chest	Air trapping (hyperinflation)	Treat underlying cause—e.g., asthma
Posterior and lateral curvature of spine	Kyphoscoliosis	Bronchial hygiene treatment
Arterial Blood Gases—Ventilatory		
pH↑, $Paco_2$↓, HCO_3^-↓	Acute alveolar hyperventilation	Treat underlying cause
pH N, $Paco_2$↓, HCO_3^-↓↓	Chronic alveolar hyperventilation	Generally none
pH↓, $Paco_2$↑, HCO_3^-↑	Acute ventilatory failure	Mechanical ventilation*
pH N, $Paco_2$↑, HCO_3^-↑↑	Chronic ventilatory failure	Low-flow oxygen, bronchial hygiene
Sudden Ventilatory Changes on Chronic Ventilatory Failure (CVF)		
pH↑, $Paco_2$↑, HCO_3^-↑↑, Pao_2↓	Acute alveolar hyperventilation on CVF	Treat underlying cause
pH↓, $Paco_2$↑↑, HCO_3^-↑ Pao_2↓	Acute ventilatory failure on CVF	Mechanical ventilation*
Metabolic		
pH↑, $Paco_2$N, or ↑, HCO_3^-↑, Pao_2N	Metabolic alkalosis	Give potassium*—Hypokalemia Give chloride*—Hypochloremia
pH↓, $Paco_2$N or ↓, HCO_3^-↓, Pao_2↓	Metabolic acidosis	Give oxygen—Lactic acidosis
pH↓, $Paco_2$N or ↓, HCO_3^-↓, Pao_2N	Metabolic acidosis	Give insulin*—Ketoacidosis
pH↓, $Paco_2$N or ↓, HCO_3^-↓, Pao_2N	Metabolic acidosis	Renal therapy*

Continued

TABLE 9–1   **Clinical Manifestations, Assessments, and Treatment Selections Commonly Made by the Respiratory Care Practitioner—cont'd**

Clinical Data (indicators)	Assessments	Treatment Selections
Indication for Mechanical Ventilation		
$pH\uparrow$, $Paco_2\downarrow$, $HCO_3^-\downarrow$, $Pao_2\downarrow$	Impending ventilatory failure	Mechanical ventilation
$pH\downarrow$, $Paco_2\uparrow$, $HCO_3^-\uparrow$, $Pao_2\downarrow$	Ventilatory failure	
$pH\downarrow$, $Paco_2\uparrow$, $HCO_3^-\uparrow$, $Pao_2\downarrow$	Apnea	
Oxygenation Status		
$Pao_2 < 80$ mm Hg	Mild hypoxemia	Oxygen treatment and treat underlying cause
$Pao_2 < 60$ mm Hg	Moderate hypoxemia	
$Pao_2 < 40$ mm Hg	Severe hypoxemia	
Oxygen Transport Status		
$\downarrow Pao_2$, anemia, $\downarrow$ cardiac output	Inadequate oxygen transport	Oxygen treatment and treat underlying cause

*These procedures should be performed only as ordered by the physician.

The Top Four Respiratory Protocols

The following four commonly used "assess and treat" respiratory protocol algorithms provide the essential foundation of a successful TDP program:

- Oxygen Therapy Protocol (Protocol 9-1)
- Bronchopulmonary Hygiene Therapy Protocol (Protocol 9-2)
- Hyperinflation Therapy Protocol (Protocol 9-3)
- Aerosolized Medication Therapy Protocol (Protocol 9-4)

The vast majority of the daily work performed by the respiratory practitioner involves assessments and treatments associated with these four protocols. Most patients with respiratory problems require care found in one or more of these protocols. These four respiratory protocols are the essential cornerstones of a good TDP program. For example, a patient experiencing an asthmatic episode would likely demonstrate a variety of objective clinical indicators to justify the assessments that call for the administration of *oxygen therapy* (e.g., to treat hypoxemia), an *aerosolized bronchodilator* (e.g., to treat bronchospasm), and *bronchial hygiene therapy* (e.g., to mobilize the thick white secretions associated with asthma).

As shown in the algorithms in Protocols 9-1 through 9-4, a step-by step, branching logic process directs the practitioner to (1) gather clinical data (clinical indicators), (2) make assessment decisions based on the clinical data, and (3) either start, up-regulate, down-regulate, or discontinue a treatment modality. In fact, the primary reason a good TDP program works is because a specific treatment modality cannot be started, stopped, or modified unless there are specific—and measurable—clinical indicators identified to justify the assessment and treatment decision.

It is important to point out, moreover, that the treatment selections outlined in each of the above protocols are based on the AARC's Clinical Practice Guidelines (CPGs), which provide the most recent scientific evidence that justifies the administration of a specific treatment modality. Using the evidence-based method mandated by the scientific community, CPGs provide the indications, contraindications, hazards and complications, assessment of need, assessment of outcome, and appropriate monitoring techniques used for specific therapy modalities. In other words, the CPGs are the *"gold standards"* used by the respiratory care practitioner to start, adjust, or discontinue a specific treatment modality. In Box 9-1, p. 141, excerpts from the AARC's CPG on *oxygen therapy for adults in the acute care facility* provide a representative example of a CPG—and, more important, the scientific basis for the Oxygen Therapy Protocol (Protocol 9-1, p. 137).*

Several different treatment selections are listed under each of the protocols. In essence, the various treatment selections serve as a "therapy selection menu." When the patient demonstrates the clinical indicators associated with any of the aforementioned protocols, the respiratory therapist is expected to select and administer the *most efficient* and *most cost-effective* treatment to the patient. As already discussed, the treatment selection decision and the frequency with which the therapy is to be administered are based on (1) the identification of the appropriate clinical indicators, (2) the severity suggested by the clinical information, (3) the patient's ability to perform or tolerate the therapy, and (4) the patient's response to the therapy.

---

*See http://www.aarc.org/(Clinical Practice Guidelines) for the most recent and complete list of clinical practice guidelines.

TABLE 9-2 Respiratory Care Protocol Severity Assessment

Item	0 Points	1 Points	2 Points	3 Points	4 Points	Total
Respiratory history	Negative for smoking or history not available	Smoking history <1 pack a day	Smoking history >1 pack a day	Pulmonary disease	Severe or exacerbation	
Surgery history	No surgery	General surgery	Lower abdominal	Thoracic or upper abdominal	Thoracic with lung disease	
Level of consciousness	Alert, oriented, cooperative	Disoriented, follows commands	Obtunded, uncooperative	Obtunded	Comatose	
Level of activity	Ambulatory	Ambulatory with assistance	Nonambulatory	Paraplegic	Quadriplegic	
Respiratory pattern	Normal rate 8-20	Respiratory rate 20-25	Patient complains of dyspnea	Dyspnea, use of accessory muscles, prolonged expiration	Severe dyspnea, use of accessory muscles, respiratory rate >25, and/or swallow	
Breath sounds	Clear	Bilateral crackles	Bilateral crackles and rhonchi	Bilateral wheezing, crackles, and rhonchi	Absent and/or diminished bilaterally and/or severe wheezing, crackles, or rhonchi	
Cough	Strong, spontaneous, nonproductive	Excessive bronchial secretions and strong cough	Excessive bronchial secretions but weak cough	Thick bronchial secretions and weak cough	Thick bronchial secretions but no cough	
Chest X-ray	Clear	One lobe: infiltrates, atelectasis, consolidation, or pleural effusion	Same lung, two lobes: infiltrates, atelectasis, consolidation, or pleural effusion	One lobe in both lungs: infiltrates, atelectasis, consolidation, or pleural effusion	Both lungs, more than one lobe: infiltrates, atelectasis, consolidation, or pleural effusion	
Arterial blood gases and/or oxygen saturation measured by pulse oximeter (SpO_2)	Normal	Normal pH and $Paco_2$ but Pao_2 60-80 and/or Spo_2 91-96%	Normal pH and $Paco_2$ 40-60 and/or Spo_2 85-90%	Acute respiratory alkalosis, Pao_2<40 and/or Spo_2 80-84%	Acute respiratory failure, Pao_2<80 and/or Spo_2<80%	

Severity Index

Total Score	Severity Assessment	Treatment Frequency
1-5	Unremarkable	As needed
6-15	Mild	Two or three times a day
16-25	Moderate	Four times a day or as needed
Greater than 26	Severe	Two to four times a day and as needed
		Alert attending physician

136

OXYGEN THERAPY PROTOCOL

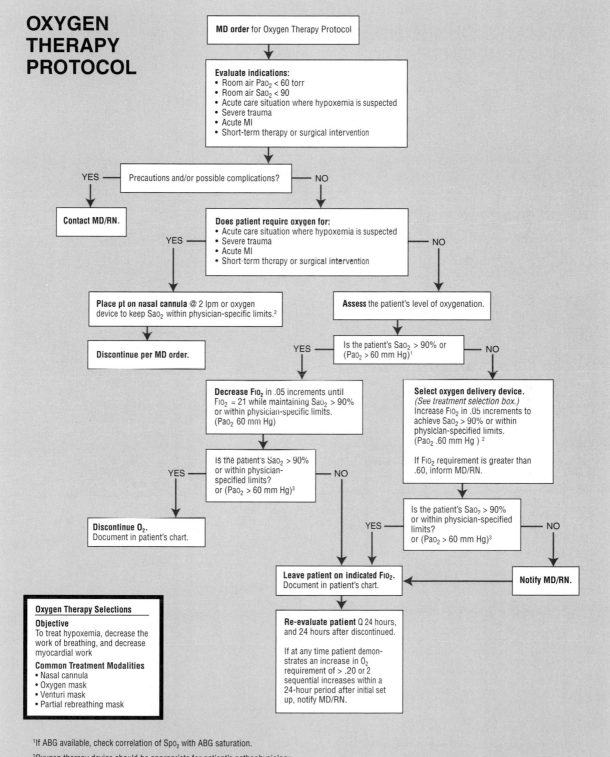

MD order for Oxygen Therapy Protocol

Evaluate indications:
- Room air $Pao_2 < 60$ torr
- Room air $Sao_2 < 90$
- Acute care situation where hypoxemia is suspected
- Severe trauma
- Acute MI
- Short-term therapy or surgical intervention

YES ← Precautions and/or possible complications? → NO

Contact MD/RN.

Does patient require oxygen for:
- Acute care situation where hypoxemia is suspected
- Severe trauma
- Acute MI
- Short-term therapy or surgical intervention

YES → **Place pt on nasal cannula** @ 2 lpm or oxygen device to keep Sao_2 within physician-specific limits.[2]

NO → **Assess** the patient's level of oxygenation.

Discontinue per MD order.

Is the patient's $Sao_2 > 90\%$ or $(Pao_2 > 60$ mm Hg$)$[1]

YES → **Decrease Fio_2** in .05 increments until $Fio_2 = 21$ while maintaining $Sao_2 > 90\%$ or within physician-specific limits. $(Pao_2\ 60$ mm Hg$)$

NO → **Select oxygen delivery device.** *(See treatment selection box.)* Increase Fio_2 in .05 increments to achieve $Sao_2 > 90\%$ or within physician-specified limits. $(Pao_2\ .60$ mm Hg $)$ [2]

If Fio_2 requirement is greater than .60, inform MD/RN.

Is the patient's $Sao_2 > 90\%$ or within physician-specified limits? or $(Pao_2 > 60$ mm Hg$)$[3]

YES → **Discontinue O_2.** Document in patient's chart.

NO ↓

Is the patient's $Sao_2 > 90\%$ or within physician-specified limits? or $(Pao_2 > 60$ mm Hg$)$[3]

YES → **Leave patient on indicated Fio_2.** Document in patient's chart.

NO → **Notify MD/RN.**

Re-evaluate patient Q 24 hours, and 24 hours after discontinued.

If at any time patient demonstrates an increase in O_2 requirement of > .20 or 2 sequential increases within a 24-hour period after initial set up, notify MD/RN.

Oxygen Therapy Selections

Objective
To treat hypoxemia, decrease the work of breathing, and decrease myocardial work

Common Treatment Modalities
- Nasal cannula
- Oxygen mask
- Venturi mask
- Partial rebreathing mask

---

[1]If ABG available, check correlation of Spo_2 with ABG saturation.

[2]Oxygen therapy device should be appropriate for patient's pathophysiology.

[3]Acceptable Fio_2 may vary with the clinical situation or physician.

Protocol 9-1

BRONCHOPULMONARY HYGIENE THERAPY PROTOCOL

MD order for Bronchopulmonary Hygiene Therapy Protocol

↓

Evaluate indications:
- Difficulty with secretion clearance with sputum production > 25 ml/day
- Evidence of retained secretions
- Mucus plug induced atelectasis
- Foreign body in airway
- Diagnosis of cystic fibrosis, bronchiectasis, or cavitating lung disease

↓

YES —— Does contraindication or potential hazard exist? —— NO

Address any immediate need and contact MD/RN.

Select method based on:
- Patient preference/comfort/pain avoidance
- Observation of effectiveness with trial
- History with documented effectiveness

Method may include:
(See treatment selection box.)
- Manual chest percussion and positioning
- External chest wall vibration
- Intrapulmonary percussion

↓

Administer therapy no less than QID and PRN, supplemented by suctioning for all patients with artificial airways.

↓

Re-evaluate pt every 24 hours, and 24 hours after discontinued.

↓

Assess Outcomes — Goals Achieved?
- Optimal hydration with sputum production > 25 ml/day
- Breath sounds from diminished to adventitious with rhonchi cleared by cough.
- Patient subjective impression of less retention and improved clearance
- Resolution/improvement in chest X-ray
- Improvement in vital signs and measures of gas exchange
- If on ventilator, reduced resistance and improved compliance

↓

Care Plan Considerations:
- Discontinue therapy if improvement is observed and sustained over a 24-hour period.
- Patients with chronic pulmonary disease who maintain secretion clearance in their home environment should remain on treatment no less than their home frequency.
- Hyperinflation Protocol (9-3) should be considered for patients who are at high risk for pulmonary complications as listed in the indications for Hyperinflation Protocol.

Bronchial Hygiene Therapy Selections

Objective
To enhance mobilization of bronchial secretions

Common Treatment Modalities
- Increased bronchial hydration
    - Increased fluid intake
        - (6-10 glasses of water a day)
    - Bland aerosol therapy
    - Ultrasonic nebulization (USN)
- Cough and deep breathing (C & DB)
    - Techniques used to enhance C & DB
        - Incentive spirometry (IS)
        - Intermittent positive-pressure breathing (IPPB)
        - Positive expiratory pressure (PEP) therapy
        - Flutter valve
- Chest physical therapy (CPT)
- Postural drainage (PD)
- Percussion and vibration with postural drainage
- Suctioning
- Mucolytic therapy (see Protocol 9-4)
    - Acetylcysteine (Mucomyst)—often in combination with a bronchodilator
    - Recombinant human deoxyribonuclease (DNase, Pulmozyme)
    - Sodium bicarbonate (2% solution)
- Assist physician in bronchoscopy

Protocol 9-2

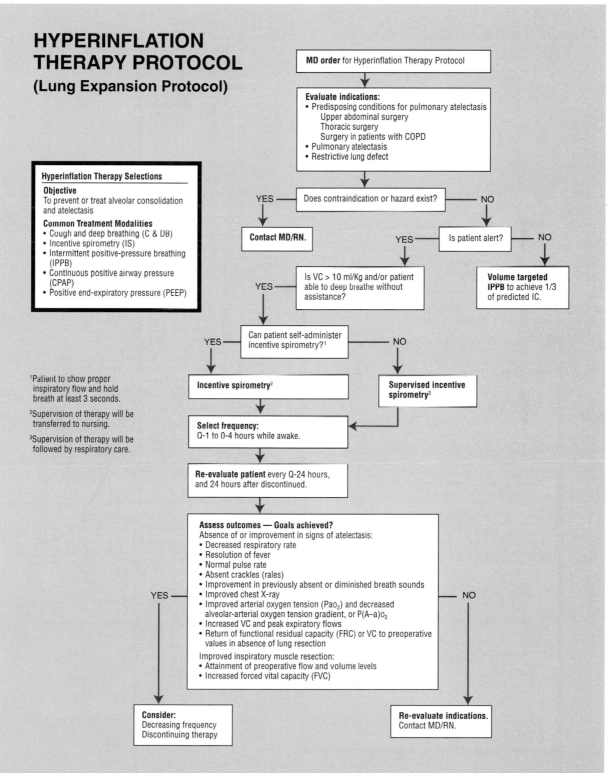

HYPERINFLATION THERAPY PROTOCOL
(Lung Expansion Protocol)

MD order for Hyperinflation Therapy Protocol

Evaluate indications:
- Predisposing conditions for pulmonary atelectasis
  Upper abdominal surgery
  Thoracic surgery
  Surgery in patients with COPD
- Pulmonary atelectasis
- Restrictive lung defect

Hyperinflation Therapy Selections

Objective
To prevent or treat alveolar consolidation and atelectasis

Common Treatment Modalities
- Cough and deep breathing (C & DB)
- Incentive spirometry (IS)
- Intermittent positive-pressure breathing (IPPB)
- Continuous positive airway pressure (CPAP)
- Positive end-expiratory pressure (PEEP)

YES ← Does contraindication or hazard exist? → NO

Contact MD/RN.

YES — Is patient alert? — NO

Is VC > 10 ml/Kg and/or patient able to deep breathe without assistance? — YES

Volume targeted IPPB to achieve 1/3 of predicted IC.

Can patient self-administer incentive spirometry?[1] — NO → YES

Incentive spirometry[2]

Supervised incentive spirometry[3]

Select frequency:
Q-1 to 0-4 hours while awake.

[1] Patient to show proper inspiratory flow and hold breath at least 3 seconds.

[2] Supervision of therapy will be transferred to nursing.

[3] Supervision of therapy will be followed by respiratory care.

Re-evaluate patient every Q-24 hours, and 24 hours after discontinued.

Assess outcomes — Goals achieved?
Absence of or improvement in signs of atelectasis:
- Decreased respiratory rate
- Resolution of fever
- Normal pulse rate
- Absent crackles (rales)
- Improvement in previously absent or diminished breath sounds
- Improved chest X-ray
- Improved arterial oxygen tension (Pao_2) and decreased alveolar-arterial oxygen tension gradient, or $P(A–a)o_2$
- Increased VC and peak expiratory flows
- Return of functional residual capacity (FRC) or VC to preoperative values in absence of lung resection

Improved inspiratory muscle resection:
- Attainment of preoperative flow and volume levels
- Increased forced vital capacity (FVC)

YES ← → NO

Consider:
Decreasing frequency
Discontinuing therapy

Re-evaluate indications.
Contact MD/RN.

Protocol 9-3

AEROSOLIZED MEDICATION THERAPY PROTOCOL

MD order for Aerosol Medication Therapy Protocol

↓

Evaluate indications:
The primary general indication for aerosolized bronchodilator therapy is reversible reactive airway disease. This condition is detected through the following symptoms:
• C/O dyspnea
• Wheezing
• Hyperinflation
• Reduction in airflow (peak flow, FEV$_1$, FVC, prolonged expiration)

↓

Does contraindication or potential hazard exist?

YES ←——— ———→ NO

Respond to immediate need and contact MD/RN.

Select aerosols for bronchospasm:
• Sympathomimetic agent
• Combine with anti-inflammatory if history of COPD (if used on a daily basis)
• Anticholinergics

Select device:
Meter Dose Inhaler (MDI) with accessory device is the preferred delivery method, unless the medication is not available in MDI, or the patient is unable to use the device with proper coaching and instruction. In which case a small volume nebulizer with equivalent dose may be used.

↓

Administer therapy no less than Q4 and PRN.
*Note that MDI dose may be titrated upward to a total of 16 puffs (with 1 minute between activations) if the patient continues to be symptomatic without dose-limiting side effects.

↓

Re-evaluate patient every 24 hours, and 24 hours after discontinued.

↓

Assess outcomes — Goals achieved?
• Diminished wheezing and the volume of air moved is increased
• Improvement in airflow (peak flow, PFT)
• Improved vital signs and measures of gas exchange
• Improved patient appearance with decreased use of accessory muscles

↓

Care Plan Considerations:
Discontinue therapy if improvement is observed and sustained over a 24-hour period. Patients with COPD or asthma who maintain aerosol bronchodilators in their home environment should remain on treatment no less than their home regimen.

Aerosolized Medication Therapy Selections

AEROSOLIZED BRONCHODILATORS
Objective
Sympathomimetics and parasympatholytics are used to offset bronchial smooth muscle constriction. Common treatment modalities are:

Sympathomimetics
Short-to-Intermediate-Acting
• Metaproterenol (Alupent, Metaprel)
• Terbutaline (Brethine, Brethaire)
• Pirbuterol (Maxair)
• Albuterol (Ventoline, Proventil)
• Levalbuterol (Xopenex)
Long-Acting
• Salmeterol (Serevent)
• Formoterol (Foradil)

Parasympatholytics (anticholinergics)
• Atropine sulfate (Dey-Dose Atropine Sulfate)
• Ipratropium bromide (Atrovent)
• Tiotroprium (Spirva)
• Ipratropium bromide and Albuterol (Combivent)

MUCOLYTIC AGENTS
Objective
Mucolytic agents are used to enhance the mobilization and thinning of bronchial secretions. Common treatment modalities are:

• Acetylcysteine (Mucomyst)
• Dornase alpha (Pulmozyme, rhDNase, DNase)
• Sodium bicarbonate (2% solution)

ANTIINFLAMMATORY AGENTS
Objective
Aerosolized corticosteroids are used to suppress bronchial inflammation and edema. They also are used for their ability to enhance the responsiveness of B$_2$ receptor sites to sympathomimetic agents. Common modalities are:

• Beclomethasone dipropionate (Beclovent, Vanceril)
• Triamcinolone acetonide (Azmacort)
• Flunisolide (AeroBid, AeroBid-M)
• Fluticasone propionate (Flovent)
• Budesonide (Pulmicort Turbuhaler, Pulmicort Respules)
• Fluticasone propionate and Salmeterol (Advair Diskus)

*Note that this protocol is for simple bronchodilator administration for non-ventilated patients. There are a variety of other options such as continuous bronchodilator administration, acute maximum titration of dose, and multiple delivery devices that can be incorporated within this protocol or as a separate protocol depending on site-specific preference.

Protocol 9-4

BOX 9–1

Oxygen Therapy for Adults in the Acute Care Facility

AARC Clinical Practice Guideline (Excerpts)*

INDICATIONS
- Documented hypoxemia. Defined as a decreased Pao_2 in the blood below normal range.
  - $Pao_2 < 60$ mm Hg or $Sao_2 < 90\%$ in subjects breathing room air
- Acute care situations in which hypoxemia is suspected
- Severe trauma
- Acute myocardial infarction
- Short-term therapy or surgical intervention (e.g., postanesthesia recovery, hip surgery)

CONTRAINDICATIONS
- No specific contraindications to oxygen therapy exist when indications are present.

PRECAUTIONS AND/OR POSSIBLE COMPLICATIONS
- $Pao_2 > 60$ mm Hg may depress ventilation in some patients with elevated $Paco_2$.
- $Fio_2 > 0.5$, may cause absorption atelectasis, oxygen toxicity, and/or ciliary or leukocyte depression.
- Supplemental oxygen should be administered with caution to patients with paraquat poisoning or to those receiving bleomycin.
- During laser bronchoscopy, minimal Fio_2 should be used to avoid intratracheal ignition.
- Fire hazard is increased in the presence of increased oxygen concentration.
- Bacterial contamination associated with nebulizers or humidifiers is a possible hazard.

ASSESSMENT OF NEED
- Need is determined by measurement of inadequate oxygen tension and/or saturation, by invasive or noninvasive methods, and/or the presence of clinical indicators.

ASSESSMENT OF OUTCOME
- Outcome is determined by clinical and physiologic assessment to establish adequacy of patient response to therapy.

MONITORING
- Patient
- Clinical assessment including cardiac, pulmonary, and neurologic status
- Assessment of physiologic parameters (Pao_2, Sao_2, Spo_2) in conjunction with the initiation of therapy or:
  - Within 12 hours of initiation with $Fio_2 < 40$
  - Within 8 hours with $Fio_2 >$ or $= 0.40$ (including postanesthesia recovery)
  - Within 72 hours in acute myocardial infarction
  - Within 2 hours for any patient with principal diagnosis of COPD
- Equipment
  - All oxygen delivery systems should be checked at least once per day.
- More frequent checks are needed in systems:
  - Susceptible to variation in oxygen concentration (e.g., hood, high-flow blending systems)
  - Applied to patients with artificial airways
  - Delivering a heated gas mixture
  - Applied to patients who are clinically unstable or who require $Fio_2 > 0.50$.
- Care should be taken to avoid interruption of oxygen therapy in situations including ambulation or transport for procedure.

From *Respir Care* 47(6):717-720, 2002. See this article for the complete guidelines.

For example, the implementation of the Hyperinflation Therapy Protocol would likely be indicated after thoracic surgery to prevent, or correct, atelectasis. However, if the patient were unconscious or unable to follow directions, a continuous positive airway pressure (CPAP) mask would be a more appropriate treatment selection (under the Hyperinflation Therapy Protocol) than, say, incentive spirometry—even though both are designed to treat or prevent atelectasis. In this example, the CPAP mask therapy would be more expensive but more appropriate than the less expensive incentive spirometry. Remember, the treatment portion of a protocol is based on the therapy that will *best* work to correct or offset the anatomic alterations and pathophysiologic mechanisms caused by the respiratory disorder in a timely and cost-efficient manner.

Mechanical Ventilation Protocol—the Fifth Protocol

Even when the patient is transferred to the intensive care unit, intubated, and placed on a mechanical ventilator, the respiratory care practitioner must usually still administer one or more of the four respiratory therapy treatment protocols (e.g., Hyperinflation Therapy Protocol via CPAP or positive end-expiratory pressure [PEEP] or an in-line aerosolized medication such as a bronchodilator). For the purpose of this textbook, the authors have chosen to refer to a Mechanical Ventilation Protocol as the Fifth Protocol (Protocol 9-5). The high-technology, high-risk, high-visibility portion of respiratory care work is clearly embedded in ventilator management. Much of the success of the TDP movement has occurred because of the dramatic ways in which standardized, data-driven algorithms have improved patient outcomes. Most dramatic are hastened ventilator weaning times, reduction of nosocomial infections, and reduced complication rates of mechanical ventilation (e.g., barotrauma). Table 9-3 provides an overview of common ventilatory management strategies and good starting points used to treat specific pulmonary disorders.

Overview Summary of a Good TDP Program

Figure 9-5 provides an overview of the essential components of a good TDP program. As illustrated, the implementation of every respiratory care plan must be directly linked to (1) a physician's order, (2) the identification and documentation of specific clinical indicators (obtained from both the patient's chart and physical examination), (3) a bedside respiratory assessment and severity assessment, (4)

a treatment selection that is both therapeutic and cost efficient, and (5) the re-evaluation of the patient's response to the treatment.

This step-by-step process mandates that the respiratory care practitioner (1) have a strong knowledge base of the major respiratory disorders, and (2) be competent in the actual assessment process (see Figure 9-4). Figure 9-6 provides an assessment form with common examples for each category (i.e., clinical indicators, respiratory assessments, and treatment plans). The examples shown in Figure 9-6 can easily be transferred to the *subjective-objective-assessment-plan (SOAP)* format. The SOAP format used in the assessment of respiratory diseases is discussed in more detail in Chapter 10.

Common Anatomic Alterations of the Lungs

Although the respiratory care practitioner may treat one or two cases of every respiratory disorder presented in this book, most of the respiratory care practitioner's professional career will be spent caring for only a few of them. For example, the *diagnosis-related-group (DRG)* and *ICD-10* identification systems show that more than 80% of the respiratory care practitioner's work is concerned with intelligent assessment and treatment selection for a relatively short list of respiratory illnesses (Table 9-4).

Therefore the most common anatomic alterations of the lungs treated by the respiratory care practitioner can be derived by recognizing the most common DRG respiratory disorders identified in Table 9-4. The major anatomic alterations include (1) *atelectasis* (which occurs from mucus plugging, upper abdominal surgery, or pneumothorax), (2) *consolidation* (e.g., pneumonia), (3) *increased alveolar-capillary membrane thickness* (e.g., acute respiratory distress syndrome [ARDS], pneumoconiosis, or pulmonary edema), (4) *bronchospasm* (e.g., asthma), (5) *excessive bronchial secretions* (e.g., chronic bronchitis, asthma, pulmonary edema), and (6) *distal airway and alveolar weakening* (e.g., emphysema). Each of these anatomic alterations of the lung in turn leads to a chain of events that can be summarized in the following clinical scenarios.

CLINICAL SCENARIOS ACTIVATED BY COMMON ANATOMIC ALTERATIONS OF THE LUNGS

Specific anatomic alterations of the lung (such as the ones listed previously) lead to the activation of specific and predictable pathophysiologic mechanisms, and to their effects. The more common pathophysiologic

(Text continued on p. 149)

MECHANICAL VENTILATION PROTOCOL

Patient meets criteria for Mechanical Ventilation Protocol.

Clinical indications for Mechanical Ventilation Protocol:
• Acute ventilatory failure
• Apnea
• Impending ventilatory failure
• Conditions that may require mechanical ventilation
  Acute exacerbation of COPD
  Neuromuscular disorders
  Cardiac or respiratory arrest
  Postoperative patients requiring ongoing sedation

Reversal of underlying conditions

Adjustment of ventilatory support to meet patient's physical condition:
• Airway establishment (intubation) and management
• Cuff management
• Ventilatory management
  Respiratory rate (frequency), tidal volume
  Oxygen concentration (Fio_2) (see Protocol 9-1)
Ventilator System Pressure
  Peak pressure
  Mean airway pressure (MAP)
  Continuous positive airway pressure (CPAP)
Ventilator Mode
  Assist control (A/C)
  Intermittent mandatory ventilation (IMV)
  Synchronized intermittent mechanical ventilation (SIMC)
  Pressure support (PS)
  Pressure regulated control (PRVC)

Ventilatory weaning protocol

Daily assessment of readiness to undergo Spontaneous Breathing Trial (SBT):
• Improvement or resolution of underlying condition
• Fio_2: < 50% with Spo_2 > 90%
• PEEP: < 8 cm H_2O
• Hemodynamic status: normal or near normal without vasopressors
• Hb: > 8 g%
• Core temperature: < 38.5°C
• Nutrition status: normal or near normal serum albumin levels

Rapid shallow breathing index < 100 ← **One minute SBT to determine readiness for prolonged SBT** → Rapid shallow breathing index > 100

SBT of 30 to 120 minutes as tolerated until patient can tolerate full 120 minutes SBT

Slow, progressive withdrawal of pressure support until able to tolerate 120 minutes SBT

Extubation

Protocol 9-5

TABLE 9-3 Common Ventilatory Management Strategies Used to Treat Specific Disorders (Good Starting Points)

Disorder	Disease Characteristics	Ventilator Mode	Tidal Volume and Respiratory Rate	Flow Rate	I:E Ratio	FIO₂	General Goals and/or Concerns
Normal Lung Mechanics	Normal compliance & airway resistance	Volume ventilation in the AC or SIMV mode.	10-12 ml/kg of ideal body weight	60-80 L/min	1:2	Low to moderate	Care to ensure plateau pressure of 30 cm H₂O or less.
But patient has apnea			10-12 bpm or slower rates (6-10 bpm) when SIMV mode is used				Small tidal volumes (< 7 ml/kg) should be avoided, since atelectasis can develop
(e.g., drug overdose or abdominal surgery)		Or pressure ventilation—either PRVC or PC					
Chronic Obstructive Pulmonary Disease	High lung compliance and high airway resistance	Volume ventilation in the AC or SIMV mode	Good starting point: 10 ml/kg and a rate of 10 to 12 bpm	60 L/min	1:2 or 1:3	Low to moderate	Air trapping and auto-PEEP can occur when expiratory time is too short. The preferred method of managing auto-PEEP is to increase expiratory time.
(e.g., chronic bronchitis or emphysema)		Or pressure ventilation—either PRVC or PC	A smaller tidal volume (8-10 ml/kg) and slightly slower rate (8-10 bpm) with increased flow rates to allow adequate expiratory time	60-100 L/min			In severe cases, the development of auto-PEEP may be inevitable. With controlled ventilation, a small amount of PEEP to offset auto-PEEP may be cautiously applied.
		Noninvasive positive pressure ventilation (NPPV) by nasal or full face mask is a good alternative during acute exacerbation					Inspiratory flow up to 100 L/min may be helpful in decreasing inspiratory time and increasing expiratory time

Condition	Pathophysiology	Mode	Tidal Volume/Rate	Flow	I:E Ratio	FIO₂	Special Considerations
Acute Asthmatic Episode	High airway resistance (bronchospasm and excessive thick airway secretions)	The SIMV mode is recommended to avoid patient triggering at an increased rate—leading to a decrease in expiratory time and further air trapping	Good starting point: 8 to 10 ml/kg and rate of 10-12 bpm. When air trapping is extensive, a lower tidal volume (5-6 ml/kg) and slower rate may be required	60 L/min	1:2 or 1:3	Start at 100% and titrate downward as pulse oximetric findings and arterial blood gas values permit	Tidal volume or rate may be decreased to reduce inspiratory and increasing expiratory time. Care to avoid overventilating COPD patients with chronically high $Paco_2$ levels. In severe cases, the development of auto-PEEP may be inevitable. With controlled ventilation, a small amount of PEEP to offset auto-PEEP may be cautiously applied.
Acute Respiratory Distress Syndrome	Diffuse, uneven alveolar injury	Volume ventilation in the AC or SIMV mode. Or pressure ventilation—either PRVC or PC	Typically started at low tidal volumes and higher respiratory rate. Initial tidal volume set at 8 ml/kg and adjusted downward to 6 ml/kg. May be as low as 4 ml/kg. Respiratory rates as high as 35 bpm may be required	60-80 L/min	1:1 or 1:2. Do what is necessary to meet a rapid respiratory rate	Fio_2 less than 0.6 if possible	The goal is to limit transpulmonary pressure and the resultant barotraumas caused by overdistending portions of the lungs. Maintaining a plateau pressure of 30 cm H_2O or less is preferred. PEEP is usually required with a low tidal volume to prevent atelectasis. The $Paco_2$ may be allowed to increase (permissive hypercapnia). The hypercapnia is not a therapeutic goal, it is a tradeoff and may be accepted as a lung protective strategy when lower airway pressures are necessary.

Continued

TABLE 9-3 Common Ventilatory Management Strategies Used to Treat Specific Disorders (Good Starting Points)—cont'd

Disorder	Disease Characteristics	Ventilator Mode	Tidal Volume and Respiratory Rate	Flow Rate	I:E Ratio	Fio$_2$	General Goals and/or Concerns
Postoperative Ventilatory Support (e.g., coronary artery bypass surgery, heart valve and replacement)	Often normal compliance and airway resisitance	SIMV with pressure support or AC volume ventilation are acceptable modes Or pressure ventilation— either PRVC or PC	Good starting point: 10 to 12 ml/kg and a rate of 10 to 12 bpm However, a larger tidal volume (12-15 ml/kg) and slower rate (6-10 bpm) may be used to maintain lung volume	60 L/min	1:2	Low to moderate	PEEP or CPAP of 3 to 5 cm H$_2$O may be applied to offset the development of atelectasis
Neuromuscular Disorder (e.g., myasthenia gravis or Guillain-Barre syndrome)	Normal compliance and airway resistance	Volume ventilation in the AC or SIMV mode Or pressure ventilation— either PRVC or PC	Good starting point: 12 to 15 ml/kg and a rate of 10 to 12 bpm	60 L/min	1:2	Low to moderate	PEEP of 3 to 5 cm H$_2$O may be applied to offset the development of atelectasis

AC, Assist-control; *SIMV*, synchronous intermittent mandatory ventilation; *PRVC*, pressure regulated volume control; *PC*, pressure control; *CPAP*, continous positive airway pressure; *bpm*, breaths per minute.

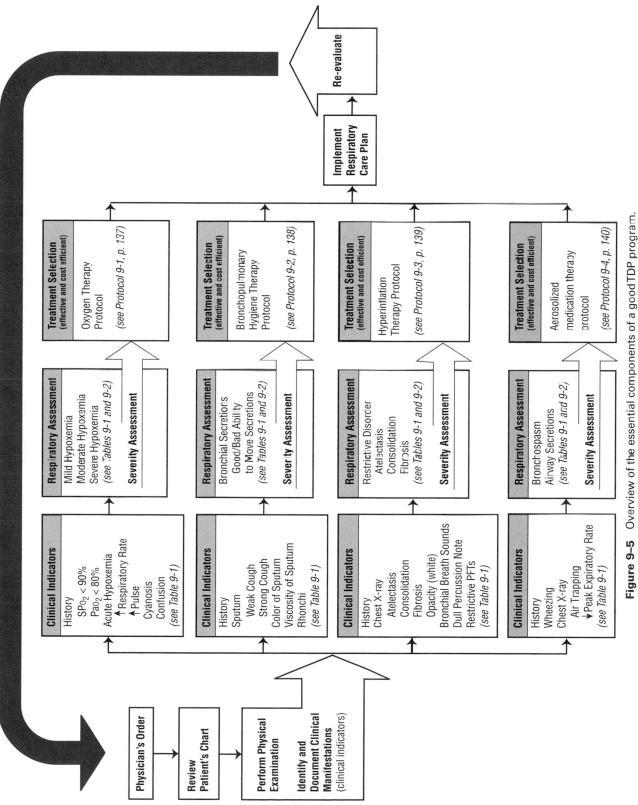

Figure 9–5 Overview of the essential components of a good TDP program.

Patient Identification Box	Date:_____	Admitting Diagnosis:_____
	Time:_____	Attending Physician:_____

Clinical Indicators (see Table 9-1)			
Oxygen Therapy	Bronchial Hygiene Therapy	Hyperinflation Therapy	Aerosolized Medication

Examples:
 	
☐ History
☐ Spo$_2$ <80%
☐ Pao$_2$ <80 mm Hg
☐ Acute hypoxemia
  ☐ ↑Respiratory rate
  ☐ ↑Pulse
  ☐ Cyanosis
  ☐ Confusion
  ☐ Other
	Examples:
	
	☐ History
	☐ Sputum
	  ☐ Weak cough
	  ☐ Color of sputum
	  ☐ Viscosity of sputum
	  ☐ Rhonchi
		Examples:
		
		☐ History
		☐ Chest X-ray
		  ☐ Atelectasis
		  ☐ Consolidation
		  ☐ Fibrosis
		  ☐ Opacity (white)
		☐ Bronchial breath sounds
		☐ Restrictive PFT values
			Examples:
			
			☐ History
			☐ Wheezing
			☐ Chest X-ray
			  ☐ Air trapping
			☐ Obstructive PFT values

Respiratory Assessments (see Tables 9-1 and 9-2)			
Oxygen Therapy	Bronchial Hygiene Therapy	Hyperinflation Therapy	Aerosolized Medication
Examples: ☐ Mild hypoxemia ☐ Moderate hypoxemia ☐ Severe hypoxemia Severity Score:_____	Examples: ☐ Excessive sputum production ☐ Thick secretions ☐ Weak cough Severity Score:_____	Examples: ☐ Atelectasis ☐ Consolidation ☐ Weak diaphragm Severity Score:_____	Examples: ☐ Bronchospasm ☐ Thick secretions ☐ Bronchial edema Severity Score:_____

Treatment Plans			
Oxygen Therapy (see Protocol 9-1)	Bronchial Hygiene Therapy (see Protocol 9-2)	Hyperinflation Therapy (see Protocol 9-3)	Aerosolized Medication (see Protocol 9-4)
Examples: ☐ Nasal cannula ☐ Oxygen mask ☐ 28% Venturi mask Frequency:_____	Examples: ☐ Deep breath and cough ☐ Chest physical therapy ☐ Postural drainage Frequency:_____	Examples: ☐ Incentive spirometry ☐ CPAP ☐ PEEP Frequency:_____	Examples: ☐ Metaproterenol ☐ Albuterol ☐ Acetylcysteine Frequency:_____

Reevaluation Date:_____	Therapist Signature:_____

Figure 9–6 Respiratory care protocol program assessment form.

TABLE 9–4 Common Respiratory Disorders

Respiratory Disorder	DRG Number*	ICD-10 Code†
Chronic bronchitis	088	491.1, 491.9
Emphysema	088	492.8
Asthma	096	493.0
Acute pneumonia	079, 089, 090	(see below)
Aspiration pneumonia	079	507.0
Atelectasis	101/102	518.89
Adult respiratory distress syndrome	099/102	518.82
Interstitial fibrosis	089	515.0
Pulmonary edema/congested heart failure	127	402.91
Acute respiratory failure	087	518.81
Respiratory failure with ventilatory support	475	96.7
Respiratory failure/tracheostomy/ventilatory support	483	96.72/31.1

*Respiratory disorders can be identified by their respective diagnosis-related group (DRG). DRG is an identification system used to categorize and document diseases, primarily for use in health care reimbursement (such as Medicaid and Medicare). Patients are routinely assigned a DRG based on their admitting diagnosis, and each DRG communicates information about patients. Because the use of DRGs is prevalent, respiratory care practitioners should recognize and understand the DRGs that they will commonly encounter.
†The ICD-10 code numbers are used for reimbursement with other third party payers. The ICD-10 system is more specific than the DRG system. For example, pneumococcal pneumonia is listed as ICD # 418.0, *Haemophilus influenzae* is ICD # 482.2, etc.

mechanisms are listed in Box 9-2. The pathophysiologic mechanisms in turn activate specific and predictable clinical manifestations (see Figure 9-3). For the purposes of this text, the authors have chosen to refer to the interrelationship among the major anatomic alterations of the lung, the pathophysiologic mechanisms, and the clinical manifestations that result as *"clinical scenarios."* To enhance the reader's knowledge and understanding of commonly encountered respiratory disorders, clinical scenarios for the anatomic alterations presented in the following paragraphs are provided.*

Atelectasis

Figure 9-7 shows the pathophysiologic mechanisms caused by atelectasis (such as that occurring after thoracic surgery), the clinical manifestations that result, and the treatment protocols used to offset them. The hypoxemia that results from atelectasis is caused by capillary shunting. This type of hypoxemia is often refractory to oxygen therapy. Therefore the implementation of the Hyperinflation Therapy

---

*The Case Study Discussion Section at the end of each respiratory disease chapter often refers the reader back to these clinical scenarios—correlating various clinical manifestations to specific pathophysiologic mechanisms and anatomic alterations of the lungs.

BOX 9–2

Pathophysiologic Mechanisms Commonly Activated in Respiratory Disorders

- Decreased ventilation/perfusion ($\dot{V}/\dot{Q}$) ratio
- Alveolar diffusion block
- Decreased lung compliance
- Stimulation of oxygen receptors
- Deflation reflex
- Irritant reflex
- Pulmonary reflex
- Increased airway resistance
- Air trapping and alveolar hyperinflation

Protocol may be more beneficial in the treatment of hypoxemia than the Oxygen Therapy Protocol in such a patient.

Alveolar Consolidation

Figure 9-8 shows the pathophysiologic mechanisms caused by alveolar consolidation (e.g., pneumonia), the clinical manifestations that result, and the treatment protocols used to offset them. The hypoxemia that develops as a result of consolidation is caused by capillary shunting. This type of hypoxemia is often *refractory* to oxygen therapy.

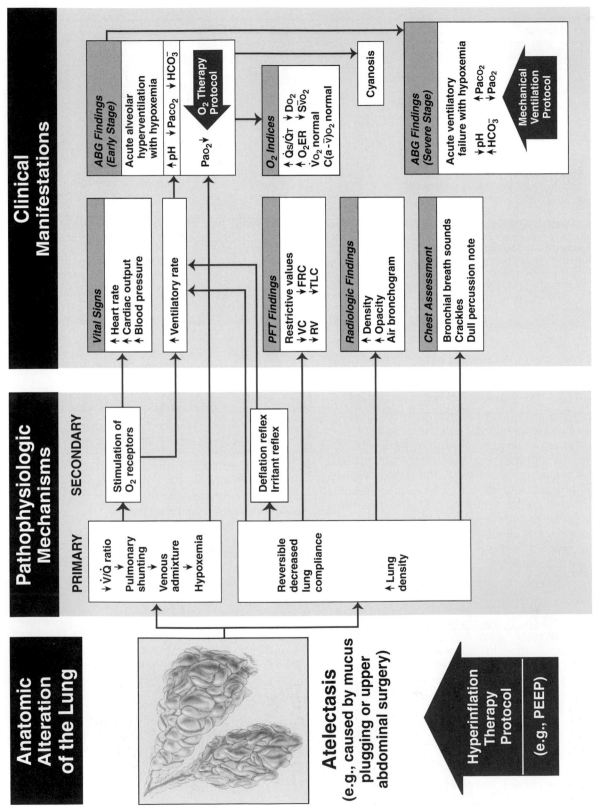

Figure 9–7 Atelectasis Clinical Scenario.

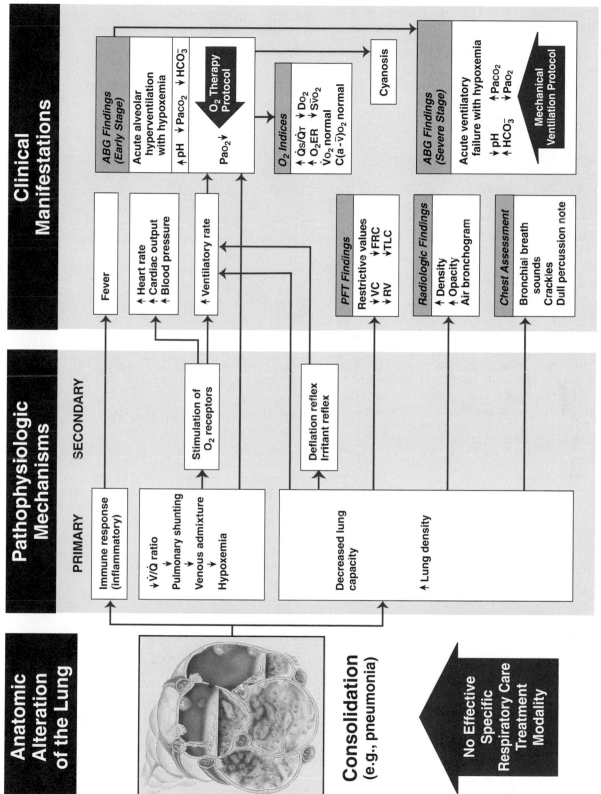

Figure 9-8 Alveolar Consolidation Clinical Scenario.

Depending on the severity of the alveolar consolidation, the Hyperinflation Therapy Protocol or the Oxygen Therapy Protocol may be beneficial. In general, however, there is no effective, specific respiratory care treatment modality for alveolar consolidation. With pneumonia the great temptation for the respiratory care practitioner is to do too much, such as instituting hyperinflation therapy, bronchodilator therapy, and bronchopulmonary hygiene therapy. Such treatment protocols generally are not indicated, especially during the early stages of the disease process. Appropriate antibiotics (prescribed by the physician), bed rest, fluids, and supplementary oxygen are all that is usually needed. When pneumonia is in its resolution stage, however, the patient may experience excessive secretions and atelectasis, accompanied by bronchoconstriction. At this time, other treatment modalities may be indicated.

Increased Alveolar-Capillary Membrane Thickness

Figure 9-9 illustrates the major pathophysiologic mechanisms caused by increased alveolar-capillary membrane thickness (e.g., postoperative ARDS, pulmonary edema, asbestosis, chronic interstitial lung disease), the clinical manifestations that develop, and the treatment protocols used to offset them. The hypoxemia that develops as a result of an increased alveolar-capillary membrane thickness is caused by an alveolar diffusion block. This type of hypoxemia often responds favorably to oxygen therapy.

Bronchospasm

Figure 9-10 shows the major pathophysiologic mechanisms activated by bronchospasm (e.g., asthma), the clinical manifestations that result, and the appropriate treatment protocols used to offset them. The Aerosolized Medication Therapy Protocol (Bronchodilator Therapy) is the primary treatment modality used to offset the anatomic alterations of bronchospasm (the original cause of the pathophysiologic chain of events). The *Oxygen Therapy Protocol* and *Mechanical Ventilation Protocol* are secondary treatment modalities used to offset the mild, moderate, or severe clinical manifestations associated with bronchospasm. In other words, when the patient responds favorably to the *Aerosolized Medication Therapy Protocol,* the need for the *Oxygen Therapy Protocol* may be minimal and the *Mechanical Ventilation Protocol* may not be necessary at all.

Excessive Bronchial Secretions

Figure 9-11 illustrates the major pathophysiologic mechanisms caused by excessive bronchial secretions

Key to Abbreviations in Figs. 9-7 through 9-12

ABG	=	Arterial blood gas
ARDS	=	Adult respiratory distress syndrome
CPAP	=	Continuous positive airway pressure
CPT	=	Chest physical therapy
DO_2	=	Total oxygen delivery
ERV	=	Expiratory reserve volume
FEF	=	Forced expiratory flow, mid-expiratory phase
FEV_1	=	Forced expiratory volume in 1 second
FEV_T	=	Forced expiratory volume, timed
FRC	=	Functional residual capacity
FVC	=	Forced vital capacity
IC	=	Inspiratory capacity
MVV	=	Maximum voluntary ventilation
O_2ER	=	Oxygen extraction ratio
PD	=	Postural drainage
PEEP	=	Positive end-expiratory pressure
PEFR	=	Peak expiratory flow rate
PFT	=	Pulmonary function test
$\dot{Q}s/\dot{Q}t$	=	Shunt fraction
RV	=	Residual volume
$S\bar{v}_{O_2}$	=	Mixed venous oxygen saturation
TLC	=	Total lung capacity
VC	=	Vital capacity
$\dot{V}/\dot{Q}$	=	Ventilation/perfusion ratio

(e.g., chronic bronchitis, asthma), the clinical manifestations that result, and the appropriate treatment protocols used to correct them. When the patient demonstrates chronic ventilatory failure during the advanced stages of respiratory disorders associated with chronic excessive airway secretions (e.g., chronic bronchitis), caution must be taken not to overoxygenate the patient.

Distal Airway and Alveolar Weakening

Figure 9-12 illustrates the major pathophysiologic mechanisms caused by distal airway and alveolar weakening (e.g., emphysema), the clinical manifestations that result, and the appropriate treatment protocols used to offset them. Pulmonary rehabilitation and oxygen therapy may be all the practitioner can provide to treat disorders associated with distal airway and alveolar weakening. When the patient demonstrates chronic ventilatory failure during the advanced stages of the disorder, caution must be taken with the *Oxygen Therapy Protocol* not to overoxygenate the patient.

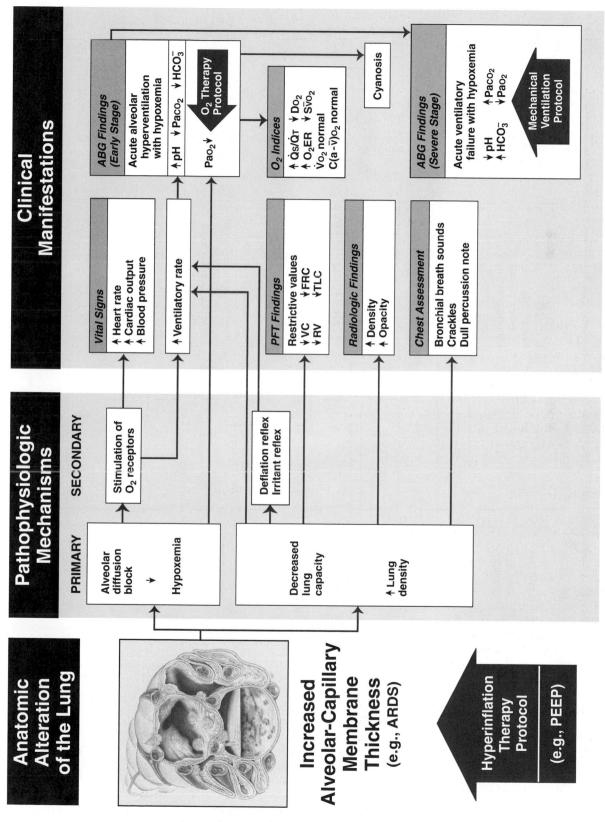

Figure 9–9 Increased Alveolar-Capillary Membrane Thickness Clinical Scenario.

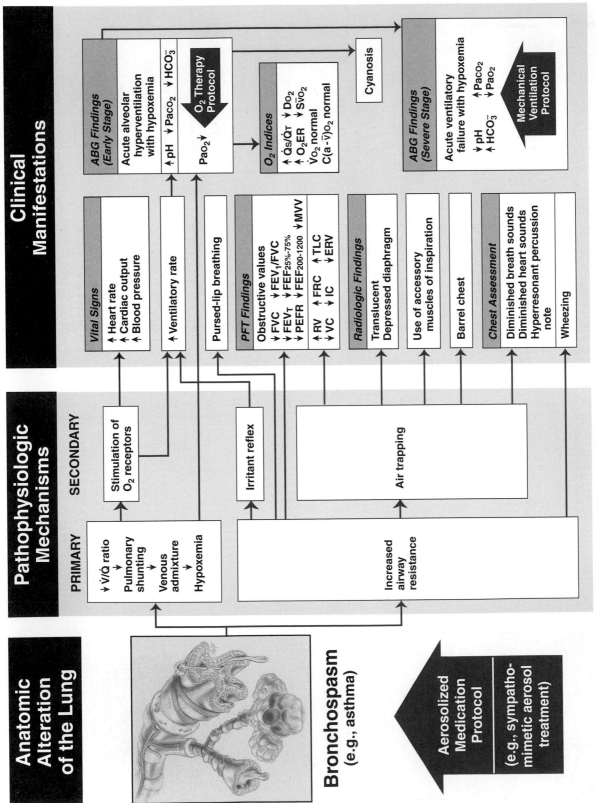

Figure 9–10   Bronchospasm Clinical Scenario.

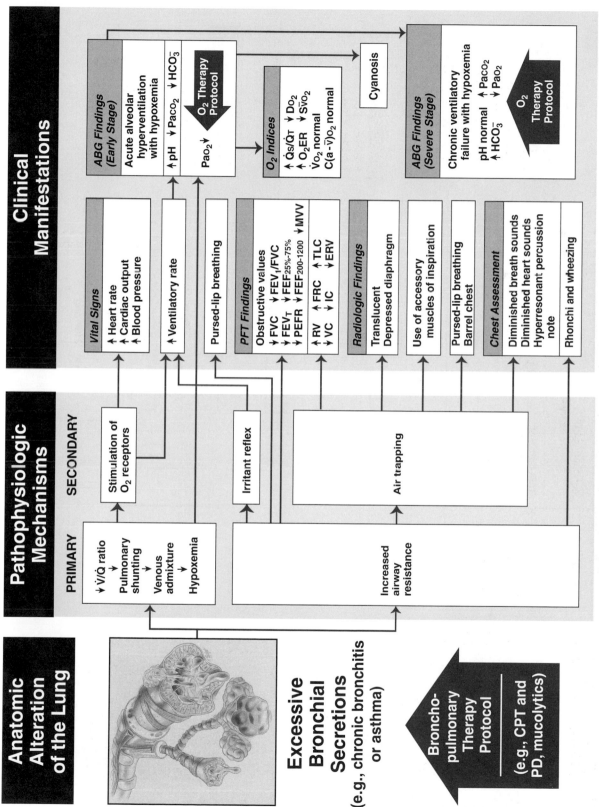

Figure 9-11 Excessive Bronchial Secretions Clinical Scenario.

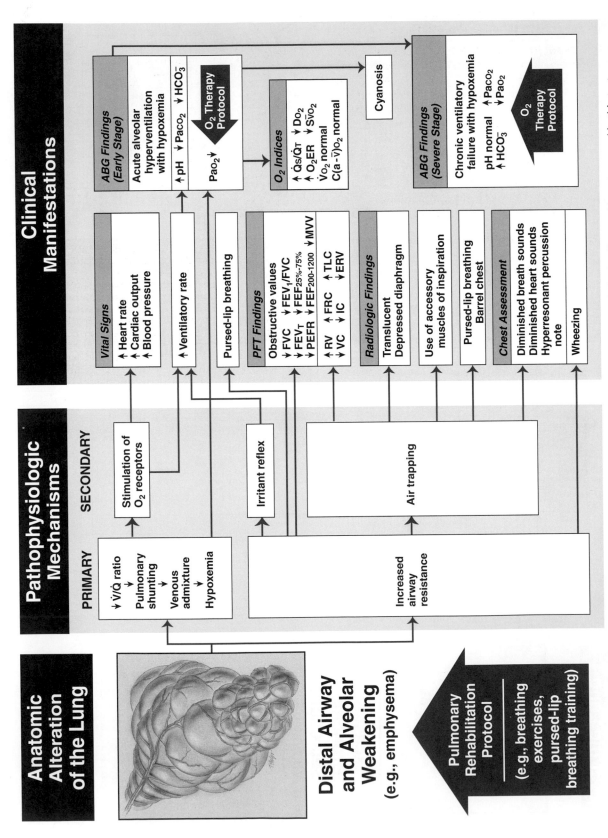

Figure 9–12   Distal Airway and Alveolar Weakening Clinical Scenario. The Pulmonary Rehabilitation Protocol is not covered in this text.

Overview of Common Anatomic Alterations Associated With Respiratory Disorders

When the respiratory therapy practitioner knows and understands the chain of events (clinical scenarios) that develop in response to common anatomic alterations of the lungs, an assessment and an appropriate treatment protocol can be easily determined. Table 9-5 provides an overview of the most common anatomic alterations associated with the respiratory disorders presented in this textbook.

Figure 9-13 provides a three-component overview model of a prototype airway to further enhance the reader's visualization of anatomic alterations of the lungs commonly associated with the obstructive respiratory disorders (e.g., asthma, bronchitis, or emphysema) and the treatment plans commonly used to offset them.

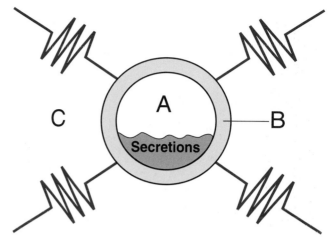

Figure 9-13 A three-component model of a prototype airway. Therapy may be directed to any or all components. *A*, Airway lumen; *B*, airway wall; *C*, supporting structures. Therapy for *A* includes deep breathing and coughing, smoking cessation, suctioning, mucolytics, bland aerosols, systemic and parenteral hydration, and therapeutic bronchoscopy. Therapy for *B* includes bronchodilators, aerosolized antiinflammatory agents, aerosolized antibiotics, and aerosolized decongestants. Therapy for *C* includes pursed-lip breathing exercises and removal of external factors compressing the airway (bullae, pleural effusion, pneumothorax, tumor masses).

TABLE 9–5 Common Anatomic Alterations of the Lungs Associated With Respiratory Disorders

Respiratory Disorder	Atelectasis	Alveolar Consolidation	Increased Alveolar-Capillary Membrane Thickness	Bronchospasm	Excessive Bronchial Secretion	Distal Airway Weakening
Chronic bronchitis				X*	X*	
Emphysema	X			X	X*	X
Bronchiectasis		X		X	X	
Asthma				X	X*	
Pneumonia		X	X		X	
Lung abscess		X	X			
Tuberculosis		X	X			
Fungal diseases		X	X			
Pulmonary edema	X				X	
Pulmonary embolism	X			X		
Flail chest	X	X				
Pneumothorax	X					
Pleural diseases	X					
Kyphoscoliosis	X		X		X*	
Pneumoconiosis				X	X	
Cancer of the lung	X	X	X			
Adult respiratory distress syndrome	X*	X	X			
Chronic interstitial lung diseases			X	X*		
Guillain-Barré syndrome	X*	X*			X*	
Myasthenia gravis	X*	X*			X*	
Meconium aspiration syndrome	X	X			X	
Transient tachypnea of newborn			X		X	
Infant respiratory distress syndrome	X	X			X	
Pulmonary air leak syndromes	X					
Respiratory syncytial virus	X	X			X	
Bronchopulmonary dysplasia	X		X		X	
Diaphragmatic hernia	X					
Cystic fibrosis	X*	X	X	X*	X	
Near drowning	X	X	X	X		
Smoke inhalation and thermal injuries	X			X		
Postoperative atelectasis	X					

*Common secondary anatomic alterations of the lung associated with this disorder

SELF-ASSESSMENT QUESTIONS

Complete the Following

1. The respiratory care practitioner with good assessment skills must first have a strong knowledge base of the major respiratory disorders. List the four components of this knowledge base.

   A.
   B.
   C.
   D.

2. The respiratory care practitioner with good assessment skills also must be competent in performing the assessment process. List the four components of this process.

   A.
   B.
   C.
   D.

3. List the top four treatment protocol categories that are the foundation of a successful TDP program.

   A.
   B.
   C.
   D.

Answers appear in Appendix XI.

CHAPTER 10

Recording Skills: The Basis for Data Collection, Organization, Assessment Skills, and Treatment Plans

Because all health-care workers share information through written or electronic communication, the respiratory care practitioner must understand the way to document and use the patient's medical records effectively and efficiently. The process of adding documentary information to the patient's chart is called *charting, recording,* or *documenting.* Good charting should provide the basic clinical information necessary for critical thinking, or assessment skills—that is, good charting should be an effective way to summarize pertinent clinical data, analyze and assess it (i.e., determine the cause of the clinical data), record the formulation of an appropriate treatment plan, and document the adjustments of the treatment plan (in response to its effectiveness) after it has been implemented.

Good charting enhances communication and continuity of care among all members of the health-care team. There is a definite and direct relationship between effective charting (communication) and the quality of patient care. Good charting also provides a permanent record of past and current assessment data, treatment plans, therapy given, and the patient's response to various therapeutic modalities. This information may be used by various governmental agencies and accreditation teams to evaluate the hospital's patient care and prove that care was given appropriately. Accurate and legible records are the only means by which hospitals can prove that they are providing appropriate care and meeting established standards.

In addition, many health-care reimbursement plans (e.g., Medicare and Medicaid) are based on diagnosis related groups (DRGs). Under these plans, remuneration is based on disease diagnoses. Many private insurance companies use similar illness categories when setting hospital payment rates. Before providing reimbursement, insurance companies carefully review the patient's medical record when assessing whether appropriate and efficient care was given.

Finally, the patient's chart is a legal document that can be called into court. Even though the physician or hospital owns the original record, the patient, lawyers, and courts can gain access to it. As an instrument of continuous patient care and as a legal document, the patient's chart therefore should contain all pertinent respiratory care assessments, planning, interventions, and evaluations.

Types of Patient Records

Three basic methods are used to record assessment data: the traditional chart, the problem-oriented medical record (POMR), and computer documentation.

TRADITIONAL CHART

The traditional record (also called *block chart* or *source-oriented record*) is divided into distinct areas or blocks, with emphasis placed on specific information. The traditional record is commonly seen in the patient's chart as full-colored sheets of block information. Typical blocks of information include the admission sheet, physician's order sheet, progress notes, history and physical examination data, medication sheet, nurses' admission information, nursing care plans, nursing notes, graph/flowsheets, laboratory and X-ray reports, and discharge summary. The order, content, and number of blocks vary among institutions. The traditional chart makes recording easier, but it also makes it more difficult to review a particular event readily and efficiently or to follow the overall progress of the patient.

PROBLEM-ORIENTED MEDICAL RECORD

The organization of the POMR is based on an objective, scientific, problem-solving method. The POMR is one of the most important medical records used by the health-care practitioner to (1) systematically gather clinical data, (2) formulate an assessment (i.e., the cause of the clinical data), and (3) develop an appropriate treatment plan. A number of good POMR methods are available for recording assessment data. Regardless of the method selected, it is essential that one method be adopted and used consistently.

A good POMR method should take a systematic approach in documenting the following:

- The subjective and objective information collected
- An assessment based on the subjective and objective data
- The treatment plan (with measurable outcomes)
- An evaluation of the patient's response to the treatment plan
- A section to record any adjustments made to the original treatment plan.

One of the most common POMR methods is the SOAPIER progress note—often abbreviated in the clinical setting to a SOAP progress note. *SOAPIER* is an acronym for seven specific aspects of charting that systematically review one health problem.

S *Subjective* information refers to information about the patient's feelings, concerns, or sensations presented by the patient:
"I coughed hard all night long."
"My chest feels very tight."
"I feel very short of breath."
Only the patient can provide subjective information. Some cases may not have subjective information. For instance, a comatose, intubated patient on a mechanical ventilator is unable to provide subjective data.

O *Objective* information is the data the respiratory care practitioner can measure, factually describe, or obtain from other professional reports or test results. Objective data include the following:

- Heart rate
- Respiratory rate
- Blood pressure
- Temperature
- Breath sounds
- Cough effort
- Sputum production (volume, consistency, color, and odor)
- Arterial blood gas and pulse oximetry data
- Pulmonary function study results
- X-ray reports
- Hemodynamic data
- Chemistry results

A *Assessment* refers to the practitioner's professional conclusion about the cause of the subjective and objective data presented by the patient. In the patient with a respiratory disorder, the cause is usually related to a specific anatomic alteration of the lung. The assessment, moreover, provides the specific reason as to why the respiratory care practitioner is working with the patient. For example, the presence of wheezes are objective data (the clinical indicator) to verify the assessment (the cause) of bronchial smooth muscle constriction; an arterial blood gas with a pH of 7.18, a $Paco_2$ of 80 mm Hg, an HCO_3^- of 29 mm/L, and a Pao_2 of 54 mm Hg are the objective data to verify the assessment of acute ventilatory failure with moderate hypoxemia. The presence of rhonchi is a clinical indicator to verify the assessment of secretions in the large airways.

P *Plan* is the therapeutic procedure(s) selected to remedy the cause identified in the assessment. For example, an assessment of bronchial smooth muscle constriction justifies the administration of a bronchodilator; the assessment of acute ventilatory failure justifies mechanical ventilation.

I *Implementation* is the actual administration of the specific therapy plan. It documents exactly what was done, when, and by whom.

E *Evaluation* is the collection of measurable data regarding the effectiveness of the therapy plan and the patient's response to it. For example, an arterial blood gas may reveal that the patient's Pao_2 did not increase to a safe level in response to oxygen therapy.

R *Revision* refers to any changes that may be made to the original therapy plan in response to the evaluation. For example, if the Pao_2 does not increase appropriately after the implementation of oxygen therapy, the respiratory care practitioner might continue to increase the patient's Fio_2 until the desired Pao_2 is reached.

For the new practitioner, a predesigned SOAP form is especially useful in (1) the rapid collection and systematic organization of important clinical data, (2) the formulation of an assessment (i.e., the cause of the clinical data), and (3) the development of a treatment plan. For example, consider the case example and SOAP progress note at the bottom of this page and on p. 163 (Figure 10-1).

Although the SOAP form may initially appear long and time-consuming, the experienced respiratory care practitioner and assessor can typically condense and abbreviate SOAP information in a few minutes (primarily at the patient's bedside), in just a few short statements. Typically, a written SOAP only uses 1 to 3 inches of space in the patient's chart. For example, the information presented in Figure 10-1

may actually be documented in the patient's chart in the following abbreviated form:

S—"It feels like someone is standing on my chest. I can't take a deep breath."

O—Use of acc. mus. of insp.; HR 111, BP 170/110, RR 28 & shallow, pursed-lip; hyperresonance; exp. whz; diaph. & alv. hyperinfl.; PEFR 165; wk. cough; lg. amt. thick/white sec., pH 7.27; $Paco_2$ 62; HCO_3^- 25; Pao_2 49.

A—Bronchospasm; hyperinflation; poor ability to mob. tk. sec.; acute vent. fail. with severe hypox.

P—Bronchodilator Tx/pro., CPT & PD/pro., mucolytic/pro., mech. vent/pro., ABG 30 min.

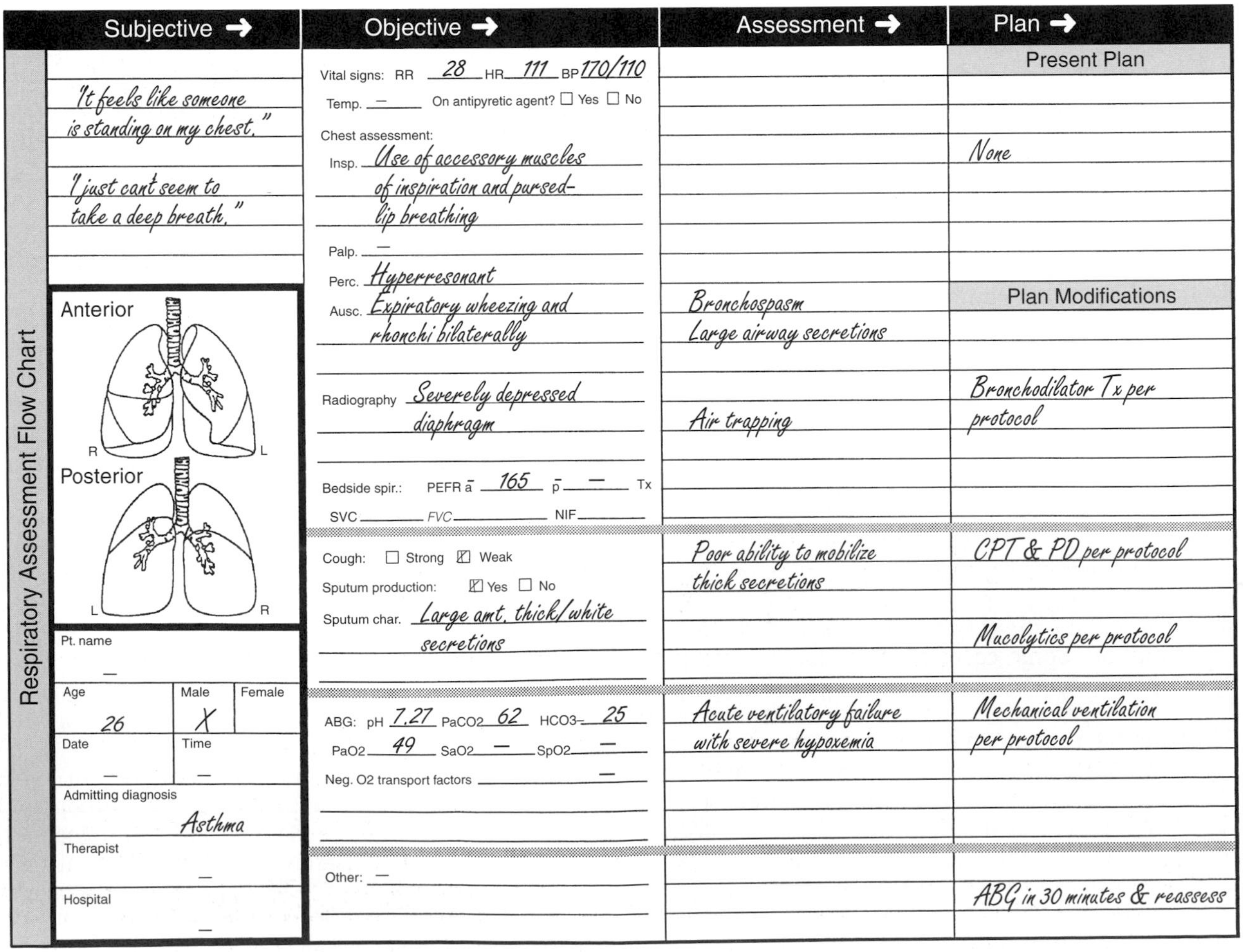

Figure 10–1 Completed predesigned SOAP form.

After the treatment has been administered, another abbreviated SOAP note should be made to determine whether the treatment plan needs to be up-regulated or down-regulated. For example, if the arterial blood gas obtained after the implementation of the plan (outlined in the SOAP) showed that the patient's Pao_2 was still too low, it would be appropriate to revise the original treatment plan by increasing the Fio_2 on the mechanical ventilator. Figure 10-2 illustrates objective data, assessments, and treatment plans commonly associated with respiratory disorders.

SOAP CASE EXAMPLE*

A **26-year-old male** arrived in the emergency room with a **severe asthmatic episode**. On observation, his arms were fixed to the bed rails, he was using his **accessory muscles of inspiration**, and he was using **pursed-lip breathing**. The patient stated that **"it feels like someone is standing on my chest. I just can't seem to take a deep breath."** His **heart rate** was **111 beats per minute** and his **blood pressure** was **170/110**. His **respiratory rate** was **28 and shallow**. **Hyperresonant notes** were produced on percussion. **Auscultation** revealed **expiratory wheezing** and **rhonchi bilaterally**. His **chest X-ray** revealed a **severely depressed diaphragm** and **alveolar hyperinflation**. His **peak expiratory flow** was **165 L/min**. Even though his **cough effort** was **weak**, he produced a **large amount** of **thick white secretions**. His **arterial blood gases** showed a **pH of 7.27**, a **$Paco_2$ of 62**, an **HCO_3^-** of 25, and a **Pao_2 of 49** (on room air) (see Figure 10-1).

*Subjective and objective data presented in bold.

A — RESPIRATORY CARE POCKET PROTOCOL CARD

Objective Data: Clinical manifestations (clinical indicators) that commonly develop in response to respiratory disease — Chest Assessment: Inspection	Palpation	Percussion	Auscultation	Chest Radiograph	Bedside Spirometry	ASSESSMENT: COMMON CAUSES/SEVERITY OF CLINICAL INDICATORS	Plan: TREATMENT SELECTI[ON] (PHYSICIAN ORDERE[D])
• Barrel chest • Use of accessory muscles • Pursed-lip breathing • Cyanosis	May show ↓chest excursion	May be hyperresonant	• Wheezes • Prolonged exhalation	May be normal	↓ PEFR ↓ FEV_1 SVC > FVC	BRONCHOSPASM e.g., Asthma EXCESSIVE BRONCHIAL SECRETIONS e.g., Bronchitis or Cystic Fibrosis BRONCHIAL TUMOR	Bronchodilator therapy Bronchial hygiene therapy General management/comfort
• Dyspneic • Cyanosis	Usually normal	Usually normal	Inspiratory stridor	Laryngeal narrowing	Not indicated	LARYNGEAL EDEMA e.g., Croup or Postextubation Edema	Cool, bland aerosol therapy Racemic epinephrine
Sputum production	May be normal	May be normal	Rhonchi	May be normal	↓ PEFR ↓ FEV_1	LARGE AIRWAY SECRETIONS e.g., Bronchitis or Cystic Fibrosis	Bronchial hygiene therapy
• Use of accessory muscles of • inspiration • Pursed-lip breathing • Barrel chest Cyanosis	↓Tactile and vocal fremitus	Hyperresonant	• ↓Breath sounds • ↓Heart sounds • Prolonged exhalation	• ↓Diaphragm • Translucency • Over expanded	↓ PEFR ↓ FVC ↓ FEV_1/FVC	AIRTRAPPING (Hyperinflation) e.g., COPD • Asthma • Bronchitis • Emphysema	Treat underlying cause, if possible, e.g., • Bronchospasm • Airway secretions
• May appear dyspneic • Cyanosis	↑Tactile and vocal fremitus	Dull	• Bronchial breath • sounds • Crackles Whispered pectoriloquy	• Opacity	↓VC	CONSOLIDATION e.g., Pneumonia ATELECTASIS e.g., Post-op or mucus plugs INFILTRATION e.g., Pneumoconiosis	• Antibiotic agents • Lung hyperinflation Tx • Bronchial hygiene therapy -when atelectasis is caused by mucus accumulation/mucus plugs.
• Rapid shallow breath • Cyanosis • Frothy pink secretions	Usually normal	Dull	• Crackles • May be: wheezes/rhonchi	• Enlarged heart • Infiltrates "Butterfly"	↓VC	PULMONARY EDEMA • Left heart failure	• Lung hyperinflation Tx • Positive inotropic agents • Diuretics
• Cyanosis • Rapid shallow breath • Unilateral expansion	• Usually normal • Tracheal shift	Hyperresonant	Absent or ↓breath sounds	• Pneumothorax • Translucency • Mediastinum shift • ↓Diaphragm	Not indicated	AIR PRESSURE IN INTRAPLEURAL SPACE GREATER THAN ATMOSPHERE • Tension pneumothorax	Chest tube to evacuate air Lung hyperinflation Tx
• Cyanosis • Rapid shallow breath • Unilateral expansion	• Usually normal • May be tracheal shift	Dull	↓ Breath sounds	• Opacity • Obscured diaphragm	↓VC	FLUID IN INTRAPLEURAL SPACE • Pleural effusion • Empyema	• Treat underlying cause • Thoracentesis Lung hyperinflation Tx
Paradoxical chest movement	Tender	Not indicated	Varies	• Rib fractures • Opacity (e.g., ARDS and/or atelectasis)	Not possible	DOUBLE FRACTURES OF THREE OR MORE ADJACENT RIBS • Flail chest	• Stabilization of chest- • mechanical ventilation Lung Hyperinflation Tx

ISBN: 0-9659350-0-0 To order: 319-557-5846

Figure 10–2 Respiratory care protocol guide. (Used by permission of Simon & Kolz Publishing, 1997, 1631 Main Street, Dubuque, IA 52001 [call toll-free 888-870-0483 to order].)

(Continued)

RESPIRATORY CARE POCKET PROTOCOL CARD   **B**

Objective Data (Clinical manifestations or clinical indicators)	ASSESSMENT COMMON CAUSES/SEVERITY	Plan TREATMENT SELECTION (PHYSICIAN ORDERED*)
Cough effort: ○ Strong ○ Weak Sputum production: ○ No ○ Yes Sputum characteristics: • Amount: > 30ml/24hrs. • White & translucent sputum ____ • Yellow/opaque sputum ____ • Green sputum ____ • Brown sputum ____ • Red sputum ____ • Frothy secretion ____	Patient's ability to mobilize secretions: ○ Good ○ Poor • Excessive bronchial secretions ____ • Normal sputum ____ • Acute airway infection ____ • Old, retained secretions & infections ____ • Old blood ____ • Fresh blood ____ • Pulmonary edema ____	Bronchial hygiene therapy • Bronchial hygiene therapy • None • Treat underlying cause • Bronchial hygiene therapy • Bronchial hygiene therapy • Notify physician • Treat underlying cause, e.g., CHF
Arterial blood gas status - Ventilatory • pH↑, PaCO₂↓, HCO₃↓ • pH normal, PaCO₂↓, HCO₃↓↓ ____ • pH↓, PaCO₂↑, HCO₃↑ pH normal, PaCO₂↑, HCO₃↑↑ ____	• Acute alveolar hyperventilation ____ • Chronic alveolar hyperventilation ____ • Acute ventilatory failure ____ • Chronic ventilatory failure ____	• Treat the underlying cause, if possible. Ex: pneumonia, pain. • Generally none (occurs normally at high altitude) • Mechanical ventilation • Low flow oxygen, bronchial hygiene, nocturnal ventilation
Sudden ventilatory changes or chronic ventilatory failure: • pH↓, PaCO₂↑, HCO₃↑↑, PaO₂↓ ____ • pH↓, PaCO₂↑↑, HCO₃↑, PaO₂↓ ____	• Acute alveolar hyperventilation on chronic ventilatory failure ____ • Acute ventilatory failure on chronic ventilatory failure ____	• Treat the underlying cause, if possible. Ex: pneumonia • Mechanical ventilation
Indicators for mechanical ventilation: • pH↓, PaCO₂↓, HCO₃↓, PaO₂↓ but pt is fatigued ____ • pH↓, PaCO₂↑, HCO₃↑, PaO₂↓ hypoventilation ____ • pH↑, PaCO₂↑, HCO₃↑, PaO₂↓ apnea ____	• Impending ventilatory failure • Ventilatory failure • Apnea	• Mechanical ventilation

Metabolic
• pH↑, PaCO₂ normal or ↑, HCO₃↑, PaO₂ normal ____
 	
• pH↓, PaCO₂ normal or ↓, HCO₃↓, PaO₂↓ ____
• pH↓, PaCO₂ normal or ↓, HCO₃↓, PaO₂ normal ____
• pH↓, PaCO₂ normal or ↓, HCO₃↓, PaO₂ normal ____
	• Metabolic alkalosis:
	  • Hypokalemia ____
	  • Hypochloremia ____
	• Metabolic acidosis:
	  • Lactic acidosis ____
	  • Ketoacidosis ____
	  • Renal failure ____
		• Potassium administration
		• Chloride administration
		
		• Oxygen administration, cardiovascular support
		• Insulin administration
		• Renal failure management

Ventilatory and metabolic: • pH↓, PaCO₂↑, HCO₃↓ ____ • pH↑, PaCO₂↓, HCO₃↑ ____	• Combined metabolic and respiratory acidosis • Combined metabolic and respiratory alkalosis	• Mechanical ventilation • Treat the underlying cause of metabolic acidosis (see above) • Treat the underlying cause for acute alveolar hyperventilation • Treat the underlying cause for metabolic alkalosis (see above)
Oxygenation status: • PaO₂ < 80mm Hg ____ • PaO₂ < 60mm Hg ____ • PaO₂ < 40mm Hg ____	• Mild hypoxemia • Moderate hypoxemia • Severe hypoxemia	• Oxygen therapy • Treat the underlying cause of hypoxemia
Negative oxygen transport indicators: ○ ↓PaO₂ ○ Anemia ○ Blood loss ○ ↓Cardiac output ○ CO poisoning ○ Abnormal Hb	Oxygen transport status: ○ Adequate ○ Inadequate	Treat the underlying cause, if possible, e.g., ○ Oxygen therapy ○ Blood replacement ○ Positive inotropic agents

Adapted with permission from DESJARDINS, CLINICAL MANIFESTATIONS & ASSESSMENT OF RESPIRATORY DISEASE, 3RD ED. (MOSBY, 1995).

Figure 10–2   Cont'd—see p. 163 for legend.

COMPUTER DOCUMENTATION

Computer documentation (the so-called paperless medical record) is increasing in popularity in the hospital setting. This technology can save time in the storage and retrieval of patient information. Common uses of computer documentation include ordering supplies and services for the patient; storing admission data; writing and storing patient care plans; listing medications, treatments, and procedures; and storing and retrieving diagnostic test results.

Computer documentation allows easy access to patient data. It eliminates the need to make phone calls to other departments to order patient supplies or services and the need to read through the entire chart to evaluate patient progress or review data such as medication listings, treatments, diagnostic test results, and procedures. The patient's clinical information is permanently recorded, and other health-care departments can review it and communicate with one another.

Basic computer knowledge and skills are usually taught through the hospital's in-service education department. Each nursing station usually has a computer screen to display information, a keyboard to enter or retrieve data, and possibly a printer to produce printed copy. The entire patient record or just a part of it may be retrieved and printed.

Good charting skills are essential to critical thinking and patient assessment—they provide the basic means to collect clinical data, analyze it, assess it, and formulate a treatment plan. Furthermore, good charting skills document the effectiveness of patient care and adjustments of the treatment plan in response to its effectiveness. Without good charting skills, the practitioner merely administers health care without a predetermined (and recorded) goal.

Historically, respiratory care practitioners have focused on treating patients with specific disease entities and implementing physicians' orders. Little planning was done by respiratory care practitioners to individualize their treatments for a specific patient. Today a systematic problem-solving approach to respiratory care, based on broad theoretical knowledge combined with technical expertise and communication skills, is crucial.

Health Insurance Portability and Accountability Act

In 2003 the Department of Health and Human Services (HHS) proposed national rules that outlined the ways in which a patient's medical files should be used or shared with others. These rules were adopted as federal standards after the passage of the *Health Insurance Portability and Accountability Act (HIPAA)*. Today the HIPAA requires that all health-care practitioners who have access to patient medical records must prove that they have a plan to protect the privacy of the records. In essence, the HIPAA regulations protect the patient's privacy with specific rules outlining when, how, and what type of health-care information can be shared. HIPAA gives the patient the right to know about—and to control—how their personal medical records will be used. The following provides a general overview of the HIPAA regulations:

- Both the health-care provider and a representative of the insurance company must explain to the patient how they plan to disclose any medical records.
- Patients may request copies of all their medical information and make appropriate changes to it. Patients may also ask for a history of any unusual disclosures.

- The patient must give formal consent should anyone want to share any health information.
- The patient's health information is to be used only for health purposes. Without the patient's consent, medical records cannot be used by either (1) a bank to determine whether to give the patient a loan or (2) a potential employer to determine whether to hire the patient.
- When the patient's health information is disclosed, only the minimum necessary amount of information should be released.
- A patient's psychotherapy records get an extra level of protection.
- The patient has the right to complain to HHS about violations of HIPAA rules.

One disadvantage of the HIPAA regulations, according to many health-care practitioners, is that the health-care provider must allocate large sums of money to comply with the HIPAA rules—dollars that might be better spent elsewhere. Critics also argue that this cost will likely be passed on to the consumer. In addition, many health-care providers believe that the quality of patient care will be compromised as a result of HIPAA, making it more difficult for various health-care practitioners to obtain vital information regarding patient care. For example, consider the potential HIPAA-related problems for a health-care team in a Miami, Florida, hospital that is trying to obtain the pharmaceutical history—in a timely fashion—of an elderly, unconscious car accident victim whose medical records are in a Detroit, Michigan, hospital. Proponents of the HIPAA regulations argue that this is the trade-off made to ensure the privacy of an individual's health-care information. Regardless of the pros or cons of the HIPAA regulations, the respiratory therapy practitioner—like all other health-care providers—must comply with the current HIPAA regulations.

SELF-ASSESSMENT QUESTIONS

Multiple Choice

1. What is the process of adding written information to the patient's chart called?

       I. Recording
       II. Critical thinking
       III. Documenting
       IV. Charting

   a. II only
   b. IV only
   c. I and III only
   d. I, III, and IV only
   e. I, II, III, and IV

2. Good charting should be an effective way to do the following:

   A. _____

   B. _____

   C. _____

   D. _____

3. The admission sheet, physician's order sheet, and history sheet are all what type of patient records?

       I. Source-oriented record
       II. Problem-oriented medical record
       III. Block chart
       IV. Traditional chart

   a. I only
   b. II only
   c. IV only
   d. III and IV only
   e. I, III, and IV only

4. Which of the following is based on an objective, scientific, problem-solving method?

       I. Source-oriented record
       II. Problem-oriented medical record
       III. Block chart
       IV. Traditional chart

   a. I only
   b. II only
   c. IV only
   d. III and IV only
   e. I, III, and IV only

5. A good problem-oriented medical record (POMR) should include a systematic approach that documents the following:

   A. _____

   B. _____

   C. _____

   D. _____

   E. _____

6. One of the most common POMR methods is the SOAPIER progress note, often abbreviated in the clinical setting to a SOAP progress note. Define the following components of a SOAP progress note and give one or more examples.

   S _____

       Example(s): _____

   O _____

       Example(s): _____

   A _____

       Example(s): _____

   P _____

       Example(s): _____

7. Bronchial breath sounds and dull percussion notes are associated with which of the following clinical assessments?

    I. Air trapping
    II. Bronchospasm
    III. Atelectasis
    IV. Consolidation

    a. I only
    b. II only
    c. III only
    d. I and II only
    e. III and IV only

8. List the three major indicators for mechanical ventilation.

    A. _____
    B. _____
    C. _____

9. A patient is placed on a mechanical ventilator with arterial blood gas values that reveal a pH of 7.56, a $Paco_2$ of 24, an HCO_3^- of 20, and a Pao_2 of 52. Write the indicators for mechanical ventilation that justify placing the patient on a mechanical ventilator with these arterial blood gas values.

    A. _____
    B. _____
    C. _____

10. CASE:
    A 36-year-old female is in the emergency room in respiratory distress. Her heart rate is 136 beats per minute, and her blood pressure is 165/120. Her respiratory rate is 32, and her breathing is labored. The patient states that "It feels like a rope is around my neck." Expiratory wheezing and rhonchi are auscultated bilaterally. Her arterial blood gas values reveal a pH of 7.56, a $Paco_2$ of 28, HCO_3^- of 21, and a Pao_2 of 47 mm Hg (on room air). Her cough effort is strong, and she is producing a moderate amount of thin white secretions. Her peak expiratory flow rate is 185 L/min, and her chest X-ray demonstrates a moderately depressed diaphragm and alveolar hyperinflation.

    With this clinical information, provide SOAP documentation for the patient (use Figure 10-2 for assistance).

    S _____
    O _____
    A _____
    P _____

Answers appear in Appendix XI.

PART II

Obstructive Airway Diseases

Introduction

Chronic obstructive pulmonary disease (COPD) is a term applied to a group of common chronic pulmonary disorders that are characterized by a variety of pathologic conditions—such as bronchial inflammation, excessive airway secretions and mucus plugging, bronchospasm, and distal airway weakening—that cause a reduction of airflow into and out of the lungs. The decreased airflow is worse on expiration.

Chronic bronchitis, emphysema, and *asthma* are the most common respiratory disorders categorized as COPD. Although chronic bronchitis, emphysema, and asthma may appear alone, they often appear in combination. For example, chronic bronchitis and emphysema commonly occur together as one disease complex. Patients who have both chronic bronchitis and emphysema are often broadly categorized as having COPD. Asthma is usually more acute and intermittent than COPD. However, asthma can be chronic. In addition, bronchiectasis is sometimes classified as a COPD. Thus as the following illustrations shows, the respiratory care practitioner should be aware that *COPD* is a general term used to describe any one of the following disorders:

- Chronic bronchitis
- Emphysema
- Asthma
- Chronic bronchitis, emphysema, and asthma in any combination
- Bronchiectasis (less commonly)

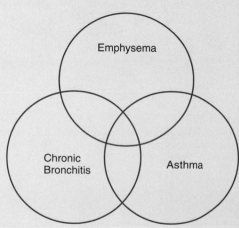

Chronic obstructive pulmonary disease (COPD). Chronic bronchitis, emphysema, and asthma are the most common COPDs. They may occur alone or in combination. Bronchiectasis is sometimes classified as COPD.

CHAPTER 11

Chronic Bronchitis

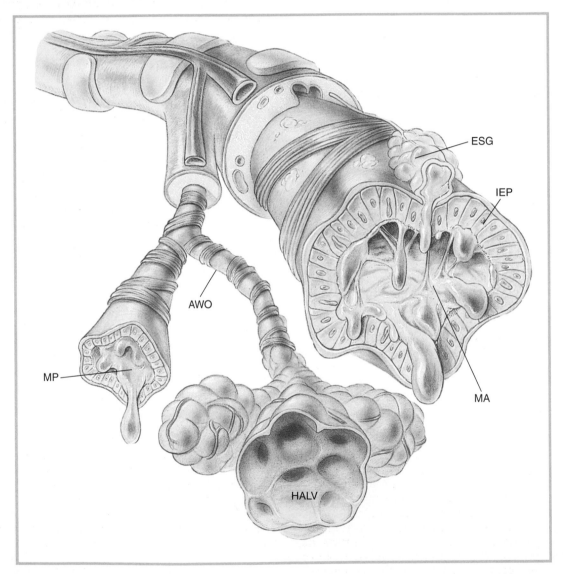

Figure 11–1 Chronic bronchitis, one of the most common airway diseases. *ESG,* Enlarged submucosal gland; *IEP,* inflammation of epithelium; *MA,* mucus accumulation; *MP,* mucus plug; *AWO,* airway obstruction; *HALV,* hyperinflation of alveoli (distal to airway obstruction). See also Plate 2.

Anatomic Alterations of the Lungs

The conducting airways (particularly the peripheral airways) are the primary structures that undergo change in chronic bronchitis. As a result of chronic inflammation the bronchial walls are narrowed by vasodilation, congestion, and mucosal edema. This condition often leads to secondary bronchial smooth muscle constriction. In addition, continued bronchial irritation causes the submucosal bronchial glands to enlarge and the number of goblet cells to increase, resulting in excessive mucus production. The number and function of cilia lining the tracheobronchial tree are diminished, and the peripheral bronchi are often partially or totally occluded by inflammation and mucus plugs, which in turn leads to hyperinflated alveoli (Figure 11-1).

The following major pathologic or structural changes are associated with chronic bronchitis:

- Chronic inflammation and swelling of the peripheral airways
- Excessive mucus production and accumulation
- Partial or total mucus plugging
- Hyperinflation of alveoli (air trapping)
- Smooth muscle constriction of bronchial airways (bronchospasm)

Etiology

It is estimated that approximately 14 million Americans suffer from chronic bronchitis. Although the exact causes of chronic bronchitis vary, the following are known to be important etiologic factors.

CIGARETTE SMOKING

Cigarette smoking clearly plays a major etiologic role in chronic bronchitis. Individuals who smoke are much more prone to develop chronic bronchitis than nonsmokers. Inhaled cigarette smoke contains thousands of particles, many of which are irritants that cause bronchial inflammation and destruction of ciliary activity. The excess mucus that accumulates because of decreased ciliary activity increases the patient's vulnerability to secondary bronchial infections, further compromising the already inflamed bronchial mucosa.

ATMOSPHERIC POLLUTANTS

Common atmospheric pollutants such as sulfur dioxide, the nitrogen oxides, and ozone play a significant etiologic role in chronic bronchitis. Prolonged exposure to ozone, present in petrochemical smog, is a respiratory tract irritant. Epidemiologic data reveal an increased morbidity from lung disease in areas of high air pollution. Occupational bronchitis risk factors include excessive exposure to various lung irritants, such as cotton, flax, or hemp dust, or exposure to chemical fumes from ammonia, strong acids, chlorine, hydrogen sulfide, sulfur dioxide, or bromine. Occupational bronchitis often disappears when the individual is no longer exposed to these substances.

INFECTION

The same viruses that cause "colds" often lead to acute bronchitis. Although the role of infection is uncertain, evidence suggests that individuals who have repeated respiratory tract infections during childhood are likely to develop chronic bronchitis later in life. Because of the inability of the tracheobronchial tree to clear the excess mucus associated with chronic bronchitis, additional infections compromise the already damaged bronchial tree, and a vicious cycle develops. *Haemophilus influenzae* and *Streptococcus pneumoniae* organisms are commonly cultured from the sputum of patients who have chronic bronchitis.

GASTROESOPHAGEAL REFLUX DISEASE

Gastroesophageal reflux disease (GERD) is a disorder that results from stomach acid moving backward from the stomach into the esophagus (acid reflux or regurgitation). GERD usually develops because the lower esophageal sphincter does not close properly. When stomach acid comes in contact with the esophagus, it causes a burning sensation, or heartburn. Although most people experience this sensation from time to time, with GERD it happens more frequently and causes more discomfort. Over time, the reflux of stomach acid can damage the tissue lining of the esophagus, causing significant inflammation and pain. In addition, the patient is at risk of aspirating some of the stomach acid, which in turn can lead to an inflammation of the tracheobronchial tree. Some factors that may cause GERD include alcohol use, obesity, pregnancy, and smoking. A variety of foods may also contribute to GERD, including citrus fruits, chocolate, caffeine, fatty and fried foods, garlic and onions, spicy foods, and tomato-based foods (e.g., spaghetti sauce, chili, and pizza).

OVERVIEW

of the Cardiopulmonary Clinical Manifestations Associated with CHRONIC BRONCHITIS*

The following clinical manifestations result from the pathophysiologic mechanisms caused (or activated) by **Excessive Bronchial Secretions** (see Figure 9-11) and **Bronchospasm** (see Figure 9-10)—the major anatomic alterations of the lungs associated with chronic bronchitis (see Figure 11-1).

CLINICAL DATA OBTAINED AT THE PATIENT'S BEDSIDE

The Physical Examination

Vital Signs

Increased respiratory rate (see page 31 ◆▸)
Several pathophysiologic mechanisms operating simultaneously may lead to an increased respiratory rate:
- Stimulation of peripheral chemoreceptors (hypoxemia)
- Decreased lung compliance/increased ventilatory rate relationship (when the lungs are hyperinflated)
- Anxiety

Increased heart rate (pulse), cardiac output, and blood pressure (see pages 11 and 99 ◆▸)

Use of Accessory Muscles During Inspiration
(see page 40 ◆▸)

Use of Accessory Muscles During Expiration
(see page 42 ◆▸)

Pursed-Lip Breathing (see page 42 ◆▸)

Increased Anteroposterior Chest Diameter (Barrel Chest) (see page 45 ◆▸)

Cyanosis (see page 45 ◆▸)

Digital Clubbing (see page 46 ◆▸)

Peripheral Edema and Venous Distention
(see page 47 ◆▸)

Because polycythemia and cor pulmonale are associated with chronic bronchitis, the following may be seen:[†]
- Distended neck veins
- Pitting edema
- Enlarged and tender liver

Cough, Sputum Production, and Hemoptysis
(see page 47 ◆▸)

---

*Chronic bronchitis and pulmonary emphysema frequently occur together as a disease complex referred to as *chronic obstructive pulmonary disease (COPD)*. Patients with COPD typically demonstrate clinical manifestations of both chronic bronchitis and emphysema.

[†]Patients with COPD and cor pulmonale are often cyanotic and edematous and have been referred to as "blue bloaters."

The American Thoracic Society's definition of chronic bronchitis is based on the major clinical manifestations of the disease. The definition states that chronic bronchitis is characterized by a daily, productive cough for at least 3 consecutive months each year for 2 years in a row. Common bacteria found in the bronchial secretions of patients with chronic bronchitis are *Streptococcus pneumoniae*, *M. catarrhalis*, and *Haemophilus influenzae.* In more complicated cases, *Klebsiella*, other gram-negatives, and even *Pseudomonas aeruginosa* and multi-resistant enterobacter species may be present. Because of the chronic airway inflammation, cough, and infection associated with chronic bronchitis, rupture of the superficial blood vessels of the bronchi and hemoptysis occasionally may be seen.

Chest Assessment Findings
(see page 22 ◆▸)

- Hyperresonant percussion note
- Diminished breath sounds
- Diminished heart sounds
- Decreased tactile and vocal fremitus
- Crackles/rhonchi/wheezing

CLINICAL DATA OBTAINED FROM LABORATORY TESTS AND SPECIAL PROCEDURES

Pulmonary Function Study Findings

Expiratory Maneuver Findings (see page 62 ◆▸)

FVC	FEV_T	$FEF_{25\%-75\%}$	$FEF_{200-1200}$
↓	↓	↓	↓
PEFR	MVV	$FEF_{50\%}$	$FEV_{1\%}$
↓	↓	↓	↓

Lung Volume and Capacity Findings
(see page 66 ◆▸)

V_T	RV	FRC	TLC
N or ↑	↑	↑	N or ↑
VC	IC	ERV	RV/TLC ratio
↓	N or ↓	N or ↓	↑

Arterial Blood Gases

Mild to Moderate Chronic Bronchitis
Acute Alveolar Hyperventilation with Hypoxemia
(see page 70 ◆▸)

pH	$Paco_2$	HCO_3^-	Pao_2
↑	↓	↓(Slightly)	↓

OVERVIEW
of the Cardiopulmonary Clinical Manifestations Associated with
CHRONIC BRONCHITIS (Continued)

Severe Chronic Bronchitis
Chronic Ventilatory Failure with Hypoxemia
(see page 73 ◆▶)

pH	$Paco_2$	HCO_3^-	Pao_2
Normal	↑	↑(Significantly)	↓

Acute Ventilatory Changes Superimposed on Chronic Ventilatory Failure (see page 75 ◆▶)

Because acute ventilatory changes frequently are seen in patients with chronic ventilatory failure, the respiratory care practitioner must be familiar with and alert for (1) acute alveolar hyperventilation superimposed on chronic ventilatory failure and (2) acute ventilatory failure superimposed on chronic ventilatory failure.

Oxygenation Indices (see page 82 ◆▶)

$\dot{Q}_S/\dot{Q}_T$	Do_2*	$\dot{V}o_2$	$C(a-\bar{v})o_2$
↑	↓	Normal	Normal

O_2ER	$S\bar{v}o_2$		
↑	↓		

*The Do_2 may be normal in patients who have compensated to the decreased oxygenation status with (1) an increased cardiac output, (2) an increased hemoglobin level, or (3) a combination of both. When the Do_2 is normal, the O_2ER is usually normal

Hemodynamic Indices (Severe Chronic Bronchitis) (see page 99)

CVP	RAP	PA	PCWP
↑	↑	↑	Normal
CO	SV	SVI	CI
Normal	Normal	Normal	Normal
RVSWI	LVSWI	PVR	SVR
↑	Normal	↑	Normal

ABNORMAL LABORATORY TESTS AND PROCEDURES

Hematology
• Increased hematocrit and hemoglobin
Electrolytes
• Hypochloremia (chronic ventilatory failure)

• Increased serum bicarbonate (chronic ventilatory failure)
Sputum examination
• Increased white blood cells (WBCs)
• *Streptococcus pneumoniae*
• *Haemophilus influenzae*
• *Moraxella catarrhalis*

RADIOLOGIC FINDINGS

Chest Radiograph
• Translucent (dark) lung fields
• Depressed or flattened diaphragms
• Long and narrow heart (pulled downward by diaphragms)
• Enlarged heart

Chronic bronchitis is not a radiologic diagnosis. No radiograph abnormalities may be present in chronic bronchitis if only the large bronchi are affected. If the more peripheral bronchi are involved, however, substantial air trapping may occur. In the advanced stages of chronic bronchitis, the density of the lungs decreases, and consequently the resistance to X-ray penetration is not as great. This is revealed on X-ray film as areas of translucency or areas that are darker in appearance. Alternatively, or even coincidentally, bronchial wall thickening may result in increased, diffuse, fibrotic-appearing lung markings, sometimes referred to as a "dirty chest" X-ray. Because of the increased functional residual capacity, the diaphragms may be depressed or flattened and are seen as such on the radiograph (Figure 11-2). Finally, because right and left ventricular enlargement and failure often develop as a secondary problem during the advanced stages of chronic bronchitis, an enlarged heart may be seen on the chest radiograph.

BRONCHOGRAM

• Small spikelike protrusions

Small spikelike protrusions ("train tracks" appearance of airways) from the larger bronchi are often seen on bronchograms of patients with chronic bronchitis. It is believed that the spikes result from pooling of the radiopaque medium in the enlarged ducts of the mucous glands (Figure 11-3). In clinical practice, bronchograms are rarely performed on patients with chronic bronchitis.

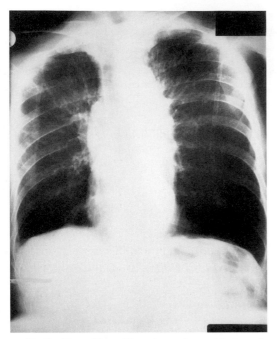

Figure 11–2   Chest X-ray film of a patient with chronic bronchitis. Note the translucent (dark) lung fields, depressed diaphragms, and long and narrow heart.

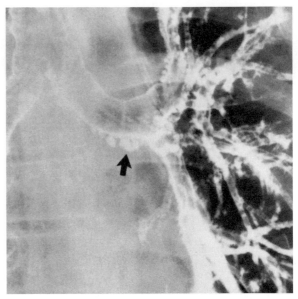

Figure 11–3   Chronic bronchitis. Bronchogram with localized view of left hilum. Rounded collections of contrast lie adjacent to bronchial walls and are particularly well seen below the left main stem bronchus *(arrow)* in this film. They are caused by contrast in dilated mucous gland ducts. (From Armstrong P, Wilson AG, Dee P: *Imaging of diseases of the chest*, St. Louis, 1990, Mosby.)

General Management of Chronic Bronchitis

PATIENT AND FAMILY EDUCATION

Both the patient and the patient's family should be instructed about the disease and its effects on the body. They also should be instructed in home care therapies, the objectives of these therapies, and the way to administer medications. As with emphysema patients, the services of a pulmonary rehabilitation team are sometimes necessary in the management of patients with chronic bronchitis. Such teams include a respiratory care practitioner, physical therapist, respiratory nurse specialist, occupational therapist, dietitian, social worker, and psychologist. A physician trained in respiratory rehabilitation usually outlines and orchestrates the patient's therapeutic program.

BEHAVIORAL MANAGEMENT

Avoidance of Smoking and Inhaled Irritants

Patients with chronic bronchitis must be strongly encouraged to stop smoking. A smoking-cessation clinic with techniques designed to disrupt and break the patient's smoking behaviors (e.g., nicotine polacrilex [nicotine gum], transdermal nicotine patches, and drugs such as bupropion hydrochloride [Wellbutrin] combined with counseling) may be helpful. Patients with chronic bronchitis should be instructed to avoid inhaled irritants such as dust, fumes, mist, and toxic gases.

Avoidance of Infections

Patients with chronic bronchitis should avoid contact with people with contagious respiratory tract infections, especially influenza. Immunization against influenza is usually performed annually, and immunization with pneumococcal vaccine is administered once every 5 years.

RESPIRATORY CARE TREATMENT PROTOCOLS

Oxygen Therapy Protocol

Oxygen therapy is used to treat hypoxemia, decrease the work of breathing, and decrease myocardial work. The hypoxemia that develops in chronic bronchitis is usually caused by the alveolar hypoventilation and shuntlike effect associated with chronic bronchitis. Hypoxemia caused by a shuntlike effect generally can be completely corrected by oxygen therapy. When the patient demonstrates chronic ventilatory failure (during the advanced stages of chronic bronchitis), caution must be taken not to overoxygenate the patient (see Oxygen Therapy Protocol, Protocol 9-1).

Bronchopulmonary Hygiene Therapy Protocol

Because of the excessive mucus production and accumulation associated with chronic bronchitis, a number of bronchial hygiene treatment modalities may be used to enhance the mobilization of bronchial secretions (see Bronchopulmonary Hygiene Therapy Protocol, Protocol 9-2).

Aerosolized Medication Protocol

Both sympathomimetic and parasympatholytic agents are commonly used in chronic bronchitis to induce bronchial smooth muscle relaxation (see Aerosolized Medication Protocol, Protocol 9-4 and Appendix II). In some cases, mucolytic agents also may be used.

Mechanical Ventilation Protocol

Mechanical ventilation may be needed to provide and support alveolar gas exchange and eventually return the patient to spontaneous breathing. Because acute ventilatory failure superimposed on chronic ventilatory failure is seen often in patients with severe chronic bronchitis, continuous mechanical ventilation may be required. Continuous mechanical ventilation is justified when the acute ventilatory failure is thought to be reversible (see Mechanical Ventilation Protocol, Protocol 9-5).

The Global Initiative for Chronic Obstructive Lung Disease (GOLD)

In 2002, the American College of Physicians (ACP), the American Society of Internal Medicine (ASIM), and the American College of Chest Physicians (ACCP) formally developed and endorsed the most current guidelines (the GOLD standards) for the management of acute exacerbations of COPD* and

the management of stable COPD*. The International Guidelines Center for Evidence-Based Practice provides respiratory care practitioners the following executive summary for the management of chronic obstructive pulmonary disease (available as a Pocketcard Guideline)[†]:

Acute Exacerbations (ACCP/ACP-ASIM)

- Chronic obstructive pulmonary disease (COPD) is characterized by chronic airflow obstruction with acute exacerbations (dyspnea, cough, and sputum production). Acute exacerbations may be triggered by tracheobronchial infections or environmental exposures.
- Nearly half of patients discharged from hospitals after acute exacerbations are re-admitted more than once within 6 months. Identifying patients at high risk for relapse should help guide decisions about hospital admissions and follow-up appointments.
- Inhaled bronchodilators and systemic corticosteroids are recommended for acute exacerbations of COPD. Systemic corticosteroids should not be used for more than 2 weeks.
- Appropriate use of antibiotics in an acute exacerbation of COPD is imperative to help control the emergence of multidrug-resistant organisms.

See Figure 11-4 for a guideline algorithm regarding acute exacerbations of COPD.

Components of Management of Stable COPD (GOLD)

1. Assess and monitor disease.
   - Perform spirometry in patients who have chronic cough and dyspnea with history of exposure to risk.
   - Diagnose by spirometry: COPD defined as $FEV_1/FVC < 70\%$ and a postbronchodilator $FEV_1 < 80\%$.

---

*Management of Acute Exacerbations of COPD: Adapted from Snow V, Lascher S, Mottur-Pilson C, for the Joint Expert Panel on Chronic Obstructive Pulmonary Disease of the American College of Chest Physicians and the American College of Physicians—American Society of Internal Medicine. Evidence base for management of acute exacerbations of chronic obstructive pulmonary disease. *Ann Intern Med* 134 (7):595-599, 2001. *Chest* 119: 1185-1189, 2001.

*Management of Stable COPD: Adapted from the Global Initiative for Chronic Obstructive Lung Disease (GOLD) Guidelines, *Global Strategy for the Diagnosis, Management, and Prevention of Chronic Obstructive Pulmonary Disease: NHLBI/WHO Workshop Report*. National Heart, Lung, and Blood Institute, National Institutes of Health; April 2001. NIH Publication 2701.

†Modified from the following resource: Pocketcard Guidelines are a product of International Guidelines Center, 5740 Executive Drive Suite 208, Baltimore, MD 21228. Telephone: 410-869-3332. Fax: 410-744-2150. E-mail: guidelines@MyGuidelinesCenter.com

Exacerbations of COPD (AECOPD): Guideline Algorithm (ACCP/ACP-ASIM)

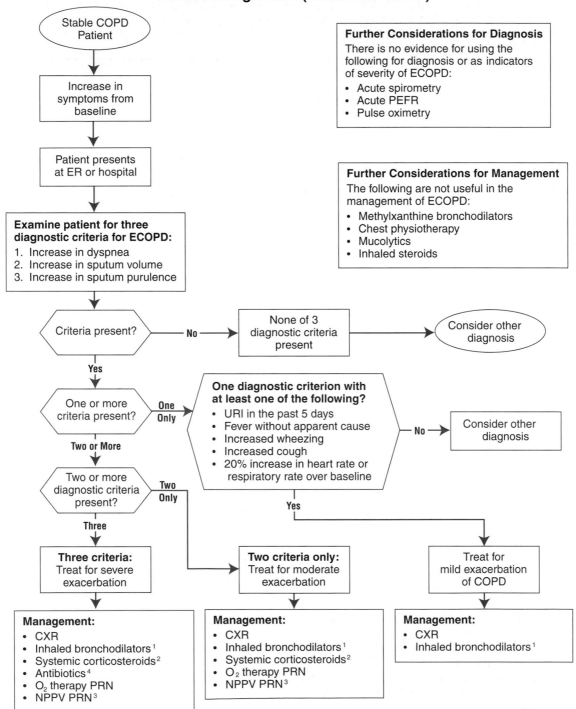

¹Inhaled anticholinergic bronchodilators or inhaled short-acting β₂-agonists are beneficial in the treatment of patients presenting to the hospital with exacerbation of COPD. Since the inhaled anticholinergic bronchodilators have fewer and more benign side effects, consider these agents first. Only after the initial bronchodilator is at maximum dose is the addition of a second inhaled bronchodilator beneficial.
²Dosing regimen used in SCCOPE trial: 3 days intravenous methylprednisolone, 125 mg every 6 hours followed by oral prednisone, taper to complete the 2-week course (60 mg/day on days 4-7, 40 mg/day on days 8-11, and 20 mg/day on days 12-15).
³Noninvasive positive pressure ventilation should be administered under the supervision of a trained physician.
⁴If evidence of bronchitis, use narrow-spectrum antibiotics; the agents favored in the trials were amoxicillin, trimethoprim-sulfamethoxazole, and tetracycline.

Figure 11–4   Acute exacerbation of COPD (AECOPD): Guideline algorithm (ACCP/ACP-ASIM). *CXR*, Chest X-ray; *NPPV*, noninvasive positive pressure ventilation; *PEFR*, peak expiratory flow rate; *URI*, upper respiratory infection. (From *GUIDELINES Pocketcard: Managing Chronic Obstructive Pulmonary Disease*, Baltimore, 2004, Version 4.0, International Guidelines Center.)

◄———

- Monitor arterial blood gases if FEV1 is < 40% predicted or signs of respiratory failure or failure of the right heart are evident.
- Monitor disease progression.
- Reduce risk factors such as exposure to second-hand tobacco smoke, occupational dust and chemicals, and indoor and outdoor pollutants.

2. Initiate and monitor patient's smoking cessation program.
3. Initiate therapy.

- Administer bronchodilator therapy for symptom management; inhaled forms of therapy are preferred.
- The choice among β_2-agonists, anticholinergics, and theophylline* therapy depends on availability and individual response to symptom relief and side effects.
- Prescribe on as-needed basis or on regular basis.
- Long-acting bronchodilators are more convenient if drug therapy is required on a regular basis.
- Combining drugs with different mechanisms and durations of action might increase the degree of bronchodilation for equivalent or lesser side effects. A combination of a short-acting β_2-agonist and anticholinergic drugs such as ipratropium or tiotropium in stable COPD produces greater and more sustained improvements in FEV_1 than does either drug alone and does not produce evidence of tachyphyasis over 90 days of treatment.
- In patients with moderately severe symptoms, administer inhaled glucocorticosteroids if significant symptoms and lung function response so indicate; administer them to patients in stage II and III (see Table 11-2) if symptoms, lung function response, or repeated exacerbations so indicate.

4. Manage exacerbations (see discussion of acute exacerbations in previous section).

———————————

*Theophylline is effective in stable COPD, but because of its potential toxicity, inhaled bronchodilators are preferred.

Recommendations

ACUTE EXACERBATIONS (ACCP/ACP-ASIM)*

1. An admission chest radiograph may be useful; studies show that up to 23% of patients admitted had changes in management related to findings on chest radiography (e.g., pneumonia). Chest radiography in patients visiting the emergency department may also be useful. To date, there is no evidence for or against the utility of chest radiography in the office setting.
2. For patients hospitalized with an acute exacerbation of COPD, spirometry should not be used to diagnose an exacerbation or assess its severity.
3. Inhaled anticholinergic bronchodilators or inhaled short-acting β_2-agonists are beneficial in the treatment of patients with acute exacerbation of COPD. Because the inhaled anticholinergic bronchodilators have fewer and more benign side effects, consider these agents first. Only after the initial bronchodilator is at maximum dose is the addition of a second inhaled bronchodilator beneficial.
4. In the treatment of patients presenting to the hospital with moderate or severe acute exacerbation of COPD, the following therapeutic options are beneficial:

- Systemic corticosteroids given for up to 2 weeks in patients who are not receiving long-term therapy with oral steroids
- Noninvasive positive pressure ventilation (NPPV) administered under the supervision of a trained physician
- Oxygen, with caution, in hypoxemic patients

5. In patients with severe exacerbations of COPD, narrow-spectrum antibiotics are reasonable first-line agents. The superiority of newer, more broad-spectrum antibiotics has not been established.

———————————

*Adapted from Snow V, Lascher S, Mottur-Pilson C, for the Joint Expert Panel on Chronic Obstructive Pulmonary Disease of the American College of Chest Physicians and the American College of Physicians—American Society of Internal Medicine. Evidence base for management of acute exacerbations of chronic obstructive pulmonary disease. *Ann Intern Med* 134(7):595-599, 2001.

6. In the treatment of patients with acute exacerbations of COPD, the following therapeutic options are not beneficial: mucolytic medications, chest physiotherapy, and methylxanthine bronchodilators. In fact, the latter two options may be harmful.
7. No reliable methods of risk stratification for relapse or inpatient mortality are currently available.

MANAGEMENT (GOLD)*

1. Bronchodilator medications are central to the symptomatic management of COPD. They are given on an as-needed basis or on a regular basis to prevent or reduce symptoms.
2. The principal bronchodilator treatments are β_2–agonists, anticholinergics, theophylline,[†] and a combination of one or more of these drugs. Long-acting inhaled bronchodilators are more convenient.
3. Combining bronchodilators may improve efficacy and decrease the risk of side effects compared with increasing the dose of a single bronchodilator.

Finally, Table 11-1 provides a definition of mild, moderate, and severe exacerbation of COPD.

Table 11-2 shows recommended therapy at each state of COPD. Table 11-3 presents anticholinergic and anticholinergic combination bronchodilators. Table 11-4 lists common short-acting and long-acting sympathomimetic brochodilators used to treat patients with COPD, and Table 11-5 provides a list of inhaled corticosteroids commonly used to treat patients with COPD.

Additional Treatment Considerations for COPD

The following treatment considerations may make the patient feel more comfortable, speed recovery time, and prevent complication:

- Plenty of bed rest
- Lots of fluids
- Use of a room humidifier
- Nonprescription cough medicine
- Avoidance of irritants
- Use of a mask when the air is polluted

TABLE 11–1	Definition of Exacerbations of COPD			
	Mild	**Moderate**	**Severe**
Three Cardinal Symptoms of Exacerbation of COPD* • Worsening of dyspnea • Increase in sputum purulence • Increase in sputum volume	One of three cardinal symptoms, as well as one of the following: upper respiratory tract infection in past 5 days; fever without other apparent cause; increased wheezing, increased cough; increase in respiratory rate or heart rate by 20% above baseline	Two of three cardinal symptoms	All three cardinal symptoms

*Outlined by Anthonisen NR, Manfreda J, Warren CP, et al: Antibiotic therapy in exacerbations of chronic obstructive pulmonary disease. *Ann Intern Med* 106:193-204, 1987.
Adapted from Bach PB, Brown C, Gelfand SE, McCrory DC: Management of acute exacerbation of chronic obstructive pulmonary disease: A summary and appraisal of published evidence. *Ann Intern Med* 134(7):600-620, 2001.

*Adapted from the Global Initiative for Chronic Obstructive Lung Disease (GOLD) Guidelines, Global Strategy for the Diagnosis, Management, and Prevention of Chronic Obstructive Pulmonary Disease: NHLBI/WHO Workshop Report. National Heart, Lung, and Blood Institute, National Institutes of Health; April 2001. NIH Publication 2701.
[†]Theophylline is effective in stable COPD, but because of its potential toxicity, inhaled bronchodilators are preferred.

TABLE 11–2 Therapy at Each Stage of COPD (GOLD)

Stage	Characteristics	Recommended Treatment
0: At risk	Chronic symptoms (cough, sputum) Exposure to risk factors Normal spirometry	Avoidance of risk factors, smoking cessation program Influenza vaccination (if no contraindication), pneumococcal vaccination Exercise, patient education
I: Mild COPD	$FEV_1/FVC < 70\%$ $FEV_1 \geq 80\%$ predicted With or without symptoms	Add short-acting bronchodilator when needed
II: Moderate COPD	$FEV_1/FVC < 70\%$ $50\% \leq FEV_1 < 80\%$ predicted With or without symptoms	Add regular treatment with 1 or more long-acting bronchodilators Add pulmonary rehabilitation
III: Severe COPD	$FEV_1/FVC < 70\%$ $30\% \leq FEV_1 < 50\%$ predicted With or without symptoms	Add inhaled glucocorticosteroids if repeated exacerbations Treatment of complications
IV: Very severe COPD	$FEV_1/FVC < 70\%$ $FEV_1 < 30\%$ predicted OR Presence of respiratory failure or right heart failure Quality of life appreciably impaired; exacerbations may be life threatening	Add long-term oxygen therapy if: – Room air $Pao_2 \leq 55$ mm Hg or $Sao_2 \leq 88\%$ OR – Pao_2 56-60 mm Hg with pulmonary hypertension, cor pulmonale, or polycythemia Consider lung volume reduction surgery or lung transplantation in carefully selected patients

In *GUIDELINES Pocketcard: Managing chronic obstructive pulmonary disease*, Baltimore, 2004, Version 4.0, International Guidelines Center.

TABLE 11–3 Anticholinergic and Anticholinergic-Sympathomimetic Combination Bronchodilators

Drug	Route of Administration	Usual Adult Dosage	Maximum Daily Dose
Short Acting			
Ipratropium bromide **MDI:** 18 μg/actuation (*Atrovent*)	Inh	2 Inh (36 μg) qid	12 Inh
Sol for Inh: 0.02% (500 μg/vial) (*Atrovent, various*)	Inh	500 μg tid-qid by nebulization	2000 μg
Ipratropium bromide and albuterol sulfate **MDI:** 18 μg ipratropium and 103 μg albuterol/actuation (*Combivent*)	Inh	2 Inh qid	12 Inh
Sol for Inh: (0.017%) 0.5 mg ipratropium bromide and (0.083%) 2.5 mg albuterol sulfate (3 mL/Vial) (*DuoNeb*)	Inh	3 mL qid by nebulization	18 mL
Long Acting			
Tiotropium bromide **DPI:** 18 μg capsule (*Spiriva Handihaler*)	Inh	1 Inh daily	1 Inh

DPI, Dry powder for inhalation; *Inh*, inhalation, *MDI*, metered dose inhaler; *Sol*, Solution.
Compiled from *Drug Facts and Comparisons*, 2004, St. Louis, 2003, Facts and Comparisons; *Physicians' Desk Reference*, ed 58, Montvale, NJ, 2004, Medical Economics Company. In *GUIDELINES Pocketcard: Managing chronic obstructive pulmonary disease*, Baltimore, 2004, Version 4.0, International Guidelines Center.

TABLE 11–4 Sympathomimetic Bronchodilators

Drug*	Adrenergic Receptor Activity	Route of Administration	Usual Adult Dose[1,2]	Maximum Recommended Daily Dose
Short Acting				
Albuterol (salbuterol)	$\beta_1 < \beta_2$			
Tablet: 2 mg, 4 mg (*Proventil, Ventolin, generics*)		PO	2 or 4 mg tid or qid	32 mg in DD
Tablets, extended release: 4 mg (*Proventil Repetabs, Volmax*) 8 mg (*Volmax*)		PO	4-8 mg q 12 h	16 mg q 12 h
Syrup: 2 mg/5 ml (*Proventil, Ventolin, generics*)		PO	2 or 4 mg tid or qid[3]	8 mg qid
MDI: 90 µg/actuation (*Proventil HFA, Ventolin HFA, generics*)		Inh	1-2 inh q 4-6 h	
Sol for Inh: 0.083% (0.83 mg/ml) and 0.5% (5 mg/ml) (*Proventil, Ventolin, Nebules, generics*)		Inh	2.5 mg tid or qid by nebulization over 5-15 min. **Note:** 0.5% solution must be diluted to total 3 ml volume with sterile normal saline before nebulization	
Capsules for Inh: 200 µg (*Ventolin Rotacaps*)		Inh	200 µg inh q 4-6 h using *Rotahaler* device[4]	Two 200 µg capsules q 4-6 h
Bitolterol	$\beta_1 < \beta_2$			
MDI: 0.8%, 0.37 mg/actuation (*Tornalate*)		Inh	2 inh tid	3 inh q 6 h or 2 inh q 4 h
Sol for Inh: 0.2% (*Tornalate*)		Inh	0.5-1 ml (1-2 mg) tid by intermittent flow nebulization **Note:** Dilute to total of 2-4 ml volume with saline	8 mg (intermittent flow) 14 mg (continuous flow)
Levalbuterol HCl	$\beta_1 < \beta_2$			
Sol for Inh: 0.31, 0.63, 1.25 mg/3 ml (*Xopenex*)		Inh	0.63-1.25 mg tid (every 6-8 h) by nebulization	
Metaproterenol	$\beta_1 < \beta_2$			
Tablets: 10, 20 mg (*generics*)		PO	20 mg tid or qid[6]	
Syrup: 10 mg/5 ml (*Alupent, generics*)		PO	2 tsp (10 ml) tid or qid[6]	
MDI: 0.65 mg/actuation (*Alupent*)		Inh	2-3 inh q 3-4 h	12 inh
Sol for Inh: 0.4%, 0.6%, 5% (*Alupent, generics*)		Inh	0.2-0.3 ml (5% sol) diluted to 2.5 ml with diluent, given by IPPB device, tid-qid ($\geq$ 4 h apart)	
Pirbuterol	$\beta_1 < \beta_2$			
MDI: 0.2 mg/actuation (*Maxair*)		Inh	2 inh (0.4 mg) q 4-6 h	12 inh
Terbutaline	$\beta_1 < \beta_2$			
Tablets: 2.5, 5 mg (*Brethine*)		PO	5 mg tid during waking hours (6 h intervals)[5]	15 mg
Injection: 1 mg/ml (*Brethine*)		SC	0.25 mg in lateral deltoid; may repeat once in 15-30 min if clinical improvement does not occur	0.5 mg in 4 h
Long Acting				
Formoterol	$\beta_1 < \beta_2$			
12 µg capsules for Inh (*Foradil Aerolizer*)		Inh	1 capsule (12 µg) inhaled q 12 h	24 µg/d in DD

TABLE 11-4 Sympathomimetic Bronchodilators—cont'd

Drug*	Adrenergic Receptor Activity	Route of Administration	Usual Adult Dose[1,2]	Maximum Recommended Daily Dose
Salmeterol	$\beta_1 < \beta_2$			
MDI: 21 µg/actuation *(Serevent)*		Inh	2 inh (42 µg) bid (q 12 h)	
DPI: 50 µg *(Serevent Diskus)*		Inh	1 inh (50 µg) bid (q 12 h)	

DD, Divided dose; *DPI*, dry powder for inhalation; *Inh*, inhalation; *IPPB*, intermittent positive pressure breathing; *MDI*, metered-dose inhaler; *SC*, subcutaneous, *Sol*, solution.

*Table is not inclusive of all available products or product strengths. Refer to specific product labeling for detailed product information.

[1]Dose for adults and children ≥12 years unless otherwise noted. [2]Dose for asthma/bronchospasm listed when specific dosing recommendations for bronchospasm associated with COPD not available. [3]Adults and children > 14 years. [4]Adults and children > 4 years. [5]Adults and children > 15 years. [6]Adults and children > 9 years or > 60 lb.

Compiled from *Drug Facts and Comparisons, 2004*, St. Louis, 2003, Facts and Comparisons; *Physicians' Desk Reference*, ed 58, Montvale, N.J., 2004, Medical Economics Company, Inc. In *GUIDELINES Pocketcard: Managing Chronic Obstructive Pulmonary Disease*, Baltimore, 2004, Version 4.0, International Guidelines Center.

TABLE 11-5 Inhaled Corticosteroids

Drug	Adult Dosing* Starting	Adult Dosing* Maximum
Beclomethasone MDI: 40, 80 µg/actuation *(QVAR HFA)*	40-80 µg bid[1] 40-160 µg bid[2]	320 µg bid[1] 320 µg bid[2]
Budesonide DPI: 200 µg/actuation *(Pulmicort Turbuhaler)*	200-400 µg bid[1,2] 400-800 µg bid[3]	400 µg bid[1] 800 µg bid[2,3]
Suspension for Inh: 0.25, 0.5 mg/2 ml *(Pulmicort Respules)*	0.5 mg qd or bid in DD[1-3]	0.5 mg,[1] 1.0 mg[2,3]
Flunisolide MDI: ≈250 µg/actuation *(AeroBid, AeroBid-M)*	500 µg (2 Inh) bid	1 mg (4 Inh) bid
Fluticasone MDI: 44, 110, 220 µg/actuation *(Flovent HFA)*	88 µg bid[1] 88-220 µg bid[2] 880 µg bid[3]	440 µg bid[1,2] 880 µg bid[3]
DPI: 50, 100, 250 µg/actuation *(Flovent Rotadisk)*	100 µg bid[1] 100-250 µg bid[2] 500-1000 µg bid[3]	500 µg bid[1,2] 1000 µg bid[3]
Fluticasone and Salmeterol DPI: 100/50, 250/50, 500/50 µg actuation *(Advair Diskus)*	100/50 µg	500/50 µg bid[2]
Mometasone MDI: 220 µg/actuation *(Asmanex Twisthaler)* Inh	220 µg qd pm[1] 220 µg qd pm[2] 440 µg bid[3]	440 µg qd pm[1] 440 µg qd pm[2] 880 µg[3]
Triamcinolone acetonide MDI: ≈100 µg/actuation *(Azmacort)* (60 mg as acetonide)	200 µg tid-qid **or** 400 µg bid	1600 µg in DD

DD, Divided dose; *DPI*, dry powder inhaler; *Inh*, inhalation; *MDI*, metered-dose inhaler.

*See prescribing information for dose recommendations in patients < 16 years.

[1]Used with inhaled bronchodilators only. [2]For patients currently on inhaled corticosteroids. [3]For patients currently receiving chronic oral corticosteroid therapy.

Compiled from *Drug Facts and Comparisons, 2004*, St. Louis, 2003, Facts and Comparisons; *Physicians' Desk Reference*, ed 58, Montvale, N.J., 2004, Medical Economics Company, Inc. In *GUIDELINES Pocketcard: Managing Chronic Obstructive Pulmonary Disease*, Baltimore, 2004, Version 4.0, International Guidelines Center.

Case Study: CHRONIC BRONCHITIS

Admitting History and Physical Examination

This 58-year-old man has worked in a cotton mill in South Carolina for the past 37 years. He has a 120 pack/year (3 packs/day for 40 years) history of cigarette smoking, and he also chews tobacco regularly. He sought medical assistance in the chest clinic because of a chronic cough. He described it as a "smoker's cough" and stated that it was present about 4 to 5 months of the year. For the past 3 years, his cough produced grayish-yellow sputum during the winter months. The sputum was mostly mucoid in nature, and only occasionally was it thicker and yellow. He stated that he was slightly more short of breath than in the past but attributed this to "getting older."

The patient had not been taking any pulmonary medications, and upon physical examination the patient was in no distress. He was obese. He generated a strong cough occasionally during the visit, but the cough was not productive. Breath sounds were diminished. The expiratory phase of respiration was prolonged. Auscultation of the chest revealed occasional moist rhonchi. The chest radiograph was read as "suggestive of increased markings in the lower lung fields bilaterally." Some pulmonary hyperinflation was noticed. Pulmonary function test showed a decrease in FVC (70% of predicted), FEV_1 (50% of predicted), and PEFR (30% of predicted). The respiratory care practitioner's assessment at this time was documented in the patient's chart as follows:

Respiratory Assessment and Plan

S   "Smoker's cough," episodic mucopurulent sputum production, mild dyspnea

O   Few rhonchi at lung bases. Strong nonproductive cough. Chest radiograph: increased markings at bases and hyperinflation. PFTs: decreased FVC, FEV_1, and PEFR.

A   • Probable moderate chronic bronchitis (history and physical exam)
   • Obstructive pathology (decreased FVC, FEV_1, and PEFR)
   • Mild to moderate airway secretions (rhonchi)
   • Good ability to mobilize secretions (strong cough)

P   Bronchopulmonary Hygiene Therapy Protocol (cough and deep breathing, PRN). Patient education on smoking. Refer to Smoking Cessation Clinic.

The patient was advised to stop smoking and seek medical assistance if his sputum became thick and yellow or his dyspnea became worse. The physician also prescribed a pneumococcal vaccine. Approximately 2 weeks later, influenza prophylaxis was performed (vaccine). The Smoking Cessation Clinic prescribed slow-release nicotine patches, and the patient attended a week-long smoking cessation program. Anti-anxiety medication for use as needed also was prescribed. The patient did well, and at the 6-month follow-up visit he was no longer smoking. The patient stated that he had not had his "smoker's cough" or produced any sputum in weeks.

• • • • •

A year later, however, the patient arrived in the emergency room and was clearly not doing well. He had been unwilling or unable to give up smoking, and he was back to his 3-packs-per-day cigarette smoking habit. He had been physically inactive and gained 30 pounds. His cough was more troublesome in the early morning and now was productive of 3 to 4 tablespoons of thick yellow sputum daily. He complained of moderate exertional dyspnea (e.g., stair climbing produced shortness of breath), and he periodically noted his own wheezing. He denied hemoptysis, chest pain, orthopnea, fever, chills, or leg edema to the respiratory care team.

Vital signs were as follows: blood pressure 165/90, heart rate 116 beats per minute, and a respiratory rate of 26 breaths per minute. He was mildly cyanotic. Auscultation of the chest revealed bilateral posterior basilar crackles, scattered expiratory wheezes, and occasional sibilant rhonchi, which partially cleared with coughing. Expectorated sputum was purulent. A bedside spirometry showed an FEV_1/FVC of 65%. On room air, his arterial blood gas values were pH 7.51, $Paco_2$ 51, HCO_3^- 39, Pao_2 41. His resting Spo_2 on room air was 83% and improved to 89% on 2 L/minute of O_2, after two metered dose inhaler (MDI) treatments with albuterol. His chest X-ray was reported as "typical of COPD," without acute infiltrate. His white blood cell count was 7800 cells/cc, and his hemoglobin was 17.8 g%. At this time, the respiratory care practitioner reported the following SOAP note in the patient's chart:

Respiratory Assessment and Plan

S   Complains of productive cough and exertional dyspnea (history)

O   Bibasilar crackles, wheezing, rhonchi, cyanosis, obesity. Spo_2 on room air 83%. Vital signs: HR 115, BP 165/90, RR 26/min. CXR: COPD, no acute infiltrate. WBC 7800. Hemoglobin

17.8 g%; ABG: pH 7.51, Pa_{CO_2} 51, HCO_3^- 40, Pa_{O_2} 41. Sp_{O_2} improves to 89% on 2 L/min O_2 after MDI. FEV_1/FVC 65%.

A • Acute exacerbation of chronic bronchitis (history, physical examination)
   • Excessive mucus accumulation (sputum, rhonchi)
   • Bronchospasm (wheezing)
   • Acute alveolar hyperventilation superimposed on chronic ventilatory failure with moderate to severe hypoxemia (ABG, Sp_{O_2})
   • Impending ventilatory failure
   • Tobacco addiction (history)

P • Aerosolized Medication Therapy Protocol (MDI with Combivent [combined albuterol and ipratropium] 2 puffs QID). Bronchopulmonary Hygiene Therapy Protocol (cough and deep breathing under supervision QID, cautious trial of CPT with postural drainage to lower lobes, 3 times a day). Call physician about impending ventilatory failure, and check to see whether the doctor wants to schedule complete pulmonary function test. Recheck Sp_{O_2} on room air. Again, advise and facilitate smoking cessation program.

Discussion

In the first portion of this case study, some of the clinical manifestations of **Excessive Airway Secretions** (see Figure 9-11) and air trapping were present, even though the patient had a nonproductive cough at the time. These findings were clearly documented in the first SOAP note when the therapist charted the presence of nonproductive cough, rhonchi, and diminished breath sounds and pulmonary function symptoms that indicated airway obstruction. The findings on the chest X-ray also suggested hyperinflation of the lungs with air trapping, which can occur in bronchitis, emphysema, or the two in combination—chronic obstructive pulmonary disease (COPD).

The first part of this case also illustrates a definite role for the modern respiratory care practitioner. Such a professional may well be working in outpatient settings that necessitate the evaluation and treatment of patients such as this one. The history of productive cough and the findings of expiratory prolongation and rhonchi in a smoker who is not seriously ill suggest a diagnosis of chronic bronchitis. The pulmonary function data and chest X-ray confirm this suspicion. The physician's prescription of influenza prophylaxis, pneumococcal vaccine, and slow-release nicotine patches speaks to the key elements of preventive therapy in chronic bronchitis—namely, avoidance of irritant fumes and particles; influenza and pneumococcal vaccines for prevention of those two common complicating diseases; and the need for continued follow-up.

In the second part of this case study, the more classic clinical manifestations of chronic bronchitis were presented. For example, the patient's **Excessive Bronchial Secretions** (see Figure 9-11) and **Bronchospasm** (see Figure 9-10) not only resulted in hypoxia and cyanosis secondary to a decreased $\dot{V}/\dot{Q}$ ratio and pulmonary shunting but also produced increased airway resistance that resulted in wheezes, rhonchi, alveolar hyperinflation (as shown on the chest X-ray), and a decreased FEV_1/FVC ratio. In addition, the second part of this case study started with the patient's failure to stop smoking and with increased symptoms and worsening of his obstructive pulmonary disease (dyspnea and productive cough). His pulmonary function was worsening, and he had acute alveolar hyperventilation superimposed on chronic ventilatory failure with moderate to severe hypoxemia. Impending ventilatory failure was a serious concern.

In addition to treating the acute symptoms with a simple MDI bronchodilator regimen (see Aerosolized Medication Therapy Protocol, Protocol 9-4) and Bronchopulmonary Hygiene Therapy Protocol (see Protocol 9-2) in the form of cough and deep breathing, a cautious trial of chest physiotherapy, and postural drainage, the respiratory therapist does not give up on the longer-term but extremely important goal of modifying behavior (smoking cessation) in the patient. A complete pulmonary function test in the near future would further define the patient's disease process, both in its nature and severity. Such data are often helpful to the patient's understanding of just how ill he is and may constitute a "teachable moment" for the physician and therapist. Although the patient was discharged from the hospital 5 days later, he unfortunately died from another acute exacerbation of chronic bronchitis, ventilatory failure, and cardiac arrest 7 months later.

SELF-ASSESSMENT QUESTIONS

Multiple Choice

1. In chronic bronchitis:
   - I. The bronchial walls are narrowed because of vasoconstriction
   - II. The bronchial glands are enlarged
   - III. The number of goblet cells is decreased
   - IV. The number of cilia lining the tracheobronchial tree is increased

   a. I only
   b. II only
   c. III only
   d. III and IV only
   e. II, III, and IV only

2. Which of the following is/are believed to play a major etiologic role in chronic bronchitis?
   - I. Ozone
   - II. Nitrous oxide
   - III. Sulfur dioxide
   - IV. Nitrogen oxides

   a. I only
   b. II only
   c. III only
   d. II and IV only
   e. I, III, and IV only

3. Which of the following common bacteria are found in the tracheobronchial tree of patients with chronic bronchitis?
   - I. *Staphylococcus*
   - II. *Haemophilus influenzae*
   - III. *Klebsiella*
   - IV. *Streptococcus*

   a. I only
   b. II only
   c. III and IV only
   d. II and IV only
   e. I, II, and IV only

4. In chronic bronchitis, the patient commonly demonstrates which of the following?
   - I. Increased FVC
   - II. Decreased ERV
   - III. Increased VC
   - IV. Decreased RV

   a. II only
   b. III only
   c. I and III only
   d. III and IV only
   e. I, III, and IV only

5. The patient with severe chronic bronchitis usually has which of the following arterial blood gas values?
   - I. Decreased pH
   - II. Increased HCO_3^-
   - III. Decreased Pa_{CO_2}
   - IV. Increased Pa_{O_2}

   a. I only
   b. II only
   c. III only
   d. I and II only
   e. III and IV only

6. Sympathomimetic agents commonly are prescribed for patients with chronic bronchitis to offset bronchial smooth muscle spasm. What is the trade name of the sympathomimetic agent albuterol?
   - I. Proventil
   - II. Ventolin
   - III. Vanceril
   - IV. Brethine

   a. I only
   b. IV only
   c. I and II only
   d. II and IV only
   e. II, III, and IV only

7. The patient with severe chronic bronchitis commonly demonstrates which of the following oxygenation indices?
   - I. Decreased $C(a-\bar{v})_{O_2}$
   - II. Increased O_2ER
   - III. Decreased D_{O_2}
   - IV. Increased $\dot{V}_{O_2}$

   a. I only
   b. III only
   c. IV only
   d. II and III only
   e. I, III, and IV only

8. The patient with severe chronic bronchitis commonly demonstrates which of the following hemodynamic indices?
   - I. Increased PCWP
   - II. Decreased RAP
   - III. Increased PA
   - IV. Decreased CO

   a. I only
   b. III only
   c. IV only
   d. I and III only
   e. I, III, and IV only

9. Parasympatholytic agents are often used to offset the bronchial smooth muscle constriction associated with chronic bronchitis. What is the trade name of the parasympatholytic agent ipratropium bromide?

   a. Theophylline
   b. Atropine sulfate
   c. Atrovent
   d. Guaifenesin
   e. Erythromycin

10. Patients with severe chronic bronchitis may demonstrate which of the following?

    I. Peripheral edema
    II. Distended neck veins
    III. An elevated hemoglobin concentration
    IV. An enlarged liver

    a. I only
    b. III only
    c. II and IV only
    d. II, III, and IV only
    e. I, II, III, and IV

Answers appear in Appendix XI.

CHAPTER 12

Emphysema

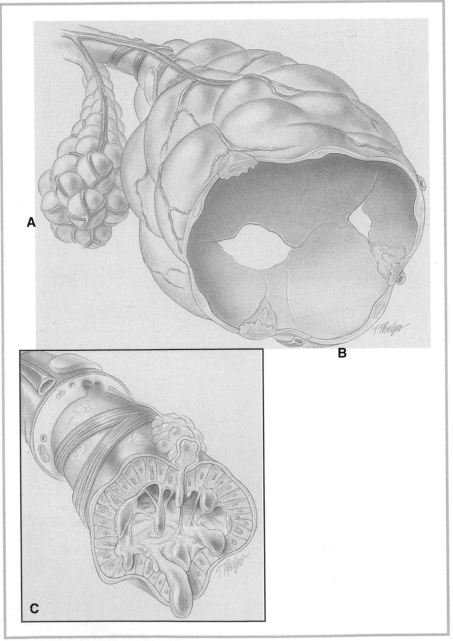

Figure 12–1 Panlobular emphysema. **A,** Normal alveoli for comparison purposes. **B,** Panlobular emphysema: abnormal weakening and enlargement of all air spaces distal to the terminal bronchioles. **C,** Excessive bronchial secretions from bronchitis, a common secondary anatomic alteration of the lungs. See also Plate 3.

Anatomic Alterations of the Lungs

Emphysema is characterized by a weakening and permanent enlargement of the air spaces distal to the terminal bronchioles and by destruction of the alveolar walls. As these structures enlarge and the alveoli coalesce, many of the adjacent pulmonary capillaries also are affected, and this results in a decreased surface area for gas exchange. Furthermore, the distal airways, weakened in the process, collapse during expiration in response to increased intrapleural pressure. This traps gas in the alveoli. There are two major types of emphysema: panacinar (panlobular) emphysema and centriacinar (centrilobular) emphysema.

In *panlobular emphysema* there is an abnormal weakening and enlargement of all air spaces distal to the terminal bronchioles, including the respiratory bronchioles, alveolar ducts, alveolar sacs, and alveoli. The alveolar-capillary surface area is significantly decreased (Figure 12-1). Panlobular emphysema commonly is found in the lower parts of the lungs and often is associated with a deficiency of α_1-protease inhibitor (previously called α_1-antitrypsin).

Centrilobular emphysema primarily involves the respiratory bronchioles in the proximal portion of the acinus. The respiratory bronchiolar walls enlarge, become confluent, and are then destroyed. A rim of parenchyma remains relatively unaffected (Figure 12-2). Centrilobular emphysema is the most common form of emphysema and often is associated with chronic bronchitis.

The following are the major pathologic or structural changes associated with emphysema:

- Permanent enlargement and destruction of the air spaces distal to the terminal bronchioles
- Destruction of pulmonary capillaries
- Weakening of the distal airways, primarily the respiratory bronchioles
- Bronchospasm (with concomitant bronchitis)
- Hyperinflation of alveoli (air trapping)

Etiology

According to estimates, approximately 2 million Americans suffer from emphysema. The following are known to be important etiologic factors.

CIGARETTE SMOKING

Cigarette smoking is the major cause of emphysema, accounting for more than 80% of all cases. In addition, cigarette smoke contains numerous irritants that stimulate mucus production and ultimately impair

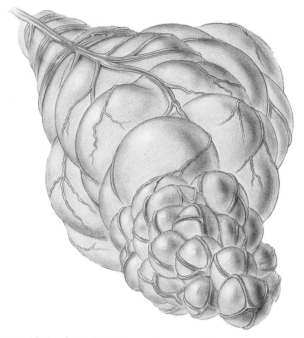

Figure 12–2 Centrilobular emphysema. Abnormal weakening and enlargement of the respiratory bronchioles in the proximal portion of the acinus. See also Plate 4.

or destroy ciliary transport. The excess mucus that accumulates as a result of decreased ciliary activity increases the patient's vulnerability to respiratory tract infections. Cigarette smoking also causes bronchospasm, which in turn increases airway resistance and further impedes tracheobronchial clearance. Men are affected more often than women. However, the incidence of women with emphysema is rapidly rising. Cigar and pipe smokers and individuals exposed to secondhand (passive) smoke are also at risk, although less so than cigarette smokers.

GENETIC PREDISPOSITION

It has been known for many years that panlobular emphysema occurs with unusual frequency in certain families, where it primarily affects young adults. It is known now that genetic α_1-protease inhibitor (α_1PI) deficiency (most commonly called **alpha-1-antitrypsin deficiency**—or α_1-antitrypsin deficiency) is the key to the high incidence of panlobular emphysema in these families. α_1PI is a serum glycoprotein that inhibits several proteolytic enzymes. It is synthesized and secreted by the liver. When old white blood cells are destroyed in the lungs, an elastase is released that in turn may destroy elastic tissue. α_1PI is the substance responsible for inactivating the elastase.

The normal level of α_1PI is 200 to 400 mg/dl. Patients with normal levels of α_1PI are referred to genetically as having an MM or simply an M phenotype (homozygote). The phenotype associated with severely lower serum concentration is ZZ, or simply Z. The heterozygous offspring of parents with the M and Z phenotypes have the phenotype MZ. The MZ phenotype results in an intermediate deficiency of α_1PI. The precise effect of the intermediate level of α_1PI is unclear. It is strongly recommended, however, that individuals with this phenotype not smoke or work in areas having significant environmental air pollution.

OCCUPATIONAL EXPOSURE TO CHEMICAL IRRITANTS

Individuals who breathe certain chemicals at work or the dust from grain, cotton, wood, or mining

projects are at risk of developing emphysema. The risk is greater in those individuals who smoke.

EXPOSURE TO ATMOSPHERIC POLLUTIONS

Common atmospheric pollutants such as sulfur dioxide, the nitrogen oxides, and ozone may have an etiologic role in emphysema. Sulfur dioxide is known to increase airway resistance, and ozone, present in urban air pollution (smog), is a respiratory tract irritant. Epidemiologic data support the observation that there is an increased incidence of obstructive lung disease in areas of high air pollution.

OVERVIEW
of the Cardiopulmonary Clinical Manifestations Associated with EMPHYSEMA*

The following clinical manifestations result from the pathophysiologic mechanisms caused (or activated) by **Distal Airway and Alveolar Weakening** (see Figure 9-12)—the major anatomic alteration of the lungs associated with emphysema (see Figures 12-1 and 12-2).

CLINICAL DATA OBTAINED AT THE PATIENT'S BEDSIDE

The Physical Examination

Vital Signs

Increased respiratory rate (see page 31 ◆▶)
Several pathophysiologic mechanisms operating simultaneously may lead to an increased ventilatory rate:
- Stimulation of peripheral chemoreceptors (hypoxemia)
- Anxiety

Increased heart rate (pulse), cardiac output, and blood pressure (see pages 11 and 99 ◆▶)

Use of Accessory Muscles During Inspiration (see page 40 ◆▶)

Use of Accessory Muscles During Expiration (see page 42 ◆▶)

Pursed-Lip Breathing (see page 42 ◆▶)

Increased Anteroposterior Chest Diameter (Barrel Chest) (see page 45 ◆▶)

Cyanosis (see page 45 ◆▶)

Digital Clubbing (see page 46 ◆▶)

Peripheral Edema and Venous Distention (see page 47 ◆▶)

Because polycythemia and cor pulmonale are associated with severe emphysema, the following may be seen:[†]
- Distended neck veins
- Pitting edema
- Enlarged and tender liver

Cough, Sputum Production, and Hemoptysis (see page 47 ◆▶)

Because emphysema often is accompanied by chronic bronchitis—a disease complex referred to as *COPD*—a productive cough frequently is seen. Common bacteria found in the bronchial secretions of patient with chronic bronchitis are *Streptococcus pneumoniae* and *Haemophilus influenzae*. Because of the chronic airway inflammation, cough, and infection associated with chronic bronchitis, rupture of the superficial blood vessels of the bronchi and hemoptysis may be seen.

Chest Assessment Findings (see page 22 ◆▶)
- Hyperresonant percussion note
- Wheezing
- Diminished breath sounds
- Diminished heart sounds
- Decreased tactile and vocal fremitus
- Crackles and rhonchi (when accompanied by acute or chronic bronchitis)

*Pulmonary emphysema and chronic bronchitis frequently occur together as COPD; therefore patients with COPD typically demonstrate clinical manifestations related to both emphysema and chronic bronchitis.
[†]Patients with COPD and cor pulmonale are often cyanotic and edematous and have been referred to as "blue bloaters."

CLINICAL DATA OBTAINED FROM LABORATORY TESTS AND SPECIAL PROCEDURES

Pulmonary Function Study Findings

Expiratory Maneuver Findings (see page 62 ◆►)

FVC	FEV_T	$FEF_{25\%-75\%}$	$FEF_{200-1200}$
↓	↓	↓	↓
PEFR	MVV	$FEF_{50\%}$	$FEV_{1\%}$
↓	↓	↓	↓

Lung Volume and Capacity Findings
(see page 66 ◆►)

VT	RV	FRC	TLC
N or ↑	↑	↑	N or ↑
VC	IC	ERV	RV/TLC ratio
↓	N or ↓	N or ↓	↑

Decreased Diffusion Capacity (DL_{co})
(see page 67 ◆►)

Arterial Blood Gases

Mild to Moderate Emphysema
Acute Alveolar Hyperventilation with Hypoxemia
(see page 70 ◆►)

pH	$Paco_2$	HCO_3^-	Pao_2
↑	↓	↓(Slightly)	↓

Severe Emphysema (End-Stage)
Chronic Ventilatory Failure with Hypoxemia
(see page 73 ◆►)

pH	$Paco_2$	HCO_3^-	Pao_2
Normal	↑	↑(Significantly)	↓

Acute Ventilatory Changes Superimposed on Chronic Ventilatory Failure (see page 75)
Because acute ventilatory changes frequently are seen in patients with chronic ventilatory failure, the respiratory care practitioner must be familiar with and alert for (1) acute alveolar hyperventilation superimposed on chronic ventilatory failure and (2) acute ventilatory failure superimposed on chronic ventilatory failure.

Oxygenation Indices (see page 82 ◆►)

$\dot{Q}_s/\dot{Q}_T$	Do_2	$\dot{V}o_2$	$C(a-\bar{v})o_2$
↑	↓	Normal	Normal
O_2ER	$S\bar{v}o_2$		
↑	↓		

Hemodynamic Indices (Severe Emphysema)
(see page 99 ◆►)

CVP	RAP	PA	PCWP
↑	↑	↑	Normal
CO	SV	SVI	CI
Normal	Normal	Normal	Normal
RVSWI	LVSWI	PVR	SVR
↑	Normal	↑	Normal

ABNORMAL LABORATORY TESTS AND PROCEDURES

Hematology
- Increased hematocrit and hemoglobin

Electrolytes
- Hypochloremia (chronic ventilatory failure)

Sputum examination (when accompanied by chronic bronchitis)
- *Streptococcus pneumoniae*
- *Haemophilus influenzae*

RADIOLOGIC FINDINGS

Chest Radiograph

- Translucent (dark) lung fields
- Depressed or flattened diaphragms
- Long and narrow heart (pulled downward by diaphragms)
- Enlarged heart (when pulmonary hypertension is present)
- Increased retrosternal air space (lateral radiograph)

Because of the decreased lung recoil and air trapping in emphysema, the functional residual capacity increases and the radiographic density of the lungs decreases. Consequently, the resistance to X-ray penetration is not as great. This resistance is revealed on X-ray films as areas of translucency or areas that are darker in appearance. Because of the increased functional residual capacity, the diaphragm is depressed or flattened and the heart is often long and narrow (Figure 12-3). The lateral chest radiograph characteristically shows an increased retrosternal air space (more than 3.0 cm from the anterior surface of the aorta to the back of the sternum measured 3.0 cm below the manubriosternal junction) and flattened diaphragms (Figure 12-4). Finally, because right ventricular enlargement and failure often develop as secondary problems during the advanced stages of emphysema, an enlarged heart may be seen on the chest radiograph (Figure 12-5).

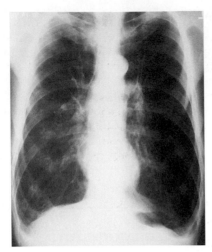

Figure 12–3   Chest X-ray of a patient with emphysema. The heart often appears long and narrow as a result of being drawn downward by the descending diaphragm.

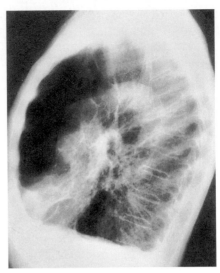

Figure 12–4   Emphysema. Lateral chest radiograph demonstrates a characteristically large retrosternal radiolucency with increased separation of the aorta and sternum measuring 4.6 cm, 3 cm below the angle of Louis and extending down to within 3 cm of the diaphragm anteriorly. Both costophrenic angles are obtuse, and both hemidiaphragms are flat. (From Armstrong P et al, editors: *Imaging of diseases of the chest*, ed 2, St. Louis, 1995, Mosby.)

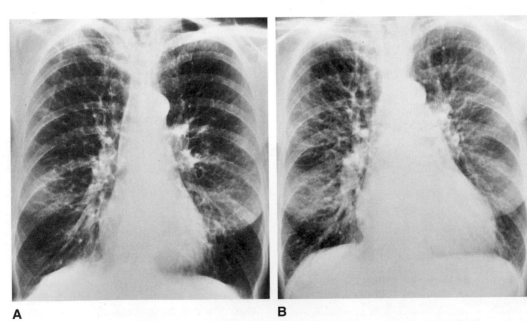

A   **B**

Figure 12–5   Cor pulmonale. **A,** A 50-year-old male with chronic airflow obstruction. Lungs are large in volume, the diaphragm is flat, and vascular attenuation is evident at the right apex. These features suggest emphysema, and this diagnosis was supported by a low CO diffusion capacity. Lung "markings" are increased peripherally, particularly in the left midzone. **B,** The patient became chronically hypoxic and, with respiratory infections, hypercapnic. One of these episodes was associated with cor pulmonale when the patient became edematous, and the heart and hilar and pulmonary parenchymal vessels became enlarged. The emphysematous right upper zone shows fewer vascular markings and is relatively transradient. The diaphragm is less depressed and more curved than before. (From Armstrong P et al, editors: *Imaging of diseases of the chest*, ed 2, St. Louis, 1995, Mosby.)

General Management of Emphysema

There is no cure for emphysema. However, early intervention may prevent further damage to the distal structures of the tracheobronchial tree. The general management of emphysema is essentially the same as that of chronic bronchitis—which makes sense given that emphysema commonly appears as a disease complex with chronic bronchitis. The patient with emphysema should receive (1) patient and family education; (2) behavioral management in regard to the avoidance of smoking, inhaled irritants, and infection; and (3) instruction in proper nutrition. Similar to chronic bronchitis, the *GOLD standard guidelines* for the management of chronic obstructive pulmonary disease should be closely followed for the general emphysema treatment plan (see page 179). Common respiratory care treatment modalities include the following.

RESPIRATORY CARE TREATMENT PROTOCOLS

Oxygen Therapy Protocol

Oxygen therapy is used to treat hypoxemia, decrease the work of breathing, and decrease myocardial work. The hypoxemia that develops in emphysema is usually caused by the hypoventilation and shuntlike effect associated with emphysema. Hypoxemia caused by a shuntlike effect can generally be partially corrected by oxygen therapy. When the patient demonstrates chronic ventilatory failure (during the advanced stages of emphysema), caution must be taken not to overoxygenate the patient (see Oxygen Therapy Protocol, Protocol 9-1).

Bronchopulmonary Hygiene Therapy Protocol

Because of the excessive mucus production and accumulation associated with COPD, a number of bronchial hygiene treatment modalities may be used to enhance the mobilization of bronchial secretions (see Bronchopulmonary Hygiene Therapy Protocol, Protocol 9-2).

Aerosolized Medication Protocol

Both sympathomimetic and parasympatholytic agents are commonly used to induce bronchial smooth muscle relaxation (see Aerosolized Medication Therapy Protocol, Protocol 9-4 and Appendix II).

Mechanical Ventilation Protocol

Mechanical ventilation may be needed to provide and support alveolar gas exchange and eventually return the patient to spontaneous breathing. Because acute ventilatory failure superimposed on chronic ventilatory failure is often seen in patients with severe emphysema, continuous mechanical ventilation may be required. Continuous mechanical ventilation is justified when the acute ventilatory failure is thought to be reversible (see Mechanical Ventilation Protocol, Protocol 9-5).

ADDITIONAL TREATMENT CONSIDERATIONS FOR EMPHYSEMA

Antibiotics

Broad-spectrum antibiotics such as ampicillin, tetracycline, erythromycin, and cephalosporin are often used to combat periodic respiratory infections that frequently complicate emphysema.

Inoculations Against Influenza and Pneumonia

Patients with emphysema should receive an annual influenza (flu) injection and a pneumonia injection every 5 to 7 years.

α-Antitrypsin Therapy

In patients with emphysema caused by a deficiency of α_1-antitrypsin, the weekly infusions of the material (e.g., Prolastin) may slow the deterioration of the lungs.

Lung Volume Reduction Surgery

In a procedure called *lung volume reduction surgery*, or *lung shaving*, small sections of damaged tissue from both lungs may be removed. Usually, about 20% to 30% of each lung is removed. The reduced lung size allows the diaphragm to return to a more normal position and contract and relax more effectively, thus improving gas exchange. The surgical removal of lung tissue is still considered somewhat experimental.

Lung Transplantation

A lung transplant may be considered in patients with severe emphysema. Usually, just one donor lung is transplanted.

Case Study: EMPHYSEMA

Admitting History and Physical Examination

This 27-year-old man was admitted to the hospital with the chief complaint of dyspnea on exertion. He had a 3-year history of recurrent respiratory problems that had required several hospitalizations of several days' duration. Recently, his respiratory status deteriorated to the point where he had to stop working. He had been employed for several years as a cook in a fast-food restaurant, where he was continuously exposed to a smoky environment. He had never smoked.

On questioning, the patient related that he had been very short of breath for the past 6 weeks. During the week before admission, he was unable to walk up one flight of stairs without stopping, and his walking tolerance had decreased to about 100 yards. At 2 days before admission, he noticed that his ankles were swollen and that he had gained 8 pounds in 1 week. He also stated that he had been coughing up small amounts of thick, rust-colored sputum. His cough was strong.

On physical examination, this anxious, profusely sweating man in moderate respiratory distress had the following vital signs: regular heart rate of 120 beats per minute, blood pressure of 140/70, respiratory rate of 32 breaths per minute, and an oral temperature of 100° F. Inspection of the chest revealed suprasternal notch retraction, with some use of the accessory muscles of inspiration. The lungs were mildly hyperresonant to percussion, and breath sounds were diminished. Tight expiratory wheezes were heard. The I:E ratio was 1:4. The chest had an increased anteroposterior diameter; the nail beds were moderately cyanotic. Pitting edema (3+) was noticed on the ankles. The patient was slightly confused. The patient was not able to cooperate well and was unable to concentrate. The chest X-ray showed a generalized increase in pulmonary markings and moderate hyperinflation of the lungs. Some infiltrates were present in the lower lung regions, and possible infiltrates were noted in the right upper lobe. The radiology report suggested the presence of a pneumonic process superimposed on chronic lung disease and mild signs of cor pulmonale.

On his third attempt, the patient was able to perform a relatively good peak expiratory flow rate (PEFR) effort, with results of 180 L/minute. His arterial blood gases while on a 3 L/minute O_2 nasal cannula were pH 7.27, $Paco_2$ 82, HCO_3^- 36, and Pao_2 of 48. The Sao_2 was 75%. Laboratory studies revealed a hemoglobin of 16.5 g/dl and a white blood count of 15,000/mm³. Sputum cultures were positive for a variety of pathogenic and nonpathogenic organisms. The serum $\alpha_1 PI$ level was 30 mg/dl (N 200 to 400 mg/dl). The remainder of the physical examination was not remarkable. The respiratory assessment read as follows:

Respiratory Assessment and Plan

S "I'm short of breath with any exercise at all." Cough for past 6 weeks.

O HR 120, BP 140/70, RR of 32, and temp of 100° F. Use of accessory muscles of inspiration, increased AP diameter, cyanosis, and pitting edema of ankles. Coughing and small amounts of thick, rusty sputum. Hyperresonant percussion note and diminished breath sounds. Lower lung infiltrates, hyperinflation of lungs, and cardiomegaly on CXR. PEFR 180. ABGs: pH 7.27, $Paco_2$ 82, HCO_3^- 36, and Pao_2 of 48. Sao_2: 75%. Elevated WBC and gram-positive organisms in the sputum, $\alpha_1 PI$ = 30 mg/dl.

A • Panacinar emphysema (history, $\alpha_1 PI$ deficiency)
   • Bronchospasm (wheezes)
   • Some airway secretions (sputum)—suggests bronchitis. Good ability to mobilize secretions (strong cough)
   • Probable pneumonitis (X-ray)
   • Mild cor pulmonale (leg edema, X-ray)
   • Acute ventilatory failure on chronic ventilatory failure with moderate hypoxemia (ABGs)

P Notify doctor about acute ventilatory failure. Aerosolized Medication Protocol (premixed albuterol, 2.0 cc in nebulizer. Oxygen Therapy Protocol (HAFOE mask at Fio_2 = 0.35). Bronchopulmonary Hygiene Therapy Protocol (cough and deep breathe Q2 hours × 6, then Q4 hours). Place intubation equipment and ventilator on standby. Monitor and evaluate per ICU standing orders (Spo_2, vital signs). Check ABG in 30 min.

The hospital course was relatively smooth. The low-flow oxygen was enough to increase the patient's Pao_2 to an acceptable level and correct the acute-on-chronic ventilatory failure. Within an hour after the low-flow oxygen was started, the patient's arterial blood gases were pH 7.36, $Paco_2$ 61, HCO_3^- 34, and Pao_2 76. The patient's heart rate, respiratory rate, and blood pressure returned to normal. Blood serologies suggested *Mycoplasma pneumoniae* infection. Intravenous antibiotics were prescribed. The patient was managed conservatively and improved steadily. When he appeared to have had the maximum benefit from the hospitalization, he was discharged with an oxygen concentrator, a portable "stroller," and an oxygen-conserving device. He was to use O_2 at 1 L/minute at rest and 2.5 L/minute with exercise for 18 to 24 hours a day. Arrangements were made to have him enroll in an α_1-antitrypsin therapy trial and attend pulmonary rehabilitation classes. He was urged to secure employment elsewhere.

Discussion

This fascinating (but fortunately rare) form of emphysema is one in which "pure" emphysema is the dominant pathology. In patients with α_1-protease inhibitor deficiency, chronic bronchitis may be present, but it is much less common than is the usual, cigarette smoking–induced COPD. In this condition the patient's lack of the protease inhibitor α_1-antitrypsin resulted in WBC-mediated protease destruction of his pulmonary parenchyma. Note the slow, insidious onset of his symptoms.

The patient's emphysema or **Distal Airway and Alveolar Weakening** (see Figure 9-12) was complicated by additional anatomic alterations of the lungs (i.e., **Alveolar Consolidation** [see Figure 9-8] and **Excessive Bronchial Secretions** [see Figure 9-11]). The alveolar consolidation was reflected in the patient's immune/inflammatory response (fever and increased WBC), alveolar infiltrates (X-ray), low Pao_2 (caused by a decreased $\dot{V}/\dot{Q}$ ratio and intrapulmonary shunting), and abnormal vital signs (see Figure 9-8).

The effects of distal airway and alveolar weakening were reflected in the patient's increased AP diameter, use of accessory muscles of inspiration, hyperresonant percussion note, diminished breath sounds, low PEFR, and the chest X-ray that showed *alveolar hyperinflation* (see Figure 9-12). Finally, *excessive bronchial secretions* (see Figure 9-11) also played a part, as shown by his cough, sputum production, hypoxemia, and reduced PEFR. These were early signs of bronchitis. When emphysema and bronchitis occur together, they collectively form the disease complex called *chronic obstructive pulmonary disease (COPD)*. Often the patient may be diagnosed only with emphysema or chronic bronchitis. As a rule of thumb, however, when treating a patient with either of these conditions, the respiratory care practitioner always should be alert for clinical manifestations associated with emphysema and chronic bronchitis (COPD).

The selection of a good program of oxygen supplementation for the patient's cor pulmonale and a trial of bronchodilator therapy were certainly indicated. Note the selection of a HAFOE mask because of his initial significant CO_2 retention. Pneumococcal and influenza prophylaxis were certainly indicated in this case. Frequent intravenous administration of α_1-antitrypsin replacement represents modern therapy in the treatment of this unusual disease, as does counseling the patient that he should not knowingly expose himself to irritants such as those present in the smoky environment of his workplace.

SELF-ASSESSMENT QUESTIONS

Multiple Choice

1. What type of emphysema creates an abnormal enlargement of all structures distal to the terminal bronchioles?

   a. Centrilobular emphysema
   b. α_1-protease inhibitor deficiency emphysema
   c. ZZ phenotype emphysema
   d. Terminal bronchiole emphysema
   e. Panlobular emphysema

2. What is the normal level of α_1-protease inhibitor?

   a. 0 to 200 mg/dl
   b. 200 to 400 mg/dl
   c. 400 to 600 mg/dl
   d. 600 to 800 mg/dl
   e. 800 to 900 mg/dl

3. The diffusion capacity of patients with emphysema is:

   a. Increased
   b. Decreased
   c. Normal

4. Patients with severe emphysema commonly demonstrate which of the following oxygenation indices?

   I. Decreased $S\bar{v}_{O_2}$
   II. Increased O_2ER
   III. Decreased D_{O_2}
   IV. Increased $C(a-\bar{v})_{O_2}$

   a. I only
   b. III only
   c. IV only
   d. I, II, and III only
   e. I, II, III, and IV

5. Which phenotype is associated with the lowest serum concentration of α_1-protease inhibitor?

   a. MM phenotype
   b. MZ phenotype
   c. ZZ phenotype
   d. M phenotype
   e. MPI phenotype

6. Which of the following pulmonary function study findings are associated with severe emphysema?

   I. Increased FRC
   II. Decreased PEFR
   III. Increased RV
   IV. Decreased FVC

   a. I and III only
   b. III and IV only
   c. II and III only
   d. II, III, and IV only
   e. I, II, III, and IV

7. The patient with severe emphysema commonly demonstrates which of the following hemodynamic indices?

   I. Decreased CVP
   II. Increased $\overline{PA}$
   III. Decreased RVSWI
   IV. Increased PVR

   a. I only
   b. III only
   c. II and IV only
   d. I and II only
   e. II, III, and IV only

8. Because acute ventilatory changes often are seen in patients with chronic ventilatory failure, the respiratory care practitioner must be alert for this problem in patients with severe emphysema. Which of the following arterial blood gas findings represent acute alveolar hyperventilation superimposed on chronic ventilatory failure?

   I. Increased pH
   II. Increased Pa_{CO_2}
   III. Increased HCO_3^-
   IV. Increased Pa_{O_2}

   a. II only
   b. II and IV only
   c. I and III only
   d. I, II, and III only
   e. I, II, III, and IV

9. The lung parenchyma in the chest radiograph of a patient with emphysema appears:

   I. Opaque
   II. White
   III. More translucent than normal
   IV. Dark

   a. I only
   b. II only
   c. I and III only
   d. II and III only
   e. III and IV only

10. What is the single most important etiologic factor in emphysema?

   a. α_1-protease inhibitor deficiency
   b. Cigarette smoking
   c. Infection
   d. Sulfur dioxide
   e. Ozone

Answers appear in Appendix XI.

CHAPTER 13

Asthma

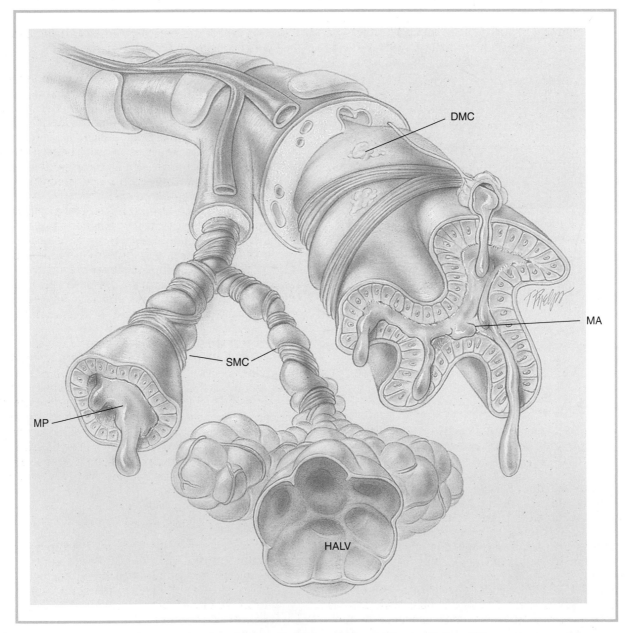

Figure 13–1 Asthma. *DMC,* Degranulation of mast cell; *SMC,* smooth muscle constriction; *MA,* mucus accumulation; *MP,* mucus plug; *HALV,* hyperinflation of alveoli. See also Plate 5.

Anatomic Alterations of the Lungs

During an asthma attack, the smooth muscles surrounding the small airways constrict in response to a particular stimulus. In time, the smooth muscle layers hypertrophy and may increase to three times their size. Goblet cells proliferate, and the bronchial mucous glands enlarge. The airways become filled with thick, whitish, tenacious mucus, and extensive mucus plugging and atelectasis may develop. The bronchial mucosa is edematous and infiltrated with eosinophils and other inflammatory cells. The cilia are damaged, and the basement membrane of the mucosa is thicker than normal. As a result of smooth muscle constriction, bronchial mucosal edema, and mucus hypersecretion, air trapping and alveolar hyperinflation develop. If chronic inflammation develops over time, these anatomic alterations become irreversible, resulting in loss of airway caliber. This process is called *airway remodeling*. A remarkable feature of bronchial asthma, however, is that many of the anatomic alterations that occur during an asthmatic attack are absent between the asthmatic episodes (Figure 13-1).

The major pathologic or structural changes observed during an asthmatic episode are as follows:

- Smooth muscle constriction of bronchial airways (bronchospasm)
- Excessive production of thick, whitish, tenacious bronchial secretions
- Hyperinflation of alveoli (air trapping)
- Mucus plugging and, in severe cases, atelectasis

Etiology

Asthma was first recognized by Hippocrates more than 2000 years ago. It remains one of the most common diseases encountered in clinical medicine. In fact, over the past decade the incidence of asthma has increased dramatically. According to estimates, approximately 15 million Americans have an asthmatic episode each year. About 500,000 Americans are hospitalized annually for severe asthma, and more than 5000 die as a result of asthma annually. According to the World Health Organization, about 180,000 people worldwide die because of asthma. Asthma is found in 3% to 5% of adults and 7% to 10% of children. Approximately 50% of people with asthma develop it before age 10. Asthma is the most common chronic illness of childhood. Among young children, asthma is more prevalent in boys than girls. After puberty, however, asthma is more common in girls.

Asthma is divided into two major types according to its precipitating factors: *extrinsic asthma*, or asthma caused by external or environmental agents; and *intrinsic asthma*, or asthma that occurs in the absence of (or without clear evidence of) an antigen-antibody reaction. Although some authorities believe that the distinction between these terms is of minimal clinical value, the terms are nevertheless widely used.

EXTRINSIC ASTHMA (ALLERGIC OR ATOPIC ASTHMA)

When an asthmatic episode clearly can be associated with exposure to a specific antigenic agent (e.g., pollen, grass and weeds, house dust, dust mites, cockroaches, animal dander, feathers, food preservatives such as sulfites), the patient is said to have *extrinsic asthma* (also called *allergic* or *atopic asthma*). Extrinsic asthma is an immediate (Type I) anaphylactic hypersensitivity reaction. It occurs in individuals who have *atopy*, a hypersensitivity condition associated with genetic predisposition and an excessive amount of IgE antibody production in response to a variety of antigens.

Between 10% and 20% of the general population are atopic and therefore have a tendency to develop an IgE-mediated allergic reaction such as asthma, hay fever, allergic rhinitis, and eczema. Such individuals develop a wheal-and-flare reaction to a variety of skin test allergens. Extrinsic asthma is family-related and usually appears in children and in adults younger than 30 years old. It often disappears after puberty.

Because extrinsic asthma is associated with an antigen–antibody-induced bronchospasm, an immunologic mechanism plays an important role. As with other organs, the lungs are protected against injury by certain immunologic mechanisms. Under normal circumstances these mechanisms function without any apparent clinical evidence of their activity. In patients susceptible to extrinsic or allergic asthma, however, the hypersensitive immune response actually creates the disease by causing acute and chronic inflammation.

The Immunologic Mechanism

1. When a susceptible individual is exposed to a certain antigen, lymphoid tissue cells form specific IgE (reaginic) antibodies. The IgE antibodies attach themselves to the surface of mast cells in the bronchial walls (Figure 13-2, *A*).
2. Reexposure or continued exposure to the same antigen creates an antigen-antibody reaction on the surface of the mast cell, which in turn causes the mast cell to degranulate and release chemical mediators such as histamine, eosinophil chemotactic factor of anaphylaxis

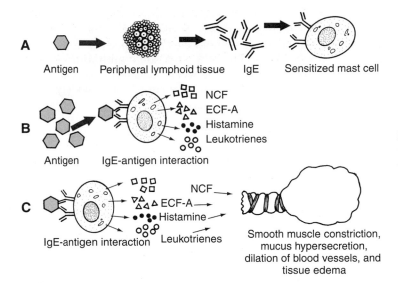

Figure 13–2 The immunologic mechanisms in asthma.

(ECF-A), neutrophil chemotactic factors (NCFs), leukotrienes (formerly known as *slow-reacting substances of anaphylaxis [SRS-A]*), prostaglandins, and platelet-activating factor (PAF; Figure 13-2, *B*).

3. The release of these chemical mediators stimulates parasympathetic nerve endings in the bronchial airways, leading to reflex bronchoconstriction and mucus hypersecretion. Moreover, these chemical mediators increase the permeability of capillaries, which results in the dilation of blood vessels and tissue edema (Figure 13-2, C).

The patient with extrinsic asthma may demonstrate an early asthmatic (allergic) response, a late asthmatic response, or a biphasic asthmatic response. The early asthmatic response begins within minutes of exposure to an inhaled antigen and resolves in approximately 1 hour. A late asthmatic response begins several hours after exposure to an inhaled antigen but lasts much longer. The late asthmatic response may or may not follow an early asthmatic response. An early asthmatic response followed by a late asthmatic response is called a *biphasic response.*

INTRINSIC ASTHMA (NONALLERGIC OR NONATOPIC ASTHMA)

When an asthmatic episode cannot be directly linked to a specific antigen, it is referred to as *intrinsic asthma* (also called *nonallergic* or *nonatopic asthma*). The etiologic factors responsible for intrinsic asthma are elusive. Individuals with intrinsic asthma are not hypersensitive or atopic to environmental antigens and have a normal serum IgE level. The onset of intrinsic asthma usually occurs after the age of 40 years, and typically there is no strong family history of allergy.

In spite of the general distinctions between extrinsic and intrinsic asthma, a significant overlap exists. Distinguishing between the two is often impossible in a clinical setting. Precipitating factors known to cause intrinsic asthma are referred to as *nonspecific stimuli.* Some of the more common nonspecific stimuli associated with intrinsic asthma are discussed in the following paragraphs (Figure 13-3).

Infections

Although bacterial infections may cause asthma, viral upper airway infections are more likely to contribute to asthma. For example, intrinsic asthma is commonly seen in children after respiratory syncytial virus, rhinovirus, or influenza virus infections.

Exercise and Cold Air Exposure

Asthma may be associated with vigorous exercise. The asthmatic episode typically occurs 5 to 10 minutes after the exercise. Exercise in cold, dry air (e.g., jogging, ice skating, cross-country skiing) also

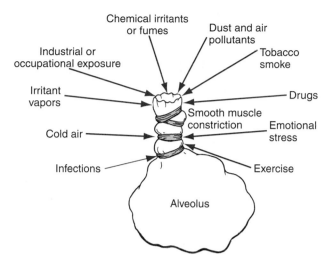

Figure 13–3 Factors triggering intrinsic asthma.

may provoke an asthmatic response in susceptible individuals.

Industrial Pollutants or Occupational Exposure

Numerous industrial pollutants are associated with occupational asthma. Atmospheric industrial pollutants known to provoke asthma include smoke, sulfur dioxide, nitrous oxide, ozone, dust, and noxious gases. Common occupational substances include isocyanate (found in polyurethane, plastics, varnish, and car spray paints), trimellitic anhydride (found in epoxy resins), and organic dusts (found in various woods and plants). Inhalation of cigarette or marijuana smoke also is associated with airway inflammation and bronchoconstriction.

Drugs, Food Additives, and Food Preservatives

Asthma is associated with the ingestion of aspirin and other nonsteroidal antiinflammatory drugs (NSAIDs). As much as 20% of the asthmatic population may be sensitive to aspirin and NSAIDs. Various β-adrenergic blocking agents used to treat hypertension and some cardiac disorders (e.g., propranolol, metoprolol) also may provoke an asthmatic episode. The yellow food coloring agent tartrazine may provoke an asthmatic episode. The ingestion of tartrazine especially is contraindicated in patients sensitive to aspirin. Bisulfites and metabisulfites, commonly used as preservatives and

antioxidants in restaurant food (e.g., salad bars, certain wines, beers, dried fruits), are known to provoke bronchoconstriction. About 5% of the asthmatic population is sensitive to food and drink that contain sulfites.

Gastroesophageal Reflux

Gastroesophageal reflux disease (GERD), or regurgitation, appears to contribute significantly to bronchoconstriction in some patients. The precise mechanism of this relationship is not known.

Sleep (Nocturnal Asthma)

Patients with asthma often have more difficulty late at night or in the early morning. Precipitating factors associated with nocturnal asthma include gastroesophageal reflux, retained airway secretions (caused by a suppressed cough reflex during sleep), exposure to irritants or allergens in the bedroom, and prolonged time between medications. Eradication of nocturnal asthma is one measure of good asthma control.

Emotional Stress

In some patients the exacerbation of asthma appears to correlate with emotional stress and other psychologic factors.

Premenstrual Asthma (Catamnemial Asthma)

The clinical manifestations associated with asthma often worsen in women during the premenstrual and menstrual periods. The peak of worsening symptoms generally occurs 2 to 3 days before menstruation begins. Premenstrual asthma correlates with the late luteal phase of ovarian activity, the phase when circulating progesterone and estrogen levels are at their lowest.

Additional Risk Factors

Researchers have identified a number of factors that may increase an individual's chances of developing asthma, including the following:

- Residence in a large urban area, especially the inner city
- Exposure to secondhand smoke
- A parent who has asthma
- Respiratory infections in childhood
- Low birth weight
- Obesity

OVERVIEW
of the Cardiopulmonary Clinical Manifestations Associated with ASTHMA

The following clinical manifestations result from the pathophysiologic mechanisms caused (or activated) by **Bronchospasm** (see Figure 9-10) and **Excessive Bronchial Secretions** (see Figure 9-11)—the major anatomic alterations of the lungs associated with an asthmatic episode (see Figure 13-1).

CLINICAL DATA OBTAINED AT THE PATIENT'S BEDSIDE

The Physical Examination

Vital Signs

Increased respiratory rate (see page 31 ◆▶)
Several pathophysiologic mechanisms operating simultaneously may lead to an increased ventilatory rate:
- Stimulation of peripheral chemoreceptors (hypoxemia)
- Decreased lung compliance/increased ventilatory rate relationship (when lungs are hyperinflated)
- Anxiety

Increased heart rate (pulse), cardiac output, and blood pressure (see pages 11 and 99 ◆▶)

Use of Accessory Muscles During Inspiration
(see page 40 ◆▶)

Use of Accessory Muscles During Expiration
(see page 42 ◆▶)

Pursed-Lip Breathing (see page 42 ◆▶)

Substernal Intercostal Retractions
(see page 43 ◆▶)
Substernal, supraclavicular, and intercostal retractions during inspiration may be seen, particularly in children

Increased Anteroposterior Chest Diameter (Barrel Chest) (see page 45 ◆▶)

Cyanosis (see page 45 ◆▶)

Cough and Sputum Production (see page 47 ◆▶)
During an asthmatic episode, the patient may produce an excessive amount of thick, whitish, tenacious mucus. Because of the presence of large numbers of eosinophils and other white blood cells, the sputum is often purulent.

Pulsus Paradoxus
When an asthmatic episode produces severe alveolar air trapping and hyperinflation, pulsus paradoxus is a classic clinical manifestation. *Pulsus paradoxus* is defined as a systolic blood pressure that is more than 10 mm Hg lower on inspiration than on expiration. This exaggerated waxing and waning of arterial blood pressure can be detected using a blood pressure cuff or, in severe cases, by palpating the strength of the pulse. Pulsus paradoxus during an asthmatic attack is believed to be caused by the major intrapleural pressure swings that occur during inspiration and expiration.

Decreased blood pressure during inspiration
During inspiration the patient frequently recruits accessory muscles of inspiration. The accessory muscles help produce an extremely negative intrapleural pressure, which in turn enhances intrapulmonary air flow. The increased negative intrapleural pressure, however, also causes blood vessels in the lungs to dilate and blood to pool. Consequently, the volume of blood returning to the left ventricle decreases. This causes a reduction in cardiac output and arterial blood pressure during inspiration.

Increased blood pressure during expiration
During expiration, the patient often activates the accessory muscles of expiration in an effort to overcome the increased airway resistance. The increased power produced by these muscles generates a greater positive intrapleural pressure. Although increased positive intrapleural pressure may help offset the airway resistance, it also works to narrow or squeeze the blood vessels of the lung. This increased pressure on the pulmonary blood vessels enhances left ventricular filling and results in an increased cardiac output and arterial blood pressure during expiration.

Chest Assessment Findings (see page 22 ◆▶)
- Expiratory prolongation
- Decreased tactile and vocal fremitus
- Hyperresonant percussion note
- Diminished breath sounds
- Diminished heart sounds
- Wheezing and rhonchi

CLINICAL DATA OBTAINED FROM LABORATORY TESTS AND SPECIAL PROCEDURES

Pulmonary Function Study Findings (During an Asthmatic Episode)

Expiratory Maneuver Findings (see page 62 ◆▶)

FVC	FEV_T	$FEF_{25\%-75\%}$	$FEF_{200-1200}$
↓	↓	↓	↓
PEFR	MVV	$FEF_{50\%}$	$FEV_{1\%}$
↓	↓	↓	↓

Lung Volume and Capacity Findings (see page 66 ◆▶)

V_T	RV	FRC	TLC
N or ↑	↑	↑	N or ↑
VC	IC	ERV	RV/TLC ratio
↓	N or ↓	N or ↓	↑

OVERVIEW

of the Cardiopulmonary Clinical Manifestations Associated with ASTHMA (Continued)

Arterial Blood Gases

Mild to Moderate Asthmatic Episode
Acute Alveolar Hyperventilation With Hypoxemia
(see page 70 ◆➤)

pH	Paco₂	HCO₃⁻	Pao₂
↑	↓	↓(Slightly)	↓

Severe Asthmatic Episode (Status Asthmaticus)
Acute Ventilatory Failure With Hypoxemia
(see page 73 ◆➤)

pH	Paco₂	HCO₃⁻*	Pao₂
↓	↑	↑(Slightly)	↓

*When tissue hypoxia is severe enough to produce lactic acid, the pH and HCO₃⁻ values will be lower than expected for a particular Paco₂ level.

Oxygenation Indices (see page 82 ◆➤)

Q̇s/Q̇т	Do₂†	V̇o₂	C(a-v̄)o₂
↑	↓	Normal	Normal

O₂ER	Sv̄o₂
↑	↓

† The Do₂ may be normal in patients who have compensated to the decreased oxygenation status with an increased cardiac output. When the Do₂ is normal, the O₂ER is usually normal.

ABNORMAL LABORATORY TESTS AND PROCEDURES

Sputum examination
- Eosinophils
- Charcot-Leyden crystals
- Casts of mucus from small airways (Kirschman spirals)
- IgE level (elevated in extrinsic asthma)

RADIOLOGIC FINDINGS

Chest Radiograph
- Increased anteroposterior diameter ("barrel chest")
- Translucent (dark) lung fields
- Depressed or flattened diaphragms

As the alveoli become enlarged during an asthmatic attack, the residual volume and functional residual capacity increase. This condition decreases the radiographic density of the lungs.

Consequently, the chest X-ray shows lung shadows that are translucent or darker than normal in appearance. Because of the increased residual volume and functional residual capacity, the diaphragm is depressed and flattened (Figure 13-4).

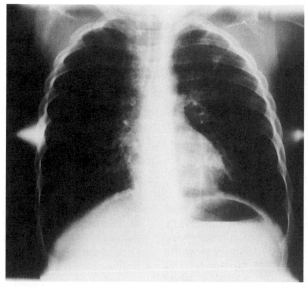

Figure 13–4   Chest X-ray of a 2-year-old patient during an acute asthma attack.

TABLE 13–1   Asthma Classification Based on Severity

Disease Category	Symptoms	Nocturnal Symptoms	Daily Medication for Long-Term Control	Medication for Quick Relief
Step 4: Severe persistent	Continual symptoms Limited physical activity Frequent exacerbations	Frequent	**Two daily medications:** Antiinflammatory agent (high-dose) inhaled glucocorticoid **and** Long-acting bronchodilator (inhaled or oral beta$_2$-agonist or theophylline) **and** Oral glucocorticoid	Short-acting, inhaled β$_2$-agoinst Daily use or increasing use indicates need for additional long-term therapy
Step 3: Moderate persistent	Daily symptoms Daily use of inhaled, short-acing β$_2$-agonist Exacerbations affect activity Exacerbations at least twice weekly and may last for days	More frequent than once weekly	**One or two daily medications:** Antiinflammatory agent (medium-dose inhaled glucocorticoid) **and/or** Medium-dose inhaled glucocorticoid plus long-acting bronchodilator	Short-acting, inhaled β$_2$-agonist Daily use or increased use indicates need for additional long-term therapy
Step 2: Mild persistent	Symptoms more frequent than twice weekly but less than once per day Exacerbations may affect activity	More frequent than twice monthly	**One-daily medication:** Antiinflammatory agent (low-dose inhaled glucocorticoid, cromolyn, or nedocromil) **or** Sustained-release theophylline NOTE: Leukotriene modifiers may be considered for individuals at least 12 yr old	Short-acting, inhaled β$_2$-agonist Daily use or increasing use indicates need for additional long-term therapy
Step 1: Mild intermittent	Symptoms no more frequent than twice weekly Asymptomatic and with normal PEFR between exacerbations Exacerbations brief (hours to days) Intensity of exacerbations varies	No more frequent than twice monthly	**No daily medication**	Short-acting, inhaled β$_2$-agonist Use more than twice weekly may indicate need to initiate long-term therapy

From McCance KL, Huether SE: *Pathophysiology: The biologic basis for disease in adults and children*, ed 4, St. Louis, 2002, Mosby. *PEFR*, Peak expiratory flow rate.

General Management of Asthma

In the United States, most guidelines used to treat asthma have been adapted from the National Heart, Lung, and Blood Institute's (NHLBI's) "stepwise approach for the management of asthma in adults and children" (Table 13-1). In general, the NHLBI provides an asthma classification system that is based on clinical severity rather than underlying pathophysiologic differences (i.e., extrinsic vs. intrinsic asthma). This "asthma classification based on severity" system is believed to correlate better with management choices and clinical outcomes). According to the NHLBI, patient self-monitoring should be performed with a peak flow meter and a daily symptom/treatment log. This management program is called an Asthma Zone Management System (Table 13-2).

TABLE 13–2 **Asthma Zone Management System**	
Green Zone (80%-100% of personal best peak expiratory flow rate [PEFR])	No asthma symptoms are present, and the routine treatment plan for maintaining control can be followed.
Yellow Zone (50%-80% of personal best PEFR)	An acute exacerbation may be present, and a temporary increase in medication may be indicated.
Red Zone (Less than 50% of the personal best PEFR)	This condition signals a medical alert: A short-acting bronchodilator should be used immediately, and the clinician should be notified if the PEFR measurements do not return immediately to, and stay in, the Yellow or Green Zones.

ENVIRONMENTAL CONTROL

The patient should make every effort to eliminate common household factors that may trigger an asthmatic episode. For example, rugs, draperies, furniture, and bed linen should be aired frequently. Foam rubber pillows should be well ventilated and kept dry. Other household members or visitors should not be allowed to smoke in the house. The heating system should be cleaned at least once a year, and temperature and humidity should be maintained at a comfortable level.

RESPIRATORY CARE TREATMENT PROTOCOLS

Oxygen Therapy Protocol

Oxygen therapy is used to treat hypoxemia, decrease the work of breathing, and decrease myocardial work. The hypoxemia that develops in asthma is usually caused by the hypoventilation and shuntlike effect associated with bronchospasm and increased airway secretions. Hypoxemia caused by a shuntlike effect can at least partly be corrected by oxygen therapy (see Oxygen Therapy Protocol, Protocol 9-1).

Bronchopulmonary Hygiene Therapy Protocol

Because of the excessive mucus production and secretion accumulation associated with asthma, a number of bronchial hygiene treatment modalities may be used to enhance the mobilization of bronchial secretions (see Bronchopulmonary Hygiene Therapy Protocol, Protocol 9-2).

Aerosolized Medication Protocol

Both sympathomimetic and parasympatholytic agents commonly are used in the treatment of asthma to induce bronchial smooth muscle relaxation (see Aerosolized Medication Protocol, Protocol 9-4 and Appendix II).

Mechanical Ventilation Protocol

When acute ventilatory failure is associated with status asthmaticus, continuous mechanical ventilation may be required to maintain an adequate ventilatory status. Status asthmaticus is defined as a severe asthmatic episode that does not respond to conventional pharmacologic therapy. When the patient becomes fatigued, the ventilatory rate decreases. Clinically, the patient demonstrates a progressive decrease in Pao_2 and pH and a steady increase in $Paco_2$ (acute ventilatory failure). If this trend is not reversed, mechanical ventilation becomes necessary (see Mechanical Ventilation Protocol, Protocol 9-5).

MEDICATIONS COMMONLY PRESCRIBED BY THE PHYSICIAN

Xanthines

Oral or intravenous xanthines such as theophylline may be prescribed for asthma patients to cause bronchial smooth muscle relaxation (see Appendix II). Inhaled bronchodilator agents, however, are the first-line bronchoconstriction hypersecretion "rescue" agents.

Corticosteroids

Corticosteroids are the first-line, antiinflammatory "preventer" or "controller" drugs. Although the exact mode of action of corticosteroids is not known, they have been shown to be highly effective in preventing and treating asthma when environmental control measures have failed (see Appendix II).

Other Antiinflammatory Agents

Some inhaled antiinflammatory agents such as cromolyn sodium (Intal) and nedocromil sodium (Tilade) are helpful and also are considered first-line "preventer" agents.

Leukotriene Inhibitors

Leukotrienes are inflammatory mediators that play a major role in the causation of asthma. They are released during the antigen-antibody reaction associated with extrinsic asthma (see Figure 13-2). Leukotrienes cause constriction of smooth muscle in the airway wall, edema, leakage from blood vessels in the airway walls, mucus gland stimulation, and secretion of mucus. Leukotrienes also attract eosinophils into the airways. Oral leukotriene inhibitor agents such as montelukast (Singulair), zafirlukast (Accolate), and zileuton (Zyflo) may be considered for Step 2 (mild persistent) patients older than 12 years. Leukotriene inhibitors also may be useful in patients who have troublesome exercise-induced asthma and in patients whose asthma is induced by aspirin and various NSAIDs.

MONITORING

Arterial blood gas determinations, pulse oximetry, and serial pulmonary function measurements such as PEFR or FEV_1 are used to assess the severity and progression of the asthmatic episode and to monitor the patient's response to treatment. Vital signs also must be monitored closely, and a chest radiograph should be obtained as soon as possible after admission to the hospital to help evaluate the degree of air trapping and identify any associated atelectasis or pneumonia.

PATIENT COMPLIANCE

Patient compliance with therapy must be monitored. Recent studies regarding the frequency and quality of use of metered dose inhalers (MDIs), particularly among children and the economically disadvantaged, show that such devices are being used incorrectly more than half of the time. Measures of patient compliance include the following:

1. Asthma-symptom/medication-use diaries
2. Serum theophylline levels
3. Carboxyhemoglobin determinations (to detect tobacco smoke exposure)
4. Total (circulating) eosinophil counts
5. No-show rates at physician offices
6. Rate of medication use
7. Frequency of emergency department visits and hospitalizations
8. Number of red zone days per month (see Table 13-2)

Case Study: ASTHMA

Admitting History and Physical Examination

A 5-year-old girl was admitted to the emergency department (ED) in severe respiratory distress. Her respiratory symptoms dated to age 1 month, when she first developed wheezing. She was hospitalized in different hospitals on a number of occasions and was usually managed satisfactorily with aerosolized albuterol, intravenous (IV) steroids, and aminophylline. She developed a cough and wheezing the night before admission and became progressively worse during the night. Her cough was nonproductive. At 8 AM, she was brought to the ED.

Physical examination revealed an extremely anxious, well-developed female child in acute respiratory distress. Her vital signs were as follows: blood pressure 152/115, pulse 220/min, and respiratory rate 62/min. Her rectal temperature was 100° F. Her extremities appeared cyanotic, and her tonsils were enlarged. She was using her accessory muscles of respiration. On auscultation, rhonchi and wheezing could be heard throughout both lung fields. Her PEFR was 50 L/min. (Her personal best was about 100 to 150 L/min.) Arterial blood gases on 2 L/min nasal cannula oxygen were pH 7.17, $Paco_2$ 71, HCO_3^- 22, and Pao_2 47. A chest X-ray was ordered but not performed. The physician ordered a respiratory care consultation and stated that she did not want to commit the patient to a ventilator at this time if possible. The physician asked that aggressive noninvasive pulmonary care be tried first. At this time, the respiratory care practitioner documented the following:

Respiratory Assessment and Plan

S Acute respiratory distress and anxiety

O Vital signs: BP 152/115, HR 220, RR 62, T 100°. Cyanotic and using accessory muscles. Wheezing and rhonchi over both lungs. PEFR: 50 L/min—Red Zone. ABGs pH 7.17, $Paco_2$ 71, HCO_3^- 22, and Pao_2 47. No CXR yet.

A • Respiratory distress (increased heart rate, blood pressure, respiratory rate)
   • Bronchospasm (wheezing, decreased PEFR, history)
   • Excessive airway secretions (rhonchi)
   • Acute ventilatory failure with moderate/severe hypoxemia (ABG)
   • Metabolic acidosis likely (both pH & HCO_3^- lower than expected for a $Paco_2$ of 71).
   • Likely caused by lactic acid (low Pao_2 47)

P Oxygen Therapy Protocol (Fio_2 80%-100% via oxygen nonrebreather mask). Monitor Spo_2

with oximeter. Aerosolized Medication Therapy Protocol (med. neb. every 30 minutes with albuterol 0.15 ml in 2.0 ml normal saline via Circulaire nebulizer). Monitor PEFR and breath sounds. Bronchopulmonary Hygiene Therapy Protocol (cough & deep breathe). Monitor breath sounds. Place endotracheal tube and mechanical ventilator on stand-by. Repeat ABG in 30 minutes. Respiratory care practitioner to remain in ED.

In addition to this plan, the patient was treated vigorously with IV aminophylline, steroids, and a beclomethasone inhaler (2 puffs every 30 minutes × 4 per emergency room standing orders for asthma) over the next 2 hours. Although the patient seemed to improve slightly, her next arterial blood gas reading showed that her $Paco_2$ had increased slightly to 79.

The respiratory therapist notified the doctor immediately. Following this, the patient was lightly sedated, paralyzed (with vecuronium [Norcuron]), intubated, and placed on a mechanical ventilator. The next morning, on an Fio_2 of 0.4 and a mechanical ventilator rate of 12 breaths per minute, her arterial blood gases were pH 7.38, $Paco_2$ 37, HCO_3^- 23, and Pao_2 124. Her vital signs were blood pressure 122/87, heart rate 93, temperature 98.8° F. Her wheezes and rhonchi had diminished but were still present. At this point, the following was recorded:

Respiratory Assessment and Plan

S N/A (patient sedated and paralyzed)

O Sedated, paralyzed, fewer wheezes & rhonchi. Vital signs: BP 122/87, HR 93, T 98.8° F. ABG: pH 7.38, $Paco_2$ 37, HCO_3^- 23, Pao_2 124 (on CMV 12, Fio_2 0.4)

A Less bronchospasm (decreased wheezing, normal ABGs)
   • Less bronchial secretions (decreased rhonchi)
   • Adequately ventilated and oxygenated on present ventilator settings (ABG)

P Discuss with physician: D/C Norcuron. Continue in-line med. nebs. IMV wean and O_2 wean as per Mechanical Ventilation Protocol. Continue to monitor O_2 saturation.

The patient remained intubated for another 24 hours, at which time her lungs were clear and when suctioned returned scant but clear secretions. She was weaned from the ventilator with ease and was extubated shortly thereafter. The patient was discharged the following day, after review of the Asthma Action Plan with her parents.

Discussion

Asthma is a potentially fatal disease—largely because its severity is often unrecognized in the home or out-patient setting. The clinical manifestations presented in this case can all be easily traced back through the **Bronchospasm** (see Figure 9-10) and **Excessive Airway Secretions** (see Figure 9-11) clinical scenarios. The patient's increased blood pressure, heart rate, and respiratory rate can all be followed back to the hypoxemia caused by the decreased $\dot{V}/\dot{Q}$ ratio, pulmonary shunting, and venous admixture (pathophysiologic mechanisms) activated by bronchospasm and excessive bronchial secretions (see Figure 13-1). The patient's anxiety and previous use of β_2-agonists also may have contributed to her abnormal vital signs.

In addition, the decreased PEFR, use of accessory muscles, diminished breath sounds, rhonchi, and wheezing reflect the increased airway resistance and air trapping caused by the **Bronchospasm** (see Figure 9-10) and **Excessive Airway Secretions** (see Fig. 9-11). The fact that the patient's arterial blood gas values showed acute ventilatory failure confirmed that the patient was in the severe stages of the asthmatic episode and that mechanical ventilation was justified, although vigorous routine respiratory care was first tried to prevent this.

After his initial assessment, the respiratory care practitioner chose a fairly aggressive approach to both the *Oxygen Therapy* (Protocol 9-1) and *Aerosolized Medication Therapy* (Protocol 9-4). Use of a non-rebreather oxygen therapy mask at initially high F_{IO_2} levels (0.8 to 1.0) allowed him to adjust the F_{IO_2} in small, precise concentration changes while not risking rebreathing of expired air. Frequent monitoring of ABGs and Sp_{O_2} levels was appropriate. Note also the frequency with which he chose to administer inhaled bronchodilators (every 30 minutes) in the Aerosolized Medication Therapy Protocol.

The manner in which any therapy modality is up-regulated may be (1) a *different* aerosolized drug or procedure, (2) a larger *dose* of a drug or therapy, or (3) *more frequent* use of such drugs or therapy. In this case, he chose the latter course, only to see it fail (the patient required intubation).

Among the lessons to be learned here is that some asthmatic episodes worsen despite vigorous therapy. This patient received optimal emergent treatment of her resistant asthma but required intubation and mechanical ventilation nonetheless. Almost continuous assessment by the respiratory care practitioner is necessary if more aggressive therapy (including induced sedation, paralysis, and mechanical ventilation) is to be effective.

The use of IV aminophylline in the emergency treatment of acute asthma in the emergency department is controversial. Care must be taken to avoid theophylline toxicity, and symptoms of toxicity often do not reflect serum concentrations of the drug. The acutely ill asthmatic requires almost continuous monitoring and frequent SOAP notes if the patient care team is to be constantly apprised of the patient's progress. The two such notes recorded here are but a small portion of the more than 14 notes that the authors found on analysis of the patient's medical record after her ED discharge alone.

SELF-ASSESSMENT QUESTIONS

Multiple Choice

1. During an asthmatic episode, the smooth muscle of the bronchi may hypertrophy as much as

   a. 2 times normal size
   b. 3 times normal size
   c. 4 times normal size
   d. 5 times normal size
   e. 6 times normal size

2. Asthma is associated with which of the following?

   I. Increase in goblet cells
   II. Decrease in cilia
   III. Increase in bronchial gland size
   IV. Decrease in eosinophils

   a. I and III only
   b. II and IV only
   c. I, II, and III only
   d. II, III, and IV only
   e. I, II, III, and IV

3. During an extrinsic-type asthma attack, the lymphoid tissue cells form which antibody?

   a. IgA
   b. IgM
   c. IgG
   d. IgE

4. When chemical mediators from mast cells are released:

   I. Bronchial dilation occurs
   II. Bronchial gland hypersecretion occurs
   III. Blood vessels constrict
   IV. Tissue edema occurs

   a. I only
   b. II only
   c. II and IV only
   d. I and III only
   e. I, III, and IV only

5. Which of the following are associated with intrinsic asthma?

   I. NSAIDs
   II. Respiratory syncytial virus
   III. Gastroesophageal reflux
   IV. Bisulfites

   a. I and IV only
   b. II and III only
   c. III and IV only
   d. II, III, and IV only
   e. I, II, III, and IV

6. When pulsus paradoxus appears during an asthma attack:

   I. Left ventricle filling is increased during inspiration.
   II. Cardiac output decreases during expiration.
   III. Left ventricle filling increases during expiration.
   IV. Cardiac output increases during inspiration.

   a. I only
   b. II only
   c. III only
   d. I and II only
   e. III and IV only

7. During an asthmatic episode, which of the following abnormal lung volume and capacity findings are found?

   I. Increased FRC
   II. Decreased ERV
   III. Increased FEV_1
   IV. Decreased RV

   a. I only
   b. II only
   c. I and II only
   d. III and IV only
   e. II, III, and IV only

8. During mast cell degranulation, which of the following chemical mediators are released?

    I. NCF
    II. ECF-A
    III. Histamine
    IV. Leukotrienes

    a. I only
    b. II only
    c. III only
    d. II and IV only
    e. I, II, III, and IV

9. Patients commonly exhibit which of the following arterial blood gas values during an acute asthmatic episode?

    I. Increased pH
    II. Increased $Paco_2$
    III. Decreased HCO_3^-
    IV. Decreased Pao_2

    a. IV only
    b. I and III only
    c. II and IV only
    d. I, II, and III only
    e. I, III, and IV only

10. The onset of intrinsic asthma usually occurs after which age?

    a. 20 years
    b. 30 years
    c. 40 years
    d. 50 years
    e. 60 years

True or False

True ☐ False ☐ 1. Pathologic alterations of the lungs are absent between moderate asthmatic episodes.

True ☐ False ☐ 2. A patient with extrinsic asthma generally demonstrates symptoms after 30 years of age.

True ☐ False ☐ 3. An antigen-antibody reaction generally is absent in intrinsic asthma.

True ☐ False ☐ 4. Extrinsic asthma is also considered an allergic disorder.

True ☐ False ☐ 5. A partial β-blockade may be responsible for the occurrence of asthma in some individuals.

True ☐ False ☐ 6. During an asthmatic attack, wheezing occurs more frequently during expiration.

Matching

Directions: On the line next to the trade name in column A, match the generic name from column B. Items in column B may be used once, more than once, or not at all.

Column A

TRADE NAME

1. _____ Vanceril
2. _____ Alupent
3. _____ Spiriva
4. _____ Serevent
5. _____ Atrovent
6. _____ Proventil
7. _____ Xopenex
8. _____ Beclovent
9. _____ Brethine
10. _____ Metaprel
11. _____ Foradil
12. _____ Ventolin
13. _____ Intal

Column B

GENERIC NAME

a. Formoterol
b. Terbutaline
c. Salmeterol
d. Metaproterenol
e. Racemic epinephrine
f. Beclomethasone
g. Theophylline
h. Albuterol
i. Levalbuterol
j. Dexamethasone
k. Ipratroprium bromide
l. Cromolyn sodium
m. Tiotropium

Answers appear in Appendix XI.

CHAPTER 14

Bronchiectasis

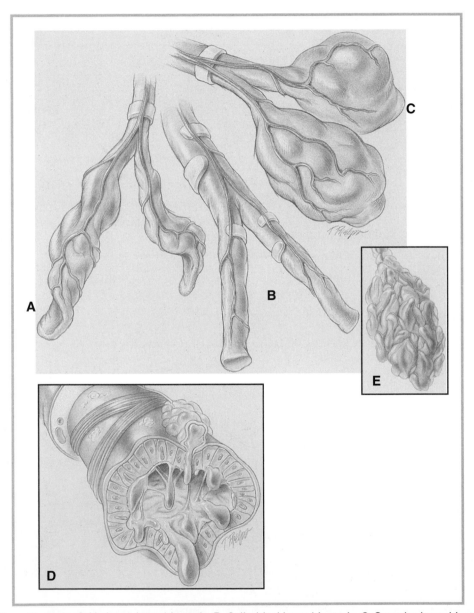

Figure 14–1   Bronchiectasis. **A,** Varicose bronchiectasis. **B,** Cylindrical bronchiectasis. **C,** Saccular bronchiectasis.
Also illustrated are excessive bronchial secretions **(D)** and atelectasis **(E),** which are both common anatomic alterations of the lungs in this disease. See also Plate 6.

Anatomic Alterations of the Lungs

Bronchiectasis is characterized by chronic dilation and distortion of one or more bronchi as a result of extensive inflammation and destruction of the bronchial wall cartilage, blood vessels, elastic tissue, and smooth muscle components. One or both lungs may be involved. Bronchiectasis is commonly limited to a lobe or segment and is frequently found in the lower lobes. The smaller bronchi, with less supporting cartilage, are predominantly affected.

Because of bronchial wall destruction, the mucociliary clearance mechanism is impaired. This results in the accumulation of copious amounts of bronchial secretions and blood that often become foul-smelling because of secondary colonization with anaerobic organisms. This condition may lead to secondary bronchial smooth muscle constriction. The small bronchi and bronchioles distal to the affected areas become partially or totally obstructed with secretions. This condition leads to one or both of the following anatomic alterations: (1) hyperinflation of the distal alveoli as a result of expiratory check-valve obstruction or (2) atelectasis, consolidation, and fibrosis as a result of complete bronchial obstruction.

Three forms or anatomic varieties of bronchiectasis have been described: *varicose (fusiform), cylindrical (tubular),* and *saccular (cystic).*

VARICOSE BRONCHIECTASIS

The bronchi are dilated and constricted in an irregular fashion similar to varicose veins, ultimately resulting in a distorted, bulbous shape (Figure 14-1, *A*).

CYLINDRICAL BRONCHIECTASIS

The bronchi are dilated and have regular outlines similar to a tube. The dilated bronchi fail to taper for six to ten generations and then appear to end abruptly because of mucus obstruction (Figure 14-1, *B*).

SACCULAR BRONCHIECTASIS

The bronchi progressively increase in diameter until they end in large, cystlike sacs in the lung parenchyma. This form of bronchiectasis causes the greatest damage to the tracheobronchial tree. The bronchial walls become composed of fibrous tissue alone—cartilage, elastic tissue, and smooth muscle are all absent (Figure 14-1, *C*).

The following are the major pathologic or structural changes associated with bronchiectasis:

- Chronic dilation and distortion of bronchial airways
- Excessive production of often foul-smelling sputum (Figure 14-1, *D*)
- Smooth muscle constriction of bronchial airways
- Hyperinflation of alveoli (air trapping)
- Atelectasis (Figure 14-1, *E*), consolidation, and parenchymal fibrosis
- Hemorrhage secondary to bronchial arterial erosion

Etiology

Bronchiectasis is not as common today as it was a few decades ago because of increased use of antibiotics for lower respiratory infections. The etiology of bronchiectasis is not always clear, but evidence indicates that the disease may be either acquired or congenital.

ACQUIRED BRONCHIECTASIS

Recurrent Pulmonary Infection

Bronchiectasis is commonly seen in individuals who have repeated and prolonged episodes of respiratory tract infections (e.g., pneumonia, tuberculosis, and fungal infections). For example, children who have frequent bouts of bronchopneumonia—because of the respiratory complications of measles, chickenpox, whooping cough, or influenza, for example—may acquire some form of bronchiectasis later in life.

Bronchial Obstruction

Bronchial obstruction caused by a foreign body, tumor, or enlarged hilar lymph nodes may result in bronchiectasis distal to the obstruction. These conditions impair the mucociliary clearance mechanism, and this impairment in turn favors the development of necrotizing bacterial infections.

CONGENITAL BRONCHIECTASIS

Kartagener's Syndrome

Kartagener's syndrome is a triad consisting of bronchiectasis, dextrocardia (having the heart on the right side of the chest), and pansinusitis. Kartagener's syndrome accounts for as much as 20% of all congenital bronchiectasis.

Hypogammaglobulinemia

Bronchiectasis is commonly seen in individuals who have inadequate regional or systemic defense mechanisms because of inherited or acquired immune deficiency disorders. These individuals have a high predisposition for recurrent episodes of respiratory infections.

Cystic Fibrosis

Because of impairment of the mucociliary clearance mechanism and the abundance of stagnant, thick mucus associated with cystic fibrosis, bronchial obstruction from mucus plugging and bronchial infections frequently results. The necrotizing inflammation that develops under these conditions often leads to secondary bronchiectasis. It is estimated that cystic fibrosis causes approximately 50% of bronchiectasis cases in the United States today.

OVERVIEW
of the Cardiopulmonary Clinical Manifestations Associated with BRONCHIECTASIS

The following clinical manifestations result from the pathophysiologic mechanisms caused (or activated) by **Atelectasis** (see Figure 9-7), **Consolidation** (see Figure 9-8), **Increased Alveolar-Capillary Membrane Thickness** (see Figure 9-9), **Bronchospasm** (see Figure 9-10), and **Excessive Bronchial Secretions** (see Figure 9-11)—the major anatomic alterations of the lungs associated with bronchiectasis (see Figure 14-1).

CLINICAL DATA OBTAINED AT THE PATIENT'S BEDSIDE

Depending on the amount of bronchial secretions and the degree of bronchial destruction and fibrosis associated with bronchiectasis, the disease may create an obstructive or a restrictive lung disorder or a combination of both. If the majority of the bronchial airways are only partially obstructed, the bronchiectasis manifests primarily as an obstructive lung disorder. If, on the other hand, the majority of the bronchial airways are completely obstructed, the distal alveoli collapse, atelectasis results, and the bronchiectasis manifests primarily as a restrictive disorder. Finally, if the disease is limited to a relatively small portion of the lung—as it often is—the patient may not have any of the following clinical manifestations.

The Physical Examination
Vital Signs

Increased respiratory rate (see page 31 ◆▶)
Several pathophysiologic mechanisms operating simultaneously may lead to an increased ventilatory rate:
- Stimulation of peripheral chemoreceptors (hypoxemia)
- Decreased lung compliance/increased ventilatory rate relationship
- Anxiety

Increased heart rate (pulse), cardiac output, and blood pressure (see pages 11 and 99 ◆▶)

Use of Accessory Muscles During Inspiration (see page 40 ◆▶)

Use of Accessory Muscles During Expiration (see page 42 ◆▶)

Pursed-Lip Breathing (see page 42 ◆▶)

Increased Anteroposterior Chest Diameter (Barrel Chest) (see page 45 ◆▶)

Cyanosis (see page 45 ◆▶)

Digital Clubbing (see page 46 ◆▶)

Peripheral Edema and Venous Distention (see page 47 ◆▶)
Because polycythemia and cor pulmonale are associated with severe bronchiectasis, the following may be seen:
- Distended neck veins
- Pitting edema
- Enlarged and tender liver

Cough, Sputum Production, and Hemoptysis (see page 47 ◆▶)
A chronic cough with production of large quantities of foul-smelling sputum is a hallmark of bronchiectasis. A 24-hour collection of sputum is usually voluminous and tends to settle into several different layers. Streaks of blood are seen frequently in the sputum, presumably originating from necrosis of the bronchial walls and erosion of bronchial blood vessels. Frank hemoptysis may also occur from time to time, but it is rarely life-threatening. Because of the excessive bronchial secretions, secondary bacterial infections are frequent. *Haemophilus influenzae, Streptococcus, Pseudomonas aeruginosa,* and various anaerobic organisms are commonly cultured from the sputum of patients with bronchiectasis.

The productive cough in bronchiectasis is triggered by the large amount of secretions that fill the tracheobronchial tree. The stagnant secretions stimulate the subepithelial mechanoreceptors, which in turn produce a vagal reflex that triggers a cough. The subepithelial mechanoreceptors are found in the trachea, bronchi, and bronchioles, but they are predominantly located in the upper airways.

OVERVIEW
of the Cardiopulmonary Clinical Manifestations Associated with
BRONCHIECTASIS (Continued)

Chest Assessment Findings (see page 22 ◆)

When the bronchiectasis is primarily obstructive in nature
- Decreased tactile and vocal fremitus
- Hyperresonant percussion note
- Diminished breath sounds
- Rhonchi and wheezing

When the bronchiectasis is primarily restrictive in nature (over areas of atelectasis and consolidation)
- Increased tactile and vocal fremitus
- Bronchial breath sounds
- Crackles
- Whispered pectoriloquy
- Dull percussion note

CLINICAL DATA OBTAINED FROM LABORATORY TESTS AND SPECIAL PROCEDURES

Pulmonary Function Study Findings

When Primarily Obstructive in Nature
Expiratory Maneuver Findings (see page 62 ◆)

FVC	FEV_T	$FEF_{25\%-75\%}$	$FEF_{200-1200}$
↓	↓	↓	↓
PEFR	MVV	$FEF_{50\%}$	$FEV_{1\%}$
↓	↓	↓	↓

Lung Volume and Capacity Findings
(see page 66 ◆)

V_T	RV	FRC	TLC
N or ↑	↑	↑	N or ↑
VC	IC	ERV	RV/TLC ratio
↓	N or ↓	N or ↓	↑

When Primarily Restrictive in Nature
Expiratory Maneuver Findings (see page 61 ◆)

FVC	FEV_T	$FEF_{25\%-75\%}$	$FEF_{200-1200}$
↓	N or ↓	N or ↓	N
PEFR	MVV	$FEF_{50\%}$	$FEV_{1\%}$
N	N or ↓	N	N or ↑

Lung Volume and Capacity Findings
(see page 62 ◆)

V_T	RV	FRC	TLC
N or ↓	↓	↓	↓
VC	IC	ERV	RV/TLC%
↓	↓	↓	N

Arterial Blood Gases

Mild to Moderate Bronchiectasis
Acute Alveolar Hyperventilation with Hypoxemia
(see page 70 ◆)

pH	$Paco_2$	HCO_3^-	Pao_2
↑	↓	↓ (Slightly)	↓

Severe Bronchiectasis
Chronic Ventilatory Failure with Hypoxemia
(see page 73 ◆)

pH	$Paco_2$	HCO_3^-	Pao_2
Normal	↑	↑ (Significantly)	↓

Acute Ventilatory Changes Superimposed on Chronic Ventilatory Failure
(see page 75 ◆)

Because acute ventilatory changes frequently are seen in patients with chronic ventilatory failure, the respiratory care practitioner must be familiar with and alert for (1) acute alveolar hyperventilation superimposed on chronic ventilatory failure and (2) acute ventilatory failure superimposed on chronic ventilatory failure.

Oxygenation Indices (see page 82 ◆)

$\dot{Q}S/\dot{Q}T$	Do_2*	$\dot{V}o_2$	$C(a-\bar{v})o_2$
↑	↓	Normal	Normal
O_2ER	Svo_2		
↑	↓		

*The Do_2 may be normal in patients who have compensated for the decreased oxygenation status with (1) an increased cardiac output, (2) an increased hemoglobin level, or (3) a combination of both. When the Do_2 is normal, the O_2ER is usually normal.

Hemodynamic Indices (Severe Chronic Bronchiectasis) (see page 99 ◆)

CVP	RAP	$\overline{PA}$	PCWP
↑	↑	↑	Normal
CO	SV	SVI	CI
Normal	Normal	Normal	Normal
RVSWI	LVSWI	PVR	SVR
↑	Normal	↑	Normal

OVERVIEW
of the Cardiopulmonary Clinical Manifestations Associated with
BRONCHIECTASIS (Continued)

ABNORMAL LABORATORY TESTS AND PROCEDURES

Hematology
* Increased hematocrit and hemoglobin

Sputum examination
* *Streptococcus pneumoniae*
* *Haemophilus influenzae*
* *Pseudomonas aeruginosa*
* Anaerobic organisms

RADIOLOGIC FINDINGS

Chest Radiograph

When the bronchiectasis is primarily obstructive in nature
* Translucent (dark) lung fields
* Depressed or flattened diaphragms
* Long and narrow heart (pulled down by diaphragms)
* Enlarged heart

When the pathophysiology of bronchiectasis is primarily obstructive in nature, the lungs become hyperinflated, the functional residual volume increases, and the radiographic density of the lungs decreases. As a result of this condition, the resistance to X-ray penetration is not as great and is revealed on the chest radiograph as areas of translucency or darker areas. Because of the increased functional residual capacity, the diaphragms may be depressed and are seen in this position on the radiograph. Finally, because right and left ventricular enlargement and failure often develop as secondary problems during the advanced stages of bronchectasis, an enlarged heart may be seen on the chest radiograph.

When the bronchiectasis is primarily restrictive in nature
* Increased opacity
* Atelectasis and consolidation
* Infiltrates (suggesting pneumonia)

When atelectasis and consolidation develop as a result of bronchiectasis, an increased opacity is seen in these areas on the radiograph.

Bronchogram

Bronchography (the injection of an opaque contrast material into the tracheobronchial tree) is occasionally performed on patients with bronchiectasis. Bronchograms may be useful in diagnosing bronchiectasis and delineating the extent and type of tracheobronchial involvement. In cylindrical bronchiectasis the bronchogram shows dilated, cylinder-shaped bronchioles. Increased bronchial markings and adjacent emphysema may be present (Figure 14-2). In saccular bronchiectasis the bronchogram shows large, saclike structures; fibrotic markings; associated atelectasis; and adjacent emphysema (Figure 14-3).

In varicose bronchiectasis the bronchogram may show bronchi that are dilated and constricted in an irregular fashion and terminate in a distorted, bulbous shape (Figure 14-4). Computed tomography (CT) of the chest has largely replaced this technique.

CT Scan

Increased bronchial wall opacity is often seen. The bronchial walls may appear as follows:
* Thick
* Dilated
* Characterized by ring lines or clusters
* Signet ring–shaped
* Flame-shaped

The CT scan changes may include many findings that are similar to the chest radiograph. The bronchial walls may appear thick, dilated, or as rings of opacities arranged in lines or clusters (Figure 14-5).

A characteristic appearance in bronchiectasis is the end-on signet ring opacity produced by the ring shadow of a dilated airway with its accompanying artery. Airways that are filled with secretions produce rounded or flame-shaped opacities that can be identified by following them through adjacent sections to unfilled airways. Bullae and cystic bronchiectasis are difficult to distinguish on the CT scan. The CT scan also confirms atelectasis, consolidation, fibrosis, scarring, and hyperinflation.

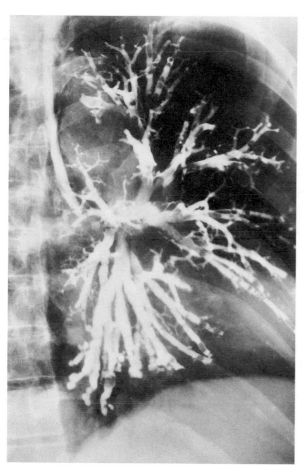

Figure 14–2   Cylindrical bronchiectasis. Left posterior oblique projection of a left bronchogram showing cylindrical bronchiectasis affecting the whole of the lower lobe except for the superior segment. Few side branches fill. Basal airways are crowded together, indicating volume loss of the lower lobe, a common finding in bronchiectasis. (From Armstrong P et al: *Imaging of diseases of the chest,* ed 2, St. Louis, 1995, Mosby.)

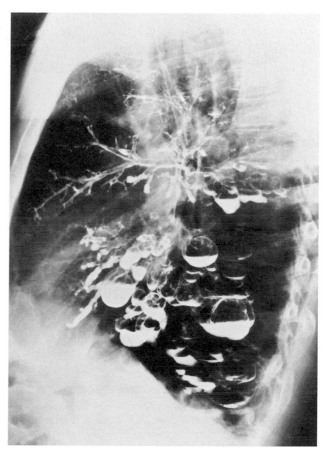

Figure 14–3   Saccular bronchiectasis. Right lateral bronchogram showing saccular bronchiectasis affecting mainly the lower lobe and posterior segment of the upper lobe. (From Armstrong P et al: *Imaging of diseases of the chest,* ed 2, St. Louis, 1995, Mosby.)

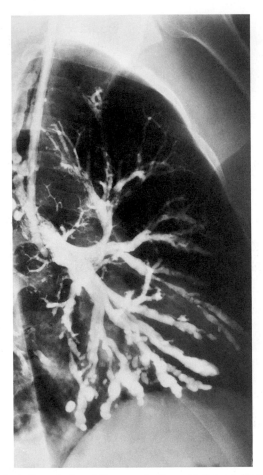

Figure 14–4 Varicose bronchiectasis. Left posterior oblique projection of left bronchogram in a patient with the ciliary dyskinesia syndrome. All basal bronchi are affected by varicose bronchiectasis. (From Armstrong P et al: *Imaging of diseases of the chest,* ed 2, St. Louis, 1995, Mosby.)

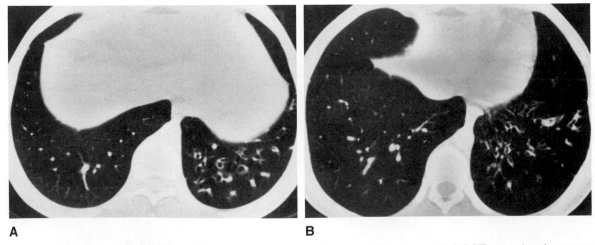

A **B**

Figure 14–5 Bronchiectasis. High-resolution thin-section (1.5-mm) computed tomographic (HRCT) scan showing numerous oval and rounded ring opacities in the left lower lobe. The right lung appears normal. The fact that the airways tend to be arranged in a linear fashion and have walls of more than hairline thickness helps distinguish these bronchiectatic airways from cysts or bullae. (From Armstrong P, Wilson AG, Dee P: *Imaging of diseases of the chest,* St. Louis, 1990, Mosby.)

General Management of Bronchiectasis

The general treatment plan is aimed at controlling pulmonary infections, airway secretions, and airway obstruction and preventing complications. Daily postural drainage and effective coughing exercises to remove bronchial secretions are routine parts of the treatment. Antibiotics, bronchodilators, and expectorants are often prescribed during periods of exacerbation. Childhood vaccinations and yearly influenza vaccination help reduce the prevalence of some infections. The avoidance of upper respiratory infections, smoking, and polluted environments also helps reduce susceptibility to pneumonia in these patients. Surgical lung resection may be indicated for those patients who respond poorly to therapy or experience massive bleeding.

RESPIRATORY CARE TREATMENT PROTOCOLS

Oxygen Therapy Protocol

Oxygen therapy is used to treat hypoxemia, decrease the work of breathing, and decrease mycocardial work. The hypoxemia that develops in bronchiectasis is usually caused by the pulmonary shunting associated with the disorder. When the patient demonstrates chronic ventilatory failure during the advanced stages of bronchiectasis, caution must be taken not to overoxygenate the patient (see Oxygen Therapy Protocol, Protocol 9-1).

Bronchopulmonary Hygiene Therapy Protocol

A number of bronchial hygiene treatment modalities may be used to enhance the mobilization of bronchial secretions (see Bronchopulmonary Hygiene Therapy Protocol, Protocol 9-2).

Hyperinflation Therapy Protocol

Attempts to keep distal lung units inflated may involve the use of deep breathing and coughing and incentive spirometry (see Hyperinflation Therapy Protocol, Protocol 9-3).

Aerosolized Medication Therapy Protocol

Both sympathomimetic and parasympatholytic agents are commonly used in bronchiectasis to induce bronchial smooth muscle relaxation (see Aerosolized Medication Therapy Protocol, Protocol 9-4 and Appendix II).

Mechanical Ventilation Protocol

Mechanical ventilation may be necessary to provide and support alveolar gas exchange and eventually return the patient to spontaneous breathing. Because acute ventilatory failure superimposed on chronic ventilatory failure is often seen in patients with severe bronchiectasis, continuous mechanical ventilation is justified when the acute ventilatory failure is thought to be reversible (see Mechanical Ventilation Protocol, Protocol 9-5).

OTHER MEDICATIONS COMMONLY PRESCRIBED BY THE PHYSICIAN

Xanthines

Xanthines are occasionally prescribed to enhance bronchial smooth muscle relaxation (see Appendix II).

Expectorants

Expectorants sometimes are ordered when oral liquids and aerosol therapy alone are not sufficient to facilitate expectoration (see Appendix II). Their clinical effectiveness is doubtful.

Antibiotic

Antibiotics commonly are administered to treat associated respiratory tract infections (see Appendix II).

Case Study: BRONCHIECTASIS

Admitting History and Physical Examination

A 31-year-old male patient consulted his physician regarding an increasingly productive cough. He reported a "bad case" of pneumonia 7 years ago and several episodes of pulmonary infection since that time. On those occasions he usually received an antibiotic, and until 6 months ago the infections responded readily to treatment. However, 6 months ago he noticed that his chronic cough had become increasingly severe, and for the first time his cough became productive. Recently, he had produced as much as a cup of thick, tenacious, yellow-white sputum per day. Within the past 2 to 3 days, he noticed some dark blood mixed with the sputum. He also noticed some dyspnea on exertion, but this had not been particularly troublesome. The past medical history revealed chronic sinusitis since adolescence but was otherwise unremarkable.

Physical examination revealed a well-developed male adult in no apparent distress. Vital signs were within normal limits. His oral temperature was 98.4° F. He coughed frequently during the examination and produced a moderate amount of thick yellow, blood-streaked sputum. Crackles and rhonchi were heard over the right lower lung fields posteriorly. His Spo_2 on room air while at rest was 85%.

Laboratory results showed a mild leukocytosis but were otherwise normal. Sputum culture indicated the presence of *H. influenzae.* A CT scan revealed saccular dilations of the right lower lobe bronchus. The respiratory care practitioner assigned to assess and treat the patient at this time recorded the following in the patient's chart:

Respiratory Assessment and Plan

S Productive cough, hemoptysis, worse in past 5 months. Mild dyspnea on exertion.

O Vital signs: normal. Afebrile. Observed moderate amount of mucopurulent, blood-streaked sputum. Crackles and rhonchi over RLL. Sputum culture: *H. influenzae.* CT scan suggests saccular dilation of RLL bronchi.

A • Postpneumonic bronchiectasis RLL (history and CT scan)
  • Excessive airway secretions and sputum production (rhonchi and sputum expectoration)
  • Acute bronchial infection and hemoptysis (yellow, blood-streaked sputum)
  • Moderate hypoxemia (Spo_2)

P Oxygen Therapy Protocol (O_2 via 2 Lpm nasal cannula). Aerosolized Medication and Bronchopulmonary Hygiene Protocols (med neb 2.0 cc 20% acetylcysteine with albuterol 0.5 cc, followed by CPT and PD, Q 6 hours).

The patient was treated vigorously with chest physiotherapy and mucolytic therapy. The physician prescribed antibiotics and administered pneumonia vaccine. The patient was discharged from the hospital after 3 days with considerable improvement. He was instructed to seek prompt medical attention for all future pulmonary infections. His wife was instructed in postural drainage techniques.

• • • • •

Approximately 6 months later, the patient arrived at the emergency department complaining of a productive cough, pain on the left side of the chest (made worse by deep breathing), shaking chills and fever

for 3 days, and noticeable swelling of both ankles. Since his previous visit, he had been performing CPT and PD only "once or twice a week," had gained 30 pounds, and had taken a new job as a painter's apprentice. He admitted to smoking an occasional cigarette. There had been no known infectious disease exposure.

Physical examination revealed a young man in obvious respiratory distress. His vital signs were blood pressure 160/100, heart rate 110 bpm and regular, respiratory rate 20/min, and oral temperature 101.5° F. His sputum was foul-smelling (a fecal odor), thick, and yellow-green. His cough was strong. Auscultation revealed sibilant rhonchi and crackles over both bases. There was early clubbing of fingers and toes, and 2 to 3+ pitting edema to midcalf. Homans' sign was negative. The physician wrote "bronchiectasis" in the diagnosis section of the patient's chart.

Although a chest X-ray had been taken, it was not yet available. The patient's WBC was 23,500 mm³, with 80% segmented neutrophils and 10% bands. EKG showed large P waves in II, III, and AVF and deep S waves across the pericardium. Room air ABG showed pH 7.51, $Paco_2$ 28 mm Hg, HCO_3^- 21, and Pao_2 45 mm Hg. His Spo_2 at rest on room air was 86%; it fell to 78% when he got out of bed to go to the bathroom. The respiratory care practitioner recorded the following note in the patient's emergency department chart:

Respiratory Assessment and Plan

S Cough, pleuritic left chest pain, chills, fever, leg swelling. Has not been doing CPT and PD on regular basis. 30# weight gain. Smoking.

O HR 110; RR 20; BP 160/100; T 101.5° F; Spo_2 (room air, rest) 86, falls to 78% with mild exertion. Sputum thick, yellow-green, foul-smelling. Rhonchi and crackles both bases. Strong cough. Clubbing of digits. 2-3+ leg edema. WBC 23,000 (80% neutrophils, 10% bands). Peaked P waves in II, III, AVF. Room air ABG; pH 7.51; $Paco_2$ 28 mm Hg; HCO_3^- 21; Pao_2 45 mm Hg.

A • Bronchiectasis (old chart record)
  • Excessive airway secretions (thick sputum, rhonchi)
  • Infection likely (fever, yellow-green sputum); good ability to mobilize secretions (strong cough)
  • Acute alveolar hyperventilation with moderate hypoxemia (ABG)
  • Cor pulmonale 2° to bronchiectasis (chronic hypoxia, EKG, leg edema)
  • Therapy and smoking cessation noncompliance (history)

P Review CXR. Oxygen Therapy Protocol (2 Lpm per nasal cannula). Aerosolized Medication and Bronchopulmonary Hygiene Protocols (med neb. 2.0 cc 20% acetylcysteine with albuterol 0.5 cc, followed by CPT and PD Q4 hours). Obtain sputum culture. Check I&O. Repeat ABG in am. Review deep breathe and cough, flutter valve, and pulmonary rehabilitation strategies with patient and his wife. Offer smoking cessation and weight reduction programs.

Discussion

The main challenge facing the respiratory care practitioner caring for the patient with bronchiectasis is one of efficient removal of excessive bronchopulmonary secretions. Over the years, postural drainage and percussion, good systemic hydration, and judicious use of antibiotics have been the hallmarks of therapy. More recently, intermittent use of mucolytics, percussive ventilation, and hyperinflation therapy has become more common. Pneumococcal prophylaxis is, of course, important, as is prompt attention to parenchymal pulmonary infections such as pneumonia. The clinical distinction between chronic bronchiectasis and cystic fibrosis is a subtle one at the bedside, and the latter condition must always be ruled out in patients with bronchiectasis. The goal of long-term therapy in bronchiectasis is prevention of lung parenchyma–destroying pulmonary infections and avoidance of frequent hospitalizations. Hemoptysis is often a sign of more deep-seated infection requiring antibiotic therapy.

The clinical manifestations throughout this case were all based on the clinical scenario associated with **Excessive Airway Secretions** (see Figure 9-11). For example, the thick yellow sputum resulted in decreased $\dot{V}/\dot{Q}$ ratios, venous admixture, and hypoxemia. These pathophysiologic mechanisms caused clinical manifestations of an increase in blood pressure and heart rate, acute alveolar hyperventilation with moderate hypoxemia, and rhonchi (see Figure 9-11).

Digital clubbing associated with hypoxemia is another clinical manifestation of bronchiectasis. Both the *Oxygen Therapy and Bronchopulmonary Hygiene Therapy Protocols* were administered appropriately (see Protocols 9-1 and 9-2). Low-flow oxygen per nasal cannula, aerosolized bronchodilators (albuterol) and mucolytic medication (acetylcysteine), chest percussion, and postural drainage therapy were selected from these protocols and applied with good results.

Finally, during the second admission, which showed the history of patient noncompliance (i.e., weight gain, resumption of smoking, employment in a dusty workplace, failure to continue CPT and P&D), early signs of pulmonary hypertension were evident, with cor pulmonale. This condition further complicated the patient's respiratory disorder. It commonly occurs as a preterminal event in chronic obstructive pulmonary disease (COPD), cystic fibrosis, end-stage pulmonary fibrosis, and bronchiectasis. Also, in the second scenario the whole respiratory care regimen was upgraded by an increase in frequency of treatments, with a strong emphasis on the patient's responsibility for his own care.

SELF-ASSESSMENT QUESTIONS

Multiple Choice

1. In which of the following forms of bronchiectasis are the bronchi dilated and constricted in an irregular fashion?

   I. Fusiform
   II. Saccular
   III. Varicose
   IV. Cylindrical

   a. I only
   b. II only
   c. III only
   d. II and IV only
   e. I and III only

2. Which of the following are common causes of acquired bronchiectasis?

   I. Hypogammaglobulinemia
   II. Pulmonary tuberculosis
   III. Kartagener's syndrome
   IV. Cystic fibrosis

   a. I only
   b. II only
   c. III only
   d. III and IV only
   e. I, III, and IV only

3. In the primarily obstructive form of bronchiectasis, the patient commonly demonstrates which of the following?

   I. Decreased FRC
   II. Increased $FEF_{25\%-75\%}$
   III. Decreased PEFR
   IV. Increased $V_{max\ 50}$

   a. I only
   b. III only
   c. I and IV only
   d. II and IV only
   e. III and IV only

4. Mucolytic agents are commonly used to enhance the mobilization of secretions in patients with bronchiectasis. Which of the following is/are classified as a mucolytic agent(s)?

   I. Acetylcysteine
   II. Cromolyn sodium
   III. Beclomethasone
   IV. rhDNase

   a. I only
   b. II only
   c. IV only
   d. II and III only
   e. I and IV only

5. Which of the following is considered the hallmark of bronchiectasis?

   a. Chronic cough and large quantities of foul-smelling sputum
   b. Abnormal bronchogram
   c. Acute ventilatory failure superimposed on chronic ventilatory failure
   d. Presentation as both a restrictive and obstructive pulmonary disorder
   e. Acute alveolar hyperventilation superimposed on chronic ventilatory failure

6. Which of the following is/are commonly cultured in the sputum of patients with bronchiectasis?

   I. *Staphylococcus aureus*
   II. *Pseudomonas aeruginosa*
   III. *Haemophilus influenzae*
   IV. *Klebsiella*

   a. I only
   b. III only
   c. IV only
   d. I, II, and III only
   e. I, II, III, and IV

7. When the pathophysiology of bronchiectasis is primarily obstructive in nature, the patient demonstrates which of the following clinical manifestations?

   I. Decreased tactile and vocal fremitus
   II. Bronchial breath sounds
   III. Dull percussion note
   IV. Crackles/rhonchi/wheezing

   a. II only
   b. III only
   c. I and IV only
   d. II and IV only
   e. II, III, and IV

8. Which of the following diagnostic procedures is/are used to diagnose bronchiectasis?

   I. Arterial blood gases
   II. Bronchography
   III. Oxygenation indices
   IV. Computed tomography

   a. II only
   b. III only
   c. I and III only
   d. II and IV only
   e. I, II, III, and IV

9. Which of the following is/are congenital causes of bronchiectasis?

    I. Pertussis
    II. Cystic fibrosis
    III. Chickenpox
    IV. Measles

    a. I only
    b. II only
    c. III and IV only
    d. I and III only
    e. I, III, and IV only

10. Which of the following hemodynamic indices is/are associated with bronchiectasis?

    I. Decreased CVP
    II. Increased PA
    III. Decreased RVSWI
    IV. Increased RAP

    a. II only
    b. III only
    c. II and IV only
    d. I and III only
    e. I, II, III, and IV

Answers appear in Appendix XI.

PART III

Infectious Pulmonary Diseases

CHAPTER 15

Pneumonia

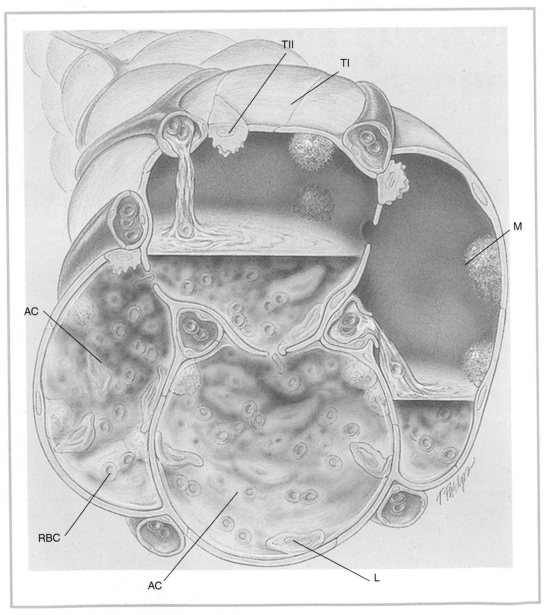

Figure 15–1 Cross-sectional view of alveolar consolidation in pneumonia. *TI,* Type I cell; *TII,* type II cell; *M,* macrophage; *AC,* alveolar consolidation; *L,* leukocyte; *RBC,* red blood cell. See also Plate 7.

Anatomic Alterations of the Lungs

Pneumonia, or pneumonitis with consolidation, is the result of an inflammatory process that primarily affects the gas exchange area of the lung. In response to the inflammation, fluid (serum) and some red blood cells (RBCs) from adjacent pulmonary capillaries pour into the alveoli. This fluid transfer is called *effusion*. Polymorphonuclear leukocytes also move into the infected area to engulf and kill invading bacteria on the alveolar walls. This process has been termed *surface phagocytosis*. Increased numbers of macrophages also appear in the infected area to remove cellular and bacterial debris. If the infection is overwhelming, the alveoli become filled with fluid, RBCs, polymorphonuclear leukocytes, and macrophages. When this occurs, the lungs are said to be *consolidated* (Figure 15-1). Atelectasis is often associated with patients who have aspiration pneumonia.

The major pathologic or structural changes associated with pneumonia are as follows:

- Inflammation of the alveoli
- Alveolar consolidation
- Atelectasis (aspiration pneumonia)

Etiology

Pneumonia is extremely common—it is the sixth leading cause of death in America. In the United States, more than 3 million people are estimated to suffer from pneumonia each year. Approximately 600,000 require hospitalization for pneumonia annually. Approximately 40,000 people die each year as a result of pneumonia. Worldwide, approximately 5 million people die as a result of pneumonia each year. As discussed in further detail below, causes of pneumonia include bacteria, viruses, fungi, tuberculosis, anaerobic organisms, aspiration, and the inhalation of irritating chemicals such as chlorine.

Involvement of an entire lobe of the lung is called *lobar pneumonia*. When both lungs are involved, it is called *double pneumonia*. Although the term *walking pneumonia* has no clinical significance it is often used to describe a mild case of pneumonia. For example, patients infected with *Mycoplasma pneumoniae*, who generally have mild symptoms and remain ambulatory, are sometimes told that they have walking pneumonia. Initially, pneumonia often mimics a common "cold" or the flu (i.e., the signs and symptoms develop quickly). For example, the patient suddenly experiences chills, shivering, high fever, sweating, chest pain (pleurisy), and a dry and nonproductive cough.

Pneumonia is often an insidious disease because the symptoms of pneumonia vary greatly depending on the patient's specific underlying condition and the type of organism causing the pneumonia. In short, what is initially thought to be a cold or the flu can, in fact, be a much more serious pulmonary infection. The early recognition and treatment of pneumonia provide the best chance of a full recovery. The major causes of pneumonia are listed in Box 15-1 and are discussed in the following paragraphs.

BACTERIAL CAUSES

Bacterial pneumonia often occurs after an individual has had an upper respiratory infection such as a cold or the flu. Early signs and symptoms include sudden chills, shaking, a high fever, sweating, chest pain, and cough (producing yellow and green sputum during the late stages). Bacterial causes are divided into *gram-positive organisms* and *gram-negative organisms*. The following are the most common.

Gram-Positive Organisms

Streptococcal Pneumonia

Streptococcus pneumoniae accounts for more than 80% of all the bacterial pneumonias. The organism is a gram-positive, nonmotile coccus that is found singly, in pairs (called *diplococci*), and in short chains (Figure 15-2). The cocci are enclosed in a smooth, thick polysaccharide capsule essential for virulence. There are more than 80 different types of *S. pneumoniae*. Serotype 3 organisms are the most virulent. Streptococci are generally transmitted by aerosol from a cough or sneeze of an infected individual. Most strains of *S. pneumoniae* are sensitive to penicillin and its derivatives. *S. pneumoniae* is commonly cultured from the sputum of patients having an acute exacerbation of chronic bronchitis.

Staphylococcal Pneumonia

There are two major groups of staphylococcus: (1) *Staphylococcus aureus*, which is responsible for most "staph" infections in humans, and (2) *Staphylococcus albus* and/or *Staphylococcus epidermidis*, which is part of the normal skin flora. The staphylococci are gram-positive cocci found singly, in pairs (called *diplococci*), and in irregular clusters (Figure 15-3). Staphylococcal pneumonia often follows a predisposing virus infection and is seen most often in children and immunosuppressed adults. *S. aureus* is commonly transmitted by aerosol from a cough or sneeze of an infected individual and indirectly via contact with contaminated floors, bedding, clothes,

BOX 15–1

Causes of Pneumonia and Classifications

Bacterial Causes
Gram-positive organisms
  Streptococcus
  Staphylococcus
Gram-negative organisms
  Haemophilus influenzae
  Klebsiella
  Pseudomonas aeruginosa
  Moraxella catarrhalis
  Escherichia coli
  Serratia species
  Enterobacter species
Atypical organisms
  Mycoplasma pneumoniae
  Legionella pneumophila
  Chlamydia psittaci
  Chlamydia pneumoniae
Anaerobic bacterial infections
  Peptostreptococcus species
  Bacteroides melaninogenicus
  Fusobacterium necrophorum
  Bacteroides asaccharolyticus
  Porphyromonas endodontalis
  Porphyromonas gingivalis

Viral Causes
  Influenza virus
  Respiratory syncytial virus
  Parainfluenza virus
  Adenovirus
  Coronavirus (SARS)

Other Causes
  Rickettsial infections
  Varicella
  Rubella
  Aspiration pneumonitis
  Lipoid pneumonitis
  Pneumocystis carinii
  Cytomegalovirus
  Tuberculosis
  Fungal infections
Acquired Pneumonia Classification
  Community-acquired pneumonia (CAP)
  Nursing home–acquired pneumonia
  Hospital-acquired pneumonia
  Ventilator-associated pneumonia

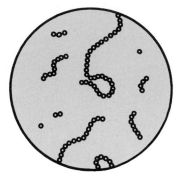

Figure 15–2   The *Streptococcus* organism is a gram-positive, nonmotile coccus that is found singly, in pairs, and in short chains.

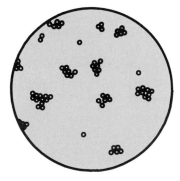

Figure 15–3   The *Staphylococcus* organism is a gram-positive, nonmotile coccus that is found singly, in pairs, and in irregular clusters.

Gram-Negative Organisms

The major gram-negative organisms responsible for pneumonia are rod-shaped microorganisms called *bacilli* (Figure 15-4). The bacilli described in the following sections are frequently seen in the clinical setting.

Haemophilus influenzae

Haemophilus influenzae is a common inhabitant of human pharyngeal flora. *H. influenzae* is one of the smallest gram-negative bacilli, measuring about 1.5 mm in length and 0.3 mm in width. It appears as coccobacilli on Gram's stain. There are six types of *H. influenzae* designated A to F—but only type B is commonly pathogenic. Pneumonia caused by *H. influenzae B* is seen most often in children between the ages of 1 month and 6 years. *H. influenzae B* is almost always the cause of *acute epiglottitis*. The organism is transmitted via aerosol or contact with contaminated objects. It is sensitive to cold and does

and the like. Staphylococci are a common cause of *hospital-acquired pneumonia* and are becoming increasingly antibiotic resistant—thus the abbreviation MDRSA: multiple drug-resistant *S. aureus* organisms.

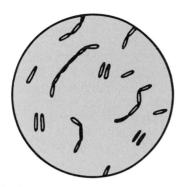

Figure 15–4 The bacilli are rod-shaped microorganisms and are the major gram-negative organisms responsible for pneumonia.

not survive long after expectoration. *H. influenzae* is commonly cultured from the sputum of patients having an acute exacerbation of chronic bronchitis. Additional risk factors for *H. influenzae* include chronic obstructive pulmonary disease (COPD), defects in B cell function, functional and anatomic asplenia, and human immunodeficiency virus (HIV) infection.

Klebsiella pneumoniae (Friedländer's Bacillus)

Klebsiella pneumoniae organisms have long been associated with lobar pneumonia, particularly in men older than 40 years, and in chronic alcoholics of both genders. *Klebsiella* is a gram-negative bacillus that is found singly, in pairs, and in chains of varying lengths. It is a normal inhabitant of the human gastrointestinal tract. The organism can be transmitted directly by aerosol or indirectly by contact with freshly contaminated articles. *K. pneumoniae* is a common nosocomial, or hospital-acquired, disease. It is typically transmitted by routes such as clothing, intravenous solutions, foods, and the hands of health-care workers. The mortality of patients with *K. pneumoniae* is quite high because septicemia is a frequent complication.

Pseudomonas aeruginosa (Bacillus pyocyaneus)

Pseudomonas aeruginosa is a highly motile, gram-negative bacillus. It colonizes the gastrointestinal tract, burns, and catheterized urinary tract and is a contaminant in many aqueous solutions. Risk factors include neutropenia, HIV infection, preexisting lung disease, endotracheal intubation, and prior antibiotic use. *P. aeruginosa* frequently is cultured from the respiratory tract of chronically ill, tracheostomized patients and is a leading cause of *hospital-acquired pneumonia*. This makes *P. aeruginosa* a particular problem to the respiratory care practitioner. Because the *Pseudomonas* organism thrives in dampness, it is frequently cultured from contaminated respiratory therapy equipment.

The organism is commonly transmitted by aerosol or by direct contact with freshly contaminated articles. The sputum from patients with *Pseudomonas* infection is frequently green and sweet smelling.

Moraxella catarrhalis

Moraxella catarrhalis is a natural inhabitant of the human pharynx. After *S. pneumoniae* and *H. influenzae*, *M. catarrhalis* is the third most common cause of acute exacerbation of chronic bronchitis.

Escherichia coli

Escherichia coli is a normal inhabitant of the intestinal tract. It is sometimes the cause of nosocomial pneumonia (see Hospital-Acquired Pneumonia, page 233).

Serratia Species

Serratia species cause about 7% of the cases of nosocomial pneumonia (see Hospital-Acquired Pneumonia, page 233).

Enterobacter Species

Enterobacter cloacae and *Enterobacter aerogenes* are sometimes the cause of pneumonia.

Atypical Organisms

Mycoplasma pneumoniae

Mycoplasma pneumoniae is a common cause of mild pneumonia. These organisms cause symptoms similar to both bacterial and viral pneumonia, although the symptoms develop more gradually and are often milder. The mycoplasma are tiny, cell wall–deficient organisms. They are smaller than bacteria but larger than viruses. The pneumonia caused by the mycoplasmal organism is described as *primary atypical pneumonia*—atypical because the organism escapes identification by standard bacteriologic tests.

M. pneumoniae is most frequently seen in people younger than 40 years of age during the late summer and early fall months. This type of pneumonia spreads easily in areas where people congregate, such as child-care centers, schools, and homeless shelters. Patients with *M. pneumoniae* often are said to have walking pneumonia because the condition is mild (i.e., slight fever, fatigue, and a characteristic dry, hacking cough) and the patient is usually ambulatory.

Legionella pneumophila

In July 1976, a severe pneumonia-like disease outbreak occurred at an American Legion convention in Philadelphia. The causative agent eluded identification for many months, despite the concerted efforts of the nation's top epidemiologic experts. When the organism finally was recovered from a patient, it was found to be an unusual and fastidious gram-negative bacillus with atypical concentrations of certain branched-chain lipids. The initial isolate was designated as *Legionella pneumophila*. More than 20 *Legionella* species have now been identified.

Most of the species are free-living in soil and water, where they act as decomposer organisms. The organism also multiplies in standing water such as contaminated mud puddles, large air-conditioning systems, and water tanks. The organism is transmitted when it becomes airborne and enters the patient's lungs as an aerosol. No convincing evidence suggests that the organism is transmitted from person to person. The organism can be detected in pleural fluid, sputum, or lung tissue by direct fluorescent antibody microscopy. Although it is rarely found outside the lungs, the organism may be found in other tissues. The disease is most commonly seen in middle-aged males who smoke.

Chlamydia psittaci (Psittacosis)

Chlamydia psittaci is a small gram-negative bacterium in the respiratory tract and feces in a variety of birds (e.g., parrots, parakeets, lorikeets, cockatoos, chickens, pigeons, ducks, pheasants, turkeys). *C. psittaci* is transmitted from birds to humans by aerosol or direct contact. The clinical manifestations of *C. psittaci* closely resemble those caused by *M. pneumoniae*.

Chlamydia pneumoniae

Chlamydia pneumoniae recently has been identified as a cause of pneumonia in adults. It has been detected in schools, military institutions, and families. It is associated with meningoencephalitis, myocarditis, endocarditis, coronary artery disease, and Guillain-Barré syndrome.

ANAEROBIC BACTERIAL INFECTIONS

The major anaerobic organisms associated with pneumonia are *Peptostreptococcus* species, *Bacteroides melaninogenicus*, *Fusobacterium necrophorum*, *Bacteroides asaccharolyticus*, *Porphyromonas endodontailis*, and *Porphyromonas gingivalis*. Aspiration of oropharyngeal secretions and gastric fluids are the major causes of anaerobic lung infections. Predisposing risk factors of aspiration include a decreased level of consciousness, impaired swallowing, poor dental hygiene, and gastrointestinal abnormalities. Aspiration pneumonia is often multimicrobial.

VIRAL CAUSES

Viruses are minute organisms not visible by ordinary light microscopy. They are parasitic and depend on nutrients inside cells for their metabolic and reproductive needs. Approximately 90% of acute upper respiratory tract infections and 50% of lower respiratory tract infections are caused by viruses. Respiratory viruses are the most common cause of pneumonia in young children, peaking between the ages of 2 and 3. By school age, *M. pneumoniae* become more prevalent (see previous section). The most common viruses that cause respiratory infections are described in the following paragraphs.

Influenza Virus

Although the virus has several subtypes, influenza A and B are the most common causes of viral respiratory tract infections. In the United States, influenza A and B commonly occur in epidemics during the winter months. Children, young adults, and older individuals are most at risk. Influenza is transmitted from person to person by aerosol droplets. Often, the first sign of an epidemic is an increase in school absenteeism. The virus survives well in conditions of low temperatures and low humidity. It also has been found in horses, swine, and birds. Influenza viruses have an incubation period of 1 to 3 days and usually cause upper respiratory tract infections.

Respiratory Syncytial Virus

The respiratory syncytial virus (RSV) is a member of the paramyxovirus group. Parainfluenza, mumps, and rubella viruses also belong to this group. The RSV is most often seen in children under 6 months of age and in older persons with underlying pulmonary disease. Approximately 25% of respiratory illnesses in children younger than 1 year of age are caused by this virus. The infection is rarely fatal in infants. The RSV often goes unrecognized but may play an important role as a forerunner to bacterial infections. The virus is transmitted by aerosol and by direct contact with infected individuals. RSV infections are most commonly seen in patients during the winter and spring months.

Parainfluenza Virus

The parainfluenza viruses also are members of the paramyxovirus group and therefore are related to mumps, rubella, and the RSVs. There are five types of parainfluenza viruses: types 1, 2, 3, 4A, and 4B. Types 1, 2, and 3 are the major causes of infections in humans. Type 1 is considered a "croup" type of virus. Types 2 and 3 are associated with severe infections. Although type 3 is seen in persons of all ages, it usually is seen in infants younger than 2 months of age; types 1 and 2 are seen most often in children between the ages of 6 months and 5 years. Types 1 and 2 typically occur in the fall, whereas type 3 infection most often is seen in the late spring and summer. Parainfluenza viruses are transmitted by aerosol droplets and by direct person-to-person contact. The parainfluenza viruses are known for their ability to spread rapidly among members of the same family.

Adenoviruses

There are more than 30 adenovirus subgroups. Serotypes 4, 7, 14, and 21 cause viral infections and pneumonia in all age groups. Serotype 7 has been related to fatal cases of pneumonia in children. Adenoviruses are transmitted by aerosol. Pneumonia caused by adenoviruses generally occurs during the fall, winter, and spring.

Severe Acute Respiratory Syndrome (SARS)

In 2002, China reported the first case of the severe acute respiratory syndrome (SARS). Shortly after this report, the disease was documented in numerous countries, including Vietnam, Singapore, and Indonesia. Both the United States and Canada have reported imported cases. Health officials believe that the cause of SARS is a newly recognized virus strain called a *coronavirus*. Other viruses, however, are still under investigation as potential causes. Coronaviruses are a group of viruses that have a halo or corona-like appearance when observed under an electon microscope. Known forms of coronavirus cause common colds and upper respiratory tract infections. SARS is highly contagious on close personal contact with infected individuals. It spreads through droplet transmission by coughing and sneezing. SARS might be transmitted through the air or from objects that have become contaminated.

The incubation period for SARS typically is between 2 and 7 days. Initially, the patient usually develops a fever (>100.4° F or >38.0° C), followed by chills, headaches, general feeling of discomfort, and body aches. Toward the end of the incubation period, the SARS patient usually develops a dry, nonproductive cough; shortness of breath; and malaise. In severe causes, hypoxemia develops. According to the Centers for Disease Control (CDC), between 10% and 20% of SARS patients require mechanical ventilation. In spite of this fact, death from SARS is rare. No specific treatment recommendations exist at this time. The CDC, however, recommends that SARS patients receive the same treatment used for any patient with serious community-acquired atypical pneumonia of unknown cause.

OTHER CAUSES

Rickettsiae

Rickettsiae are small, pleomorphic coccobacilli. Most rickettsiae are intracellular parasites possessing both ribonucleic acid (RNA) and deoxyribonucleic acid (DNA). There are several pathogenic members of the *Rickettsia* family: *Rickettsia rickettsii* (Rocky Mountain spotted fever), *Rickettsia akari* (rickettsialpox), *Rickettsia prowazekii* (typhus), and *Rickettsia burnetii*, also called *Coxiella burnetii* (Q fever).

All species of the genus *Rickettsia* are unstable outside of cells except for *R. burnetii* (Q fever), which is extremely resistant to heat and light. Q fever can cause pneumonia as well as a prolonged febrile illness, an influenza-like illness, and endocarditis. The organism is commonly transmitted by arthropods (lice, fleas, ticks, mites). It also may be transmitted by cattle, sheep, and goats and possibly in raw milk.

Varicella (Chickenpox)

The varicella virus usually causes a benign disease in children between the ages of 2 and 8 years, and complications of varicella are not common. In some cases, however, varicella has been noted to spread to the lungs and cause a serious secondary pneumonitis.

Rubella (Measles)

Measles virus spreads from person to person by the respiratory route. Respiratory complications often are encountered in measles because of the widespread involvement of the mucosa of the respiratory tract.

Aspiration Pneumonitis

Aspiration of gastric fluid with a pH of 2.5 or less causes a serious and often fatal form of pneumonia. Aspiration of oropharyngeal secretions and gastric fluids are the major causes of anaerobic lung infections (see Anaerobic Bacterial Infections above). Aspiration pneumonitis is commonly missed because acute inflammatory reactions may not begin until several hours after aspiration of the gastric fluid. The inflammatory reaction generally increases in severity for 12 to 26 hours and may progress to acute respiratory distress syndrome (ARDS), which includes interstitial and intraalveolar edema, intraalveolar hyaline membrane, and atelectasis. In the absence of a secondary bacterial infection, the inflammation usually becomes clinically insignificant in approximately 72 hours. In 1946 Mendelson first described the clinical manifestations of tachycardia, dyspnea, and cyanosis associated with the aspiration of acid stomach contents. The clinical picture he described is now known as Mendelson's syndrome and is usually confined to aspiration pneumonitis in pregnant females.

Aspiration pneumonia is broadly defined as the pulmonary result of the entry of material from the stomach or upper respiratory tract into the lower airways. There are at least three distinctive forms of aspiration pneumonia, classified according to the nature of the aspirate, the clinical presentation, and management guidelines:

1. Toxic injury to the lung (such as that caused by gastric acid)
2. Obstruction (by foreign body or fluids)
3. Infection

Aspiration is the presumed cause of nearly all cases of anaerobic pulmonary infections. Studies suggest that anaerobic bacteria are the most common causative agents of lung abscesses; they are commonly isolated in cases of empyema.

There is a difference between the aspiration of gastric contents and the aspiration of food. Aspiration of gastric contents causes initial hypoxemia regardless of the aspirate's pH level. Consequently, oximetry is a good measurement if aspiration is suspected. If the aspirate's pH is relatively high (greater than 5.9), the initial injury is rapidly reversible. Such aspiration occurs in patients who receive antacids. If the pH is low (unbuffered gastric contents normally range from 1 to 1.5), parenchymal damage may occur, with inflammation, edema, and hemorrhage. When food is aspirated, obliterative bronchiolitis with subsequent granuloma formation occurs.

Gastroesophageal reflux disease (GERD) is the regurgitation of stomach contents into the esophagus. GERD causes disruption in nerve-mediated reflexes in the distal esophagus, resulting in alteration of the primary and secondary peristaltic wave and reflux. Therefore "to-and-fro" peristalsis can result from spasticity at the distal esophageal sphincter and retropulsion of middle and upper esophageal contents. This may result in aspiration, although not necessarily.

GERD is three times more prevalent in patients with asthma than in other patients. In other words, GERD is a frequently unrecognized cause of asthma. Presumably, acid reflux into the esophagus causes vagal stimulation, resulting in a reflexive increase in bronchial tone in patients with asthma. Recent literature suggests that asymptomatic reflux does not contribute to worsening lung function. Nevertheless, GERD does cause chronic cough in 10% to 20% of patients with GERD.

Normal swallowing has four phases:

1. Oral preparatory
2. Oral
3. Pharyngeal
4. Esophageal

The first two phases are considered voluntary stages (cerebral). These phases occur as the food or liquid is prepared for entry to the pharynx and esophagus. The airway is open while food is prepared in the oral cavity. Adequate tongue function is important for the manipulation and propulsion of the prepared food or liquid (called a *bolus*) into the pharynx. Spillage of liquid into the pharynx during the chewing of food is usually not a problem in patients with good airway protection.

The pharyngeal phase (involuntary brainstem function) of swallowing involves numerous physiologic actions that direct the bolus into the esophagus:

- Elevation and retraction of the velopharyngeal port (velum closure)
- Pharyngeal muscle contraction
- Elevation and forward excursion of the larynx (epiglottic closure)
- Closure of the laryngeal vestibule, false vocal folds, and true vocal folds (laryngeal closure)
- Relaxation of the upper esophageal sphincter

Airway closure progresses inferiorly to superiorly in the larynx as the food bolus is directed laterally around the airway.

Respiration is halted during the pharyngeal phase for an approximate 1-second apneic period, although duration varies with bolus volume and viscosity. Bolus transit in the esophageal phase (under both brainstem and intrinsic neural control) lasts between 8 and 20 seconds. In this phase the upper esophageal sphincter (UES) relaxes to receive the bolus with a peristaltic wave from the pharyngeal superior constrictor muscles, forcing the bolus through the relaxed UES. The primary peristalsis propels the bolus through the esophagus and lower esophageal sphincter and into the stomach.

Six cranial nerves carry motor signals generated by cerebral and brainstem swallowing centers:

1. V (trigeminal)
2. VII (facial)
3. IX (glossopharyngeal)
4. X (vagus)
5. XI (spinal accessory [minor involvement])
6. XII (hypoglossal)

The relation between respiration and swallowing is not random. Expiration before and after the pharyngeal phase in normal swallowing is believed to serve as an inherent closure and clearance mechanism against penetration into the airway entrance.

Dysphagia is the result of an abnormal swallow that can involve the oral, pharyngeal, and esophageal phases. Penetration into the laryngeal vestibule occurs when food or liquid (or both) enters the larynx but does not pass through the vocal cords into the trachea. Aspiration is the passage of food or liquid into the trachea via the vocal cords.

Diagnostic tests for dysphagia include the modified barium swallow (MBS), videofluoroscopy, videofiberoptic endoscopy, and the modified Evan's blue dye test. The Evan's blue dye test involves instilling a deep blue dye into the gastrointestinal tract and seeing if it can be suctioned from the trachea. If it can, it suggests a communication between the two structures, such as a fistula. The MBS and videofluoroscopy tests are most definitive for identification of the particular phase of the swallow that is dysfunctional. The modified Evan's blue dye test can be unreliable (as much as 40% of the time) as a test suggesting aspiration in a tracheostomized patient. Both false-positive and false-negative tests occur.

A compromised respiratory system can cause dysphagia, and conversely, dysphagia may cause respiratory complications. COPD can result in a slowed oral and pharyngeal transit time, reduced coordination and strength of the oral and pharyngeal musculature, and reduced airway clearance by coughing.

Treatment of dysphagia is specific to the nature of the disorder. Varied methods of presentation of foods and liquids, bolus volumes and consistency, postural movements, and food temperature can affect the dynamics of the relation between respiration and swallowing. Large volumes of liquid requiring uninterrupted swallowing result in longer apneic periods and can be difficult for patients with shortness of breath and dyspnea. Small-volume bites and swallows make sense in this setting.

Unilateral cerebrovascular accidents (stroke) and hemorrhage tend to cause hypopharyngeal hemiparesis. Difficulty in swallowing (with impairment of the oral phase) and aspiration of thin fluids therefore may follow. The contralateral facial and tongue weakness can result in poor bolus control in the oral cavity.

Silent aspiration is defined as aspiration that does not evoke clinically observable adverse symptoms such as coughing, choking, and immediate respiratory distress. Some patients have silent aspiration after a stroke. Evidence also suggests that some sequelae of stroke include laryngopharyngeal sensory deficits with no subjective or objective evidence of dysphagia, such as choking, gagging or cough.

Some patients with severe and bilateral sensory deficits develop aspiration pneumonia. The clinical findings of dysphonia, dysarthria, abnormal gag reflex, abnormal volitional cough, cough after swallow, and voice change after swallow all significantly relate to aspiration and are predictors of silent aspiration. Conversely, a normal reflex cough after a stroke indicates an intact laryngeal cough reflex, a protected airway, and low risk for developing aspiration pneumonia with oral feeding. The cough reflex is significantly reduced in older patients.

Tracheostomized patients are at high risk for silent aspiration. Perhaps 55% to 70% of intubated or tracheostomized patients aspirate. A tracheostomy tube has a direct effect on the pharyngeal phase of a swallow because of the alteration of normal respiratory function (exhalation timing) as well as the anatomic alteration and the physical resistance imposed by the tracheostomy tube itself. Laryngeal elevation is reduced, particularly with the cuff inflated, which leads to inadequate airway closure and increased pharyngeal residue.

Poor sensory response to material entering the larynx contributes to the slowing of an uncoordinated laryngeal closure. The protective cough may be lessened because of the impaired laryngeal sensation. Subglottic air pressure (coordinated exhalation with swallow) helps prevent entry of material into the trachea and is reduced in patients with a tracheostomy. An inflated cuffed tracheostomy can cause complications that can anchor the larynx to the anterior wall of the neck and desensitize the pharynx. Delayed triggering of the swallowing response and increased pharyngeal residue are prevalent.

Recommendations for oral feeding include considerations of dietary consistency, specifically defined for solids and liquids; skilled supervision with oral intake; safe swallowing strategies; positioning requirements; cuff deflation; and tracheal occlusion issues. It may be necessary to coordinate mealtime with ventilator weaning attempts to optimize more positive pressure generation to aid in expelling laryngeal residue and creating subglottic pressure.

Partial or complete cuff deflation during meals promotes laryngeal elevation, allows expectoration of secretions, reduces the effect of friction on the tracheoesophageal wall, and enhances the senses of taste and smell. If an uncuffed tracheostomy is in place, possible placement of a Passey Muir valve or capping of a fenestrated trach will aid in subglottic negative pressure and assist in an effective swallow.

The dynamic changes a patient may experience clinically necessitate a coordinated team approach, including physical, occupational, and respiratory therapists; a speech-language pathologist; registered dietitian; and nurse. This approach allows for effective management of tracheostomized and nontracheostomized patients and avoidance of aspiration.

Lipoid Pneumonitis

The aspiration of mineral oil, used medically as a lubricant, also has been known to cause pneumonitis. The severity of the pneumonia depends on the type of oil aspirated. Oils from animal fats cause the most serious reaction, whereas oils of vegetable origin are relatively inert. When mineral oil is inhaled in an aerosolized form, an intense pulmonary tissue reaction occurs.

Pneumocystis carinii Pneumonia

Pneumocystis carinii is an opportunistic, often fatal, form of pneumonia seen in profoundly immunosuppressed patients. Although the *Pneumocystis* organism has been identified as a protozoan, recent information suggests that it is more closely related to fungi. *Pneumocystis* normally can be found in the lungs of humans, but it does not cause disease in healthy hosts, only in individuals whose immune systems are critically impaired. Currently, *Pneumocystis* pneumonia is the major pulmonary infection seen in patients with acquired immunodeficiency syndrome (AIDS).

In vulnerable hosts the disease spreads rapidly throughout the lungs. Before AIDS, *P. carinii* pneumonia was seen primarily in patients with malignancy, in organ transplant recipients, and in patients with diseases requiring treatment with large doses of immunosuppressive agents. Today, most cases of *P. carinii* pneumonia are seen in patients with AIDS. The early clinical manifestations of *Pneumocystis* in patients with AIDS are indistinguishable from any other pneumonia. Typical symptoms include progressive exertional dyspnea, a dry cough that may or may not produce mucoid sputum, difficulty in taking a deep breath (not caused by pleurisy), and fever with or without sweats. The therapist may hear normal breath sounds on auscultation or end-inspiratory crackles. The chest X-ray may be normal at first; later, it will show bilateral interstitial infiltrates, which may progress to alveolar filling and "white out" of the chest X-ray.

Cytomegalovirus

Cytomegalovirus (CMV), a member of the herpesvirus family, is the most common viral pulmonary complication of AIDS. CMV infection commonly coexists with *P. carinii* infection.

Tuberculosis

According to the World Health Organization, approximately 1 billion people will be newly infected with tuberculosis (TB) between the years 2000 and 2020 worldwide. During this period, it is estimated that about 200 million people will become ill and 35 million will die from TB. In the early 1980s the United States had the lowest TB rate in modern history. However, in 1985 the TB incidence started rising and has risen ever since. Tuberculosis is an infectious disease caused by *Mycobacterium tuberculosis*. *M. tuberculosis* is a slender, rod-shaped aerobic organism. Predisposing factors of tuberculosis include homelessness, drug abuse, and AIDS. The initial response of the lung is an inflammatory reaction that is similar to any acute pneumonia (see Chapter 17).

Fungal Infections

Because most fungi are aerobes, the lung is a prime site for fungal infections. Primary fungal pathogens include *Histoplasma capsulatum*, *Coccidioides immitis*, and *Blastomyces dermatitidis*. In addition, the opportunistic yeast pathogens *Candida albicans*, *Cryptococcus neoformans*, and *Aspergillus* also may cause pneumonia in certain patients. For example, *C. albicans*, which occurs as normal flora in the oral cavity, genitalia, and large intestine, is rarely seen in the tracheobronchial tree or lung parenchyma. In patients with AIDS, however, *C. albicans* commonly causes an infection of the mouth, pharynx, esophagus, vagina, skin, and lungs. A *C. albicans* infection of the mouth is called thrush; it is characterized by a white, adherent, patchy infection of the membranes of the mouth, gums, cheeks, and throat.

C. neoformans proliferates in pigeon droppings, which have a high nitrogen content, and readily scatters into the air and dust. Today, the highest rate of cryptococcosis occurs among patients with AIDS and persons undergoing steroid therapy. The molds of the genus *Aspergillus* may be the most pervasive of all fungi—especially *Aspergillus fumigatus*. *Aspergillus* is found in soil, vegetation, leaf detritus, food, and compost heaps. Persons who breathe the air of granaries, barns, and silos are at the greatest risk. *Aspergillus* infection usually occurs in the lungs. *Aspergillus* is almost always an opportunistic infection and lately has posed a serious threat to patients with AIDS. When fungal organisms are inhaled, the initial response of the lung is an inflammatory reaction similar to that produced by any acute pneumonia (see Chapter 18).

ACQUIRED PNEUMONIA CLASSIFICATIONS

Pneumonia is often classified according to the location or method of exposure. Common classifications are Community-Acquired Pneumonia (CAP), Hospital-Acquired Pneumonia, Ventilator-Associated Pneumonia (VAP), and Nursing Home–Acquired Pneumonia.

Community-Acquired Pneumonias (CAPs)

Community-acquired pneumonias (CAPs) are acquired outside the hospital. Two good systems are used to evaluate the severity of a CAP. For example, the American Thoracic Society (ATS) categorizes CAP according to the following severity levels*:

1. Patients 60 years of age or younger, with no comorbidity, who can be treated as outpatients
2. Patients older than 60 years of age, with comorbidity, who can be treated as outpatients
3. Patients requiring hospitalization but not in an intensive care unit
4. Severely ill patients requiring admission to an intensive care unit

On the basis of the clinical presentation, CAP can also be divided into two types, discussed in the following sections.

Community-Acquired: Acute

The most common cause of community-acquired pneumonia is *S. pneumoniae*. Other organisms include *M. pneumoniae, H. influenzae* A and B, oral anaerobic bacteria (aspiration), *L. pneumophila, C. pneumoniae,* and *M. catarrhalis.*

---

*From Niederman MS, Bass JB, Fein AM, et al: American Thoracic Society guidelines for the initial management of adults with community-acquired pneumonia: diagnosis, assessment of severity, and initial anti-microbial therapy. *Am Rev Respir Dis* 148:1418-1426, 1993.

Community-Acquired: Chronic

Community-acquired pneumonias include *M. tuberculosis, H. capsulatum, B. dermatitidis,* and *C. immitis.*

Hospital-Acquired Pneumonia

Hospital-acquired pneumonia (also called *nosocomial pneumonia*) is defined as a pneumonia that develops 48 hours or more after admission to the hospital. Nosocomial pneumonia is estimated to account for more than 15% of all respiratory infections. Nosocomial infections include *P. aeruginosa, S. aureus, K. pneumoniae, E. coli, Serratia* species, and oral anaerobes (aspiration).

Ventilator-Acquired Pneumonia (VAP)

Ventilator-acquired pneumonia (also called *ventilator-associated pneumonia*) is defined as a pneumonia that develops after 48 hours of mechanical ventilation. An International Consensus Conference provides guideline criteria for the diagnosis of ventilator-associated pneumonia (Box 15-2). Common ventilator-associated infections include *P. aeruginosa, Acinetobacter, Enterobacter, Klebsiella, Stenotrophomonas maltophilia,* and *S. aureus.*

Nursing Home–Acquired Pneumonia

Nursing home–acquired pneumonia is defined as a respiratory tract infection that develops in a long-term care facility. Common nursing home–acquired infections include mixed aerobic and anaerobic mouth flora, *S. aureus,* enteric gram-negative bacilli, influenza, and *M. tuberculosis.*

BOX 15–2

Criteria for the Diagnosis of Ventilator-Associated Pneumonia

A. **Definite pneumonia:** New or persistent pulmonary infiltrates and purulent secretions in addition to one of the following:
   1. Radiographic evidence of abscess and positive needle aspirate culture
   2. Pathogenic evidence of pneumonia on histologic examination of lung tissue obtained by open lung biopsy or postmortem plus a positive quantitative culture of lung parenchyma ($>10^4$ CFU/g of lung tissue)
B. **Probable pneumonia:** New or persistent pulmonary infiltrate (in the absence of the above) and one of the following:
   1. The presence of positive quantitative culture by protected specimen brush (PSB) or bronchoalveolar lavage (BAL)
   2. Blood culture positive for the same organisms as respiratory sample
   3. Positive pleural fluid culture as respiratory secretions

4. Pathologic evidence of pneumonia by open lung biopsy or autopsy
C. **Definitive absence of pneumonia:** One of the following:
   1. No histologic evidence of pneumonia postmortem
   2. Definitive alternate etiology
   3. Cytologic identification of nonpneumonia diagnosis
D. **Probable absence of pneumonia:** Lack of significant growth from reliable specimen in addition to one of the following:
   1. Resolution of fever, infiltrate or radiographic infiltrate without antibiotic, and a definite alternative diagnosis
   2. Persistent fever and infiltrate with alternative diagnosis

From Pingleton SK, Fagon JY, Leper KV: Patient selection for clinical investigation of ventilator associated pneumonia. *Chest* 1992; 102:553S-556S.

OVERVIEW
of the Cardiopulmonary Clinical Manifestations Associated with PNEUMONIA

The following clinical manifestations result from the pathologic mechanisms caused (or activated) by **Alveolar Consolidation** (see Figure 9-8), **Increased Alveolar-Capillary Membrane Thickness** (see Figure 9-9), and **Atelectasis** (see Figure 9-7)—the major anatomic alterations of the lungs associated with pneumonia (see Figure 15-1). During the resolution stage of pneumonia, **Excessive Bronchial Secretions** (see Figure 9-11) also may play a part in the clinical presentation.

CLINICAL DATA OBTAINED AT THE PATIENT'S BEDSIDE

The Physical Examination
Vital Signs

Increased respiratory rate (see page 31 ◆►)
Several pathophysiologic mechanisms operating simultaneously may lead to an increased ventilatory rate:
- Stimulation of peripheral chemoreceptors (hypoxemia)
- Decreased lung compliance/increased ventilatory rate relationship
- Stimulation of J receptors
- Pain/anxiety/fever

Increased heart rate (pulse), cardiac output, and blood pressure (see pages 11 and 99 ◆►)

Chest Pain/Decreased Chest Expansion
(see page 42 ◆►)

Cyanosis (see page 45 ◆►)

Cough, Sputum Production, and Hemoptysis
(see page 47 ◆►)

Initially, the patient with pneumonia usually has a nonproductive barking or hacking cough. As the disease progresses, however, the cough becomes productive. When the disease progresses to this point, the patient often expectorates small amounts of purulent, blood-streaked, or rusty sputum. This is caused by fluid moving from the pulmonary capillaries into the alveoli in response to the inflammatory process. As fluid crosses into the alveoli, some RBCs also move into the alveoli and produce the blood-streaked or rusty appearance of the fluid (see Figure 15-1). Some of the fluid that moves in the alveoli also may work its way into the bronchioles and bronchi. As the fluid accumulates in the bronchial tree, the subepithelial mechano-receptors in the trachea, bronchi, and bronchioles are stimulated and initiate a cough reflex. Because the bronchioles and the smaller bronchi are deep in the lung parenchyma, the patient with pneumonia initially has a dry, hacking cough, and fluid cannot be easily expectorated until secretions reach the larger bronchi.

OVERVIEW

of the Cardiopulmonary Clinical Manifestations Associated with PNEUMONIA (Continued)

Chest Assessment Findings (see page 22 ◆)

- Increased tactile and vocal fremitus
- Dull percussion note
- Bronchial breath sounds
- Crackles and rhonchi
- Pleural friction rub (if process extends to pleural surface)
- Whispered pectoriloquy

CLINICAL DATA OBTAINED FROM LABORATORY TESTS AND SPECIAL PROCEDURES

Pulmonary Function Study Findings

Expiratory Maneuver Findings (see page 61 ◆)

FVC	FEV_T	$FEF_{25\%-75\%}$	$FEF_{200-1200}$
↓	N or ↓	N or ↓	N
PEFR	MVV	$FEF_{50\%}$	$FEV_{1\%}$
N	N or ↓	N	N or ↑

Lung Volume and Capacity Findings (see page 62 ◆)

V_T	RV	FRC	TLC
N or ↓	↓	↓	↓
VC	IC	ERV	RV/TLC%
↓	↓	↓	N

Arterial Blood Gases

Mild to Moderate Pneumonia
Acute Alveolar Hyperventilation with Hypoxemia (see page 70 ◆)

pH	$Paco_2$	HCO_3^-	Pao_2
↑	↓	↓(Slightly)	↓

Severe Pneumonia
Acute Ventilatory Failure with Hypoxemia (see page 73 ◆)

pH	$Paco_2$	HCO_3^-*	Pao_2
↓	↑	↑(Slightly)	↓

*When tissue hypoxia is severe enough to produce lactic acid, the pH and HCO_3^- values will be lower than expected for a particular $Paco_2$ level.

Oxygenation Indices (see page 82)

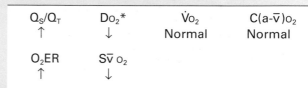

Q_S/Q_T	Do_2*	$\dot{V}o_2$	$C(a-\bar{v})o_2$
↑	↓	Normal	Normal
O_2ER	$S\bar{v}o_2$		
↑	↓		

*The Do_2 may be normal in patients who have compensated to the decreased oxygenation status with an increased cardiac output. When the Do_2 is normal, the O_2ER is usually normal

ABNORMAL LABORATORY TESTS AND PROCEDURES

Sputum examination (see etiology in this chapter, page 225)

- Gram-positive organisms
  Streptococcus
  Staphylococcus
- Gram-negative organisms
  Klebsiella
  Pseudomonas aeruginosa
  Haemophilus influenzae
  Legionella pneumophila

RADIOLOGIC FINDINGS

Chest Radiograph

- Increased density (from consolidation and atelectasis)
- Air bronchograms
- Pleural effusions

The radiographic signs vary considerably depending on the causative agent. In general, pneumonia (alveolar consolidation) appears as an area of increased density that may involve a small lung segment, a lobe, or one or both lungs (Figure 15-5). The process may appear patchy or uniform throughout the area. As the alveolar consolidation intensifies, alveolar density increases and air bronchograms may be seen (Figure 15-6). A pleural effusion may be identified on the chest radiograph (see Chapter 23).

CT Scan

- Alveolar consolidation and air bronchograms also can be seen on the CT scan (Figure 15-7).

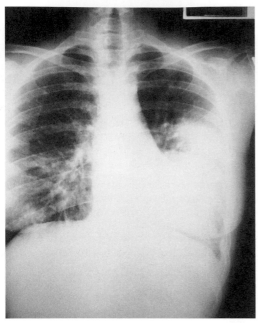

Figure 15–5   Chest X-ray film of a 20-year-old woman with severe pneumonia of the left lung.

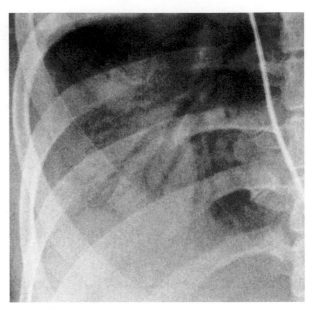

Figure 15–6   Air bronchogram. The branching linear lucencies within the consolidation in the right lower lobe are particularly well demonstrated in this example of staphylococcal pneumonia. (From Armstrong P et al: *Imaging of diseases of the chest,* ed 2, St. Louis, 1995, Mosby.)

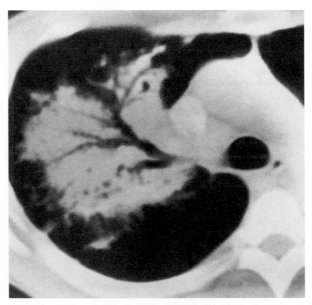

Figure 15–7   Air bronchogram shown by CT in a patient with pneumonia. (From Armstrong P et al: *Imaging of diseases of the chest,* ed 2, St. Louis, 1995, Mosby.)

General Management of Pneumonia

RESPIRATORY CARE TREATMENT PROTOCOLS

Oxygen Therapy Protocol

Oxygen therapy is used to treat hypoxemia, decrease the work of breathing, and decrease myocardial work. Because of the hypoxemia associated with pneumonia, supplemental oxygen may be required. The hypoxemia that develops in pneumonia is most commonly caused by alveolar consolidation and capillary shunting associated with the disorder. Hypoxemia caused by capillary shunting is at least partially refractory to oxygen therapy (see Oxygen Therapy Protocol, Protocol 9-1).

Bronchopulmonary Hygiene Therapy Protocol

Because of the airway secretions associated with the resolution stage of pneumonia, a number of bronchopulmonary hygiene treatment modalities may be used to enhance the mobilization of bronchial secretions. In addition, because of food particles in the aspirate, the bronchopulmonary hygiene protocol is useful in the treatment of aspiration pneumonia (see Bronchopulmonary Hygiene Therapy Protocol, Protocol 9-2).

Hyperinflation Therapy Protocol

Hyperinflation techniques are occasionally administered to offset (at least temporarily) the atelectasis associated with pneumonia (see Hyperinflation Therapy Protocol, Protocol 9-3).

MEDICATIONS AND PROCEDURES COMMONLY PRESCRIBED BY THE PHYSICIAN

Antibiotics

Antibiotics are commonly administered to combat the infective agents that cause pneumonia (see Appendix II).

Analgesic Agents

Analgesics may be ordered to relieve pleuritic pain. As the pain decreases, the depth of inspiration and cough efforts should improve.

Ribavirin Aerosol

Ribavirin (Virazole) has been shown to be effective in treating children with RSV infection. Ribavirin is supplied as 6 g of lyophilized powder in a 100-ml vial, which is reconstituted in 300 ml of sterile water, making a 2% (20 mg/ml) strength solution. The solution is aerosolized and delivered to the patient by means of a device called a *small particle aerosol generator (SPAG)*. The aerosol is administered continuously for 12 to 18 hours per day, for 3 to 7 days, through an oxygen hood, face tent, or oxygen tent.

Aerosolized Pentamidine

Pentamidine has been found to be effective against *P. carinii* in patients with HIV infection. Pentamidine can be administered parenterally or as an inhaled aerosol. When given by inhaled aerosol, pentamidine reaches a much higher concentration in the lungs than when given intravenously.

Thoracentesis

Therapeutically, a thoracentesis may be used to treat pleural effusion. Fluid samples may be examined for the following:

- Color
- Odor
- RBC count
- Protein
- Glucose
- Lactic dehydrogenase (LDH)
- Amylase
- pH
- Wright's, Gram's, and acid-fast bacillus (AFB) stains
- Aerobic, anaerobic, tuberculosis, and fungal cultures
- Cytology

Case Study: PNEUMONIA

Admitting History and Physical Examination

A 47-year-old male was hunting in northern Michigan with some friends. They spent considerable time outdoors in inclement weather and indulged freely in alcoholic beverages during the afternoons and evenings. Previously, the man had been essentially healthy. He smoked 1 pack of cigarettes a day.

Returning home, he felt listless and thought that he was "coming down with a cold." That night, he noticed a mild, nonproductive cough. He had a headache and some pain in the right side of his chest on deep inspiration and noticed that he was somewhat short of breath when he climbed one flight of stairs. During the night, he woke up and felt very chilled, then very warm. His wife put her hand on his forehead and was certain that he had a "high fever." Because he felt miserable, they went to the emergency room of the nearest hospital.

On physical examination, his vital signs were as follows: blood pressure 150/88, pulse 116/min, respiratory rate 28/min, and temperature (oral) 39.9° C. He was in moderate distress. Percussion of the chest revealed dullness on the right lower side, and on inspiration there were fine crackles heard in that area. The breath sounds were described as "bronchial." The chest radiograph showed pneumonic consolidation of the right lower lung field. On room air, his arterial blood gas values were pH 7.53, $Paco_2$ 27, HCO_3^- 21, and Pao_2 72. The respiratory therapist assigned to assess and treat the patient charted the following SOAP note:

Respiratory Assessment and Plan

S "I feel miserable." Mild exertional dyspnea.

O Alert, cooperative, acutely ill. Mild nonproductive cough. Vital signs: T 39.9° C, BP 150/88, P 116, RR 28. Dull to percussion over RLL, where crackles are heard. CXR: Pneumonic consolidation RLL. AGB on room air: pH 7.53, $Paco_2$ 27, HCO_3^- 21, and Pao_2 72

A • RLL consolidation (pneumonia presumed)
   • Acute alveolar hyperventilation with mild hypoxemia (ABG)

P Oxygen Therapy Protocol: Monitor Spo_2. (Titrate O_2 per NC as needed to keep $Spo_2 \geq 90\%$).
The patient was started on oxygen (2 L/min) via a nasal cannula. The physician prescribed intravenous antibiotic therapy.

• • • • •

Over the next 72 hours, the patient steadily improved, although he had been nauseated and vomiting times three. On the fourth hospital day, however, the patient complained of increased shortness of breath. He started to cough up large amounts (3 to 4 tablespoons every 2 hours) of foul-smelling, greenish-yellow sputum. He also complained of a bitter taste in his mouth, belching, mild substernal discomfort, and chills.

On physical examination, the patient appeared anxious. His vital signs were blood pressure 120/82, pulse 140 bpm, respiratory rate 20/min, and oral temperature 40.0° C. His sputum was thick, yellow-green, and foul smelling. His cough was strong. He had bronchial breath sounds, rhonchi, and nonclearing crackles in the right middle of the anterior chest and over both lower lobes posteriorly. There was mild cyanosis of the nail beds. The abdominal examination was unremarkable. There was no peripheral edema. A chest X-ray showed a new infiltrate in the right middle lung field and left lung base. The opaque infiltrate obstructed the view of the heart and was described by the radiologist as consolidation. On 2 L/min O_2 nasal cannula, his ABGs were as follows: pH 7.50, $Paco_2$ 29, HCO_3^- 20, Pao_2 36, and Sao_2 69%. At this time the respiratory therapist charted this SOAP progress note:

S Increased dyspnea. Symptoms of belching and substernal chest pain.

O Anxious appearance. BP 120/82, HR 140, RR 20, T 40.0° C. Cyanotic. Strong productive cough (sputum foul-smelling, yellow-green). Bronchial breath sounds, rhonchi, persistent crackles in right middle anterior chest and both bases. CXR: RML and LLL infiltrate, persistent RLL infiltrate. ABG (on 2 LPM): pH 7.50, $Paco_2$ 29, HCO_3^- 20, Pao_2 36, and Sao_2 69%.

A • Aspiration complicating community-acquired pneumonia, involving RML, both lower lobes (history, CXR)
   • Alveolar consolidation (CXR)
   • Excessive airway secretions (thick, yellow-green sputum)
   • Good ability to mobilize secretions (strong cough)
   • Acute alveolar hyperventilation with severe hypoxemia (ABG)

P Oxygen Therapy Protocol: (increase FIo_2 to 0.60 via HAFOE mask). Bronchopulmonary Hygiene Protocol: (DB&C instruction, prn oropharyngeal suctioning. Trial P&D to lower lobes and RML q shift as tolerated).

Aerosolized Medication Protocol: (2.0 cc 10% acetylcysteine (Mucomyst) with 0.5 cc albuterol q 4 hours). ABG in 1 hour

Discussion

A history of cold exposure in conjunction with the use of alcoholic beverages before the onset of pneumonia is not uncommon. The first part of this case begins with a classic presentation for community-acquired pneumonia with **Alveolar Consolidation** (see Figure 9-8). For example, the fever and tachycardia represent a normal functioning immune response, and the tachycardia and tachypnea reflect the body's response to shunt-induced hypoxemia. The auscultation of crackles and bronchial breath sounds also reflects the patient's pulmonary consolidation. An attempt at improving his oxygenation, though not successful, was certainly in order. It was hoped that by providing an oxygen-enriched gas to both normal and partially consolidated alvcoli, the effects of pulmonary shunting would be at least partially offset.

The **second SOAP** presents the complication of the patient's community-acquired pneumonia with aspiration pneumonitis. Alcoholics frequently have gastritis or esophagitis, and the patient's eructus (belching) and pyrosis ("heartburn") were clues to the development of that complication. At this time there were new clinical manifestations associated with **Excessive Bronchial Secretions** (see Figure 9-11). For example, the patient demonstrated a cough, sputum, rhonchi, and crackles. Bronchopulmonary Hygiene Therapy (e.g., mucolytic with a bronchodilator, DB&C, suctioning, and P&D) was appropriate. A trial of volume expansion therapy was not given in this case. However, **Atelectasis** often complicates aspiration pneumonia, and such a trial would not have been inappropriate (see Figure 9-7).

In cases of pneumonia, respiratory care practitioners are often tempted to do too much. Typically, volume expansion therapy, bronchodilator aerosol therapy, and bland aerosol therapy have all been ordered for these patients, even in the acute, consolidative stage of their pneumonia. Often, however, all that is needed is the appropriate selection of antibiotics, rest, fluids, and supplementary oxygen. When the pneumonia "breaks up" (resolution stage) or is complicated by aspiration (as in this case), excessive airway secretions and even bronchoconstriction may appear. When this happens, use of other modalities is necessary.

SELF-ASSESSMENT QUESTIONS

Multiple Choice

1. Which of the following is also known as Friedländer's bacillus?

   a. *Haemophilus influenzae*
   b. *Pseudomonas aeruginosa*
   c. *Legionella pneumophila*
   d. *Klebsiella*
   e. *Streptococcus*

2. Of the six types of *Haemophilus influenzae,* which type is most frequently pathogenic?

   a. Type A
   b. Type B
   c. Type C
   d. Type D
   e. Type E
   f. Type F

3. Which of the following is associated with Q fever?

   a. *Mycoplasma pneumoniae*
   b. *Rickettsia*
   c. Ornithosis
   d. Varicella
   e. Respiratory syncytial virus

4. Mendelson's syndrome is associated with which of the following?

   a. Lipoid pneumonitis
   b. Rubella
   c. Varicella
   d. Aspiration pneumonia
   e. *Rickettsia*

5. Which of the following is/are commonly seen in patients with AIDS?

   I. *Aspergillus*
   II. *Cryptococcus*
   III. *Pneumocystis carinii*
   IV. Cytomegalovirus

   a. I only
   b. III only
   c. II and IV only
   d. II, III, and IV only
   e. I, II, III, and IV

6. Ribavirin aerosol has been shown to be effective in treating children with which of the following?

   a. *Klebsiella*
   b. *Haemophilus influenzae B*
   c. Respiratory syncytial virus
   d. *Pseudomonas aeruginosa*
   e. *Streptococcus*

7. Which of the following is almost always the cause of acute epiglottitis?

   a. *Haemophilus influenzae B*
   b. *Klebsiella*
   c. *Streptococcus*
   d. *Mycoplasma pneumoniae*
   e. Parainfluenza virus

8. Which of the following is most associated with "croup"?

   a. *Streptococcus*
   b. Parainfluenza virus
   c. *Mycoplasma pneumoniae*
   d. Adenovirus
   e. *Chlamydia psittaci*

9. In the absence of a secondary bacterial infection, lung inflammation caused by the aspiration of gastric fluids usually becomes insignificant in approximately how many days?

   a. 2
   b. 3
   c. 5
   d. 7
   e. 10

10. Which of the following is/are associated with pneumonia?

    I. Decreased tactile and vocal fremitus
   II. Increased $C(a-\bar{v})_{O_2}$
  III. Decreased PEFR
  IV. Increased VC

    a. I only
    b. III only
    c. II and IV only
    d. I and III only
    e. II and III only

Answers appear in Appendix XI.

CHAPTER 16

Lung Abscess

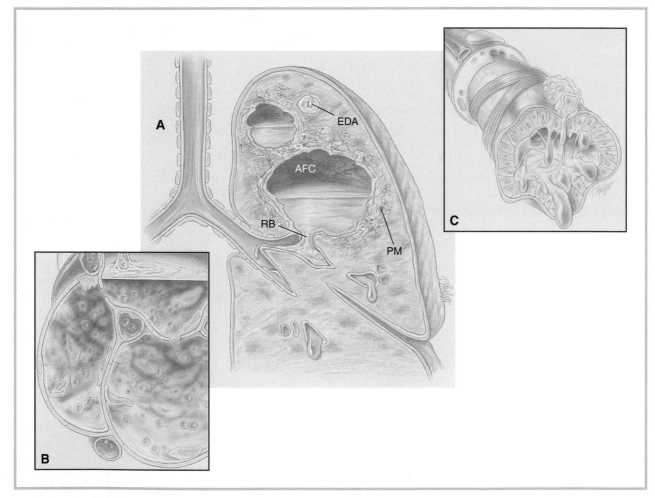

Figure 16–1 Lung abscess. **A,** Cross-sectional view of lung abscess. *AFC,* Air-fluid cavity; *RB,* ruptured bronchus (and drainage of the liquified contents of the cavity); *EDA,* early development of abscess; *PM,* pyogenic membrane. Consolidation **(B)** and excessive bronchial secretions **(C)** are common secondary anatomic alterations of the lungs. See also Plate 8.

Anatomic Alterations of the Lungs

A *lung abscess* is defined as a necrosis of lung tissue that, in severe cases, leads to a localized air- and fluid-filled cavity. The fluid in the cavity is a collection of purulent exudate that is composed of liquefied white blood cell remains, proteins, and tissue debris. The air- and fluid-filled cavity is encapsulated in a so-called pyogenic membrane that consists of a layer of fibrin, inflammatory cells, and granulation tissue.

During the early stages of a lung abscess, the pathology is indistinguishable from that of any acute pneumonia. Polymorphonuclear leukocytes and macrophages move into the infected area to engulf any invading organisms. This action causes the pulmonary capillaries to dilate, the interstitium to fill with fluid, and the alveolar epithelium to swell from the edema fluid. In response to this inflammatory reaction, the alveoli in the infected area become consolidated (see Figure 15-1).

As the inflammatory process progresses, tissue necrosis involving all the lung structures occurs. In severe cases the tissue necrosis ruptures into a bronchus and allows a partial or total drainage of the liquefied contents into the cavity. An air- and fluid-filled cavity also may rupture into the intrapleural space via a bronchopleural fistula and cause pleural effusion and empyema. This may lead to inflammation of the parietal pleura, chest pain, atelectasis, and decreased chest expansion. After a period of time, fibrosis and calcification of the tissues around the cavity encapsulate the abscess (Figure 16-1).

The major pathologic or structural changes associated with a lung abscess are as follows:

- Alveolar consolidation
- Alveolar-capillary and bronchial wall destruction
- Tissue necrosis
- Cavity formation
- Fibrosis and calcification of the lung parenchyma
- Bronchopleural fistulae and empyema
- Atelectasis
- Excessive airway secretions

Etiology

Pneumonia caused by aspiration, *Klebsiella,* or *Staphylococcus* is the most common cause of abscess formation. The formation of a lung abscess is often associated with anaerobic organisms. In humans, anaerobic organisms normally inhabit the intestinal tract and are even found in the saliva. They often colonize in the small grooves and spaces between the teeth and gums in patients with poor oral hygiene (anaerobic organisms are commonly associated with gingivitis and dead or abscessed teeth). As a general rule, anaerobic organisms enter the lungs when an individual aspirates gastrointestinal fluids that contain the organisms. Anaerobic organisms found in gastrointestinal fluids and saliva include *Peptococcus, Peptostreptococcus, Bacteroides,* and *Fusobacterium.*

Predisposing factors that often lead to the aspiration of gastrointestinal fluids (and anaerobes) include (1) alcohol abuse, (2) seizure disorders, (3) general anesthesia, (4) head trauma, (5) cerebrovascular accident, and (6) swallowing disorders. The incidence of lung abscesses caused by anaerobic organisms is also high in patients with poor oral hygiene.

Although less frequent, aerobic organisms such as *Streptococcus pyogenes, Klebsiella pneumoniae,* and *Escherichia coli* also can cause significant tissue destruction with the formation of a lung abscess. On rare occasions a lung abscess also may be caused by *Streptococcus pneumoniae, Pseudomonas aeruginosa,* or *Legionella pneumophila.* Typically, more than one type of bacterium is involved, as in an infection with anaerobic organisms mixed with aerobic ones.

Other organisms that may lead to a lung abscess are *Mycobacterium tuberculosis* (including the atypical organisms *Mycobacterium kansasii* and *Mycobacterium avium-intracellulare*) and fungal organisms such as *Histoplasma capsulatum, Coccidioides immitis, Blastomyces,* and *Aspergillus fumigatus.* Some parasites such as *Paragonimus westermani, Echinococcus,* and *Entamoeba histolytica* also may cause lung abscess formation.

Finally, a lung abscess may develop as a result of (1) bronchial obstruction with secondary cavitating infection (e.g., distal to bronchogenic carcinoma, or aspirated foreign body), (2) vascular obstruction with tissue infarction (e.g., septic embolism, vasculitis), (3) interstitial lung disease with cavity formation (e.g., pneumoconiosis [silicosis], Wegener's granulomatosis, and rheumatoid nodules), (4) bullae or cysts that become infected (e.g., congenital or bronchogenic cysts), or (5) penetrating chest wounds that lead to an infection (e.g., bullet wound).

Anatomically, a lung abscess most commonly forms in the superior segments of the lower lobes and the posterior segments of the upper lobes. The tendency for an abscess to form in these areas is because of the effect of gravity and the dependent position of the tracheobronchial tree at the time of aspiration, which commonly occurs while the patient is in the supine position. The right lung is more commonly involved than the left.

OVERVIEW
of the Cardiopulmonary Clinical Manifestations Associated with LUNG ABSCESS

The following clinical manifestations result from the pathological mechanisms caused (or activated) by **Alveolar Consolidation** (see Figure 9-8) and, when the abscess is draining, by **Excessive Bronchial Secretions** (see Figure 9-11)—the major anatomic alterations of the lungs associated with lung abscess (see Figure 16-1).

CLINICAL DATA OBTAINED AT THE PATIENT'S BESIDE

The Physical Examination
Vital Signs

Increased respiratory rate (see page 31 ◆)
Several pathophysiologic mechanisms operating simultaneously may lead to an increased ventilatory rate:

- Stimulation of peripheral chemoreceptors (hypoxemia)
- Decreased lung compliance/increased ventilatory rate relationship
- Stimulation of J receptors
- Pain/anxiety/fever

Increased heart rate (pulse), cardiac output, and blood pressure (see pages 11 and 99 ◆)

Chest Pain/Decreased Chest Expansion (see page 42 ◆)

Cyanosis (see page 45 ◆)

Cough, Sputum Production, and Hemoptysis (see page 47 ◆)
During the early stages, when the lung abscess is in the inflammatory pneumonia-like phase, the patient generally has a nonproductive barking or hacking cough. If the abscess progresses into an air- and fluid-filled cavity and ruptures through a bronchus, the patient may suddenly cough up large amounts of sputum. Foul-smelling brown or gray sputum indicates a putrid infection that is caused by numerous organisms, including anaerobes. An odorless green or yellow sputum indicates a nonputrid infection caused by a single aerobic organism. Blood-streaked sputum is common in patients with a lung abscess. Occasionally, frank hemoptysis is seen.

Chest Assessment Findings (see page 22 ◆)

- Increased tactile and vocal fremitus
- Crackles and rhonchi
- The following may be noted directly over the abscess:
  - Dull percussion note
  - Bronchial breath sounds
  - Diminished breath sounds

- Whispered pectoriloquy
- Pleural friction rub (if abscess is near pleural surface)

CLINICAL DATA OBTAINED FROM LABORATORY TESTS AND SPECIAL PROCEDURES

Pulmonary Function Study Findings (Severe and Extensive Cases)

Expiratory Maneuver Findings (see page 61 ◆)

FVC	FEV_T	$FEF_{25\%-75\%}$	$FEF_{200-1200}$
↓	N or ↓	N or ↓	N
PEFR	**MVV**	$FEF_{50\%}$	$FEV_{1\%}$
N	N or ↓	N	N or ↑

Lung Volume and Capacity Findings (see page 62 ◆)

V_T	RV	FRC	TLC
N or ↓	↓	↓	↓
VC	**IC**	**ERV**	**RV/TLC%**
↓	↓	↓	N

Arterial Blood Gases

Mild to Moderate Lung Abscess
Acute Alveolar Hyperventilation with Hypoxemia (see page 70 ◆)

pH	$Paco_2$	HCO_3^-	Pao_2
↑	↓	↓ (Slightly)	↓

Severe Lung Abscess
Acute Ventilatory Failure with Hypoxemia (see page 73 ◆)

pH	$Paco_2$	HCO_3^-*	Pao_2
↓	↑	↑ (Slightly)	↓

*When tissue hypoxia is severe enough to produce lactic acid, the pH and HCO_3^- values will be lower than expected for a particular $Paco_2$ level.

Oxygenation Indices (see page 82 ◆)

$\dot{Q}_S/\dot{Q}_T$	Do_2†	$\dot{V}o_2$	$C(a-\bar{v})o_2$
↑	↓	Normal	Normal
O_2ER	$S\bar{v}o_2$		
↑	↓		

†The Do_2 may be normal in patients who have compensated to the decreased oxygenation status with an increased cardiac output. When the Do_2 is normal, the O_2ER is usually normal.

OVERVIEW

of the Cardiopulmonary Clinical Manifestations Associated with
LUNG ABSCESS—(Continued)

ABNORMAL LABORATORY TESTS AND PROCEDURES

Sputum examination (see etiology in this chapter, page 243 ◆▸)

Gram-positive organisms:
- *Staphylococcus*

Anaerobic organisms:
- *Peptococcus*
- *Peptostreptococcus*
- *Bacteroides*
- *Fusobacterium*

RADIOLOGIC FINDINGS

Chest Radiograph
- Increased opacity
- Cavity formation
- Cavity with air-fluid levels
- Fibrosis and calcification
- Pleural effusion

The chest radiograph typically reveals localized consolidation during the early stages of lung abscess formation. The characteristic radiographic appearance of a lung abscess appears after (1) the infection ruptures into a bronchus, (2) tissue destruction and necrosis have occurred, and (3) partial evacuation of the purulent contents has occurred. The abscess usually appears on the radiograph as a circular radiolucency that contains an air-fluid level surrounded by a dense wall of lung parenchyma (Figure 16-2).

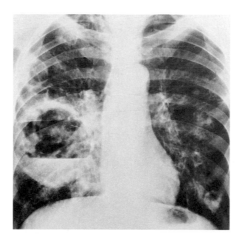

Figure 16–2 Reactivation tuberculosis with a large cavitary lesion containing an air-fluid level in the right lower lobe. Smaller cavitary lesions are seen in other lobes. (From Armstrong P et al: *Imaging of diseases of the chest,* ed 2, St. Louis, 1995, Mosby.)

General Management of Lung Abscess

When treated properly, most patients with a lung abscess show improvement. In acute cases, the size of the abscess quickly decreases and eventually closes altogether. In severe or chronic cases, the patient's improvement may be slow or insignificant, even with appropriate therapy.

RESPIRATORY CARE TREATMENT PROTOCOLS

Oxygen Therapy Protocol

Oxygen therapy is used to treat hypoxemia, decrease the work of breathing, and decrease myocardial work. The hypoxemia that develops in lung abscess is usually caused by pulmonary capillary shunting. Hypoxemia caused by capillary shunting is at least partially refractory to oxygen therapy (see Oxygen Therapy Protocol, Protocol 9-1).

Bronchopulmonary Hygiene Therapy Protocol

Because of the excessive mucus production and accumulation associated with a ruptured lung abscess, a number of bronchial hygiene treatment modalities may be used to enhance the mobilization of bronchial secretions (see Bronchopulmonary Hygiene Therapy Protocol, Protocol 9-2). Modalities used may include bland or ultrasonic aerosol therapy, cough and deep breathing maneuvers, incentive spirometry, chest physical therapy and postural drainage, deep tracheal suctioning, and mucolytic aerosol therapy. Bronchoscopy may be used to identify possible bronchogenic carcinoma and obtain deep lung specimens for culture.

Hyperinflation Therapy Protocol

Because of the alveolar consolidation and atelectasis associated with conditions such as a lung abscess, hyperinflation may be used to offset the pathophysiologic effects of these anatomic alterations of the lungs (see Hyperinflation Therapy Protocol, Protocol 9-3).

MEDICATIONS AND PROCEDURES COMMONLY PRESCRIBED BY THE PHYSICIAN

Antibiotics

Antibiotics are the primary treatment for a lung abscess. Penicillin or semisynthetic penicillin analogs are usually the first drugs of choice. For patients who have serious penicillin hypersensitivity, clindamycin, lincomycin, erythromycin, streptomycin, or tetracycline may be used. Methicillin, nafcillin, or vancomycin are used to treat lung abscesses caused by *Staphylococcus aureus*. When *Klebsiella* is the causative agent, kanamycin is administered. For resistant organisms, the choice of antibiotic is based on culture and sensitivity studies (see Appendix II).

Surgery

Surgical intervention for drainage or resection of the abscessed lobe or lobes may be helpful in selected, antibiotic-refractory cases.

Case Study: LUNG ABSCESS

Admitting History and Physical Examination

This 64-year-old unemployed male sought medical attention because of an increasingly severe cough that produced moderate amounts of foul-smelling sputum. He had undergone splenectomy for removal of a ruptured spleen 1 year ago. He reported that on several occasions recently he had a slight fever and that his appetite was poor; he has lost about 6 pounds. For the past 3 days he had noticed some right-sided chest pain, and his cough had become very productive. The patient denied cigarette smoking.

Physical examination showed a small and poorly nourished male in moderate distress, coughing throughout the interview. The patient's vital signs were blood pressure 160/90, heart rate 120/min, respiratory rate 22/min, and oral temperature of 100.6° F. There was brawny discoloration of the legs below the knees. His teeth were in deplorable condition, and he had marked halitosis. Examination of the chest revealed dullness, crackles, rhonchi, and bronchial breath sounds in the right lower lobe.

His frequent cough produced large amounts of foul-smelling brown and gray sputum. His cough was strong. The chest X-ray showed a 4-cm diameter cavity in the right lower lobe with a clear air-fluid level. Patches of alveolar consolidation surrounded the cavity. There was no evidence of air trapping. Sputum for a culture and sensitivity study was obtained, but the results were still pending. His arterial blood gas values were as follows: pH 7.51, $Paco_2$ 29, HCO_3^- 22, and Pao_2 61 on room air. The respiratory care practitioner assigned to his case recorded the following:

Respiratory Assessment and Plan

S "I can't stop coughing." Complains of low-grade fever, loss of appetite, weight loss (6 pounds).

O Cachectic. BP 160/90, HR 120, RR 22, T 100.6° F orally. Teeth carious. Flat to percussion over RLL. Crackles, rhonchi, and bronchial breath sounds over RLL. CXR: 4-cm diameter cavity with fluid level and consolidation RLL. ABGs: pH 7.51, $Paco_2$ 29, HCO_3^- 22, and Pao_2 61. Excessive amount of foul-smelling, thick brown and gray sputum.

A • Malnourished (inspection)
- Lung abscess and consolidation (CXR)
- Acute alveolar hyperventilation with mild hypoxemia (ABG)

- Excessive and thick airway secretions (sputum, rhonchi)
- Good ability to mobilize secretions (strong cough)

P Oxygen Therapy Protocol: (2 Lpm per nasal cannula. Spo_2 spot check to verify appropriateness of O_2 therapy. O_2 titration if necessary). Bronchopulmonary Hygiene Therapy Protocols: (Deep breathe and cough, with postural drainage to right lower lobe q 6 hours). Aerosolized Medication Protocol: (Trial period of med nebs: 2.0 cc acetylcysteine with 0.5 cc L-albuterol (Xopenex) ½ hour before postural drainage × 3 days, then reevaluate).

• • • • •

After reviewing the results of sputum culture sensitivity studies, the physician adjusted the patient's antibiotic therapy. Over the next 5 days, the patient's general condition improved. His cough and sputum production decreased remarkably but not completely. The sputum produced was no longer thick. His Pao_2 increased to 86 mm Hg, and he no longer had acute alveolar hyperventilation. A chest radiograph revealed that his lung abscess was slightly reduced in size compared with the chest radiograph taken on the day of his admission, and his pneumonia had improved significantly. A complete pulmonary function test (PFT) study revealed a mild reduction in lung volumes, capacities, and expiratory flow rates. Social Service worked with him on two occasions during his hospitalization and scheduled a follow-up appointment at his home 4 weeks after discharge. An oral surgery consultation was obtained and extraction of the patient's carious teeth was scheduled. The patient was instructed on deep-breathing and coughing techniques and general bronchial hygiene and was discharged on the morning of the sixth day. He was discharged on a month-long course of oral antibiotics.

Discussion

This case illustrates some of the classic clinical manifestations of a lung abscess. For example, the **Alveolar Consolidation** (see Figure 9-8), which was identified on the chest X-ray surrounding the abscess, likely played a role in producing the patient's fever and increased heart rate, blood pressure, and respiratory rate. In addition, the pneumonic consolidation also contributed to the patient's alveolar hyperventilation and hypoxemia, bronchial breath sounds, and reduced lung volumes and capacities and flow rates identified on his PFT. In addition, the clinical manifestations associated with **Excessive Bronchial Secretions** (see Figure 9-11) also were seen in this case. Not only did the excessive airway secretions contribute to the patient's hypoxemia, secondary to the decreased $\dot{V}/\dot{Q}$ ratio and pulmonary shunting, but it also contributed to the increased airway resistance (caused by the secretions) that resulted in the rhonchi, sputum production, and reduced flow rates.

The main respiratory therapy treatments ordered by the respiratory care practitioner were directed to the patient's excessive secretions. Pulmonary hyperinflation therapy was not employed in this case. One could argue that it should have been, given the chest X-ray infiltrates that could have represented atelectasis just as well as pneumonia.

The appropriate respiratory care of patients with lung abscesses closely resembles that of those with bronchiectasis (see Chapter 14). Identification of this patient's lung abscess in the right lower lobe allowed targeted chest physical therapy to be practiced. The suggestion that a Social Service representative see the patient was entirely appropriate to instruct him on his personal hygiene. Finally, extraction of his carious teeth was suggested by the Dental Service.

SELF-ASSESSMENT QUESTIONS

Multiple Choice

1. Which of the following is/are anaerobic organisms?

    I. *Klebsiella*
    II. *Peptococcus*
    III. *Coccidioides immitis*
    IV. *Bacteroides*

    a. I and II only
    b. II and IV only
    c. III and IV only
    d. II, III, and IV only
    e. I, III, and IV only

2. Which of the following is/are predisposing factors to the aspiration of gastrointestinal fluids (and anaerobes)?

    I. Seizure disorders
    II. Head trauma
    III. Alcoholic binges
    IV. General anesthesia

    a. I and III only
    b. II and IV only
    c. II and III only
    d. II, III, and IV only
    e. I, II, III, and IV

3. Which of the following aerobic organisms is/are associated with the formation of a lung abscess?

    I. *Fusobacterium*
    II. *Staphylococcus aureus*
    III. *Klebsiella*
    IV. *Streptococcus pyogenes*

    a. I only
    b. III only
    c. II and IV only
    d. II, III, and IV only
    e. I, II, III, and IV

4. Anatomically, a lung abscess most commonly forms in which part(s) of the lung?

    I. Posterior segment of the upper lobe
    II. Lateral basal segment of the lower lobe
    III. Anterior segment of the upper lobe
    IV. Superior segment of the lower lobe

    a. I only
    b. III only
    c. I and IV only
    d. II and III only
    e. II, III, and IV only

5. Which of the following pulmonary function findings may be associated with a severe and extensive lung abscess?

    I. Decreased FVC
    II. Increased PEFR
    III. Decreased RV
    IV. Increased FRC

    a. I only
    b. III only
    c. II and IV only
    d. III and IV only
    e. I and III only

True or False

True ☐ False ☐ **1.** Penicillin or semisynthetic penicillin analogs are usually the first drugs of choice in treating a lung abscess.

True ☐ False ☐ **2.** Odorless green or yellow sputum indicates a putrid infection that is caused by numerous organisms.

True ☐ False ☐ **3.** In humans, anaerobic organisms normally inhabit the intestines and are found in the saliva.

True ☐ False ☐ **4.** Some parasites such as *Echinococcus* are associated with lung abscesses.

True ☐ False ☐ **5.** A lung abscess is more commonly found in the left lung than in the right lung.

Answers appear in Appendix XI.

CHAPTER 17

Tuberculosis

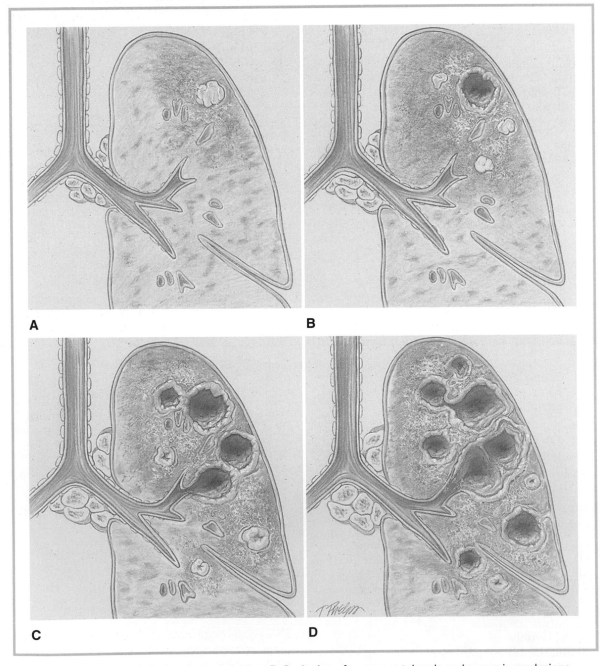

Figure 17–1   Tuberculosis. **A,** Early primary infection. **B,** Cavitation of a caseous tubercle and new primary lesions developing. **C,** Further progression and development of cavitations and new primary infections. Note the subpleural location of some of these lesions. **D,** Severe lung destruction caused by tuberculosis. See also Plate 9.

Anatomic Alterations of the Lungs

Tuberculosis (TB) is a chronic bacterial infection that primarily affects the lungs, although it may involve almost any part of the body. Clinically, TB is separated into three categories: primary TB, postprimary TB, and disseminated TB.

PRIMARY TUBERCULOSIS

Primary TB (also called the *primary infection stage*) follows the patient's first exposure to the pathogen. Primary TB begins when inhaled bacilli implant in the alveoli. As the bacilli multiply over a 3- to 4-week period, the initial response of the lungs is an inflammatory reaction that is similar to any acute pneumonia (see Figure 15-1). In other words, a large influx of polymorphonuclear leukocytes and macrophages move into the infected area to engulf (but not fully kill) the bacilli. This action also causes the pulmonary capillaries to dilate, the interstitium to fill with fluid, and the alveolar epithelium to swell from the edema fluid. Eventually, the alveoli become consolidated (i.e., filled with fluid, polymorphonuclear leukocytes, and macrophages). Clinically, this phase of TB coincides with a positive tuberculin reaction (positive PPD skin test).

Unlike pneumonia, however, the lung tissue that surrounds the infected area slowly produces a protective cell wall called a *tubercle,* or *granuloma,* that surrounds and encases the bacilli (Figure 17-1, *A*). A tubercle consists of a central core containing TB bacilli and enlarged macrophages with an outer wall composed of fibroblasts, lymphocytes, and neutrophils. A tubercle takes about 2 to 10 weeks to form. Although the formation of a tubercle works to prevent further spread of infection, it also carries the potential for more damage. For example, the center of the tubercle frequently breaks down and fills with necrotic tissue that resembles dry cottage cheese. When this occurs, the tubercle is called a *caseous lesion,* or *caseous granuloma* (Figure 17-1, *B*).

If the bacilli are controlled (either by the patient's immunologic defense system or by antituberculous drugs), fibrosis and calcification of the lung parenchyma ultimately replace the tubercle during the healing process. As a result of the fibrosis and calcification, the lung tissue retracts and becomes scarred. Because of the destruction and calcification, fibrosis, distortion, and dilation of the bronchi (bronchiectasis) are commonly seen.

POSTPRIMARY TUBERCULOSIS

Postprimary TB (also called *secondary* or *reinfection TB*) is a term used to describe the reactivation of TB months or even years after the initial infection has been controlled. Even though most patients with primary TB recover completely from a clinical standpoint, it is important to note that live tubercle bacilli can remain dormant for decades. Because of this long dormancy, a positive tuberculin reaction generally persists even after the primary infection stage has been controlled. At any time, tuberculosis may become reactivated, especially in patients with weakened immunity. If the infection is uncontrolled, cavitation of the caseous tubercle develops. In severe cases a deep tuberculous cavity may rupture and allow air and infected material to flow into the pleural space or the tracheobronchial tree. Pleural complications are common in tuberculosis (Figure 17-1, *C*).

DISSEMINATED TUBERCULOSIS

Disseminated TB (also called *extrapulmonary TB*) refers to infection from bacilli that escape from a tubercle and rapidly disseminate to sites other than the lungs by means of the pulmonary lymphatic system or bloodstream. In general, the bacilli that gain entrance to the bloodstream usually gather and multiply in portions of the body that have a high tissue oxygen tension. The most common location is the apex of the lungs. Other oxygen-rich areas in the body include the regional lymph nodes, kidneys, ends of long bones, genital tract, brain, and meninges. When a large number of bacilli are freed into the bloodstream, they can produce a condition called *miliary TB* (i.e., the presence of numerous small tubercles, about the size of a pinhead, scattered throughout the body).

TB is primarily a chronic restrictive pulmonary disorder. The major pathologic or structural changes of the lungs associated with TB (mainly postprimary TB) are as follows:

- Alveolar consolidation
- Alveolar-capillary destruction
- Caseous tubercles or granulomas
- Cavity formation
- Fibrosis and secondary calcification of the lung parenchyma
- Distortion and dilation of the bronchi
- Increased bronchial airway secretions

Etiology

TB is one of the oldest diseases known to man and remains one of the most widespread diseases in the world. Characteristic TB changes have been found in the remains of skeletons from 4000 BC. TB was a common disease in Egypt circa 1000 BC. In early writings, the disease was commonly called "consumption," "Captain of the Men of Death," and "white plague." In the nineteenth century, the disease was named *tuberculosis*, a term that derives mainly from the tubercle formation evident during postmortem examinations of victims of the disease. Today, between 10 and 15 million people in the United States are estimated to be currently infected with TB. Approximately 17,000 new cases of TB are reported each year in the United States. Worldwide, TB infects approximately 8 to 10 million people annually. The World Health Organization estimates that between the years 2000 and 2020 nearly 1 billion people will be newly infected with TB, about 200 million will become ill, and about 35 million will die of the disease.

In humans, TB is primarily caused by *Mycobacterium tuberculosis*. The mycobacteria are long, slender, straight, or curved rods. Approximately 50 different mycobacteria species have been identified, several of which can cause tuberculosis in humans (e.g., *Mycobacterium bovis, Mycobacterium ulcerans, Mycobacterium kansasii,* and *Mycobacterium avium-intracellulare*). The *M. tuberculosis* organism enters humans in the following three ways: the respiratory tract, the gastrointestinal tract, and an open wound in the skin. Most TB infections, however, are contracted via the airborne route (e.g., inhalation of aerosol droplets containing organisms of the tubercle bacillus from an infected individual).

The mycobacteria are highly aerobic organisms and thrive best in areas of the body with high oxygen tension—especially in the apex of the lung. When stained, the hard outer layer of the tubercle bacilli resists decolorization by acid or alcohol; therefore the bacilli are called *acid-fast bacilli.* In addition, the hard outer coat of the tubercle bacillus also protects the organism against killing and digestion by phagocytes and renders the bacilli more resistant to antituberculous drugs.

The tubercle bacillus is almost exclusively transmitted within aerosol droplets produced by the coughing, sneezing, or laughing of an individual with active TB. In fact, in fine dried aerosol droplets, the tubercle bacillus can remain suspended in air for several hours after a cough or sneeze. When inhaled, some of the tubercle bacilli may be trapped in the mucus of the nasal passages and removed. The smaller bacilli, however, can easily be inhaled as an aerosol into the bronchioles and alveoli. People living in closed, small rooms with limited access to sunlight and fresh air are especially at risk. The aerosol is composed of organisms contained in small particles known as *droplet nuclei.*

Although the factors responsible for postprimary TB are not fully understood, conditions that weaken local and systemic body defenses seem to play a major role. Such conditions include acquired immunodeficiency syndrome (AIDS), diabetes mellitus, surgery, childbirth, puberty, treatment with immunosuppressive drugs, alcoholism, nutritional deficiency, chronic debilitating disorders, and old age. TB in patients with AIDS is currently at near-epidemic levels in certain areas of the world.

Diagnosis

The most frequently used diagnostic methods for TB are the tuberculin skin test, acid-fast stain and sputum cultures, and chest radiographs.

INTRADERMAL (MANTOUX) TUBERCULIN SKIN TESTING

The tuberculin skin test measures the delayed hypersensitivity (cell mediated, type IV) that follows exposure to tuberculoproteins. The most commonly used tuberculin test is the Mantoux test, which consists of an intradermal injection of a small amount of a *purified protein derivative* (PPD) of the tuberculin bacillus. In the Mantoux test, 0.1 ml of PPD is injected into the forearm to produce an immediate small bleb. The skin is then observed for induration (wheal) after 48 hours and 72 hours. An induration less than 5 mm is negative. An induration between 5 mm and 9 mm is considered suspicious, and retesting is required. An induration of 10 mm or greater is considered positive. A positive reaction is fairly sound evidence of recent or past infection or disease. It should be stressed, however, that a positive reaction does not necessarily confirm that a patient has active TB, only that the patient has been exposed to the bacillus and has developed cell-mediated immunity to it.

ACID-FAST STAIN AND SPUTUM CULTURE

An acid-fast stain of sputum is commonly used to establish the diagnosis of infection with *M. tuberculosis.* Several variations of the acid-fast stain are currently in use. The Ziehl-Neelsen stain reveals bright red acid-fast bacilli (AFB) against a blue background. Another technique involves a fluorescent acid-fast stain that reveals luminescent yellow-green bacilli against a dark brown background. The fluorescent acid-fast stain is becoming the acid-fast test of choice because it is easier to read and provides a striking contrast. Expectorated sputum is positive in as many as 30% of patients with cavitary disease. When the patient is coughing productively, collection of three deep cough morning sputum samples is more likely to produce positive smears and cultures than randomly collected specimens. Failing this, the use of inhaled warm hypertonic saline may help induce cough and sputum production.

A culture is necessary to differentiate *M. tuberculosis* from other acid-fast organisms. Culture results can take as long as 6 to 8 weeks to obtain. Culturing also identifies drug-resistant bacilli and their sensitivity to antibiotic therapy. The sputum specimen should be obtained from deep in the lungs early in the morning. Saliva or nasal secretions are not acceptable.

IDENTIFICATION OF MYCOBACTERIUM SPECIES

Quick identification of organisms in expectorated or bronchoscopically obtained sputum can be done by a deoxyribonucleic acid (DNA) probe in a technique called the *polymerase chain reaction (PCR)*. Specificity as to precise organism identification is quite good. The technique currently is used only on acid-fast bacillus smear–positive specimens, and the results are available within 24 hours.

NONTUBERCULOSIS MYCOBACTERIA

Mycobacterial infections caused by species other than *M. tuberculosis* are called *nontuberculosis Mycobacteria* (NTM); they also are called *mycobacteria other than tuberculosis* (*MOTT*) or *atypical mycobacterial infections*. These organisms are found in soil and water. The mode of transmission is not clear. Many cases of NTM are reported in smokers with chronic obstructive pulmonary disease (COPD), silicosis, malignancy, cystic fibrosis, and human immunodeficiency virus (HIV) infections. In patients with COPD, the following mycobacterial infections are often seen: *Mycobacterium avium-intracellulare* (MAI) and *Mycobacterium kansasii*.

OVERVIEW
of the *Cardiopulmonary Clinical Manifestations Associated with TUBERCULOSIS*

The following clinical manifestations result from the pathophysiologic mechanisms caused (or activated) by **Alveolar Consolidation** (see Figure 9-8) and **Increased Alveolar-Capillary Membrane Thickness** (see Figure 9-9)—the major anatomic alterations of the lungs associated with tuberculosis (see Figure 17-1).

CLINICAL DATA OBTAINED AT THE PATIENT'S BEDSIDE

The Physical Examination
Vital Signs

Increased respiratory rate (see page 31 ◆)
Several pathophysiologic mechanisms operating simultaneously may lead to an increased ventilatory rate:
- Stimulation of peripheral chemoreceptors
- Decreased lung compliance/increased ventilatory rate relationship
- Pain/anxiety/fever

Increased heart rate (pulse), cardiac output, and blood pressure (see pages 11 and 99 ◆)

Chest Pain/Decreased Chest Expansion (see page 42 ◆)

Cyanosis (see page 45 ◆)

Digital Clubbing (see page 46 ◆)

Peripheral Edema and Distention (see page 47 ◆)

Because polycythemia and cor pulmonale are associated with severe TB, the following may be seen:
- Distended neck veins
- Pitting edema
- Enlarged and tender liver

Cough, Sputum Production, and Hemoptysis (see page 47 ◆)

Chest Assessment Findings (see page 22 ◆)
- Increased tactile and vocal fremitus
- Dull percussion note
- Bronchial breath sounds
- Crackles, rhonchi, and wheezing
- Pleural friction rub (if process extends to pleural surface)
- Whispered pectoriloquy

CLINICAL DATA OBTAINED FROM LABORATORY TESTS AND SPECIAL PROCEDURES

Pulmonary Function Study Findings

Expiratory Maneuver Findings (see page 61 ◆)

FVC	FEV_T	$FEF_{25\%-75\%}$	$FEF_{200-1200}$
↓	N or ↓	N or ↓	N
PEFR	MVV	$FEF_{50\%}$	$FEV_{1\%}$
N	N or ↓	N	N or ↑

OVERVIEW

of the Cardiopulmonary Clinical Manifestations Associated with TUBERCULOSIS (Continued)

Lung Volume and Capacity Findings (see page 62 ◆▷)

V_T	RV	FRC	TLC
N or ↓	↓	↓	↓
VC	IC	ERV	RV/TLC%
↓	↓	↓	N

Arterial Blood Gases

Mild to Moderate Tuberculosis
Acute Alveolar Hyperventilation with Hypoxemia
(see page 70 ◆▷)

pH	$Paco_2$	HCO_3^-	Pao_2
↑	↓	↓ (Slightly)	↓

Extensive Tuberculosis with Pulmonary Fibrosis
Chronic Ventilatory Failure with Hypoxemia
(see page 73 ◆▷)

pH	$Paco_2$	HCO_3^-	Pao_2
Normal	↑	↑ (Significantly)	↓

Acute Ventilatory Changes Superimposed on Chronic Ventilatory Failure (see page 75 ◆▷)
Because acute ventilatory changes frequently are seen in patients with chronic ventilatory failure, the respiratory care practitioner must be familiar with and alert for (1) acute alveolar hyperventilation superimposed on chronic ventilatory failure and (2) acute ventilatory failure superimposed on chronic ventilatory failure.

Oxygenation Indices (see page 82 ◆▷)

Q_S/Q_T	Do_2*	$\dot{V}o_2$	$C(a-\bar{v})o_2$
↑	↓	Normal	Normal
O_2ER*	$S-\bar{v}o_2$		
↑	↓		

*The Do_2 may be normal in patients who have compensated to the decreased oxygenation status with (1) an increased cardiac output, (2) an increased hemoglobin level, or (3) a combination of both. When the Do_2 is normal, the O_2ER is usually normal.

Hemodynamic Indices (Severe Tuberculosis) (see page 99 ◆▷)

CVP	RAP	$\overline{PA}$	PCWP
↑	↑	↑	Normal
CO	SV	SVI	CI
Normal	Normal	Normal	Normal
RVSWI	LVSWI	PVR	SVR
↑	Normal	↑	Normal

ABNORMAL LABORATORY TESTS AND PROCEDURES

Positive tuberculosis skin test (PPD)
Positive acid-fast bacillus stain of sputum and sputum culture

RADIOLOGIC FINDINGS

Chest Radiograph
- Increased opacity
- Ghon's complex
- Cavity formation
- Pleural effusion
- Calcification and fibrosis
- Retraction of lung segments or lobe
- Right ventricular enlargement

Chest radiography is most valuable in the diagnosis of pulmonary TB. During the initial primary infection stage, peripheral pneumonic infiltrates can be identified. As the disease progresses, the combination of tubercles and the involvement of the lymph nodes in the hilar region (the Ghon complex) can be seen. In severe cases, cavity formation and pleural effusion are quite evident (Figure 17-2). Healed lesions appear fibrotic or calcified. Retraction of the healed lesions or segments also is revealed on chest radiographs. In patients with postprimary TB of the lungs, lesions involving the apical and posterior segments of the upper lobes are often seen. Finally, because right-sided heart failure may develop as a secondary problem during the advanced stages of TB, an enlarged heart may be seen on the chest radiograph.

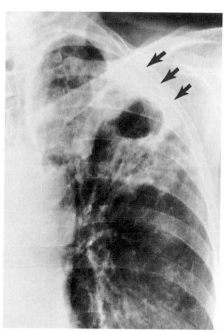

Figure 17–2 Cavitary reactivation TB showing a left upper lobe cavity and localized pleural thickening *(arrows).* (From Armstrong P et al: *Imaging of diseases of the chest,* ed 2, St. Louis, 1995, Mosby.)

General Management of Tuberculosis

Because the tubercle bacillus can exist in open cavitary lesions, in closed lesions, and within the cytoplasm of macrophages, a drug that may be effective in one of these environments may be ineffective in another. In addition, some of the TB bacilli are often drug-resistant. Because of this problem, several drugs usually are prescribed concurrently for individuals with tuberculosis. Because toxicity is associated with some antituberculosis drugs, frequent examinations are performed to identify toxicity manifested in the kidneys, liver, eyes, and ears. In noncompliant patients the drug may need to be administered under the direct supervision of a health-care worker.

PHARMACOLOGIC AGENTS USED TO TREAT TUBERCULOSIS

The standard pharmacologic agents used to treat *M. tuberculosis* consist of two to four drugs for 6 to 12 months. Isoniazid (INH) and rifampin (Rifadin) are first-line agents prescribed for the entire 9 months. Isoniazid is considered to be the most effective first-line antituberculosis agent. Rifampin is bactericidal and is most commonly used with isoniazid. During the initial period, isoniazid and rifampin generally are supplemented with ethambutol, streptomycin, or pyrazinamide. This period is called the induction phase. When laboratory results are available in 6 to 8 weeks, ineffective drugs will be stopped or replaced with other drugs.

Although patients with TB usually are not contagious after a few weeks of treatment, a full course of treatment is necessary to kill all the bacteria. "Standard therapy" changes rapidly, depending on the presence or absence of drug-resistant organisms in the area. Drug resistance is not considered probable when the patient is not foreign-born or has not traveled in a country with a high incidence of drug-resistant TB, has not had previous antituberculous drug therapy, and has not been exposed to another patient with drug-resistant TB. The prophylactic use of isoniazid is often prescribed as a daily dose for 1 year in individuals who have been exposed to the TB bacilli or who demonstrate a positive tuberculin reaction (even when the acid-fast stain is negative).

RESPIRATORY CARE TREATMENT PROTOCOLS

Oxygen Therapy Protocol

Oxygen therapy is used to treat hypoxemia, decrease the work of breathing, and decrease myocardial work. Because of the hypoxemia associated with TB, supplemental oxygen may be required. It should be noted, however, that because of the alveolar consolidation and destruction caused by TB, capillary shunting is present. Hypoxemia caused by capillary shunting is often refractory to oxygen therapy. In addition, when the patient demonstrates chronic ventilatory failure during the advanced stages of tuberculosis, caution must be taken not to over-oxygenate the patient (see Oxygen Therapy Protocol, Protocol 9-1).

Bronchopulmonary Hygiene Therapy Protocol

Because of the excessive mucus production and accumulation sometimes associated with severe TB, a number of bronchial hygiene treatment modalities may be used to enhance the mobilization of bronchial secretions (see Bronchopulmonary Hygiene Therapy Protocol, Protocol 9-2).

Hyperinflation Therapy Protocol

Because of the atelectasis sometimes associated with TB, hyperinflation therapy is occasionally used to prevent or treat alveolar atelectasis and consolidation (see Hyperinflation Therapy Protocol, Protocol 9-3).

Mechanical Ventilation Protocol

Mechanical ventilation may be necessary to provide and support alveolar gas exchange and eventually return the patient to spontaneous breathing. Because acute ventilatory failure superimposed on chronic ventilatory failure is often seen in patients with severe TB, continuous mechanical ventilation may be required. Continuous mechanical ventilation is justified when the acute ventilatory failure is thought to be reversible (see Mechanical Ventilation Protocol, Protocol 9-5).

Case Study: TUBERCULOSIS

Admitting History and Physical Examination

This 60-year-old male patient had been in good health until about 4 months before admission, when he first noted the onset of night sweats, occasionally accompanied by chills. About 3 months ago he noted that his appetite was decreasing, and he lost about 25 pounds since that time.

Approximately 3 weeks before his admission, he noted that his "smoker's cough" of long standing had become more productive. For the past 2 weeks, his daily sputum production had increased to about a cup of thick yellow sputum with an occasional fleck or two of blood. There was a concomitant increase in dyspnea. About 10 days ago, he had a gradual onset of moderately sharp left-sided chest pain. It was aggravated by deep breathing but did not radiate.

The past history gave little useful information. The last time he sought medical assistance was 35 years ago, when he suffered a broken arm in an industrial accident. At that time he was told that he had a positive TB skin test but that he had no pulmonary problems. Since that time, he has had several chest X-rays in mobile chest X-ray units, once for an insurance application. The last X-ray was 5 years ago.

For the past 35 years, he was employed in a foundry as a "cone maker" and "shaker." He volunteered the information that he worked in a "dusty" environment and that he had worn a protective mask only for the past few months. His family history was noncontributory. He and his wife lived in the same house with his married daughter and two young granddaughters.

Physical examination revealed a thin man who appeared to be both chronically and acutely ill. His vital signs were blood pressure 132/90, heart rate 116/min, respiratory rate 32/min, and oral temperature 102.4° F. His room air Spo_2 was 90%. There was marked dullness to percussion in both apical areas and diffuse inspiratory crackles and expiratory rhonchi in the right upper and middle lobes. A chest X-ray demonstrated extensive bilateral apical calcification with cavity formation in the right upper lobe and diffuse infiltrate and consolidation in the right middle lobe. He was admitted to the hospital. This initial respiratory assessment was entered into the patient's chart:

Respiratory Assessment and Plan

S Productive cough, slight hemoptysis; moderate dyspnea. History of left-sided chest pain for 10 days.

O Febrile to 102.4° F. RR 32; HR 116, BP 132/90. Room air Spo_2 90%. Productive cough: large amounts yellow sputum. Crackles and rhonchi in right upper and middle lobes. CXR: Apical calcification; RUL cavity; RML infiltrate/consolidation.

A • Probable tuberculosis (patient possibly infectious)

- Excessive airway secretions (yellow sputum, cough)
- Mild hypoxemia (Spo_2 90%)

P Flag chart: Respiratory isolation pending smear results and obtain sputum for routine, anaerobic, and acid-fast cultures and cytology—induce if necessary. Obtain baseline ABG on room air. Bronchopulmonary Hygiene Therapy Protocol: C&DB q 2 hr. Based on ABG results, titrate oxygen therapy per protocol. Discuss need for bedside spirogram with physician.

Discussion

TB is currently at near-epidemic proportions in many parts of the United States. In almost every hospital of any size, the number of acute TB cases admitted per year is increasing. Much of this epidemic is associated with the presence of multiple–drug resistant organisms in patients who have not completed initial courses of chemotherapy. Another significant percentage of these cases are patients with HIV or other immune system disorders. Older patients who live in crowded quarters, including those in nursing homes and convalescent hospitals, also are at risk. The diagnosis of TB is first made on the basis of a strong clinical suspicion, particularly in these settings. The history of a positive tuberculin reaction, fever, cough, hemoptysis, and an apical infiltrate with abscess formation strongly suggests a diagnosis of TB.

The inpatient respiratory care of such patients is made slightly more complex by the recent Occupational Safety and Health Administration (OSHA) guidelines requiring at least six room air changes an hour, particulate scrubbers, and protective masks to be worn by all health-care workers. The decision by the respiratory care practitioner (who was the first person on the ward to see the patient) to place him in isolation pending smear results was entirely appropriate. Had there been difficulty obtaining a sputum specimen, sputum induction, postural drainage, induction with hypertonic saline, or even bronchoscopy may have been necessary.

Two primary clinical scenarios were activated in this case. First, the **Alveolar Consolidation** identified on the chest X-ray reflected the patient's challenged immune response. This was further manifested by the objective data noted at the patient's bedside—fever, dull percussion notes, and increased heart rate, blood pressure, and respiratory rate. In addition, the alveolar consolidation undoubtedly contributed to the patient's pulmonary shunting and mild hypoxemia (see Figure 9-8). Clinical manifestations associated with **Excessive Bronchial Secretions** (see Figure 9-11) also presented in this case as a daily cough, yellow sputum production, crackles, and rhonchi.

His oxygen desaturation was mild (Spo_2 = 90%), and a room air ABG and subsequent oxygen titration (presumably with low-flow oxygen by nasal cannula) were appropriate. As expected, the patient produced sputum containing acid-fast organisms. The attending physician prescribed isoniazid, rifampin, and streptomycin for 2 months, followed by an outpatient course of isoniazid and rifampin for 4 months. The patient also was instructed in several different bronchial hygiene techniques to perform at home. The patient did well through 1 year of follow-up.

SELF-ASSESSMENT QUESTIONS

Multiple Choice

1. What is the first stage of tuberculosis known as?

    I. Reinfection tuberculosis
    II. Primary tuberculosis
    III. Secondary tuberculosis
    IV. Primary infection stage

    a. I only
    b. II only
    c. III only
    d. I and III only
    e. II and IV only

2. What is the name of the protective cell wall that surrounds and encases lung tissue infected with tuberculosis?

    I. Miliary tuberculosis
    II. Reinfection tuberculosis
    III. Granuloma
    IV. Tubercle

    a. I only
    b. III only
    c. IV only
    d. III and IV only
    e. II and III only

3. The tubercle bacillus is:

    I. Highly aerobic
    II. Acid-fast
    III. Capable of surviving for months outside of the body
    IV. Rod-shaped

    a. I only
    b. II only
    c. IV only
    d. II and III only
    e. I, II, III, and IV

4. At which size wheal is a tuberculin skin test considered to be positive?

    a. Greater than 4 mm
    b. Greater than 6 mm
    c. Greater than 8 mm
    d. Greater than 10 mm
    e. Greater than 12 mm

5. Which of the following is often prescribed as a daily dose for 1 year in individuals who have been exposed to the tuberculosis bacilli?

    a. Streptomycin
    b. Ethambutol
    c. Isoniazid
    d. Rifampin
    e. Pyrazinamide

True or False

True ☐ False ☐ **1.** Pleural space complications such as empyema and pneumothorax are common in patients with tuberculosis.

True ☐ False ☐ **2.** A positive reaction to the tuberculin skin test confirms that a patient has active tuberculosis.

True ☐ False ☐ **3.** Tuberculosis commonly develops in the apices of the lungs.

True ☐ False ☐ **4.** The tuberculin skin test measures the delayed hypersensitivity that follows exposure to the tubercle bacillus.

True ☐ False ☐ **5.** Miliary tuberculosis presents as a small, isolated tubercle lesion.

Answers appear in Appendix XI.

CHAPTER 18

Fungal Diseases of the Lung

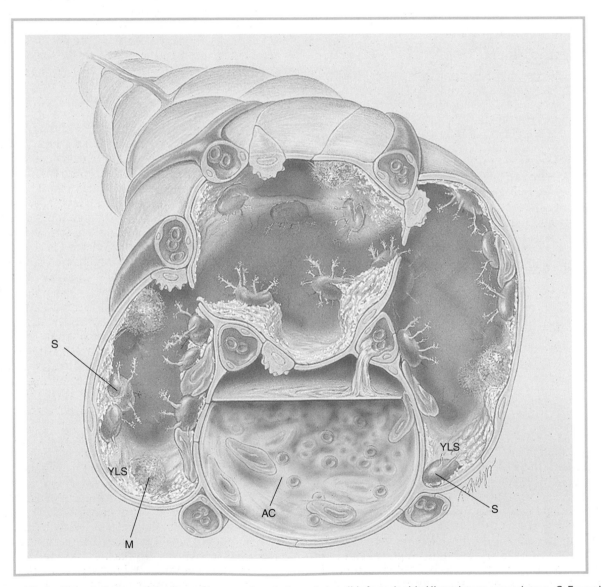

Figure 18–1　Fungal disease of the lung. Cross-sectional view of alveoli infected with *Histoplasma capsulatum. S,* Fungal spore; *YLS,* yeastlike substance; *AC,* alveolar consolidation; *M,* alveolar macrophage. See also Plate 10.

Anatomic Alterations of the Lungs

When fungal spores are inhaled, they may reach the lungs and germinate. When this happens, the spores produce a frothy, yeastlike substance that leads to an inflammatory response. Polymorphonuclear leukocytes and macrophages move into the infected area and engulf the fungal spores. The pulmonary capillaries dilate, the interstitium fills with fluid, and the alveolar epithelium swells with edema fluid. Regional lymph node involvement commonly occurs during this period. Because of the inflammatory reaction, the alveoli in the infected area eventually become consolidated. Airway secretions may also develop at this time (Figure 18-1).

In severe cases, tissue necrosis, granulomas, and cavity formation may be seen. During the healing process, fibrosis and calcification of the lung parenchyma ultimately replace the granulomas. In response to the fibrosis and occasionally calcification, the lung tissue retracts and becomes firm. The apical and posterior segments of the upper lobes are most commonly involved. The anatomic changes of the lungs caused by fungal diseases are similar to those seen in tuberculosis.

Fungal diseases of the lung cause a chronic restrictive pulmonary disorder. The major pathologic or structural changes of the lungs associated with fungal diseases of the lungs are as follows:

- Alveolar consolidation
- Alveolar-capillary destruction
- Caseous tubercles or granulomas
- Cavity formation
- Fibrosis and secondary calcification of the lung parenchyma
- Bronchial airway secretions

Etiology

Fungal spores are widely distributed throughout the air, soil, fomites, and animals, and even exist in the normal flora of humans. As many as 300 fungal species may be linked to disease in animals. In plants, fungal disease is the most common cause of death and destruction. In humans, most exposures to fungal pathogens do not lead to overt infection because humans have a relatively high resistance to them. Human fungal disease (also called *mycotic disease* or *mycosis*) can be caused, however, by "primary" or "true" fungal pathogens that exhibit some degree of virulence or by "opportunistic" or "secondary" pathogens that take advantage of a weakened immune defense system (e.g., in acquired immunodeficiency syndrome [AIDS]).

Primary Pathogens

HISTOPLASMOSIS

Histoplasmosis is the most common fungal infection in the United States. It is caused by the dimorphic fungus *Histoplasma capsulatum.* In the United States, the incidence of histoplasmosis is estimated to be approximately 500,000 cases per year, with several thousand cases requiring hospitalization. A small number of cases result in death. The prevalence of histoplasmosis is especially high along the major river valleys of the Midwest (e.g., Ohio, Michigan, Illinois, Mississippi, Missouri, Kentucky, Tennessee, Georgia, and Arkansas). In fact, on the basis of skin test surveys it is estimated that 80% to 90% of the population throughout these areas show signs of previous infection. Histoplasmosis is often called *Ohio Valley fever.*

H. capsulatum is commonly found in soils enriched with bird excreta, such as the soil near chicken houses, pigeon lofts, barns, and trees where starlings and blackbirds roost. The birds themselves, however, do not carry the organism, although the *H. capsulatum* spore may be carried by bats. Generally, an individual acquires the infection by inhaling the fungal spores that are released when the soil from an infected area is disturbed (e.g., children playing in dirt).

When the *H. capsulatum* organism reaches the alveoli, at body temperature it converts from its mycelial form (mold) to a parasitic yeast form. The clinical manifestations of histoplasmosis are strikingly similar to those of tuberculosis. The incubation period for the infection is approximately 17 days. Only about 40% of those infected demonstrate symptoms, and only about 10% of these patients are ill enough to consult a physician. Depending on the individual's immune system, the disease may take on one of the following forms: *asymptomatic primary histoplasmosis, acute symptomatic pulmonary histoplasmosis, chronic histoplasmosis,* and *disseminated histoplasmosis.*

Asymptomatic histoplasmosis is the most common form of histoplasmosis. Normally, it produces no signs or symptoms in otherwise healthy individuals who become infected. The only residual sign of infection may be a small, healed lesion of the lung parenchyma or calcified hilar lymph nodes. The patient has a positive histoplasmin skin test.

Acute symptomatic pulmonary histoplasmosis tends to occur in otherwise healthy individuals who have had an intense exposure to *H. capsulatum.* Depending on the number of spores inhaled, the individual signs and symptoms may range from a mild to serious illness. Mild signs and symptoms include fever, muscle and joint pain, headache, dry hacking cough, chills, chest pain, weight loss, and sweats. People who have inhaled a large number of spores may develop a severe acute pulmonary syndrome, a potentially life-threatening condition in which the individual becomes extremely short of breath. The acute pulmonary syndrome is often referred to as *spelunker's lung* because it frequently develops after excessive exposure to bat excrement stirred up by individuals exploring caves. During this phase of the disease, the patient's chest radiograph generally shows single or multiple infection sites, resembling those associated with pneumonia.

Chronic pulmonary histoplasmosis is characterized by infiltration and cavity formation in the upper lobes of one or both lungs. This type of histoplasmosis often affects people with an underlying lung disease such as emphysema. It is most commonly seen in middle-aged Caucasian men who smoke. Signs and symptoms include fatigue, fever, night sweats, weight loss, a productive cough, and hemoptysis—similar to signs and symptoms of tuberculosis. Often, the infection is self-limiting. In some patients, however, progressive destruction of lung tissue and dissemination of the infection may occur.

Disseminated histoplasmosis may follow either self-limited histoplasmosis or chronic histoplasmosis. It is most often seen in very young or very old patients with compromised immune systems (e.g., patients with AIDS). Even though the macrophages can remove the fungi from the bloodstream, they are unable to kill the fungal organisms. As a result, disseminated histoplasmosis can affect nearly any part of the body, including eyes, liver, bone marrow, skin, adrenal glands, and intestinal tract. Depending on which body organs are affected, the patient may develop anemia; pneumonia; pericarditis; meningitis; adrenal insufficiency; and ulcers of the mouth, tongue, or intestinal tract. If untreated, disseminated histoplasmosis is usually fatal.

Screening and Diagnosis

Fungal Culture

The fungal culture test is considered the gold standard for detecting histoplasmosis. A small amount of blood, sputum, or tissue from a lymph node, lung, or bone marrow is cultured. The disadvantage of this test is that it takes time for the fungus to grow— 4 weeks or longer. For this reason, it is not the test of choice for cases of disseminated histoplasmosis. Treatment delays in these patients may prove fatal.

Fungal Stain

In the fungal stain test, a tissue sample, which may be obtained from sputum, bone marrow, lungs, or a skin lesion, is stained with dye and examined under a microscope for *H. capsulatum*. A positive test result is 100% accurate. The disadvantage of this test is that obtaining a sputum sample can be difficult, and obtaining a sample from other sites requires invasive procedures.

Serology

A blood serology test checks blood serum for antigens and antibodies. When an individual is exposed to histoplasmosis spores (antigens), the body's immune system produces antibodies (proteins) to react to the histoplasmosis antigens. Tests that check for histoplasmosis antigen/antibody reactions are relatively fast and fairly accurate. False-negative results, however, may occur in people who have compromised immune systems or who are infected with other types of fungi.

COCCIDIOIDOMYCOSIS

Coccidioidomycosis is caused by inhaling the spores of *Coccidioides immitis,* which are spherical fungi carried by wind-borne dust particles. The disease is endemic in hot, dry regions. Approximately 100,000 new cases are estimated to occur annually. In the United States, coccidioidomycosis is especially prevalent in California, Arizona, Nevada, New Mexico, Texas, and Utah. About 80% of the people in the San Joaquin Valley are coccidioidin skin test positive. Because the prevalence of coccidioidomycosis is high in these regions, the disease is also known as *California disease, desert fever, San Joaquin Valley disease,* or *valley fever.* The fungus has been isolated in these regions from soils, plants, and a large number of vertebrates (e.g., mammals, birds, reptiles, amphibians).

When *C. immitis* spores are inhaled, they settle in the lungs, begin to germinate, and form round, thin-walled cells called *spherules.* The spherules, in turn, produce endospores that make more spherules (the spherule-endospore phase). The disease usually takes the form of an acute, primary, self-limiting pulmonary infection with or without systemic involvement. Some cases, however, progress to a disseminated disease.

Clinical manifestations are absent in about 60% of the people who have a positive skin test. In the remaining 40%, most of the patients demonstrate coldlike symptoms such as fever, chest pain, cough, headaches, and malaise. In uncomplicated cases, patients generally recover completely and enjoy lifelong immunity. In approximately 1 out of 200 cases, however, the primary infection does not resolve and progresses with varied clinical manifestations. *Chronic progressive pulmonary disease* is characterized by nodular growths called *fungomas* and cavity formation in the lungs. *Disseminated coccidioidomycosis* occurs in about one out of 6000 exposed persons. When this condition exists, the lymph nodes, meninges, spleen, liver, kidney, skin, and adrenals may be involved. The skin lesions (e.g., bumps on the face and chest) are commonly accompanied by arthralgia or arthritis, especially in the ankles and knees. This condition is commonly called *desert bumps, desert arthritis,* or *desert rheumatism.* Death is most commonly caused by meningitis.

Screening and Diagnosis

The diagnosis of coccidioidomycosis can be made by the direct visualization of distinctive spherules in microscopy of the patient's sputum, tissue exudates, biopsies, or spinal fluid. The diagnosis can be further supported by blood tests that detect antibodies to the fungus or a culture of the organism from infected fluid or tissue.

BLASTOMYCOSIS

Blastomycosis (also called *Chicago disease, Gilchrist's disease,* and *North American blastomycosis*) is caused by *Blastomyces dermatitidis.* Blastomycosis is most common in North America. In general, blastomycosis is seen from southern Canada to southern Louisiana and from Minnesota to the Carolinas and Georgia. Cases also have been reported in Central America, South America, Africa, and the Middle East. *B. dermatitidis* inhabits areas high in organic matter, such as forest soil, decaying wood, animal manure, and abandoned buildings. Blastomycosis is most common among pregnant women and middle-aged African-American males. The disease also is found in dogs, cats, and horses.

The primary portal of entry of *B. dermatitidis* is the lungs. The acute clinical manifestations resemble those of acute histoplasmosis, including fever, cough, hoarseness, aching of the joints and muscles, and, in some cases, pleuritic pain. Unlike histoplasmosis, however, the cough is frequently productive, and the sputum is purulent. Acute pulmonary infections may be self-limiting or progressive. When the condition is progressive, nodules and abscesses develop in the lungs. Extrapulmonary lesions commonly involve the skin, bones, reproductive tract, spleen, liver, kidney, or prostate gland. The skin lesions may, in fact, be the first signs of the disease. It often begins on the face, hands, wrists, or legs as subcutaneous nodules that erode to the skin surface. Dissemination of the yeast also may cause arthritis and osteomyelitis, and involvement of the central nervous system causes headache, convulsions, coma, and mental confusion. Standardized testing procedures for blastomycosis are not available. The diagnosis of blastomycosis can be made from direct visualization of the yeast in sputum smears. Culture of the fungus also can be performed. An accurate blastomycin skin test is not available.

OPPORTUNISTIC PATHOGENS

Opportunistic yeast pathogens such as *Candida albicans, Cryptococcus neoformans,* and *Aspergillus* also are associated with lung infections in certain patients.

C. albicans occurs as normal flora in the oral cavity, genitalia, and large intestine. *C. albicans* infection of the mouth is characterized by a white, adherent, patchy infection of the mouth, gums, cheeks, and throat. In patients with AIDS, *C. albicans* often causes infection of the mouth, pharynx, vagina, skin, and lungs.

C. neoformans proliferates in the high nitrogen content of pigeon droppings and is readily scattered into the air and dust. Today, *Cryptococcus* is most often seen among patients with AIDS and persons undergoing steroid therapy.

Aspergillus may be the most pervasive of all fungi—especially *Aspergillus fumigatus. Aspergillus* is found in soil, vegetation, leaf detritus, food, and compost heaps. Persons breathing the air of granaries, barns, and silos are at greatest risk. *Aspergillus* infection usually occurs in the lungs. It is almost always an opportunistic infection and poses a serious threat to patients with AIDS.

OVERVIEW

of the Cardiopulmonary Clinical Manifestations Associated with FUNGAL DISEASES OF THE LUNGS

The following clinical manifestations result from the pathophysiologic mechanisms caused (or activated) by **Alveolar Consolidation** (see Figure 9-8) and, in severe cases, with fibrosis, **Increased Alveolar-Capillary Membrane Thickness** (see Figure 9-9)—the major anatomic alterations of the lungs associated with fungal diseases of the lungs (see Figure 18-1).

CLINICAL DATA OBTAINED AT THE PATIENT'S BEDSIDE

The Physical Examination

Vital Signs

Increased respiratory rate (see page 31 ◆▶)
Several pathophysiologic mechanisms operating simultaneously may lead to an increased ventilatory rate:
- Stimulation of peripheral chemoreceptors (hypoxemia)
- Decreased lung compliance/increased ventilatory rate relationship
- Stimulation of J receptors
- Pain/anxiety/fever

Increased heart rate (pulse), cardiac output, and blood pressure (see pages 11 and 99 ◆▶)

Chest Pain/Decreased Chest Expansion (see page 42 ◆▶)

Cyanosis (see page 45 ◆▶)

Digital Clubbing (see page 46 ◆▶)

Peripheral Edema and Venous Distention (see page 47 ◆▶)
Because polycythemia and cor pulmonale are associated with severe fungal disease, the following may be seen:
- Distended neck veins
- Pitting edema
- Enlarged and tender liver

Cough, Sputum Production, and Hemoptysis (see page 47 ◆▶)

Chest Assessment Findings (see page 22)
- Increased tactile and vocal fremitus
- Dull percussion note
- Bronchial breath sounds
- Crackles, rhonchi, and wheezing
- Pleural friction rub (if process extends to pleural surface)
- Whispered pectoriloquy

CLINICAL DATA OBTAINED FROM LABORATORY TESTS AND SPECIAL PROCEDURES

Pulmonary Function Study Findings

Expiratory Maneuver Findings (see page 61 ◆▶)

FVC	FEV_T	$FEF_{25\%-75\%}$	$FEF_{200-1200}$
↓	N or ↓	N or ↓	N
PEFR	MVV	$FEF_{50\%}$	$FEV_{1\%}$
N	N or ↓	N	N or ↑

Lung Volume and Capacity Findings (see page 62 ◆▶)

V_T	RV	FRC	TLC
N or ↓	↓	↓	↓
VC	IC	ERV	RV/TLC%
↓	↓	↓	N

Arterial Blood Gases

Mild to Moderate Fungal Disease
Acute Alveolar Hyperventilation with Hypoxemia (see page 70 ◆▶)

pH	Pa_{CO_2}	HCO_3^-	Pa_{O_2}
↑	↓	↓ (Slightly)	↓

Severe Fungal Disease with Pulmonary Fibrosis
Chronic Ventilatory Failure with Hypoxemia (see page 73 ◆▶)

pH	Pa_{CO_2}	HCO_3^-	Pa_{O_2}
Normal	↑	↑(Significantly)	↓

Acute Ventilatory Changes Superimposed on Chronic Ventilatory Failure (see page 75 ◆▶)
Because acute ventilatory changes are frequently seen in patients with chronic ventilatory failure, the respiratory care practitioner must be familiar with and alert for (1) acute alveolar hyperventilation superimposed on chronic ventilatory failure and (2) acute ventilatory failure superimposed on chronic ventilatory failure.

OVERVIEW

of the Cardiopulmonary Clinical Manifestations Associated with
FUNGAL DISEASES OF THE LUNGS (Continued)

Oxygenation Indices (see page 82)

$\dot{Q}_S/\dot{Q}_T$	DO_2*	$\dot{V}O_2$	$C(a-\bar{v})O_2$
↑	↓	Normal	Normal

O_2ER*	$S\bar{v}O_2$		
↑	↓		

*The DO_2 may be normal in patients who have compensated to the decreased oxygenation status with (1) an increased cardiac output, (2) an increased hemoglobin level, or (3) a combination of both. When the DO_2 is normal, the O_2ER is usually normal.

Hemodynamic Indices (Severe Fungal Disease) (see page 99)

CVP	RAP	$\overline{PA}$	PCWP
↑	↑	↑	Normal
CO	SV	SVI	CI
Normal	Normal	Normal	Normal
RVSWI	LVSWI	PVR	SVR
↑	Normal	↑	Normal

ABNORMAL LABORATORY TESTS AND PROCEDURES (SEE ETIOLOGY AND PRIMARY PATHOGEN SECTIONS IN THIS CHAPTER, PAGE 261)

RADIOLOGIC FINDINGS

Chest Radiograph

- Increased opacity
- Cavity formation
- Pleural effusion
- Calcification and fibrosis
- Right ventricular enlargement

During the early stages of many pulmonary fungal infections, localized infiltration and consolidation with or without lymph node involvement are commonly seen (Figure 18-2). Single or numerous spherical nodules may be seen (Figure 18-3). During the advanced stages, bilateral cavities in the apical and posterior segments of the upper lobes are often seen (Figure 18-4). In disseminated disease a diffuse bilateral micronodular pattern and pleural effusion may be seen. Fibrosis and calcification of healed lesions can be identified. Finally, because right-sided heart failure may develop as a secondary problem during the advanced stages of fungal disease, an enlarged heart may be seen on the chest radiograph.

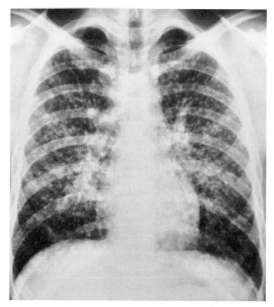

Figure 18–2 Acute inhalational histoplasmosis in an otherwise healthy patient. This young man developed fever and cough after tearing down an old barn. The study shows bilateral hilar adenopathy. (From Armstrong P et al: *Imaging of diseases of the chest,* ed 2, St. Louis, 1995, Mosby.)

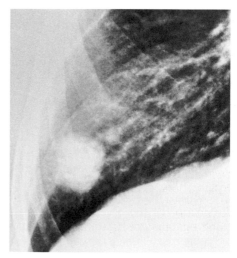

Figure 18–3 Histoplasmoma, showing a well-defined spherical nodule. The central portion of the nodule shows calcification. (From Armstrong P et al: *Imaging of diseases of the chest,* ed 2, St. Louis, 1995, Mosby.)

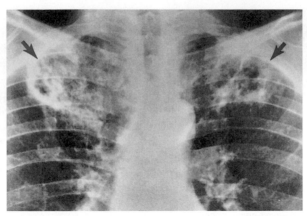

Figure 18–4   Chronic cavitary histoplasmosis. Note the striking upper zone predominance of the shadows. Numerous large cavities *(arrows)* are present, resembling tuberculosis. (From Armstrong P et al: *Imaging of diseases of the chest,* ed 2, St. Louis, 1995, Mosby.)

General Management of Fungal Disease

Drugs commonly used to treat fungal diseases of the lungs include amphotericin B (Fungizone) and itraconazole (Sporanox). In general, the IV administration of amphotericin B is the drug of choice for individuals with disseminated histoplasmosis or severe disease. Itraconazole alone may be effective in mild cases of disseminated histoplasmosis as well as in chronic pulmonary dieases. Although itraconazole does not work as quickly as amphotericin B, it has fewer side effects and can be taken in oral form. Fluconazole (Diflucan) also may be used in patients who are unable to tolerate itraconazole. However, fluconazole is not as effective as itraconazole, and the patient is more likely to experience a relapse with this medication.

RESPIRATORY CARE TREATMENT PROTOCOLS

Oxygen Therapy Protocol

Oxygen therapy is used to treat hypoxemia, decrease the work of breathing, and decrease myocardial work. Because of the hypoxemia associated with the fungal pulmonary condition, supplemental oxygen may be required. Because of the alveolar consolidation produced by a fungal disorder, capillary shunting may be present. Hypoxemia caused by capillary shunting is often refractory to oxygen therapy. In addition, when the patient demonstrates chronic ventilatory failure during the advanced stages of fungal disease, caution must be taken not to overoxygenate the patient (see Oxygen Therapy Protocol, Protocol 9-1).

Bronchopulmonary Hygiene Therapy Protocol

Because of the excessive mucus production and accumulation sometimes associated with fungal disease, a number of bronchial hygiene treatment modalities may be used to enhance the mobilization of bronchial secretions (see Bronchial Hygiene Therapy Protocol, Protocol 9-2).

Hyperinflation Therapy Protocol

Because of the atelectasis occasionally associated with fungal disease, hyperinflation therapy may be used to prevent or treat alveolar atelectasis and consolidation (see Hyperinflation Therapy Protocol, Protocol 9-3).

Mechanical Ventilation Protocol

Mechanical ventilation may be necessary to provide and support alveolar gas exchange and eventually return the patient to spontaneous breathing. Because acute ventilatory failure superimposed on chronic ventilatory failure is seen occasionally in patients with severe fungal disease, continuous mechanical ventilation may be required. Continuous mechanical ventilation is justified when the acute ventilatory failure is thought to be reversible (see Mechanical Ventilation Protocol, Protocol 9-5).

Case Study: FUNGAL DISEASES OF THE LUNGS

Admitting History

A 56-year-old cattle driver was admitted to the arthritis clinic of a small hospital just outside Phoenix because of joint pain. The man stated that the tenderness in his joints prevented him from riding his horse for any extended period. He was born on a cattle ranch in New Mexico and spent most of his adult life working as a cattle driver in Arizona, New Mexico, and Colorado. He had always considered himself an "outdoors" kind of man. He loved the range, wide open spaces, clear air, and beauty of the desert.

In his early 20s he traveled to the East Coast to attend college. While there, he became withdrawn and depressed and felt confined. After 1 year he dropped out of college and returned to New Mexico. Shortly after returning home, his symptoms of depression disappeared. He worked on a large cattle ranch, made several new friends, and was content with the fact that he "belonged on the open range." He never married or settled down in one place he could call home. He often said that the great outdoors was his home. He never owned an automobile. In fact, he often said that the only things of real value he owned were a roan quarter horse and a saddle.

The hospital had no past medical record on the patient. The man reported, however, that although he was rarely ill, he had gone to see a doctor while in Colorado about a year ago for severe "cold" symptoms, which included fever, cough, chest pain, headaches, and a general feeling of fatigue. He was a nonsmoker, although he did chew tobacco for a short time in his teens. The patient verified that he consumed alcohol regularly on Friday and Saturday nights. The man estimated that on average he consumed between 6 and 10 beers per outing and sometimes more.

Despite the patient's somewhat rugged living conditions and alcohol consumption, he was not overweight and was in reasonably good physical condition.

Physical Examination

The patient appeared to be a well-developed, well-nourished white man in moderate respiratory distress. He complained of soreness and stiffness in all his joints. He also stated that he thought he had a "bad cold" and that he was short of breath.

The patient's knees and ankle joints were warm, swollen, and tender to the touch. Although his skin appeared weathered and tan, his lips and nail beds were cyanotic. He demonstrated a frequent cough productive of a moderate amount of thick, yellow sputum. Although the cough was strong, he experienced difficulty raising sputum during each coughing episode. His vital signs were as follows: blood pressure 160/90, heart rate 90 bpm, respiratory rate 18/min, and oral temperature 37.8° C (100° F). Palpation revealed a few erythematous lesions on his anterior chest, of which he was unaware. In addition, a walnut-size erythematous lesion was present on the patient's left cheek. Percussion of the chest was not remarkable. Auscultation revealed bilateral crackles and rhonchi in the lung apices.

The patient's chest X-ray showed scattered infiltrates consistent with fibrosis and calcification and multiple spherical nodules throughout both lungs. In the upper lobes of both lungs, two to three small, 1- to 3-cm cavities were visible (Figure 18-5). On room air the patient's arterial blood gas values (ABGs) were as follows: pH 7.51, $Paco_2$ 29 mm Hg, HCO_3^- 22 mmol/L, and Pao_2 64 mm Hg. Concerned about the patient's respiratory status, the physician requested

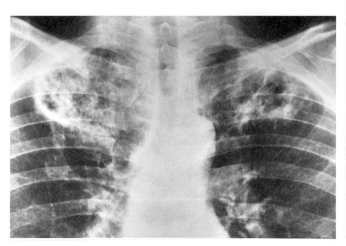

Figure 18–5　Chest X-ray of a 56-year-old man with a fungal disease of the lungs.

a respiratory care consult. On the basis of these clinical data, the following SOAP was documented:

Respiratory Assessment and Plan

S "I feel short of breath, and my joints are swollen and painful."

O Cyanosis; cough: frequent and strong, producing moderate amounts of thick, yellow sputum; vital signs: BP 160/90, HR 90, RR 18, T 37.8° C (100° F); palpation: red lesions on anterior chest and left cheek; auscultation: bilateral crackles and rhonchi in lung apices; CXR: bilateral fibrosis and calcification and spherical nodules; two to three 1- to 3-cm cavities in both upper lobes; ABGs (room air): pH 7.51, $Paco_2$ 29, HCO_3^- 22, Pao_2 64

A • Moderate respiratory distress (cyanosis, vital signs)
   • Large amounts of thick, yellow secretions (sputum, rhonchi)
   • Infection likely (yellow sputum)
   • Pulmonary fibrosis, calcification, and cavities (CXR)
   • Acute alveolar hyperventilation with mild hypoxemia (ABGs)

P Initiate Oxygen Therapy Protocol (2 lpm per nasal cannula) and Bronchopulmonary Hygiene Therapy Protocol (C&DB instruction, PD to both upper lobes q shift × 3 days). Order sputum culture (routine, AFB, and fungal). Encourage fluid intake. Monitor (oximeter, I&O).

• • • • •

5 Days After Admission

After microscopy of the patient's sputum and a spherulin skin test, the diagnosis of coccidioidomycosis was written in the patient's chart. The patient had been receiving amphotericin B intravenously for 2 days. A complete pulmonary function study revealed a moderate-to-severe restrictive disorder, with a moderate obstructive component as well.

When the respiratory practitioner entered the patient's room, the man was sitting up in bed, appearing cyanotic, short of breath, and fatigued. He stated that he was becoming tired of people in white outfits coming in and out of his room, day and night, with "needles, pills, and bills." He further stated that he still could not get a good breath of air. In fact, he said it was more difficult for him to breathe today than it had been on the day he entered the hospital.

The patient still had a frequent, strong cough productive of moderate amounts of thick, opaque sputum. His vital signs were as follows: blood pressure 165/95,

heart rate 96 bpm, respiratory rate 24/min, and temperature 37° C (98.6° F). Auscultation revealed persistent bilateral tight wheezes, and bilateral crackles and rhonchi in the apices of both lungs. A current chest X-ray was not available. His hemoglobin oxygen saturation measured by pulse oximetry (Spo_2) was 88%. His ABGs were as follows: pH 7.54, $Paco_2$ 27 mm Hg, HCO_3^- 21 mmol/L, and Pao_2 55 mm Hg. At this time, the following SOAP was charted:

Respiratory Assessment and Plan

S "I still can't get a good breath of air."

O Respiratory distress: cyanotic, short of breath; positive spherulin skin test; coccidioidomycosis organisms seen in sputum smear; frequent strong cough: moderate amount of thick, opaque sputum; vital signs: BP 165/95, HR 96, RR 24, T normal; bilateral crackles and rhonchi in the lung apices; Spo_2 88%; ABGs: pH 7.54, $Paco_2$ 27, HCO_3^- 21, Pao_2 55.

A • Coccidioidomycosis (positive spherulin skin test, sputum smear)
   • Continued respiratory distress (cyanosis, vital signs)
   • Excessive amounts of thick bronchial secretions (sputum, rhonchi)
   • Acute alveolar hyperventilation with moderate hypoxemia (worsening ABGs)

P Increase Oxygen Therapy Protocol (3 lpm nasal cannula). Add Aerosolized Medication Protocol; up-regulate Bronchopulmonary Hygiene Therapy Protocol (2 cc 10% acetylcysteine with 0.2 cc albuterol q 6 h followed by C&DB and PD to both upper lobes). Add supervised use of flutter valve 2 times per shift. Request repeat CXR. Continue to monitor and reevaluate.

• • • • •

10 Days After Admission

On this day, the respiratory therapist found the patient walking up and down the corridor talking to various staff members and patients. The man appeared to be in no respiratory distress. He stated that he was breathing much better and was ready to ride his horse a long distance in any direction away from the hospital.

No spontaneous cough was noted. When asked to generate a cough, the patient produced a strong, nonproductive cough. His vital signs were as follows: blood pressure 135/88, heart rate 80 bpm, respiratory rate 14/min, and normal temperature. Auscultation revealed persistent bilateral crackles in the apices of both lungs. A recent chest X-ray was not available. His pulse oximetry on room air showed an Spo_2 of 91%. His ABGs were as follows: pH 7.44, Paco$_2$ 34 mm Hg, HCO$_3^-$ 23 mmol/L, and Pao$_2$ 71 mm Hg. On the basis of these clinical data, the following SOAP note was written:

Respiratory Assessment and Plan

S "I'm breathing much better."

O No obvious respiratory distress; no spontaneous cough; strong, nonproductive cough on request; vital signs: BP 135/88, HR 80, RR 14, T normal; bilateral crackles in the lung apices; Spo$_2$ 91%; ABGs: pH 7.44, Paco$_2$ 34, HCO$_3^-$ 23, Pao$_2$ 71

A • Adequate bronchial hygiene status (nonproductive cough, absence of rhonchi, crackles expected in lung fibrosis)
  • Normal acid-base status with mild hypoxemia (ABGs)

P Discontinue Oxygen Therapy Protocol. Recheck Spo$_2$ on room air ("spot check") in 1 hour. Discontinue Bronchopulmonary Hygiene Therapy Protocol. Instruct patient in trial use of Combivent (albuterol/ipratropium) MDI. Reevaluate the patient when he is off all therapy modalities but on self-administered MDI in AM; then sign off.

Discussion

Respiratory care practitioners (RCPs) who work in the Southwest, where coccidioidomycosis is endemic, would probably anticipate this diagnosis in the patient with bilateral pulmonary infiltrates, swollen tender joints, and the skin rash typical of this lesion. Others could not be blamed if they missed this fact until the coccidioidal skin test came back positive and the sputum fungal smear demonstrated the presence of the coccidioidomycosis organism. In this case, the patient demonstrated the clinical manifestations associated with the following two anatomic alterations of the lungs: **Increased Alveolar-Capillary Membrane Thickness** (e.g., bilateral fibrosis and calcification; see Figure 9-9) and **Excessive Bronchial Secretions** (e.g., cough, sputum, and rhonchi; see Figure 9-11).

The **first assessment**—that the patient is hypoxemic despite alveolar hyperventilation and that he has alveolar fibrosis and cavity formation—is correct. For the hypoxemia, oxygen therapy is appropriate and should be started with a nasal oxygen cannula at 1 to 2 L/min and then regulated with a pulse oximeter. In treating this case, as with any other pneumonia, the assessing RCP should quickly obtain a sputum, Gram stain, and acid-fast bacillus and fungal preparations; this step was appropriately done in this case. The treating RCP would do well to understand the use of tuberculin and fungal testing in such patients and to understand, as with other pneumonic infiltrates, that the therapist's impact once that is done would probably be minimal.

In the **second assessment**, the offending organism has been isolated and appropriate therapy with intravenous amphotericin-B started. The patient is still hypoxemic, and up-regulation of his oxygen therapy (perhaps to 3 or 4 L/min, or with a nonrebreathing mask if the former is unsuccessful) is indicated. Because the patient is still coughing up thick, opaque sputum and because his dyspnea is not relieved so far, up-regulation of the bronchopulmonary hygiene therapy program with a trial of bronchodilator therapy and mucolytic therapy is in order. Because the patient is not improving, a repeat chest X-ray appears to be indicated.

At the **last assessment** 10 days after the patient's admission to the hospital, clear improvement is noted. Oximetry reveals good peripheral oxygen saturation, and the blood gases are much improved. Now is the time for the treating therapist to reduce the intensity of the patient's respiratory care, and this step is illustrated in the appropriate response for this section of the case study. Follow-up pulmonary function testing 6 to 12 months after the abatement of acute illness would be worthwhile.

SELF-ASSESSMENT QUESTIONS

Multiple Choice

1. Which of the following is the most common fungal infection in the United States?

   a. Coccidioidomycosis
   b. Histoplasmosis
   c. San Joaquin Valley disease
   d. Blastomycosis
   e. Desert fever

2. Incidence of histoplasmosis is especially high in which of the following area(s)?

   I. Arizona
   II. Mississippi
   III. Nevada
   IV. Texas

   a. II only
   b. IV only
   c. II and IV only
   d. II and III only
   e. I, III, and IV only

3. The condition called *desert bumps, desert arthritis,* or *desert rheumatism* is associated with which fungal disorder?

   a. Ohio Valley fever
   b. Blastomycosis
   c. Coccidioidomycosis
   d. *Aspergillosis*
   e. *Candida albicans* pneumonitis

4. Which of the following is/are used to treat fungal diseases?

   I. Streptomycin
   II. Amphotericin B
   III. Penicillin G
   IV. Itraconazole

   a. I only
   b. II only
   c. IV only
   d. II and IV only
   e. I, II, and III only

5. Which of the following forms of histoplasmosis is characterized by healed lesions in the hilar lymph nodes as well as a positive histoplasmin skin test response?

   a. Disseminated infection
   b. Latent asymptomatic disease
   c. Chronic histoplasmosis
   d. Self-limiting primary disease
   e. None of the above

True or False

True ☐ False ☐ **1.** *Histoplasma capsulatum* is commonly found in soils near chicken houses and pigeon lofts.

True ☐ False ☐ **2.** It is estimated that about 50,000 new cases of coccidioidomycosis occur annually.

True ☐ False ☐ **3.** Blastomycosis also is known as *valley* or *desert fever.*

True ☐ False ☐ **4.** The diagnosis of coccidioidomycosis can be made by blood tests that detect antibodies of the fungus, or a culture of the organism from infected fluid or tissue.

True ☐ False ☐ **5.** Blastomycosis is most common in young men living in North America.

Answers appear in Appendix XI.

PART IV

Pulmonary Vascular Diseases

CHAPTER 19

Pulmonary Edema

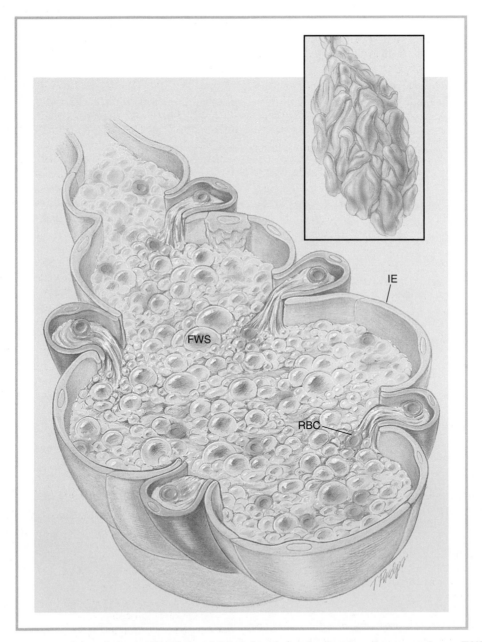

Figure 19–1 Pulmonary edema. Cross-sectional view of alveoli and alveolar duct in pulmonary edema. *FWS,* Frothy white secretions; *IE,* interstitial edema; *RBC,* red blood cell. *Inset,* Atelectasis, a common secondary anatomic alteration of the lungs. See also Plate 11.

Anatomic Alterations of the Lungs

Pulmonary edema results from excessive movement of fluid from the pulmonary vascular system to the extravascular system and air spaces of the lungs. Fluid first seeps into the perivascular and peribronchial interstitial spaces; depending on the degree of severity, fluid may progressively move into the alveoli, bronchioles, and bronchi (Figure 19-1).

As a consequence of this fluid movement, the alveolar walls and interstitial spaces swell. As the swelling intensifies, the alveolar surface tension increases and causes alveolar shrinkage and atelectasis. Moreover, much of the fluid that accumulates in the tracheobronchial tree is churned into a frothy white (sometimes blood-tinged or pink) sputum as a result of air moving in and out of the lungs. The abundance of fluid in the interstitial spaces causes the lymphatic vessels to widen and the lymph flow to increase.

Pulmonary edema is a restrictive pulmonary disorder. The major pathologic or structural changes of the lungs associated with pulmonary edema are as follows:

- Interstitial edema, including fluid engorgement of the perivascular and peribronchial spaces and the alveolar wall interstitium
- Alveolar flooding
- Increased surface tension of pulmonary surfactant
- Alveolar shrinkage and atelectasis
- Frothy white (or pink) secretions throughout the tracheobronchial tree

Etiology

The etiology of pulmonary edema can be divided into two major categories: cardiogenic and noncardiogenic.

CARDIOGENIC PULMONARY EDEMA

Cardiac pulmonary edema (also known as *congestive heart failure*) occurs when the left ventricle is not able to pump out all of the blood that it receives from the lungs. As a result, the blood pressure inside the pulmonary veins and capillaries increases. This action literally causes fluid to be pushed through the capillary walls and into the alveoli. The basic pathophysiologic mechanism for this action is described in the following sections.

Ordinarily, *hydrostatic pressure* of about 10 to 15 mm Hg tends to move fluid *out* of the pulmonary capillaries into the interstitial space. This force is normally offset by colloid osmotic forces of about 25 to 30 mm Hg that tend to keep fluid *in* the

pulmonary capillaries. The colloid osmotic pressure is referred to as *oncotic pressure* and is produced by the albumin and globulin particles in the blood. The stability of fluid within the pulmonary capillaries is determined by the balance between hydrostatic and oncotic pressure. This relationship also maintains fluid stability in the interstitial compartments of the lung.

Movement of fluid in and out of the capillaries is expressed by Starling's equation:

$$J = K (Pc - Pi) - (\pi c - \pi i)$$

where *J* is the net fluid movement out of the capillary, *K* is the capillary permeability factor, *Pc* and *Pi* are the hydrostatic pressures in the capillary and interstitial space, and πc and πi are the oncotic pressures in the capillary and interstitial space.

Though conceptually valuable, this equation has limited practical use. Of the four pressures, only the oncotic and hydrostatic pressures of blood in the pulmonary capillaries can be measured with any certainty. The oncotic and hydrostatic pressures within the interstitial compartments cannot be readily determined.

When the hydrostatic pressure within the pulmonary vascular system rises to more than 25 to 30 mm Hg, the oncotic pressure loses its holding force over the fluid within the pulmonary capillaries. Consequently, fluid starts to spill into the interstitial and air spaces of the lungs (see Figure 19-1).

Increased pulmonary capillary hydrostatic pressure is the most common cause of pulmonary edema. Box 19-1 provides common causes of cardiogenic pulmonary edema. Box 19-2 provides common risk factors for coronary heart disease (CHD).

BOX 19–1

Common Causes of Cardiogenic Pulmonary Edema

- Arrhythmias (e.g., premature ventricular contractions, bradycardia) producing low cardiac output
- Congenital heart defects
- Excessive fluid administration
- Left ventricular failure
- Mitral or aortic valve disease
- Myocardial infarction
- Pulmonary embolus
- Renal failure
- Rheumatic heart disease (myocarditis)
- Systemic hypertension

BOX 19–2

Risk Factors for Coronary Heart Disease (CHD)

- Age
  - Male ≥ 45 years old
  - Female ≥ 55 years old
- Family history of CHD
  - Male relative: < 55 years old
  - Female relative: < 65 years old
- Cigarette smoker
- Overweight
- Hypertension: (blood pressure > 140/90 mm Hg or on antihypertensive agents)
- High level of low-density lipoprotein cholesterol (LDL-C): > 130 mg/dl ("bad cholesterol")
- Low level of high-density lipoprotein cholesterol (HDL-C): < 35 mg/dl ("good cholesterol")
- High level of homocysteine: > 10 mg/dl
- High total cholesterol level (>150-200 mg/dl) and high triglyceride level (>200-300 mg/dl)
- Diabetes mellitus (Type 1 and Type 2)

NONCARDIOGENIC PULMONARY EDEMA

There are numerous noncardiogenic causes of pulmonary edema. In these conditions, fluid can readily flow from the pulmonary capillaries into the alveoli—even in the absence of the back pressure caused by an abnormal heart. The more common conditions include the following:

Increased Capillary Permeability

Pulmonary edema may develop as a result of increased capillary permeability stemming from infectious, inflammatory, and other processes. The following are some causes of increased capillary permeability:

- Alveolar hypoxia
- Acute respiratory distress syndrome (ARDS)
- Inhalation of toxic agents such as chlorine, sulfur dioxide, nitrogen dioxides, ammonia, and phosgene
- Pulmonary infections (e.g., pneumonia)
- Therapeutic radiation of the lungs
- Head injury (also known as cephalogenic pulmonary edema)

Lymphatic Insufficiency

Should the lungs' normal lymphatic drainage be decreased, intravascular and extravascular fluid begins to pool, and pulmonary edema ensues. Lymphatic drainage may be slowed because of obliteration or distortion of lymphatic vessels. The lymphatic vessels may be obstructed by tumor cells in lymphangitic carcinomatosis. Because the lymphatic vessels empty into systemic veins, increased systemic venous pressure may slow lymphatic drainage. Lymphatic insufficiency also has been observed after lung transplantation.

Decreased Intrapleural Pressure

Reduced intrapleural pressure may cause pulmonary edema. During severe airway obstruction, for example, the negative pressure exerted by the patient during inspiration may create a suction effect on the pulmonary capillaries and cause fluid to move into the alveoli. Furthermore, the increased negative intrapleural pressure promotes filling of the right side of the heart and hinders blood flow in the left side of the heart. This condition may cause pooling of the blood in the lungs and, subsequently, an elevated hydrostatic pressure and pulmonary edema. Another related kind of pulmonary edema is caused by the sudden removal of a pleural effusion. Clinically, this condition is called *decompression pulmonary edema.*

Decreased Oncotic Pressure

Although this condition is rare, if the oncotic pressure is reduced from its normal 25 to 30 mm Hg and falls below the patient's normal hydrostatic pressure of 10 to 15 mm Hg, fluid may begin to seep into the interstitial and air spaces of the lungs. Decreased oncotic pressure may be caused by the following:

- Overtransfusion and/or rapid transfusion of intravenous fluids
- Uremia
- Hypoproteinemia (e.g., severe malnutrition)
- Acute nephritis
- Polyarteritis nodosa

Although the exact mechanisms are not known, Box 19-3 provides other causes of conditions associated with noncardiogenic pulmonary edema.

BOX 19–3

Other Causes of Noncardiogenic Pulmonary Edema

- Allergic reaction to drugs
- Excessive sodium consumption
- Drug overdose (e.g., heroin, aspirin, amphetamines, cocaine, antituberculosis agents, cancer chemotherapy agents)
- Metal poisoning (e.g., cobalt, iron, lead)
- Chronic alcohol ingestion
- Aspiration (e.g., near drowning)
- Central nervous system (CNS) stimulation
- Encephalitis
- Cardiac tamponade
- High altitudes (greater than 8000 or 10,000 feet)

OVERVIEW
of the Cardiopulmonary Clinical Manifestations Associated with PULMONARY EDEMA

The following clinical manifestations result from the pathologic mechanisms caused (or activated) by **Atelectasis** (see Figure 9-7), **Increased Alveolar-Capillary Membrane Thickness** (see Figure 9-9), and, in severe cases, **Excessive Bronchial Secretions** (see Figure 9-11)—the major anatomic alterations of the lungs associated with pulmonary edema (see Figure 19-1).

CLINICAL DATA OBTAINED AT THE PATIENT'S BEDSIDE

The Physical Examination
Vital Signs
Increased respiratory rate (see page 31 ◆▶)
Several pathophysiologic mechanisms operating simultaneously may lead to an increased ventilatory rate:

- Stimulation of peripheral chemoreceptors (hypoxemia)
- Decreased lung compliance/increased ventilatory rate relationship
- Stimulation of J receptors
- Anxiety

Increased heart rate (pulse), cardiac output, and blood pressure (see pages 11 and 99 ◆▶)

Cheyne-Stokes Respiration (see page 18 ◆▶)
Cheyne-Stokes respiration may be seen in patients with severe left-sided heart failure and pulmonary edema. Some authorities have suggested that the cause of Cheyne-Stokes respiration in these patients may be related to the prolonged circulation time between the lungs and the central chemoreceptors.

Paroxysmal Nocturnal Dyspnea (PND) and Orthopnea
Patients with pulmonary edema often awaken with severe dyspnea after several hours of sleep. This condition is called *paroxysmal nocturnal dyspnea.* This condition is particularly prevalent in patients with cardiogenic pulmonary edema. While the patient is awake, more time is spent in the erect position and, as a result, excess fluids tend to accumulate in the dependent portions of the body. When the patient lies down, however, the excess fluids from the dependent parts of the body move into the bloodstream and cause an increase in venous return to the lungs. This action raises the pulmonary hydrostatic pressure and promotes pulmonary edema. The pulmonary edema in turn promotes pulmonary shunting, venous admixture, and hypoxemia. When the hypoxemia becomes severe, the peripheral chemoreceptors are stimulated and initiate an increased ventilatory rate (see Fig. 4-1). The decreased lung compliance, J receptor stimulation, and anxiety also may contribute to the paroxysmal nocturnal dyspnea commonly seen

in this disorder at night. A patient is said to have orthopnea when dyspnea increases while the patient is in a recumbent position.

Cyanosis (see page 42 ◆▶)

Cough and Sputum (Frothy and Pink in Appearance) (see page 47 ◆▶)

Chest Assessment Findings (see page 22 ◆▶)
- Increased tactile and vocal fremitus
- Crackles, rhonchi, and wheezing

CLINICAL DATA OBTAINED FROM LABORATORY TESTS AND SPECIAL PROCEDURES

Pulmonary Function Study Findings
Expiratory Maneuver Findings (see page 61 ◆▶)

FVC	FEV_T	$FEF_{25\%-75\%}$	$FEF_{200-1200}$
↓	N or ↓	N or ↓	N
PEFR	MVV	$FEF_{50\%}$	$FEV_{1\%}$
N	N or ↓	N	N or ↑

Lung Volume and Capacity Findings (see page 62 ◆▶)

V_T	RV	FRC	TLC
N or ↓	↓	↓	↓
VC	IC	ERV	RV/TLC%
↓	↓	↓	N

Decreased Diffusion Capacity (D_{LCO}) (see page 67 ◆▶)

Arterial Blood Gases

Mild to Moderate Pulmonary Edema
Acute Alveolar Hyperventilation with Hypoxemia (see page 70 ◆▶)

pH	$Paco_2$	HCO_3^-	Pao_2
↑	↓	↓ (Slightly)	↓

Severe Pulmonary Edema
Acute Ventilatory Failure with Hypoxemia (see page 73 ◆▶)

pH	$Paco_2$	HCO_3^- *	Pao_2
↓	↑	↑(Slightly)	↓

*When tissue hypoxia is severe enough to produce lactic acid, the pH and HCO_3 values will be lower than expected for a particular $Paco_2$ level.

OVERVIEW

of the Cardiopulmonary Clinical Manifestations Associated with PULMONARY EDEMA (Continued)

Oxygenation Indices (see page 82 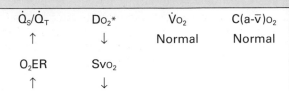)

$\dot{Q}_S/\dot{Q}_T$	Do_2*	$\dot{V}o_2$	$C(a-\bar{v})o_2$
↑	↓	Normal	Normal

O_2ER	Svo_2
↑	↓

*The Do_2 may be normal in patients who have compensated to the decreased oxygenation status with an increased cardiac output. When the Do_2 is normal, the O_2ER is usually normal.

Hemodynamic Indices (Cardiogenic Pulmonary Edema) (see page 99 ◆)

CVP	RAP	$\overline{PA}$	PCWP
↑	↑	↑	↑
CO	SV	SVI	CI
↓	↓	↓	↓
RVSWI	LVSWI	PVR	SVR
↑	↓	↑	↑

ABNORMAL LABORATORY TESTS AND PROCEDURES

- Serum potassium: low
- Serum sodium: low

Hypokalemia and hyponatremia are often seen in patients with left-sided heart failure and may result from diuretic therapy or excessive fluid retention.

RADIOLOGIC FINDINGS

Chest Radiograph

- Fluffy opacities
- Left ventricular hypertrophy
- Kerley A and B lines
- Pleural effusion

Cardiogenic Pulmonary Edema

Because X-ray densities primarily reflect alveolar filling and not early interstitial edema, by the time abnormal findings are encountered, the pathologic changes associated with pulmonary edema are advanced. Chest X-rays typically reveal dense, fluffy opacities that spread outward from the hilar areas to the peripheral borders of the lungs (Figure 19-2).

The peripheral portion of the lungs often remains clear, and this produces what is described as a "butterfly" or "batwing" distribution. Left ventricular hypertrophy and enlarged pulmonary vessels are commonly seen. Pleural effusions may be seen. Kerley A and B lines may appear earlier in the radiograph. Kerley A lines are 1- to 2-cm lines of interstitial edema extending from the hilum. Kerley B lines are short, thin, horizontal lines of interstitial edema that extend inward from the pleural surface of the lower regions of the lungs. Kerley B lines originate from the septa that separate the lung lobules. When thickened by pulmonary edema, these septa form the so-called septal lines or Kerley B lines.

Noncardiogenic Pulmonary Edema

In noncardiogenic pulmonary edema the chest radiograph commonly shows areas of fluffy densities that are usually more dense near the hilum. The density may be unilateral or bilateral. Pleural effusion is usually not present, and (most important) the cardiac silhouette is not enlarged.

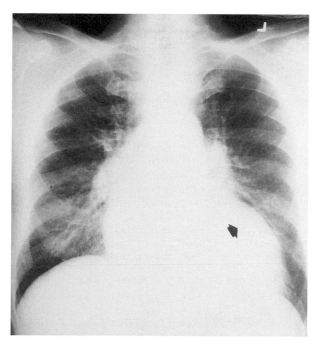

Figure 19–2 Cardiomegaly (*arrow*) and pulmonary edema in congestive heart failure.

General Management of Pulmonary Edema

The treatment of pulmonary edema is based on the underlying etiology. Common therapeutic interventions include those described in the following paragraphs.

RESPIRATORY CARE TREATMENT PROTOCOLS

Oxygen Therapy Protocol

Oxygen therapy is used to treat hypoxemia, decrease the work of breathing, and decrease myocardial work. The hypoxemia that develops in pulmonary edema is most commonly caused by the interstitial and alveolar fluid, atelectasis, and capillary shunting associated with the disorder. Hypoxemia caused by capillary shunting is at least partially refractory to oxygen therapy (see Oxygen Therapy Protocol, Protocol 9-1).

Bronchopulmonary Hygiene Therapy Protocol

Because of the excessive frothy white secretions associated with pulmonary edema, bronchial hygiene treatment modalities may be used to enhance the mobilization of bronchial secretions (see Bronchopulmonary Hygiene Therapy Protocol, Protocol 9-2).

Hyperinflation Therapy Protocol

Hyperinflation therapy is commonly prescribed to offset the fluid accumulation and alveolar shrinkage associated with pulmonary edema. For example, high-flow mask continuous positive airway pressure (CPAP) has been shown to produce a significant and rapid improvement in oxygenation and ventilatory status in patients with pulmonary edema. **Mask CPAP** improves decreased lung compliance, decreases the work of breathing, enhances gas exchange, and decreases vascular congestion in patients with pulmonary edema. In fact, mask CPAP is prescribed (at least for a trial period) for patients with pulmonary edema who have arterial blood gas values that reveal impending or acute ventilatory failure—the hallmark clinical manifestation for mechanical ventilation. Often, mask CPAP dramatically improves oxygenation and ventilatory status in these patients and eliminates the need for mechanical ventilation (see Hyperinflation Therapy Protocol, Protocol 9-3).

Aerosolized Medication Protocol

Both sympathomimetic and parasympatholytic agents are commonly used to induce bronchial smooth muscle relaxation (see Aerosolized Medication Protocol, Protocol 9-4). They often are not effective in this disorder, however.

MEDICATIONS AND PROCEDURES COMMONLY PRESCRIBED BY THE PHYSICIAN

Positive Inotropic Agents

When left-sided heart failure is present, positive inotropic drugs (e.g., digitalis, dopamine, dobutamine, and amiodarone) are commonly administered to increase cardiac output (see Appendix II).

Afterload Reduction Agents

The work of the heart can be reduced and contractility improved with afterload reduction agents. Systemic hypertension (elevated afterload) is most often acutely reduced with direct-acting vasodilators such as nitroglycerin, nitroprusside, hydralazine, and minoxidil. Afterload reducers such as the angiotensin-converting enzyme inhibitors (ACE inhibitors; e.g., lisinopril, captopril) are used in the more chronic cases.

Morphine Sulfate

Morphine sulfate is used to reduce afterload by inducing venodilation and venous pooling. It also is used for sedation and relief of anxiety.

Diuretic Agents

Diuretic agents are prescribed to promote fluid excretion (see Appendix II).

Albumin and Mannitol

Albumin or mannitol is sometimes administered to increase the patient's oncotic pressure in an effort to offset the increased hydrostatic forces of cardiogenic pulmonary edema, if the patient's osmotic pressure is low.

Alcohol (Ethanol, Ethyl Alcohol)

Because alcohol is a specific surface–active agent, it may be aerosolized into the patient's lungs to lower the surface tension of the frothy secretions. This action enhances the mobilization of secretions. Between 5 and 15 ml of 30% to 50% alcohol solution is generally administered. This is rarely used today.

Decreasing Hydrostatic Pressure

In an effort to lower hydrostatic pressure, the physician may order the following:

* Positioning the patient in Fowler's position (sitting up)
* Rotating tourniquets (rarely used)
* Phlebotomy (rarely used)

Case Study: PULMONARY EDEMA

Admitting History and Physical Examination

This 76-year-old male patient was admitted to the emergency room in obvious respiratory distress. His wife reported that her husband had gone to bed feeling well. He woke up with chest pain about 2:30 AM, very short of breath. She became concerned and called an ambulance. Neither the patient nor the wife were good historians, but they did report that the patient had been under a physician's care for some time for "heart trouble" and that he was taking "little white pills" on a daily basis. For the past 3 days, he had not taken any medication.

On admission to the emergency room, the patient was mildly disoriented and slightly cyanotic. He repeatedly tried to take the oxygen mask from his face. He complained of a feeling of suffocation. His neck veins were distended, and the skin of his extremities was mottled. On auscultation, there were coarse rhonchi and crackles in both lower lung fields and some crackles in the middle and upper lung fields.

His cough was productive of pinkish, frothy sputum. His vital signs were as follows: blood pressure 105/50, heart rate 124/min, and respiratory rate 28/min. ECG showed evidence of an old infarct, sinus tachycardia, and an occasional premature ventricular contraction. X-rays taken in the emergency room with the patient in a sitting position revealed bilateral fluffy infiltrates, more marked in the lower lung fields. The heart was enlarged. Laboratory findings were within normal limits. Blood gases on an FIO_2 of 0.30 were: pH 7.11, $Paco_2$ 72, HCO_3^- 27, and Pao_2 56. His oxygen saturation by oximetry (Spo_2) was 87%. The respiratory therapist working in the emergency room during the night shift recorded this SOAP note:

Respiratory Assessment and Plan

S Patient states . . . "a feeling of suffocation."

O Cyanosis, disorientation. Distended neck veins & mottled extremities. BP 105/50, HR 124, RR 28. ECG: sinus tach and occasional PVCs. Distended neck veins, mottled extremities, coarse rhonchi and crackles bilaterally. Frothy pink sputum. CXR: Bilateral fluffy infiltrates and an enlarged heart, ABG: pH 7.11, $Paco_2$ 72, HCO_3^- 25, and Pao_2 56 (FIO_2: 0.30). Spo_2 87%

A • Acute pulmonary edema (CXR)
 • Acute ventilatory failure with moderate hypoxemia (ABG)
 • Large and small airway secretions (rhonchi & crackles)

P Oxygen Therapy Protocol: Increase FIO_2 to 0.60 via continuous CPAP mask at 25 cm H_2O. Remain on standby for emergency endotracheal intubation and ventilator support. Continue ECG and oximetry monitoring, and repeat ABG in 30 minutes.

The patient was admitted on the cardiology service with a diagnosis of pulmonary edema—congestive heart failure. ECG monitoring and continuous oximetry were followed. Treatment consisted of intravenous furosemide, dopamine, and nitroprusside, as well as mask CPAP at 25 cm H_2O pressure with an FIO_2 of 0.6. A Foley catheter was placed.

• • • • •

Two hours later, the patient was very much improved and no longer cyanotic. Vital signs were as follows: blood pressure 126/70, heart rate 96/min, and respiratory rate 18/min. ECG revealed mild sinus tachycardia and no ectopic beats. Auscultation showed considerable improvement. There were still some basilar crackles, but the upper lung fields were clear. Cough was much reduced and no longer productive. Repeat chest X-ray at the bedside showed considerable improvement. Urine output was in excess of 600 ml/hr. The patient was calm and rational, stating that he was less short of breath and had no pain. Repeat arterial blood gases revealed pH 7.35, $Paco_2$ 46, HCO_3^- 24, and Pao_2 120 on an FIO_2 of 0.50. This respiratory therapy SOAP note was made at the time:

Respiratory Assessment and Plan

S Patient states . . . "I'm less short of breath. No pain."

O Not cyanotic. BP 126/70, HR 96, RR 18. ECG: Mild sinus tachycardia without ectopic beats. Fewer crackles; no sputum production; CXR: Improved. ABG: pH 7.35, $Paco_2$ 46, HCO_3^- 24, Pao_2 120 (FIO_2: 0.50)

A • Decreased pulmonary edema (overall impression from the data)
- No longer in ventilatory failure (ABG)
- Excessively corrected hypoxemia (ABG)
- Secretions controlled (no sputum & fewer crackles)

P Reduce O_2 per Oxygen Therapy Protocol to 2 Lpm by nasal cannula. Discontinue CPAP. Continue ECG and oximetric monitoring. Repeat ABG in 60 minutes.

Discussion

Acute pulmonary edema is a classic finding in congestive heart failure. Several clinical manifestations associated with **Increased Alveolar-Capillary Membrane Thickness** (see Figure 9-9) were present in this case. For example, the patient's decreased lung compliance was manifested in his tachycardia and tachypnea, whereas his hypoxemia reflected diffusion blockade associated with classic pulmonary edema (see Figure 9-10). His lung compliance was so reduced that he had progressed to acute ventilatory failure—the severe stage of pulmonary edema. Some **Atelectasis** (see Figure 9-7) was doubtless also present and was the rationale for CPAP therapy. In addition, the clinical scenario associated with **Excessive Bronchial Secretions** (see Figure 9-11) also was evident initially with frothy blood-tinged sputum and coarse rhonchi and crackles in both lower lung fields. The patient was too ill to allow valid pulmonary function testing, but the suspicion is that a combined obstructive and restrictive pattern may have been present at the time of the first assessment.

The *Aerosolized Medication* and *Bronchopulmonary Hygiene Therapy Protocols* were not used in this case. Often, the first-line management of pulmonary edema consists only of improving myocardial efficiency, decreasing the cardiovascular afterload, decreasing the hypervolemia, providing CPAP, and improving oxygenation. Furosemide (Lasix) is a potent loop diuretic, dopamine has direct inotropic effects, and nitroprusside is a potent peripheral vasodilator. The combination of these drugs, along with CPAP and oxygen therapy, resulted in marked improvement of the patient's myocardial activity and a rapid change in the clinical picture.

In short, this patient had an acute respiratory problem, but the basic cause was cardiac. After the cardiac condition was treated, the respiratory symptoms rapidly disappeared. CPAP and an increased FIO_2 were adequate, and this patient was spared the trauma and risk associated with intubation and mechanical ventilation. No evidence of acute myocardial infarction was found. He was discharged after 48 hours, his condition much improved. He was instructed to take his cardiac medication and diuretics without fail and to return to his family physician in 3 days.

SELF-ASSESSMENT QUESTIONS

Multiple Choice

1. In pulmonary edema, fluid first moves into the:

   I. Alveoli
   II. Perivascular interstitial space
   III. Bronchioles
   IV. Peribronchial interstitial space

   a. I only
   b. II only
   c. III only
   d. I and III only
   e. II and IV only

2. What is the normal hydrostatic pressure in the pulmonary capillaries?

   a. 5 to 10 mm Hg
   b. 10 to 15 mm Hg
   c. 15 to 20 mm Hg
   d. 20 to 25 mm Hg
   e. 25 to 30 mm Hg

3. What is the normal oncotic pressure of the blood?

   a. 5 to 10 mm Hg
   b. 10 to 15 mm Hg
   c. 15 to 20 mm Hg
   d. 20 to 25 mm Hg
   e. 25 to 30 mm Hg

4. Which of the following are causes of cardiogenic pulmonary edema?

   I. Excessive fluid administration
   II. Right ventricular failure
   III. Mitral valve disease
   IV. Pulmonary embolus

   a. III and IV only
   b. I and II only
   c. I, II, and III only
   d. II, III, and IV only
   e. I, III, and IV only

5. As a result of pulmonary edema, the patient's:

   I. RV is decreased
   II. FRC is increased
   III. VC is increased
   IV. TLC is increased

   a. I only
   b. I and IV only
   c. II and III only
   d. III and IV only
   e. II, III, and IV only

True or False

True ☐ False ☐ **1.** Morphine sulfate induces venodilation.

True ☐ False ☐ **2.** Patients with pulmonary edema frequently receive 30% to 50% aerosolized alcohol.

True ☐ False ☐ **3.** A patient is said to have orthopnea if dyspnea increases when the patient is in the upright position.

True ☐ False ☐ **4.** Kerley B lines on chest X-ray films are believed to originate from edematous interlobar septa.

True ☐ False ☐ **5.** Hypoproteinemia reduces oncotic pressure.

Fill in the Blank

1. An agent used to increase the patient's oncotic pressure to counteract the increased hydrostatic forces associated with cardiogenic pulmonary edema is _____.

Answers appear in Appendix XI.

CHAPTER 20

Pulmonary Embolism and Infarction

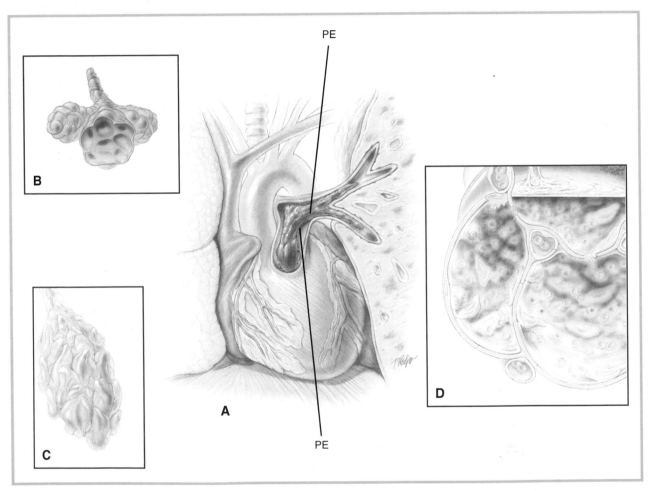

PE

PE

B

C

A

D

Figure 20–1 **A,** Pulmonary embolism *(PE)*. Bronchial smooth muscle constriction **(B)**, atelectasis **(C)**, and alveolar consolidation **(D)** are common secondary anatomic alterations of the lungs. See also Plate 12.

Anatomic Alterations of the Lungs

A pulmonary embolism occurs when a blood clot (thrombus) becomes dislodged from veins elsewhere in the body and moves (embolizes) into the pulmonary arterial circulation. If the embolism significantly disrupts pulmonary blood flow, pulmonary infarction develops and causes alveolar atelectasis, consolidation, and tissue necrosis. Bronchial smooth muscle constriction occasionally accompanies pulmonary embolism. Although the precise mechanism is not known, it is believed that the embolism causes the release of cellular mediators such as serotonin, histamine, and prostaglandins from platelets, which in turn leads to bronchoconstriction. Local areas of alveolar hypocapnia and hypoxemia also may contribute to the bronchoconstriction associated with pulmonary embolism.

Embolism may occur from one large thrombus or as a shower of small thrombi that may or may not interfere with the right side of the heart's ability to perfuse the lungs adequately. When a large embolus detaches from a thrombus and passes through the right heart, it may lodge in the bifurcation of the pulmonary artery where it forms what is known as a *saddle embolus* (partially shown in Figure 20-1). This is often fatal.

The major pathologic or structural changes of the lungs associated with pulmonary embolism are as follows:

- Blockage of the pulmonary vascular system
- Pulmonary infarction
- Alveolar atelectasis
- Alveolar consolidation
- Occasional bronchial smooth muscle constriction (bronchospasm)

Etiology

There are more than 600,000 cases of pulmonary embolism reported each year in the United States. It is estimated that more than 30,000 Americans from this group die from a pulmonary embolism annually, and approximately one third of the deaths occur within the first hour. A pulmonary embolism is the most common cause of maternal death after a live birth. The diagnosis of a pulmonary embolism is missed in about 70% of cases overall. Among patients over 70 years of age, the diagnosis of a pulmonary embolism is missed in about 90% of the patients because there is no typical clinical presentation. The classic triad of symptoms—dyspnea, hemoptysis, and pleuritic chest pain—occurs in fewer than 20% of patients. Thus any unexplained dyspnea, tachypnea, and chest pain should always raise the question of pulmonary embolism as a possible cause.

Although there are many possible sources of pulmonary emboli (e.g., fat, air, amniotic fluid, bone marrow, tumor fragments), blood clots (from venous thrombosis) are by far the most common. Most pulmonary emboli caused by blood clots originate from deep veins in the lower part of the body (i.e., the leg and pelvic veins and the inferior vena cava). A deep vein blood clot is commonly called a deep vein thrombus (DVT). When a thrombus or a piece of a thrombus breaks loose in a deep vein, the clot is carried through the venous system to the right atrium and ventricle of the heart and ultimately lodges in the pulmonary arteries or arterioles.

RISK FACTORS

The following are some of the factors predisposing to pulmonary embolism:

Venous Stasis

- Prolonged bed rest and/or immobilization
- Prolonged sitting (e.g., car or plane travel)
- Congestive heart failure
- Varicose veins
- Thrombophlebitis

Trauma

- Bone fractures (especially of the pelvis and the long bones of the lower extremities)
- Extensive injury to soft tissue
- Postoperative or postpartum states
- Extensive hip or abdominal operations
- Phlegmasia alba dolens puerperarum ("milk-leg" of pregnancy)

Hypercoagulation Disorders

- Oral contraceptives
- Polycythemia
- Multiple myeloma

Others

- Obesity
- Malignant neoplasms
- Pregnancy
- Burns

DIAGNOSIS AND SCREENING

Chest X-Ray

A chest X-ray is often normal in the patient with a pulmonary embolism. It can, however, be used to rule out conditions that mimic a pulmonary embolism—such as pneumonia or pneumothorax. In addition, infiltrate or atelectasis will be seen in about 50% of the pulmonary embolism cases, and an elevated hemidiaphragm occurs in about 40% of the cases.

Electrocardiogram (ECG)

The most common electrocardiogram (ECG) abnormality in pulmonary embolism is nonspecific ST-T wave changes. Sinus tachycardia is the most commonly seen rhythm disturbance. Atrial fibrillation and flutter may also occur. The ECG is an excellent test to rule out disorders such as pericarditis or myocardial infarction.

Ventilation/Perfusion Scan ($\dot{V}/\dot{Q}$ Scan)

A ventilation/perfusion scan ($\dot{V}/\dot{Q}$ scan) is reliable only at the extremes of interpretation (i.e., the test confirms that the lungs are normal or that there is a high probability of a pulmonary embolism). The $\dot{V}/\dot{Q}$ scan often raises more questions than it answers. This test is slowly being replaced by other more sensitive and rapid tests, such as the computed tomography (CT) scan.

Fast Computed Tomography Scan

Because of the fast turn-around time of a CT scan, it is rapidly becoming a first-choice test for patients suspected of having a pulmonary embolism. The CT scan is relatively fast and less invasive, and it eliminates the need for invasive pulmonary catheterization.

Pulmonary Angiogram

A pulmonary angiogram provides a clear image of the blood flow in the lung's arteries. It is an extremely accurate test to diagnose pulmonary embolism. However, because it is invasive (catheter insertion and dye injection) and time consuming (about 1 hour) and requires a high degree of skill to administer, it is usually performed when other tests have failed to provide a definitive diagnosis.

ADDITIONAL TESTS USED TO DETECT BLOOD CLOTS IN VEINS

In addition to the previously described tests that are used to detect a pulmonary embolism, several tests can be performed to detect a blood clot in the vein—called a *venous thromboembolism (VTE)*.

Fibrinogen Test

The fibrinogen test checks for increased levels of the protein fibrinogen—an integral component of the blood clotting process. Normal test results are actually more meaningful than abnormal results because many conditions can increase an individual's fibrinogen level. A normal result can accurately rule out the presence of a VTE. In addition, plasmin is the major clot-lysing enzyme capable of cleaving both fibrinogen and fibrin to yield various degradation products. Plasmin lysis of cross-linked fibrin generates the D-dimer fragment. Elevated D-dimer levels are found in many clinical conditions, including DVT and pulmonary embolism. D-dimer is not sensitive or specific enough to be diagnostic, but a value higher than 500 ng/ml is considered positive and can be used to supplement other clinical information.

Extremity Venography

The extremity venography test is a more complex and invasive procedure. It entails the insertion of a catheter into a vein of the patient's arm or leg. A contrast dye is injected into the vein to make it visible on an X-ray. Although venography can accurately detect a DVT, it has largely been replaced by duplex ultrasonography.

Duplex Ultrasonography (DUS)

A duplex ultrasonography (DUS) test is noninvasive, using high-frequency sound waves to detect blood clots in the thigh veins. This test is painless and takes only 30 minutes or less to perform. Although it is relatively sensitive in detecting a DVT above the knee, it is insensitive in detecting a DVT below the knee.

Magnetic Resonance Imaging (MRI)

A magnetic resonance imaging (MRI) test of the chest may be used for individuals whose kidneys may be harmed by dyes used in X-ray tests and for women who are pregnant.

OVERVIEW

of the Cardiopulmonary Clinical Manifestations Associated with PULMONARY EMBOLISM

The following clinical manifestations result from the pathological mechanisms caused (or activated) by **Atelectasis** (see Figure 9-7)—the major anatomic alteration of the lungs associated with a pulmonary embolism (see Figure 20-1). **Bronchospasm** (see Figure 9-10) also may explain some of the following findings. It occurs rarely and is of little clinical significance compared with the atelectasis and increased physiologic dead space caused by the embolism.*

CLINICAL DATA OBTAINED AT THE PATIENT'S BEDSIDE

The Physical Examination

Vital Signs

Increased respiratory rate (see page 31 ◆)

Several unique mechanisms probably work simultaneously to increase the rate of breathing in patients with pulmonary embolism.

Stimulation of peripheral chemoreceptors (hypoxemia)

When an embolus lodges in the pulmonary vascular system, blood flow is reduced or completely absent distal to the obstruction. Consequently, the alveolar ventilation beyond the obstruction is wasted, or dead space, ventilation. In other words, no carbon dioxide-oxygen exchange occurs. The $\dot{V}/\dot{Q}$ ratio distal to the pulmonary embolus is high and may even be infinite if there is no perfusion at all (Figure 20-2).

Although portions of the lungs have a high $\dot{V}/\dot{Q}$ ratio at the onset of a pulmonary embolism, this condition is quickly reversed, and a decrease in the $\dot{V}/\dot{Q}$ ratio occurs. The pathophysiologic mechanisms responsible for the decreased $\dot{V}/\dot{Q}$ ratio are as follows: In response to the pulmonary embolus, pulmonary infarction develops and causes alveolar atelectasis, consolidation, and parenchymal necrosis. In addition, the embolus is believed to activate the release of humoral agents such as serotonin, histamine, and prostaglandins into the pulmonary circulation, causing bronchial constriction. Collectively, the alveolar atelectasis, consolidation, tissue necrosis, and bronchial constriction lead to a decreased alveolar ventilation relative to the alveolar perfusion (decreased $\dot{V}/\dot{Q}$ ratio). As a result of the decreased $\dot{V}/\dot{Q}$ ratio, pulmonary shunting and venous admixture ensue.

*In an uncomplicated pulmonary embolism, none of the clinical scenarios presented in Figures 9-7 through 9-12 are activated. In these patients, "wasted" or increased alveolar dead space ventilation is the primary pathophysiologic mechanism (i.e., the ventilation of embolized [nonperfused] pulmonary subsegments, segments, or lobes).

The result of the venous admixture is a decrease in the patient's Pa_{O_2} and Ca_{O_2} (Figure 20-3). It should be emphasized that *it is not the pulmonary embolism but rather the decreased $\dot{V}/\dot{Q}$ ratio that develops from the pulmonary infarction (atelectasis and consolidation) and bronchial constriction (release of cellular mediators) that actually causes the reduction of the patient's arterial oxygen level.* As this condition intensifies, the patient's oxygen level may decline to a point low enough to stimulate the peripheral chemoreceptors, which in turn initiates an increased ventilatory rate.

Reflexes from the aortic and carotid sinus baroreceptors

If obstruction of the pulmonary vascular system is severe, left ventricular output will diminish and cause the systemic blood pressure to drop. The decreased systemic blood pressure reduces the tension of the walls of the aorta and carotid artery, which activates the baroreceptors. Activation of the baroreceptors in turn initiates an increased heart rate and an increased ventilatory rate.

Other pathophysiologic mechanisms that may increase the patient's ventilatory rate include the following (see page 40 ◆):

- Stimulation of the J receptors
- Anxiety/pain/fever

Increased heart rate (see pages 11 and 99 ◆)

The two major mechanisms responsible for the increased heart rate associated with pulmonary embolism are (1) reflexes from the aortic and carotid sinus baroreceptors and (2) stimulation of the pulmonary reflex mechanism.

For a discussion of reflexes from the aortic and carotid sinus baroreceptors, see the previous section on increased respiratory rate. The increased heart rate also may reflect an indirect response of the heart rate to hypoxic stimulation of the peripheral chemoreceptors, mainly the carotid bodies. When the carotid bodies are stimulated in this manner, the patient's ventilatory rate increases.

As a result of the increased rate of lung inflation, the pulmonary reflex mechanism is activated; this mechanism triggers tachycardia.

Systemic hypotension (decreased blood pressure)

When significant pulmonary hypertension develops in pulmonary embolic disease, systemic hypotension is nearly always present because of the decrease in the cross-sectional area of the pulmonary vascular system, which reduces cardiac return and causes a decrease in left ventricular output and results in systemic hypotension.

Cyanosis (see page 45 ◆)

OVERVIEW

of the Cardiopulmonary Clinical Manifestations Associated with PULMONARY EMBOLISM (Continued)

Cough and Hemoptysis (see page 47 ◆►)

As a result of the pulmonary hypertension, the pulmonary hydrostatic pressure, normally about 15 mm Hg, often becomes higher than the pulmonary oncotic pressure (normally about 25 mm Hg). This increase in the hydrostatic pressure permits plasma and red blood cells to move across the alveolar-capillary membrane and into alveolar spaces. If this process continues, the subepithelial mechano-receptors located in the bronchioles, bronchi, and trachea are stimulated. Such stimulation initiates a cough reflex and the expectoration of blood-tinged sputum.

Peripheral edema and venous distention

(see page 47 ◆►)
- Distended neck veins
- Swollen and tender liver

Chest pain/decreased chest expansion

(see page 42 ◆►)

Chest pain is frequently noted in patients with pulmonary embolism. The origin of the pain is obscure. It may be cardiac or pleural, but it is one of the common early findings in all forms of pulmonary embolism, even in the absence of obvious cor pulmonale or pleural involvement.

Syncope, light-headedness, and confusion

If the left ventricular output and systemic blood pressure decrease substantially, blood flow to the brain also may diminish significantly. This may cause periods of lightheadedness, confusion, and even syncope.

Abnormal heart sounds (see page 93 ◆►)
- Increased second heart sound (S_2)
- Increased splitting of the second heart sound (S_2)
- Third heart sound (or ventricular gallop)

Increased Second Heart Sound (S_2)—As a result of pulmonary embolization, abnormally high blood pressure develops in the pulmonary artery. This condition causes the pulmonic valve to close more forcefully. As a result the sound produced by the pulmonic valve (P_2) is often louder than the aortic sound (A_2), which causes a louder second heart sound, or S_2.

Increased Splitting of the Second Heart Sound (S_2)—Two major mechanisms either individually or together may contribute to the increased splitting of S_2 sometimes noted in pulmonary embolism: (1) increased pulmonary hypertension and (2) incomplete right bundle branch block.

The incomplete right bundle branch block that sometimes accompanies pulmonary embolism also may contribute to the increased splitting of S_2. In an incomplete block the electrical activity through the right heart is delayed; this delayed activity in turn slows right ventricular contraction. The blood pressure in the pulmonic valve area remains higher than normal for a longer time during right ventricular contraction. As a result, the closure of the pulmonic valve is delayed, which may further widen the S_2 split.

Third Heart Sound (Ventricular Gallop)—A third heart sound (S_3), or ventricular gallop, is sometimes heard in patients with pulmonary embolism. It occurs early in diastole, about 0.12 to 0.16 seconds after S_2. Although its precise origin is unknown, S_3 is thought to be created by cardiac wall vibrations during diastole, when the rush of blood into the ventricles is abruptly stopped by ventricular walls that have lost some of their elasticity because of hypertrophy. An S_3 generated in the right ventricle usually is best heard to the right of the apex, close to the lower sternal border during inspiration.

Other cardiac manifestations

Right Ventricular Heave or Lift—As a consequence of the elevated pulmonary blood pressure, right ventricular strain or right ventricular hypertrophy (or both) often develop. When this occurs, a sustained lift of the chest wall can be felt at the lower left side of the sternum during systole (Figure 20-4) because the right ventricle lies directly beneath the sternum.

Chest Assessment Findings (see page 22 ◆►)
- Crackles
- Wheezes
- Pleural friction rub (especially when pulmonary infarction involves the pleura)

CLINICAL DATA OBTAINED FROM LABORATORY TESTS AND SPECIAL PROCEDURES

Arterial Blood Gases

Mild to Moderate Pulmonary Embolism

Acute Alveolar Hyperventilation with Hypoxemia (see page 70 ◆►)

pH	$Paco_2$	HCO_3^-	Pao_2
↑	↓	↓ (Slightly)	↓

Extensive Pulmonary Embolism and Infarction

Acute Ventilatory Failure with Hypoxemia (see page 73 ◆►)

pH	$Paco_2$	HCO_3^-*	Pao_2
↓	↑	↑(Slightly)	↓

*When tissue hypoxia is severe enough to produce lactic acid, the pH and HCO_3^- values will be lower than expected for a particular $Paco_2$ level.

OVERVIEW

of the Cardiopulmonary Clinical Manifestations Associated with PULMONARY EMBOLISM (Continued)

Oxygenation Indices (see page 82 ◆◆)

$\dot{Q}_S/\dot{Q}_T$	DO_2	$\dot{V}O_2$	$C(a\text{-}\bar{v})O_2$
↑	↓	Normal	Normal

O_2ER	$S\bar{v}O_2$
↑	↓

Hemodynamic Indices (Extensive Pulmonary Embolism) (see page 99 ◆◆)

CVP	RAP	$\overline{PA}$	PCWP
↑	↑	↑	↓/normal

CO	SV	SVI	CI
↓	↓	↓	↓

RVSWI	LVSWI	PVR	SVR
↑	↓	↑	normal

Normally the pulmonary artery pressure is no greater than 25/10 mm Hg, with a mean pulmonary artery pressure of approximately 15 mm Hg. Most patients with a pulmonary embolism, however, have a mean pulmonary artery pressure in excess of 20 mm Hg. Three major mechanisms may contribute to the pulmonary hypertension: (1) decreased cross-sectional area of the pulmonary vascular system because of the emboli, (2) vasoconstriction induced by humoral agents, and (3) vasoconstriction induced by alveolar hypoxia.

Decreased Cross-Sectional Area of the Pulmonary Vascular System because of the Embolus—

The cross-sectional area of the pulmonary vascular system will decrease significantly if a large embolus becomes lodged in a major artery or if many small emboli become lodged in numerous small pulmonary vessels.

Vasoconstriction Induced by Humoral Agents—

One of the consequences of pulmonary embolism is the release of certain humoral agents, primarily serotonin and prostaglandin. These agents induce smooth muscle constriction of both the tracheo-bronchial tree and the pulmonary vascular system. Such smooth muscle vasoconstriction may further reduce the total cross-sectional area of the pulmonary vascular system and cause the pulmonary artery pressure to rise further.

Vasoconstriction Induced by Alveolar Hypoxia—

In response to the humoral agents liberated in pulmonary embolism, the smooth muscles of the tracheobronchial tree constrict and cause the V/Q ratio to decrease and the PaO_2 to decline. Although the precise mechanism is unclear, when the PAO_2 and PaO_2 decrease, pulmonary vasoconstriction ensues. This action appears to be a normal compensatory mechanism that offsets the shunt produced by underventilated alveoli. When the number of hypoxic areas become significant, however, generalized pulmonary vasoconstriction may develop and further contribute to the increase in pulmonary blood pressure. When the pulmonary embolism is severe, right-sided heart strain and cor pulmonale may ensue. Cor pulmonale leads to an increased CVP, distended neck veins, and a swollen and tender liver.

ABNORMAL ELECTROCARDIOGRAPHIC PATTERNS

- Sinus tachycardia
- Atrial arrhythmias
  - Atrial tachycardia
  - Atrial flutter
  - Atrial fibrillation
- Acute right ventricular strain pattern and right bundle branch block
- P-pulmonale (peaked p-waves)

In some cases, the obstruction of pulmonary blood flow produced by pulmonary emboli leads to abnormal ECG patterns. However, there is no single ECG pattern diagnostic of pulmonary embolism. Abnormal patterns merely suggest the possibility of pulmonary embolic disease. Sinus tachycardia is the most common arrhythmia seen. The sinus tachycardia and atrial arrhythmias sometimes noted also are thought to be related to the increased right-sided heart strain and cor pulmonale.

RADIOLOGIC FINDINGS

Chest Radiograph

- Increased density (in infarcted areas)
- Hyperradiolucency distal to the embolus (in noninfarcted areas)
- Dilation of the pulmonary arteries
- Pulmonary edema
- Right ventricular cardiomegaly (cor pulmonale)
- Pleural effusion (usually small)

Patients with a pulmonary embolus often demonstrate no radiographic signs. However, a density with an appearance similar to that of pneumonia may be seen if infarction has occurred. Hyperradiolucency also may be apparent distal to the embolus; it is caused by decreased vascularity (Westermark's sign). Dilation of the pulmonary artery on the affected side, pulmonary edema (common after a fat embolus), right ventricular cardiomegaly, and pleural effusions also may be seen.

OVERVIEW

of the Cardiopulmonary Clinical Manifestations Associated with PULMONARY EMBOLISM (Continued)

Ventilation-Perfusion Lung Scan Findings

Ventilation-perfusion lung scanning provides important information in this disease. The patient first breathes a gas mixture containing a small amount of radioactive gas, usually xenon-133. The presence of the xenon is detected by an external scintillation camera during a wash-in or wash-out breathing maneuver. Patients with a pulmonary embolism usually demonstrate normal ventilation in the region of their perfusion defect (Figure 20-5, A).

Next, an intravenous injection of radiolabeled particles 20 to 50 μm in diameter is injected. Particles labeled with a γ-emitting isotope, usually iodine or technetium, are injected into venous blood. The isotope accompanies the venous blood through the chambers of the right side of the heart and into the pulmonary vascular system. Because blood flow is decreased or absent distal to a pulmonary embolus, fewer radioactive particles are present in that area of the thorax. This is recorded by an external scintillation camera (Figure 20-5, B). *Areas of lung with normal ventilation and absent or reduced perfusion are suspected of having pulmonary emboli.*

Pulmonary Angiographic Findings

Pulmonary angiography is the "gold standard" used to confirm the presence of pulmonary embolism in patients with borderline or indeterminant ventilation-perfusion lung scans.

A catheter is advanced through the right side of the heart and into the pulmonary artery. A radiopaque dye is then rapidly injected into the pulmonary artery while serial roentgenograms are taken. Pulmonary embolism is confirmed by abnormal filling within the artery or a cutoff of the artery. A dark area appears on the angiogram distal to the embolization because the radiopaque material is prevented from flowing past the obstruction (Figure 20-6). The procedure generally poses no risk to the patient unless there is severe pulmonary hypertension (mean pulmonary artery pressure >45 mm Hg) or the patient is in shock or allergic to the contrast medium. The pulmonary angiogram is rarely positive if the ventilation-perfusion lung scan is normal.

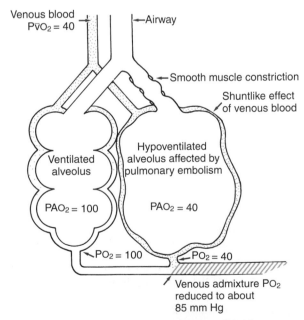

Figure 20–3 Venous admixture develops in pulmonary embolism as a result of bronchial smooth muscle constriction (shuntlike effect). Venous admixture also may occur when an embolus leads to pulmonary infarction and causes alveolar atelectasis and consolidation (true capillary shunt). Alveolar atelectasis and consolidation are not shown in this illustration.

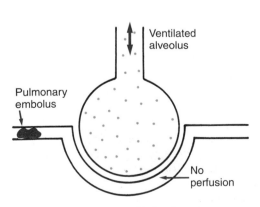

Figure 20–2 Dead-space ventilation in pulmonary embolism.

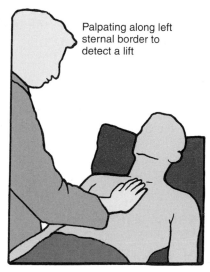

Figure 20–4   A right ventricular lift can be detected in patients with a pulmonary embolism if significant pulmonary hypertension is present.

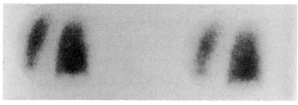

A

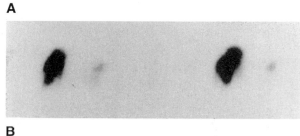

B

Figure 20–5   Abnormal ventilation and perfusion lung scans in a patient with a right main pulmonary artery embolism. **A,** A normal ventilation scan shows a uniform distribution of gas, with the dark areas reflecting the presence of the radioactive gas and, therefore, good ventilation (right lung is on viewer's left). **B,** An abnormal perfusion scan. The dark area shown in the right lung represents good blood flow. The white or light areas shown in the left lung represent decreased or completely absent blood flow (right lung is on viewer's left).

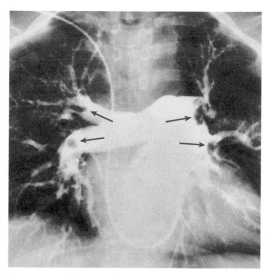

Figure 20–6   Pulmonary emboli. Pulmonary angiogram shows numerous filling defects. Trailing ends of the occluding thromboemboli are particularly well shown *(arrows).*

General Management of Pulmonary Embolism

All patients with a known or suspected pulmonary embolism should be admitted to the hospital. Initially, the patient likely will receive oxygen and a fast-acting anticoagulant *heparin* (Calciparine, Liquaemin), which works to prevent existing clots from growing and stops the formation of new ones. This is typically followed by the slow-acting anticoagulant *warfarin* (Coumadin, Panwarfin). Patients taking anticoagulant therapy should refrain from using aspirin and other *nonsteroidal antiinflammatory drugs (NSAIDs)* such as *ibuprofen* (e.g., Advil or Motrin), which also affect the blood's ability to clot.

Unfractionated heparin administered intravenously has until recently been the mainstay of treatment for patients suffering from acute pulmonary embolism, except in those with hemodynamic instability (see the following section on thrombolytic agents). *Unfractionated heparin* dosing must be governed by frequent monitoring of the *activated partial thromboplastin time (APTT),* and bleeding from *unfractionated heparin*–induced thrombocytopenia has been reported. Recently, low–molecular-weight heparin (LMWH) has recently become available (e.g., enoxaparin, dalteparin, and ardeparin) and has been shown to be safer and more effective than unfractionated heparin for prophylaxis of DVT or pulmonary emboli. It is also more cost-effective and does not require APTT monitoring.

THROMBOLYTIC AGENTS

Use of the fibrinolytic agents such as streptokinase (Kabikinase or Streptase), urokinase (Abbokinase), and the tissue plasminogen activator alteplase (Activase) actually dissolves blood clots. These agents (commonly referred to as "clot-busters") have proved beneficial in treating pulmonary embolism. These thrombolytic agents are sometimes used in conjunction with heparin. Their effect in patients with hemodynamic instability may be dramatic. Because of the excessive risk of bleeding, however, the use of fibrinolytic agents in treating pulmonary embolism has been limited.

PREVENTIVE MEASURES

Vein Filter

A filter may be surgically placed in the inferior vena cava to prevent clots from being carried into the pulmonary artery.

Heparin or Warfarin Therapy

Anticoagulants such as heparin and warfarin are often given to high-risk patients before and after surgery. Patients hospitalized for heart attack or stroke also are given anticoagulants.

Graduated Compression Stockings

Tight-fitting elastic stockings squeeze the patient's legs, helping the veins and leg muscles move blood more efficiently. They provide a safe, simple, and inexpensive way to keep blood from stagnating.

Research has shown that compression stockings used in combination with heparin are much more effective than heparin alone.

Pneumatic Compression

This treatment uses thigh-high cuffs that automatically inflate every few minutes to massage and compress the veins in a patient's legs. Studies show that this procedure can significantly decrease the risk of blood clots, especially in patients who undergo hip replacement surgery.

RESPIRATORY CARE TREATMENT PROTOCOLS

Oxygen Therapy Protocol

Oxygen therapy is used to treat hypoxemia, decrease the work of breathing, and decrease myocardial work. The hypoxemia that develops in pulmonary emboli usually is caused by wasted dead space ventilation. Hypoxemia caused by dead space ventilation is generally refractory to oxygen therapy (see Oxygen Therapy Protocol, Protocol 9-1).

Aerosolized Medication Protocol

Both sympathomimetic and parasympatholytic agents may be used to induce bronchial smooth muscle relaxation on the rare occasions when wheezing is present in patients with pulmonary emboli (see Aerosolized Medication Protocol, Protocol 9-4).

Mechanical Ventilation Protocol

Because acute ventilatory failure is commonly associated with severe pulmonary emboli, continuous mechanical ventilation may be required to maintain an adequate ventilatory status. Clinically, the patient demonstrates a progressive decrease in Pao_2 and pH and a steady increase in $Paco_2$ (acute ventilatory failure). If this trend is not reversed, mechanical ventilation becomes necessary (see Mechanical Ventilation Protocol, Protocol 9-5).

Pulmonary Embolectomy

Surgical removal of blood clots from the pulmonary circulation is generally a last resort in treating pulmonary embolism because of the mortality rate associated with the procedure and because of the availability of fibrinolytic agents to treat pulmonary embolism.

Case Study: PULMONARY EMBOLISM

Admitting History

A 32-year-old motorcycle enthusiast who smoked one pack of cigarettes per day fell asleep and fell from his bike while riding with a group of Harley "hogs" to the annual Sturgis Rally in North Dakota. Although his motorcycle sustained extensive damage, the man was conscious when the ambulance arrived. Before he was transported to the local hospital, he was treated in the field; splints and an immobilizer were applied. His injuries were thought to include a fractured pelvis, left tibia, and left knee.

En route to the hospital, a partial rebreathing oxygen mask was placed over the man's face. An intravenous infusion was started with 5% glucose solution. The patient was alert and able to answer questions. His vital signs were as follows: blood pressure 150/90, heart rate 105 bpm, and respiratory rate 20/min. Various small lacerations and scrapes on his face and left shoulder were treated. Each time the man was moved slightly or when the ambulance suddenly bounced or turned sharply as it moved over the highway, he complained of abdominal and bilateral chest pain. The emergency medical technician (EMT) crew all believed that his helmet and his youth had saved his life.

In the emergency room, a laboratory technician drew the patient's blood; several X-rays were taken, and the man was given morphine for the pain. Within an hour the patient was taken to surgery to have the broken bones in his left leg repaired. He was transferred 4 hours later to the intensive care unit (ICU) with his left leg in a cast. Thrombosis and embolism prophylaxis had been started with low-dose heparin. Busy with another surgery, the physician ordered a respiratory care consult for the patient.

Physical Examination

The respiratory care practitioner found the patient lying in bed with his left leg suspended about 25 cm (10 inches) above the bed surface. He had a partial rebreathing oxygen mask on his face and was alert. His wife and twin boys, who were 10 years of age and wearing black motorcycle jackets, were at the man's bedside. The patient stated that he was feeling much better and that his breathing was OK.

His vital signs were as follows: blood pressure 115/75, heart rate 75 bpm, and respiratory rate 12/min. He was afebrile, and his skin color appeared good. No remarkable breathing problems were noted. Palpation revealed mild tenderness over the left shoulder and left anterior chest area. Percussion was unremarkable, and auscultation revealed normal vesicular breath sounds. The chest X-ray taken earlier that morning in the emergency room was normal. His arterial blood gas values (ABGs) on a partial rebreathing mask were as follows: pH 7.40, $Paco_2$ 41 mm Hg, HCO_3^- 24 mMol/L, and Pao_2 504 mm Hg. His oxygen saturation measured by pulse oximetry (Spo_2) was 97%. On the basis of these clinical data, the following SOAP was documented:

Respiratory Assessment and Plan

S "My breathing is OK."

O No remarkable respiratory distress noted; vital signs: BP 115/75, HR 75, RR 12; afebrile; tenderness over left shoulder and left anterior chest area; normal vesicular breath sounds; CXR: normal; ABGs (partial rebreathing mask): pH 7.40, $Paco_2$ 41, HCO_3^- 24, Pao_2 504 mm Hg; Spo_2 97%.

A • No remarkable respiratory problems
  • Normal acid-base status with over-oxygenation

P Reduce oxygen therapy per protocol (2 lpm by nasal cannula). Recheck Spo_2.

3 Days After Admission

The man's general course of recovery was uneventful until the third day after his admission, when the nurses noticed swelling of the left calf while giving him a bath. A Doppler venogram revealed a left femoral vein DVT. The physician was informed. Anticoagulant therapy was started. Then, 5 hours later, the patient became short of breath and agitated. A spontaneous cough was noted, productive of a small amount of blood-tinged sputum. Concerned, the nurse called the physician and respiratory care.

When the respiratory care practitioner walked into the patient's room, the man appeared cyanotic, was extremely short of breath, and stated that he felt awful. The patient also said that he had precordial chest pain, felt lightheaded, and had a feeling of impending doom. His vital signs were as follows: blood pressure 90/45, heart rate 125 bpm, respiratory rate 30/min, and oral temperature 37.2° C (99° F). Palpation and percussion of the chest were unremarkable. Auscultation revealed faint wheezing throughout both lung fields. A pleural friction rub was audible anteriorly over the right middle lobe. A pulmonary artery catheter had been inserted.

The patient's ECG pattern alternated among a normal sinus rhythm, sinus tachycardia, and atrial flutter. His hemodynamic indices showed an increased central venous pressure (CVP), right atrial pressure (RAP), mean pulmonary artery pressure ($\overline{PA}$), right ventricular stroke work index (RVSWI), and pulmonary vascular resistance (PVR), as well as a decreased pulmonary capillary wedge pressure (PCWP), cardiac output (CO), stroke volume (SV), stroke volume index (SVI), and cardiac index (CI). The chest X-ray showed increased density in the right middle lobe consistent with atelectasis and consolidation. On an F_{IO_2} of 0.50, the ABGs were as follows: pH 7.53, Pa_{CO_2} 26 mm Hg, HCO_3^- 21 mMol/L, and Pa_{O_2} 53 mm Hg. His Sp_{O_2} was 89%. The physician started the patient on intravenous streptokinase, ordered a ventilation-perfusion lung scan, and requested that respiratory care see the patient again. On the basis of these clinical data, the following SOAP was documented:

Respiratory Assessment and Plan

S "I feel awful. I'm short of breath and lightheaded."

O Cyanosis; agitation, and dyspnea; cough productive of small amount of blood-tinged sputum; vital signs: BP 90/45, HR 125, RR 30, T 37.2° C (99° F), slight wheezing throughout both lung fields; pleural friction rub, right middle lobe; ECG: normal sinus rhythm, sinus tachycardia, atrial flutter; hemodynamic indices: increased CVP, RAP, $\overline{PA}$, RVSWI, and PVR and decreased PCWP, CO, SV, SVI, and CI; CXR: atelectasis and consolidation in the right middle lobe; on $F_{IO_2} = 0.05$, ABGs: pH 7.53, Pa_{CO_2} 26, HCO_3^- 21 mMol/L, Pa_{O_2} 53 mm Hg; Sp_{O_2} 89%.

A • Hypotension (BP)
   • Respiratory distress (cyanosis, heart rate, respiratory rate, ABGs)
   • Pulmonary embolism and infarction likely (history, vital signs, CXR, ECG, blood-tinged sputum, wheezing, pleural friction rub)
   • Bronchospasm, probably secondary to pulmonary embolism or infarction (wheezing)
   • Alveolar atelectasis and consolidation (CXR)
   • Acute alveolar hyperventilation with moderate hypoxemia (ABGs)
   • Pulmonary artery hypertension and low cardiac output probably secondary to pulmonary embolism (clinical presentation and hemodynamic data)

P Contact physician to request transfer to ICU. Increase oxygen therapy per protocol. Begin Aerosolized Medication Protocol (med. neb. with 2 cc albuterol premix qid). Monitor and reevaluate in 30 minutes (e.g., ABG). Remain on standby with mechanical ventilator available.

2 Hours Later

The ventilation-perfusion scan showed no blood flow to the right middle lobe. The patient's eyes were closed, and he no longer was responsive to questions. His skin appeared cyanotic, and his cough was productive of a small amount of blood-tinged sputum. His vital signs were as follows: blood pressure 70/35, heart rate 160 bpm, respiratory rate 25/min and shallow, and rectal temperature 37.5° C (99.2° F). Palpation of the chest was normal. Dull percussion notes were elicited over the right midlung. Wheezing was heard throughout both lung fields, and a pleural friction rub was audible over the right middle lobe.

The patient demonstrated an ECG pattern that alternated among a normal sinus rhythm, sinus tachycardia, and atrial flutter. His hemodynamic indices continued to show an increased CVP, RAP, $\overline{PA}$, RVSWI, and PVR and a decreased PCWP, CO, SV, SVI, and CI. The patient's ABGs on 100% oxygen were as follows: pH 7.25, Pa_{CO_2} 69 mm Hg, HCO_3^- 27 mMol/L, and Pa_{O_2} 37 mm Hg. His Sp_{O_2} was 64%. On the basis of these clinical data, the following SOAP was documented:

Respiratory Assessment and Plan

S N/A (patient not responsive)

O Ventilation-perfusion scan: no blood flow to right middle lobe; cyanosis; cough: small amount of blood-tinged sputum; vital signs: BP 70/35, HR 160, RR 25 and shallow, T 37.5° C (99.2° F); palpation negative; dull percussion notes over right middle lobe; wheezing over both lung fields; pleural friction rub over right middle lobe; ECG: alternating among normal sinus rhythm, sinus tachycardia, and atrial flutter; hemodynamic indices: increased CVP, RAP, $\overline{PA}$, RVSWI, and PVR and decreased PCWP, CO, SV, SVI, and CI; ABGs on 100% O_2: pH 7.25, Pa_{CO_2} 69, HCO_3^- 27, Pa_{O_2} 37; Sp_{O_2} 64%.

A • Pulmonary embolism and infarction (history, vital signs, hemodynamics, CXR, ECG, blood-tinged sputum, wheezing, pleural friction rub)
   • Continued respiratory distress (heart rate, respiratory rate, ABGs)
   • Bronchospasm (wheezing)
   • Acute ventilatory failure with severe hypoxemia (ABGs)

P Contact physician stat. Discuss acute ventilatory failure and need for intubation and mechanical ventilation. Continue Oxygen Therapy Protocol. Increase Aerosolized Medication Protocol (changing med. nebs. to IPPB to assist patient's work of breathing q 4 h).

Discussion

Risk factors for development of a fatal pulmonary embolism include immobilization, malignant disease, and a history of thrombotic disease (including venous thrombosis) congestive heart failure, and chronic lung disease. Only about 10% of patients with pulmonary emboli do not have at least one of these risk factors. The symptoms of ultimately fatal pulmonary embolism include dyspnea (in about 60% of patients), syncope (in about 25%), altered mental status, apprehension, nonpleuritic chest pain, sweating, cough, and hemoptysis (in a smaller percentage of patients).

The signs of acute pulmonary embolism include tachypnea, tachycardia, crackles, low-grade temperature, lower extremity edema, hypotension, cyanosis, gallop rhythm, diaphoresis, and clinically evident phlebitis (in a small percentage of patients).

The diagnosis of thromboembolic disease is most often made with ventilation-perfusion lung scanning, although pulmonary angiography remains the "gold standard" for diagnosis. Impedance plethysmography or duplex ultrasonography or venography of the extremities is helpful when embolic disease is suspected from venous thrombosis in the extremities.

It is interesting to note that in surgical patients at least half of the deaths caused by pulmonary embolism occur within the first week after the surgical procedure, most commonly on the third to seventh day after the operation. The remainder of the deaths, however, divide equally among the second, third, and fourth postoperative weeks. The current patient certainly had one of the obvious causes for pulmonary embolism—namely, immobilization of the left leg, which was put in a cast after surgery.

At the time of the **first assessment** the patient is not in any respiratory distress. His chest physical examination is basically unremarkable, as are the chest X-ray and arterial blood gases. The patient might well have been placed on hyperexpansion therapy, as with incentive spirometry, because his known fractures were expected to be surgically reduced. This fact is particularly important for this patient, who was on morphine and might be tempted to hypoventilate because of his left shoulder and left anterior chest pain and tenderness.

By the time of the **second assessment**, however, things had changed, and the patient demonstrated many of the signs and symptoms listed previously. The assessing therapist should recognize the seriousness of the situation from the patient's complaints, physical findings, hemodynamic parameters, and arterial blood gases. The patient's wheezing most likely was due to pulmonary embolism and infarction, as was the atelectasis. However, a trial of aerosolized bronchodilation was not inappropriate. The data were abnormal enough to prompt the therapist to suggest that the patient be transferred to the intensive care unit and to prepare for ventilator standby because acute ventilatory failure might not be far off.

Indeed, in the **last assessment**, things had progressed to the point at which the patient was in severe respiratory acidemia with severe hypoxemia, and mechanical ventilation became necessary. The treating therapist should recognize that the therapeutic options in these cases are limited by the amount of ventilation "wasted" in such patients because of their embolic disease. High minute volume ventilation may be necessary to improve (even slightly) the arterial blood gases in such patients.

One final note: Wheezing caused by pulmonary embolic disease is relatively rare, occurring in less than 2% of hospitalized patients. The outlook for this patient was extremely poor. Indeed, he died during the fifth week of his hospitalization. He remained on ventilatory support until the time of his death.

SELF-ASSESSMENT QUESTIONS

Multiple Choice

1. Most pulmonary emboli originate from thrombi in the:
   a. Lungs
   b. Right heart
   c. Leg and pelvic veins
   d. Pulmonary veins

2. The aortic and carotid sinus baroreceptors initiate which of the following in response to a decreased systemic blood pressure?
   I. Increased heart rate
   II. Increased ventilatory rate
   III. Decreased heart rate
   IV. Decreased ventilatory rate
   V. Ventilatory rate is not affected by the aortic and carotid sinus baroreceptors

   a. I and IV only
   b. II and III only
   c. III and IV only
   d. I and II only
   e. V only

3. What is the upper limit of the normal mean pulmonary artery pressure?
   a. 5 mm Hg
   b. 10 mm Hg
   c. 15 mm Hg
   d. 20 mm Hg
   e. 25 mm Hg

4. Pulmonary hypertension develops in pulmonary embolism because of which of the following?
   I. Increased cross-sectional area of the pulmonary vascular system
   II. Vasoconstriction caused by humoral agent release
   III. Vasoconstriction induced by decreased arterial oxygen pressure (Pao_2)
   IV. Vasoconstriction induced by decreased alveolar oxygen pressure (Pao_2)

   a. I and III only
   b. II and III only
   c. I, II, and III only
   d. II, III, and IV only
   e. II and IV only

5. In severe pulmonary embolism, which of the following hemodynamic indices is/are commonly seen?
   I. Decreased PVR
   II. Increased $\overline{PA}$
   III. Decreased CVP
   IV. Increased PCWP

   a. II only
   b. III only
   c. IV only
   d. I and II only
   e. II, III, and IV only

6. When humoral agents such as serotonin are released into the pulmonary circulation, which of the following occur?
   I. The bronchial smooth muscles dilate.
   II. The $\dot{V}/\dot{Q}$ ratio decreases.
   III. The bronchial smooth muscles constrict.
   IV. The $\dot{V}/\dot{Q}$ ratio increases.

   a. I only
   b. II only
   c. IV only
   d. II and III only
   e. I and IV only

7. Which of the following is a thrombolytic agent?
   I. Urokinase
   II. Heparin
   III. Warfarin
   IV. Streptokinase

   a. I only
   b. IV only
   c. II and III only
   d. I and IV only
   e. I, II, III, and IV

8. Which of the following is the most prominent source of pulmonary emboli?
   a. Fat
   b. Blood clots
   c. Bone marrow
   d. Air
   e. Malignant neoplasms

Answers appear in Appendix XI.

PART V

Chest and Pleural Trauma

CHAPTER 21

Flail Chest

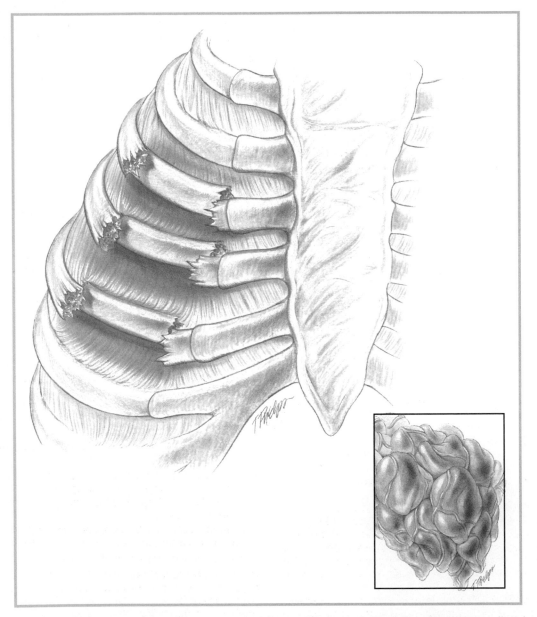

Figure 21–1   Flail chest. Double fractures of three or more adjacent ribs produce instability of the chest wall and paradoxical motion of the thorax. *Inset,* Atelectasis, a common secondary anatomic alteration of the lungs. See also Plate 13.

Anatomic Alterations of the Lungs

A flail chest is the result of double fractures of at least three or more adjacent ribs, which causes the thoracic cage to become unstable (Figure 21-1). The affected ribs cave in (flail) during inspiration as a result of the subatmospheric intrapleural pressure. This compresses and restricts the underlying lung area and promotes a number of pathologies, including atelectasis and lung collapse. In addition, the lung also may be contused under the fractured ribs.

A flail chest causes a restrictive lung disorder. The major pathologic or structural changes of the lungs associated with flail chest are as follows:

- Double fracture of numerous adjacent ribs
- Rib instability
- Lung restriction
- Atelectasis
- Lung collapse (pneumothorax)
- Lung contusion
- Secondary pneumonia

Etiology

A crushing injury to the chest is usually the cause of flail chest. Such trauma may result from the following:

- Direct compression by a heavy object
- Motor vehicle accident
- Industrial accident

OVERVIEW
of the Cardiopulmonary Clinical Manifestations Associated with FLAIL CHEST

The following clinical manifestations result from the pathologic mechanisms caused (or activated) by **Atelectasis** (see Figure 9-7) and **Pneumonic Consolidation** (see Figure 9-8)—the major anatomic alterations of the lungs associated with flail chest (see Figure 21-1).

CLINICAL DATA OBTAINED AT THE PATIENT'S BEDSIDE

The Physical Examination
Vital Signs

Increased respiratory rate (see page 31 ◄►)
Several pathophysiologic mechanisms operating simultaneously may lead to an increased ventilatory rate. These include the following:

- **Stimulation of peripheral chemoreceptors (hypoxemia)**
As a result of the paradoxical movement of the chest wall, the lung area directly beneath the broken ribs is compressed during inspiration and is pushed outward through the flail area during expiration. This abnormal chest and lung movement causes air to be shunted from one lung to another during a ventilatory cycle.

When the lung on the affected side is compressed during inspiration, gas moves into the lung on the unaffected side. During expiration, however, air from the unaffected lung moves into the affected lung. The shunting of air from one lung to another is known as *pendelluft* (Figure 21-2). In consequence of the pendelluft, the patient rebreathes dead-space gas and hypoventilates. In addition to the hypoventilation produced by the pendelluft, alveolar ventilation also may be decreased by the lung compression and atelectasis associated with an unstable chest.

As a result of the pendelluft, lung compression, and atelectasis, the V/Q ratio decreases. This leads to intrapulmonary shunting and venous admixture (Figure 21-3). Because of the venous admixture, the patient's Pao_2 and Cao_2 decrease. As this condition intensifies, the patient's oxygen level may decline to a point low enough to stimulate the peripheral chemoreceptors, which in turn initiate an increased ventilatory rate.

- **Other possible mechanisms**
  - Decreased lung compliance/increased ventilatory rate relationship
  - Activation of the deflation receptors
  - Activation of the irritant receptors
  - Stimulation of the J receptors
  - Pain/anxiety

Increased heart rate (pulse), cardiac output, and blood pressure (see page 11 and 99 ◄►)

Paradoxical Movement of the Chest Wall
When double fractures exist in at least three or more adjacent ribs, a paradoxical movement of the chest wall is seen. During inspiration the fractured ribs are pushed inward by the atmospheric pressure surrounding the chest and negative intrapleural pressure. During expiration (and particularly during forced exhalation), the flail area bulges outward when the intrapleural pressure becomes greater than the atmospheric pressure.

OVERVIEW

of the Cardiopulmonary Clinical Manifestations Associated with FLAIL CHEST (Continued)

Cyanosis (see page 45 ◆►)

Chest Assessment Findings (see page 22 ◆►)

Diminished breath sounds, both on the affected and unaffected side

CLINICAL DATA OBTAINED FROM LABORATORY TESTS AND SPECIAL PROCEDURES

Pulmonary Function Study Findings

Lung Volume and Capacity Findings (see page 61 ◆►)

V_T	RV	FRC	TLC
N or ↓	↓	↓	↓
VC	IC	ERV	RV/TLC%
↓	↓	↓	N

Arterial Blood Gases

Mild to Moderate Flail Chest

Acute Alveolar Hyperventilation with Hypoxemia (see page 70 ◆►)

pH	$Paco_2$	HCO_3^-	Pao_2
↑	↓	↓ (Slightly)	↓

Severe Flail Chest

Acute Ventilatory Failure with Hypoxemia (see page 73 ◆►)

pH*	$Paco_2$	HCO_3^-*	Pao_2
↓	↑	↑(Slightly)	↓

*When tissue hypoxia is severe enough to produce lactic acid, the pH and HCO_3 values will be lower than expected for a particular $Paco_2$ level.

Oxygenation Indices (see page 82 ◆►)

$\dot{Q}_S/\dot{Q}_T$	Do_2	$\dot{V}o_2$	$C(a-\bar{v})o_2$
↑	↓	Normal	↑
O_2ER	$S\bar{v}o_2$		
↑	↓		

Hemodynamic Indices (Severe Flail Chest) (see page 99 ◆►)

CVP	RAP	$\overline{PA}$	PCWP
↑	↑	↑	↓
CO	SV	SVI	CI
↓	↓	↓	↓
RVSWI	LVSWI	PVR	SVR
↑	↓	↑	↓

RADIOLOGIC FINDINGS

Chest Radiograph

- Increased opacity (in atelectic areas or areas with postflail pneumonia)
- Rib fractures (may need special films—rib series—to demonstrate)
- Because of the lung compression and atelectasis associated with flail chest, the density of the lungs increases. The increase in lung density is revealed on the chest radiograph as increased opacity (i.e., whiter in appearance). The chest radiograph also shows the rib fractures (Figure 21-4).

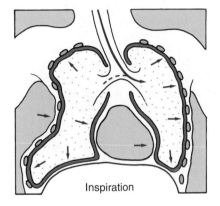

Inspiration

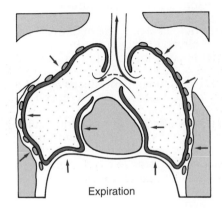

Expiration

Figure 21–2   Lateral flail chest with accompanying pendelluft.

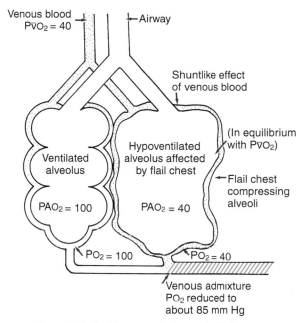

Figure 21–3 Venous admixture in flail chest.

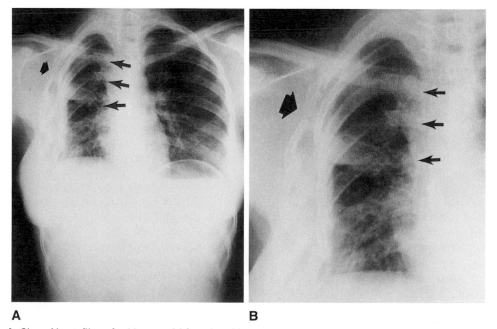

A   **B**

Figure 21–4 **A,** Chest X-ray film of a 20-year-old female with a severe right-sided flail chest. **B,** Close-up of the same X-ray film, demonstrating rib fractures *(arrows).*

General Management of Flail Chest

In mild cases, medication for pain and routine bronchial hygiene may be all that is needed. In more severe cases, however, stabilization of the chest is usually required to allow bone healing and prevent atelectasis. Today, volume controlled ventilation, accompanied by positive end-expiratory pressure (PEEP), is commonly used to stabilize a flail chest. Generally, mechanical ventilation for 5 to 10 days is an adequate time for sufficient bone healing to occur.

RESPIRATORY CARE TREATMENT PROTOCOLS

Oxygen Therapy Protocol

Oxygen therapy is used to treat hypoxia, decrease the work of breathing, and decrease myocardial work.

It should be noted, however, that the hypoxemia that develops in flail chest is most commonly caused by the alveolar atelectasis and capillary shunting associated with the disorder. Hypoxemia caused by capillary shunting is often refractory to oxygen therapy (see Oxygen Therapy Protocol, Protocol 9-1).

Hyperinflation Therapy Protocol

Hyperinflation techniques are commonly administered to offset and prevent the alveolar consolidation and atelectasis associated with flail chest (see Hyperinflation Therapy Protocol, Protocol 9-3).

Mechanical Ventilation Protocol

Because acute ventilatory failure is associated with flail chest, continuous mechanical ventilation is often required to maintain an adequate ventilatory status (see Mechanical Ventilation Protocol, Protocol 9-5).

Case Study: FLAIL CHEST

Admitting History and Physical Examination

A 40-year-old obese male truck driver was involved in a serious four-vehicle accident and was taken to the emergency department of a nearby medical center, where he was found to be markedly agitated and uncooperative. He was conscious and in obvious respiratory distress. His vital signs were as follows: blood pressure 80/62, pulse 90/min, respiration rate 42/min and shallow. Bilateral paradoxical movement of the chest wall was evident.

He had a laceration of the right eye and deep lacerations of the right thigh with rupture of the patellar tendon. There was pain and tenderness on palpation of the right posterior chest wall. The ribs moved inward with inspiration. The anteroposterior (AP) diameter of the chest was increased. Breath sounds were decreased bilaterally, and expiration was prolonged.

X-ray examination revealed posterolateral fractures of ribs 2 through 10 on the right and fractures of the necks of ribs 11 and 12 on the left. He had a 4+ hematuria, but his other laboratory findings were within normal limits.

The patient was intubated in the emergency department and placed on a mechanical ventilator with a V_T of 15 mL/kg and ventilatory rate of 12. An arterial line was placed, and the patient was taken to the operating room, where surgical repair of the eye

and thigh was performed. In the operating room, with an F_{IO_2} of 1.0, his blood gases were pH 7.48, $Paco_2$ 30, HCO_3^- 23, and Pao_2 360. The patient was transferred to the surgical intensive care unit, where the respiratory care practitioner on duty made the following assessment:

Respiratory Assessment and Plan

S N/A—patient is intubated, put on mechanical ventilator, sedated, and paralyzed (Norcuron).

O No spontaneous respirations. No paradoxical movement of chest wall on ventilator. BP 110/70, HR 100 regular, RR 12 on vent. On 100% O_2, pH 7.48, $Paco_2$ 30, HCO_3^- 23, and Pao_2 360. CXR: Bilateral rib fractures, left lung contused, no pneumothorax, no hemothorax.

A • Bilateral flail chest (history, paradoxical chest movement, CXR)
 • Acute alveolar hyperventilation with over-oxygenation (ABG)

P Mechanical ventilation protocol: Decrease V_T to correct acute alveolar hyperventilation and maintain patient on controlled ventilation per protocol until chest wall is stable. Wean oxygen per ventilator protocol (decreased to F_{IO_2} 0.4). Alert charge nurse (to request increase sedation and muscle paralysis) if the patient begins to inhale above preset mechanical ventilation rate.

Routine ABG monitoring and continuous Sao_2 monitoring. Careful chest assessment and auscultation to monitor for secondary pneumothorax and pneumonia.

Over the next 72 hours, the patient was kept intubated and ventilated with an Fio_2 of 0.4 and a mechanical ventilation rate of 12/min. However, his hospital course was stormy. His sputum rapidly became thick and yellow. Hyperinflation Therapy Protocol was started at a PEEP of 5 cm H_2O. On the second day, a right pneumothorax was demonstrated and a chest tube was inserted. A persistent air leak was present.

The next day, his pulse rose to 160/min and the pulmonary artery catheter showed evidence of left ventricular failure. His blood pressure was 142/82. His ventilator rate was 12 breaths/min and a PEEP of 10 cm H_2O. Auscultation revealed bilateral crackles. On an Fio_2 of 0.7, his ABGs were as follows: pH 7.37, $Paco_2$ 38, HCO_3^- 23, and Pao_2 58. He was rapidly diuresed, and his cardiac function improved dramatically. His Swan-Ganz catheter failed to "wedge." Over the next few days, the chest X-ray showed dense infiltrates in both lungs, and it was difficult to maintain adequate oxygenation, even with high inspired oxygen concentrations. His sputum was yellow and thick. Whenever his Sao_2 dropped below 90%, he became restless and agitated. At this time, the respiratory assessment was as follows:

Respiratory Assessment and Plan

S N/A—intubated, sedated, and paralyzed.

O Afebrile. HR 160 regular, BP 142/82, RR 12 (on vent). Right chest tube shows air leak. Crackles bilaterally. CXR: Fractures appear in line; bilateral dense infiltrates. ABG: pH 7.37, $Paco_2$ 38, HCO_3^- 23, and Pao_2 58 on Fio_2 of 0.7. Sputum thick, yellow.

A • Persistent flail chest bilaterally (CXR)
   • Bilateral dense infiltrates suggest pulmonary edema/ARDS/pneumonia (CXR)
   • Normal ventilatory status with moderate hypoxemia on present ventilatory settings. Oxygenation continues to worsen (ABG)
   • Thick, yellow bronchial secretions (sputum)
   • Pulmonary likely
   • Bronchopleural fistula on right side (chest tube bubbles)

P Mechanical ventilation and hyperinflation per protocol. Increase PEEP to 12 cm H_2O. Oxygen therapy per protocol (increase Fio_2 to 0.7).

Institute Bronchopulmonary Hygiene Therapy and Aerosolized Medication Protocols (in-line med neb with 2.0 cc premixed albuterol, followed by direct instillation of acetylcysteine q 4 h, and suction prn. Obtain sputum for Gram's stain and culture). Assist physician in the replacement of the Swan-Ganz catheter to optimize fluid therapy. Continue Sao_2 monitoring.

During the first week of his hospitalization, his BUN increased to 60 mg% and his creatinine to 1.9 mg%. Liver function tests remained within normal limits. The abnormal BUN and creatinine gradually returned to normal during the second week. The patient was slowly but successfully weaned off the ventilator over the next 2 weeks.

Discussion

This complicated case demonstrates the care of the traumatized patient with multi-organ failure. In this case, the second organ system affected was the cardiovascular system, probably secondary to fluid overload. Initial therapy included chest wall rest and internal fixation with mechanical ventilation. PEEP could have been added to his management at this point. By the time of the second assessment, the more classic clinical manifestations of pulmonary parenchymal change secondary to flail chest had developed. The clinical scenarios of **Atelectasis** (see Figure 9-7) and/or **Alveolar Consolidation** (see Figure 9-8) were well established, with oxygen-refractory pulmonary capillary shunting clearly in evidence.

Later, when what appeared to be acute respiratory distress syndrome (ARDS) supervened, PEEP was added, both for its effect on the ARDS and to stabilize the chest wall. Although these problems were dramatic enough, the therapist alertly noted the thick yellow bronchial secretions and added acetylcysteine and vigorous suctioning to deal with this problem. Aerosolized bronchodilator therapy (in this case albuterol) must always be given before or concurrently with acetylcysteine because the latter agent may cause bronchospasm if given alone. The ordering of a sputum Gram's stain and culture was appropriate.

Clearly, a patient this ill should be assessed at least once—possibly more—per shift. Because this patient was hospitalized for 40 days, more than 120 such assessments were found in his chart! As the authors of this book reviewed his case, this certainly did not seem to be excessive.

SELF-ASSESSMENT QUESTIONS

Multiple Choice

1. When the deflation reflex is activated, which of the following occurs?

   I. The lungs deflate.
   II. The expiratory time increases.
   III. The ventilatory rate increases.
   IV. The Hering-Breuer inflation reflex is activated.

   a. I only
   b. II only
   c. III only
   d. III and IV only
   e. I, III, and IV only

2. When a patient has a severe flail chest, which of the following occurs?

   I. Venous return increases.
   II. Cardiac output decreases.
   III. Systemic blood pressure increases.
   IV. Central venous pressure increases.

   a. I only
   b. III only
   c. III and IV only
   d. II and IV only
   e. I, III, and IV only

3. A flail chest consists of a double fracture of at least:

   a. Two adjacent ribs
   b. Three adjacent ribs
   c. Four adjacent ribs
   d. Five adjacent ribs
   e. Six adjacent ribs

4. As a consequence of a severe flail chest, which of the following occurs?

   I. RV increases.
   II. V_T decreases.
   III. VC increases.
   IV. FRC decreases.

   a. IV only
   b. I and III only
   c. II and IV only
   d. II, III, and IV only
   e. I, II, III, and IV

5. When mechanical ventilation is used to stabilize a flail chest, how much time generally is needed for bone healing to occur?

   a. 5 to 10 days
   b. 10 to 15 days
   c. 15 to 20 days
   d. 20 to 25 days
   e. 25 to 30 days

True or False

True ☐ False ☐ **1.** The shunting of air from one lung to another is known as *pendelluft.*

True ☐ False ☐ **2.** The fractured ribs of a severe flail chest commonly move outward during expiration.

True ☐ False ☐ **3.** In pendelluft, lung compression and atelectasis cause the $\dot{V}/\dot{Q}$ ratio to increase.

True ☐ False ☐ **4.** The irritant receptors may be stimulated in a flail chest.

True ☐ False ☐ **5.** During the advanced stages of severe flail chest, the increased HCO_3^- level in the arterial blood gases is secondary to the increased Pa_{CO_2}.

Answers appear in Appendix XI.

CHAPTER 22

Pneumothorax

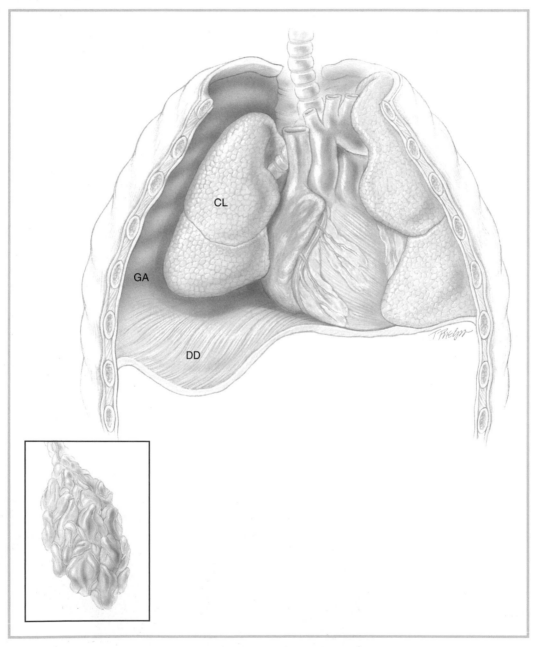

Figure 22–1   Right-side pneumothorax. *GA,* Gas accumulation; *DD,* depressed diaphragm; *CL,* collapsed lung. *Inset,* Atelectasis, a common secondary anatomic alteration of the lungs. See also Plate 14.

Anatomic Alterations of the Lungs

A pneumothorax exists when gas (sometimes called *free air*) accumulates in the pleural space (Figure 22-1). When gas enters the pleural space, the visceral and parietal pleura separate. This enhances the natural tendency of the lungs to recoil, or collapse, and the natural tendency of the chest wall to move outward, or expand. As the lung collapses, the alveoli are compressed and atelectasis ensues. In severe cases, the great veins may be compressed and cause the venous return to the heart to diminish.

A pneumothorax is a restrictive lung disorder. The major pathologic or structural changes associated with a pneumothorax are as follows:

- Lung collapse
- Atelectasis
- Chest wall expansion
- Compression of the great veins and decreased cardiac venous return

Etiology

Gas can gain entrance to the pleural space in three ways:

1. From the lungs through a perforation of the visceral pleura
2. From the surrounding atmosphere through a perforation of the chest wall and parietal pleura or, rarely, through an esophageal fistula or a perforated abdominal viscus
3. From gas-forming microorganisms in an empyema in the pleural space (rare)

A pneumothorax may be classified as either *closed* or *open* according to the way gas gains entrance to the pleural space. In a *closed pneumothorax*, gas in the pleural space is not in direct contact with the atmosphere. An *open pneumothorax,* on the other hand, implies that the pleural space is in direct contact with the atmosphere and that gas can move freely in and out. A pneumothorax in which the intrapleural pressure exceeds the intra-alveolar (or atmospheric) pressure is known as a *tension pneumothorax.* Some etiologic forms of pneumothorax are identified on the basis of origin, as follows:

- Traumatic pneumothorax
- Spontaneous pneumothorax
- Iatrogenic pneumothorax

TRAUMATIC PNEUMOTHORAX

Penetrating wounds to the chest wall from a knife, a bullet, or an impaling object in an automobile or industrial accident are common causes of traumatic pneumothorax. When this type of trauma occurs, the pleural space is in direct contact with the atmosphere, and gas can move in and out of the pleural cavity. This condition is known as a *sucking chest wound* and is classified as an *open pneumothorax* (Figure 22-2).

A piercing chest wound also may result in a closed (valvular) or tension pneumothorax through a one-way valvelike action of the ruptured parietal pleura. In this form of pneumothorax, gas enters the pleural space during inspiration but cannot leave during expiration because the parietal pleura (or more infrequently, the chest wall itself) acts as a check valve. This condition may cause the intrapleural pressure to exceed the atmospheric pressure in the affected area. Technically, this form of pneumothorax is classified as a *tension pneumothorax* (Figure 22-3). This form of pneumothorax is the most serious of all.

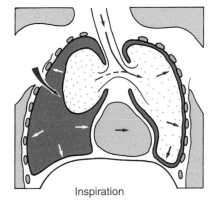
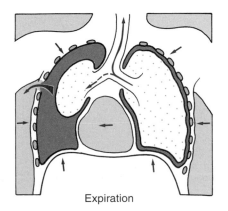

Figure 22–2 Sucking chest wound with accompanying pendelluft in an open pneumothorax.

Inspiration

Expiration

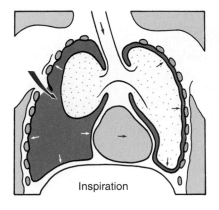

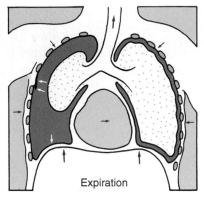

Inspiration   Expiration

Figure 22–3   Closed (tension) pneumothorax produced by a chest wall wound.

When a crushing chest injury occurs, the pleural space may not be in direct contact with the atmosphere, but the sharp end of a fractured rib may pierce or tear the visceral pleura. This may permit gas to leak into the pleural space from the lungs. Technically, this form of pneumothorax is classified as a *closed pneumothorax.*

SPONTANEOUS PNEUMOTHORAX

When a pneumothorax occurs suddenly and without any obvious underlying cause, it is referred to as a *spontaneous pneumothorax.* A spontaneous pneumothorax is secondary to certain underlying pathologic processes such as pneumonia, tuberculosis, and chronic obstructive pulmonary disease. A spontaneous pneumothorax is sometimes caused by the rupture of a small bleb or bulla on the surface of the lung. This type of pneumothorax often occurs in tall persons between the ages of 15 and 35 years. It may result from the high negative intrathoracic pressure and mechanical stresses that take place in the upper zone of the upright lung.

A spontaneous pneumothorax also may behave as a tension pneumothorax. Air from the lung parenchyma may enter the pleural space via a tear in the visceral pleura during inspiration but is unable to leave during expiration because the visceral tear functions as a check valve (Figure 22-4). This condition may cause the intrapleural pressure to exceed the intra-alveolar pressure. This form of pneumothorax is classified both as a *closed* and a *tension pneumothorax.*

IATROGENIC PNEUMOTHORAX

An iatrogenic pneumothorax sometimes occurs during specific diagnostic or therapeutic procedures. For example, a pleural or liver biopsy may cause a pneumothorax. Thoracentesis, intercostal nerve block, cannulation of a subclavian vein, and tracheostomy are possible causes of an *iatrogenic pneumothorax. An iatrogenic pneumothorax is always a hazard during positive-pressure mechanical ventilation—particularly when high tidal volumes or high system pressures are used.*

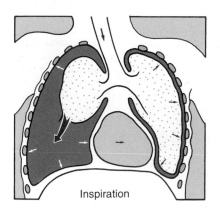

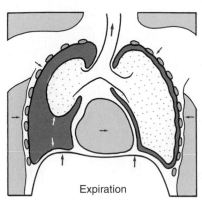

Inspiration   Expiration

Figure 22–4   Pneumothorax produced by a rupture in the visceral pleura that functions as a check valve.

OVERVIEW
of the Cardiopulmonary Clinical Manifestations Associated with PNEUMOTHORAX

The following clinical manifestations result from the pathologic mechanisms caused (or activated) by **Atelectasis** (see Figure 9-7)—the major anatomic alteration of the lungs associated with pneumothorax (see Figure 22-1).

CLINICAL DATA OBTAINED AT THE PATIENT'S BEDSIDE

The Physical Examination

Vital Signs

Increased respiratory rate (see page 31 ◆)
Several pathophysiologic mechanisms operating simultaneously may lead to an increased ventilatory rate:

- **Stimulation of peripheral chemoreceptors (hypoxemia)**
As gas moves into the pleural space, the visceral and parietal pleura separate and the lung on the affected side begins to collapse. As the lung collapses, atelectasis develops, and alveolar ventilation decreases.

If the patient has a pneumothorax as a result of a sucking chest wound, an additional mechanism also may promote hypoventilation. In other words, when a patient with this type of pneumothorax inhales, the intrapleural pressure on the unaffected side decreases. As a result the mediastinum often moves to the unaffected side, where the pressure is lower, and compresses the normal lung. The intrapleural pressure on the affected side also may decrease, and some air may enter through the chest wound and further shift the mediastinum toward the normal lung. During expiration the intrapleural pressure on the affected side rises above atmospheric pressure, and gas escapes from the pleural space through the chest wound. As gas leaves the pleural space, the mediastinum moves back toward the affected side. Because of this back-and-forth movement of the mediastinum, some gas from the normal lung may enter the collapsed lung during expiration and cause it to expand slightly. During inspiration, however, some of this "rebreathed dead space gas" may move back into the normal lung. This paradoxical movement of gas within the lungs is known as *pendelluft*. As a result of the pendelluft, the patient hypoventilates (see Figure 22-2).

Therefore when a patient has a pneumothorax, alveolar ventilation is reduced because of lung collapse and atelectasis. If the pneumothorax is accompanied by a sucking chest wound, alveolar ventilation may be further decreased by pendelluft.

As a result of the reduced alveolar ventilation, the patient's V/Q ratio decreases. This leads to intrapulmonary shunting and venous admixture (Figure 22-5). Because of the venous admixture, the Pao_2 and Cao_2 decrease. As this condition intensifies, the patient's oxygen level may decline to a point low enough to stimulate the peripheral chemoreceptors. Stimulation of the peripheral chemoreceptors in turn initiates an increased ventilatory rate.

- **Other possible mechanisms**
  - Decreased lung compliance/increased ventilatory rate relationship
  - Activation of the deflation receptors
  - Activation of the irritant receptors
  - Stimulation of the J receptors
  - Pain/anxiety

Increased heart rate (pulse), cardiac output, and blood pressure (small pneumothorax) (see pages 11 and 99 ◆)

Cyanosis (see page 45 ◆)

Chest Assessment Findings (see page 22 ◆)
- Hyperresonant percussion note over the pneumothorax
- Diminished breath sounds over the pneumothorax
- Tracheal shift
- Displaced heart sounds
- Increased thoracic volume on the affected side (particularly in tension pneumothorax)

As gas accumulates in the pleural space, the ratio of air to solid tissue increases. Percussion notes resonate more freely throughout the gas in the pleural space as well as in the air spaces within the lung (Figure 22-6). When this area is auscultated, however, the breath sounds are diminished (Figure 22-7). When intrapleural gas accumulates, and pressure is excessively high, the mediastinum may be forced to the unaffected side. If this is the case, there will be a tracheal shift and the heart sounds will be displaced during auscultation. Finally, the gas that accumulates in the pleural space enhances not only the natural tendency of the lungs to collapse but also the natural tendency of the chest wall to expand. Therefore in a large pneumothorax, the chest often appears larger on the affected side. This is especially true in patients with a severe tension pneumothorax (Figure 22-8).

OVERVIEW
of the Cardiopulmonary Clinical Manifestations Associated with
PNEUMOTHORAX (Continued)

CLINICAL DATA OBTAINED FROM LABORATORY TESTS AND SPECIAL PROCEDURES

Pulmonary Function Study Findings
Lung Volume and Capacity Findings (see page 61 ◆▶)

V_T	RV	FRC	TLC
N or ↓	↓	↓	↓
VC	IC	ERV	RV/TLC%
↓	↓	↓	N

Arterial Blood Gases
Small Pneumothorax
Acute Alveolar Hyperventilation with Hypoxemia
(see page 70 ◆▶)

pH	$Paco_2$	HCO_3^-	Pao_2
↑	↓	↓ (Slightly)	↓

Large Pneumothorax
Acute Ventilatory Failure with Hypoxemia
(see page 73 ◆▶)

pH*	$Paco_2$	HCO_3^-*	Pao_2
↓	↑	↑(Slightly)	↓

*When tissue hypoxia is severe enough to produce lactic acid, the pH and HCO_3^- values will be lower than expected for a particular $Paco_2$ level.

Oxygenation Indices (see page 82 ◆▶)

$\dot{Q}_s/\dot{Q}_T$	Do_2	$\dot{V}o_2$	$C(a\text{-}v)o_2$
↑	↓	Normal	↑(severe)
O_2ER	$S\bar{v}o_2$		
↑	↓		

Hemodynamic Indices (Large Pneumothorax)
(see page 99 ◆▶)

CVP	RAP	$\overline{PA}$	PCWP
↑	↑	↑	↓
CO	SV	SVI	CI
↓	↓	↓	↓
RVSWI	LVSWI	PVR	SVR
↑	↓	↑	↓

RADIOLOGIC FINDINGS

Chest Radiograph
- Increased translucency (darker lung fields) on the side of pneumothorax
- Mediastinal shift to unaffected side in tension pneumothorax
- Depressed diaphragm
- Lung collapse
- Atelectasis

Ordinarily, the presence of a pneumothorax is easily identified on the chest radiograph in the upright posteroanterior view (Figure 22-9). A small collection of air is often visible if the exposure is made at the end of maximal expiration because the translucency of the pneumothorax is more obvious when contrasted with the density of a partially deflated lung. The pneumothorax is usually seen in the upper part of the pleural cavity when the film is exposed while the patient is in the upright position. Severe adhesions, however, may limit the collection of gas to a specific portion of the pleural space. Figure 22-10, *A* shows the development of a tension pneumothorax in the lower part of the right lung. Figure 22-10, *B* shows progression of the same pneumothorax 30 minutes later.

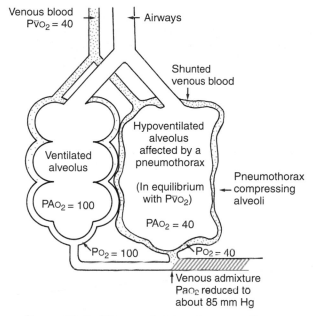

Figure 22–5 Venous admixture in pneumothorax.

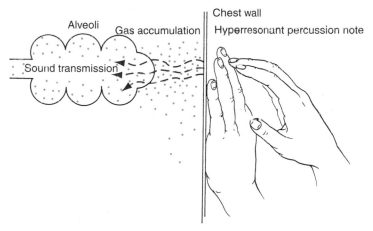

Figure 22–6 Because the ratio of extrapulmonary gas to solid tissue increases in a pneumothorax, hyperresonant percussion notes are produced over the affected area.

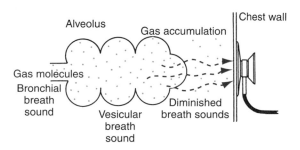

Figure 22–7 Breath sounds diminish as gas accumulates in the intrapleural space.

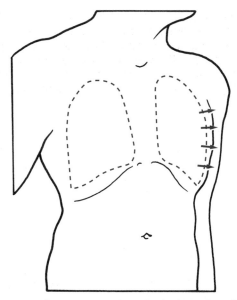

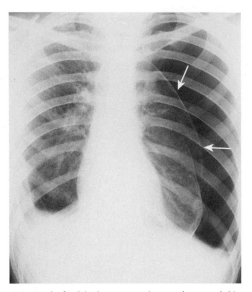

Figure 22–8   As gas accumulates in the intrapleural space, the chest diameter increases on the affected side in a tension pneumothorax.

Figure 22–9   Left-sided pneumothorax *(arrows)*. Note the shift of the heart and mediastinum to the right away from the tension pneumothorax.

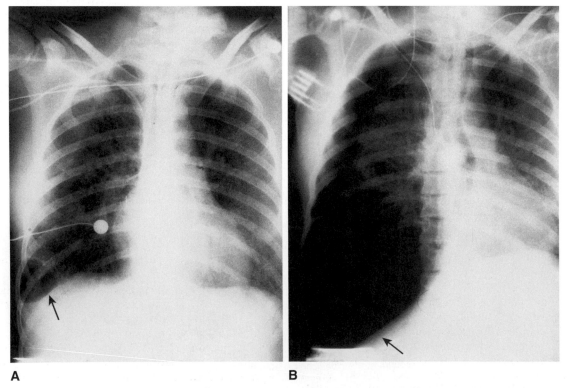

A   **B**

Figure 22–10   **A**, Development of a small tension pneumothorax in the lower part of the right lung *(arrow)*. **B**, The same pneumothorax 30 minutes later. Note the shift of the heart and mediastinum to the left away from the tension pneumothorax. Also note the depression of the right hemidiaphragm *(arrow)*.

General Management of Pneumothorax

The management of pneumothorax depends on the degree of lung collapse. When the pneumothorax is relatively small (15% to 20%), the patient may need only bed rest or limited physical activity. In such cases, resorption of intrapleural gas usually occurs within 30 days.

When the pneumothorax is larger than 20%, it should be evacuated. In less severe cases, air may simply be withdrawn from the pleural cavity by needle aspiration. In more serious cases, a chest tube attached to an underwater seal is inserted into the patient's pleural cavity. Because air rises, the tube is usually placed anteriorly near the lung's apex. Typically, a #28 to #36 French gauge thoracostomy tube is used for adults, with smaller sizes used for children. The tube permits evacuation of air and enhances the reexpansion and pleural adherence of the affected lung. The chest tube may or may not be attached to gentle negative suction. When suction is used, the negative pressure usually need not exceed −12 cm H_2O; −5 cm H_2O is generally all that is needed. After the lung has reexpanded and bubbling from the chest tube has ceased, the tube is left in place for another 24 to 48 hours.

RESPIRATORY CARE TREATMENT PROTOCOLS

Oxygen Therapy Protocol

Oxygen therapy is used to treat hypoxemia, decrease the work of breathing, and decrease myocardial work.

It should be noted, however, that the hypoxemia that develops in a pneumothorax is most commonly caused by the alveolar atelectasis and capillary shunting associated with the disorder. Hypoxemia caused by capillary shunting is often refractory to oxygen therapy (see Oxygen Therapy Protocol, Protocol 9-1).

Hyperinflation Therapy Protocol

Hyperinflation techniques are commonly administered to offset the atelectasis associated with a pneumothorax (see Hyperinflation Therapy Protocol, Protocol 9-3) in patients with chest tubes.

Mechanical Ventilation Protocol

Because acute ventilatory failure may develop with severe pneumothorax, continuous mechanical ventilation with positive end-expiratory pressure (PEEP) may be required to maintain an adequate ventilatory status (see Mechanical Ventilation Protocol, Protocol 9-5).

PLEURODESIS

On occasion, a thoracentesis may be performed before a procedure called *pleurodesis*. During this procedure, a chemical or medication (talc, tetracycline, or bleomycin sulfate) is injected into the chest cavity. The chemical or medication causes an intense inflammatory reaction over the outer surface of the lung and inside of the chest cavity. This procedure is performed to cause the surface of the lung to stick to the chest cavity, thus preventing or reducing recurrent fluid accumulation or pneumothorax.

Case Study: SPONTANEOUS PNEUMOTHORAX

Admitting History and Physical Examination

This patient was a 20-year-old male university student who was in excellent health until 5 hours before admission. He was sitting quietly in his dorm room studying for an examination when he suddenly developed a sharp pain in his left lower thoracic region. It was most acute in the anterior axillary line. The pain was exacerbated by deep inspiration and radiated anteriorly, almost to the midline. It did not radiate into the shoulder or neck. The patient became mildly dyspneic and had episodes of nonproductive cough that seemed to increase the chest pain. These symptoms worsened, and at 1 AM, his roommate drove him to the university hospital emergency department.

On examination the patient was a well-nourished, well-developed young man in moderately acute distress. His trachea was shifted to the right of the midline. His blood pressure was 150/82, pulse 96, and respirations 28 and shallow. The left chest was tympanitic to percussion, and the breath sounds were described as "distant." The patient was not cyanotic. The emergency department physician was momentarily busy with another patient and asked the respiratory therapist on duty to assess the patient's respiratory status. The respiratory care practitioner assigned to the emergency room during the night shift made the following assessments and plans:

Respiratory Assessment and Plan

S Left chest pain worsened by cough; shortness of breath.

O Normal vital signs. Left chest hyperresonant. Trachea shifted to the right. Breath sounds on left "distant."

A Probable left pneumothorax (history & objective indicators)

P Notify physician (who is in the next room). Request stat CXR & ABG. Oxygen therapy via partial rebreathing mask (F_{IO_2} 0.6 to 0.8). Obtain supplies for tube thoracostomy and place at patient's bedside.

• • • • •

The chest radiograph confirmed the diagnosis of a 50% left-sided pneumothorax, lung collapse, and mediastinal shift to the right. The arterial blood gas values on a partial rebreathing mask were pH 7.53, Pa_{CO_2} 29, HCO_3^- 21, and Pa_{O_2} 56. The physician was still busy with the patient in the next room. With this new information, the respiratory therapist charted the following:

Respiratory Assessment and Plan

S "This oxygen mask helps a little."

O Persistent symptoms as in SOAP-1 above. CXR: 50% left tension pneumothorax. Mediastinum shifted to right. ABGs: pH 7.53, Pa_{CO_2} 29, HCO_3^- 21, and Pa_{O_2} 56 (on partial rebreathing mask).

A • 50% left pneumothorax with mediastinal shift—lung collapse & atelectasis (CXR)
   • Acute alveolar hyperventilation with mild hypoxemia (ABG)

P Inform physician of previous and current assessment. Increase F_{IO_2} to 0.8 to 1.0 via a nonrebreathing mask. Stay at patient's bedside until physician arrives. Assist in placement of chest tube.

Approximately 15 minutes later, the attending physician entered the room and quickly reviewed the clinical data and assessments. Moments later, he introduced a thoracostomy tube and began underwater drainage. The respiratory therapist placed a CPAP mask on the patient's face at 5 cm H_2O. The F_{IO_2} on the mask was adjusted to 0.5. Over the next 30 minutes, the lung expanded well and the patient's ventilatory and oxygenation status quickly improved. The chest tube was removed after 48 hours. Follow-up examination after 2 weeks revealed full expansion of the left lung. There was no evidence of blebs or bullae. A tuberculin skin test was negative, and the etiology of the pneumothorax was never found.

Discussion

Few respiratory conditions persist with a "crisis" onset, and this is one of them. Other instances include foreign body aspiration, pulmonary embolism, anaphylactic shock, and some cases of asthma.

This case nicely demonstrates the signs and symptoms of **Atelectasis** and intrapulmonary shunting (see Figure 9-7). The physician and respiratory therapist could not hear crackles, however, presumably because the atelectatic segments were separated (distant) from the chest wall and the examiner's stethoscope.

Although the respiratory care administered in this case (oxygen therapy) was fairly pedestrian, the therapist's assistance in the assessment of this patient and his presence at bedside made a great difference in the speed and ease with which the patient was treated. The value of an assessing/treating therapist in this situation cannot be overestimated.

Finally, it should be noted that whenever patients are placed on mechanical ventilation, the risk of pneumothorax must always be kept in mind. This is particularly common in chronic obstructive pulmonary disease (COPD) and in human immunodeficiency virus (HIV)–related acute respiratory distress syndrome (ARDS). Indeed, when very high mean airway pressures are required to ventilate such patients, prophylactic bilateral tube thoracostomies are often mandatory.

SELF-ASSESSMENT QUESTIONS

Multiple Choice

1. When gas moves between the pleural space and the atmosphere during a ventilatory cycle, the patient is said to have a/an:
   - I. Closed pneumothorax
   - II. Open pneumothorax
   - III. Valvular pneumothorax
   - IV. Sucking chest wound

   a. I only
   b. II only
   c. III only
   d. I and III only
   e. II and IV only

2. When gas enters the pleural space during inspiration but is unable to leave during expiration, the patient is said to have a/an:
   - I. Iatrogenic pneumothorax
   - II. Valvular pneumothorax
   - III. Tension pneumothorax
   - IV. Open pneumothorax

   a. I only
   b. III only
   c. II and III only
   d. III and IV only
   e. II, III, and IV only

3. Which of the following may cause a pneumothorax?
   - I. Pneumonia
   - II. Tuberculosis
   - III. Chronic obstructive pulmonary disease
   - IV. Blebs

   a. IV only
   b. I and II only
   c. II and III only
   d. II, III, and IV only
   e. I, II, III, and IV

4. When a patient has a pneumothorax because of a sucking chest wound, which of the following occurs?
   - I. Intrapleural pressure on the unaffected side increases during inspiration.
   - II. The mediastinum often moves to the unaffected side during inspiration.
   - III. Intrapleural pressure on the affected side often rises above the atmospheric pressure during expiration.
   - IV. The mediastinum often moves to the affected side during expiration.

   a. I and IV only
   b. I and III only
   c. II and III only
   d. II, III, and IV only
   e. I, II, III, and IV

5. The increased ventilatory rate commonly manifested in patients with pneumothorax may result from which of the following?
   - I. Stimulation of the J receptors
   - II. Increased lung compliance
   - III. Increased stimulation of the Hering-Breuer reflex
   - IV. Stimulation of the irritant reflex

   a. I and IV only
   b. II and III only
   c. III and IV only
   d. II, III, and IV only
   e. I, II, III, and IV

6. The physician usually elects to evacuate the intrathoracic gas when the pneumothorax is greater than:

   a. 5%
   b. 10%
   c. 15%
   d. 20%
   e. 25%

7. When treating a pneumothorax with a chest tube and suction, the negative (suction) pressure usually need not exceed:

   a. 4 cm H_2O
   b. 6 cm H_2O
   c. 8 cm H_2O
   d. 10 cm H_2O
   e. 12 cm H_2O

8. A patient with a severe tension pneumothorax demonstrates which of the following?
   - I. Diminished breath sounds
   - II. Hyperresonant percussion note
   - III. Dull percussion notes
   - IV. Whispered pectoriloquy

   a. II only
   b. I and II only
   c. III and IV only
   d. I, II, and IV only
   e. I, II, III, and IV

9. When a patient has a large tension pneumothorax, which of the following occurs?

    I. $Paco_2$ decreases.
    II. pH increases.
    III. HCO_3^- decreases.
    IV. $Paco_2$ increases.

  a. I only
  b. IV only
  c. III and IV only
  d. II and III only
  e. I, II, and III only

10. When a patient has a large tension pneumothorax, which of the following occurs?

    I. PVR decreases.
    II. $\overline{PA}$ increases.
    III. CVP decreases.
    IV. CO increases.

  a. I only
  b. II only
  c. III only
  d. I and III only
  e. II and IV only

Answers appear in Appendix XI.

PART VI

Disorders of the Pleura and of the Chest Wall

CHAPTER 23

Pleural Diseases

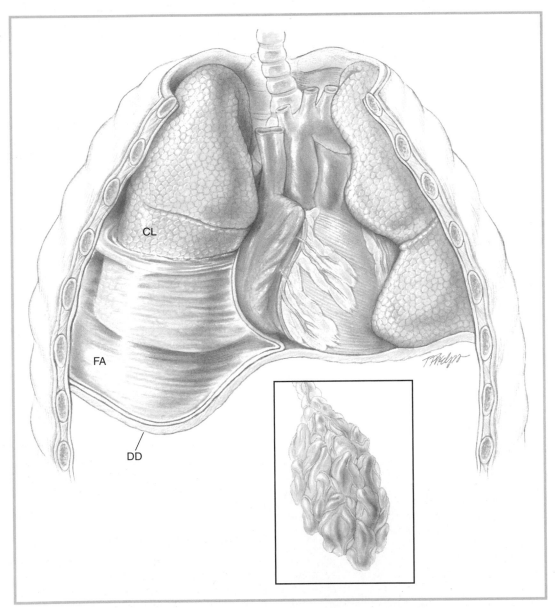

Figure 23–1 Right-sided pleural effusion. *FA,* Fluid accumulation; *DD,* depressed diaphragm; *CL,* collapsed lung (partially collapsed). *Inset,* Atelectasis, a common secondary anatomic alteration of the lungs. See also Plate 15.

Anatomic Alterations of the Lungs

A number of pleural diseases can cause fluid to accumulate in the pleural space; this fluid is called a pleural effusion (Figure 23-1). Similar to free air in the pleural space, fluid accumulation separates the visceral and parietal pleura and compresses the lungs. In severe cases, atelectasis will develop, the great veins may be compressed, and cardiac venous return may be diminished. Pleural effusion produces a restrictive lung disorder.

The major pathologic or structural changes associated with significant pleural effusion are as follows:

- Lung compression
- Atelectasis
- Compression of the great veins and decreased cardiac venous return

Etiology

A pleural effusion may be *transudative* or *exudative*. A *transudate* develops when fluid from the pulmonary capillaries moves into the pleural space. The fluid is thin and watery, containing a few blood cells and little protein. The pleural surfaces are not involved in producing the transudate.

In contrast, an *exudate* develops when the pleural surfaces are diseased. The fluid has a high protein content and a great deal of cellular debris. Exudate is usually caused by inflammation, infection, or malignancy.

MAJOR CAUSES OF A TRANSUDATIVE PLEURAL EFFUSION

Congestive Heart Failure

Congestive heart failure is probably the most common cause of pleural effusion. Both right- and left-sided heart failure can result in pleural effusion. In right-sided heart failure, an increase in the hydrostatic pressure in the systemic circulation can (1) increase the rate of pleural fluid formation and (2) decrease lymphatic drainage from the pleural space because of the elevated systemic venous pressure. In left-sided heart failure, an increase in hydrostatic pressure in the pulmonary circulation can (1) decrease the rate of pleural fluid absorption through the visceral pleura and (2) cause fluid movement through the visceral pleura into the pleural space. In general, left-sided heart failure is more likely to produce pleural effusion than right-sided heart failure.

Hepatic Hydrothorax

Occasionally, pleural effusions can develop as a complication of hepatic cirrhosis, particularly when ascitic fluid is present in the abdomen. The pleural effusion in these patients is generally right-sided.

Peritoneal Dialysis

As in the pleural effusion that occurs as a result of abdominal ascites, pleural fluid also may develop as a complication of peritoneal dialysis. When the peritoneal dialysis is stopped, the pleural effusion usually disappears rapidly.

Nephrotic Syndrome

Pleural effusion is commonly seen in patients with nephrotic syndrome. It is generally bilateral. The effusion is a result of the decreased plasma oncotic pressure that develops in this disorder.

Pulmonary Embolus

Between 30% and 50% of patients with pulmonary arterial emboli develop pleural effusion. Two distinct mechanisms are responsible. First, obstruction of the pulmonary vasculature can lead to right-sided heart failure, which in turn can lead to pleural effusion. The second mechanism involves the increased permeability of the capillaries in the visceral pleura that develops in response to the ischemia caused by the pulmonary emboli.

MAJOR CAUSES OF AN EXUDATIVE PLEURAL EFFUSION

Malignant Pleural Effusions

Metastatic disease of the pleura or of the mediastinal lymph nodes is the most common cause of exudative pleural effusions. Carcinoma of the lung and breast and lymphomas account for about 75% of malignant pleural effusions.

Malignant Mesotheliomas

Malignant mesotheliomas arise from the mesothelial cells that line the pleural cavities. Individuals with chronic asbestos exposure have a much greater risk of developing mesothelioma. The pleural fluid is exudative and generally contains a mixture of normal mesothelial cells, differentiated and undifferentiated malignant mesothelial cells, and a varying number of lymphocytes and polymorphonuclear leukocytes.

Pneumonias

As many as 40% of patients with bacterial pneumonia have an accompanying pleural effusion. Most pleural effusions associated with pneumonia resolve without any specific therapy. Approximately 10%, however, require some sort of therapeutic intervention. If appropriate antibiotic therapy is not instituted, bacteria invade the pleural fluid from the lung parenchyma. Eventually, pus will accumulate in the pleural cavity (**empyema**). Pleural effusion also can be produced by viruses, *Mycoplasma pneumoniae,* and *Rickettsia,* although the pleural effusions are usually small.

Tuberculosis

Pleural effusion may develop from a rupture of a caseous tubercle into the pleural cavity. It also is possible that the inflammatory reaction that develops in tuberculosis obstructs the lymphatic pores in the parietal pleura. This in turn leads to an accumulation of protein and fluid in the pleural space. Pleural effusion caused by tuberculosis is generally unilateral and small to moderate in size.

Fungal Diseases

Patients with fungal diseases occasionally have secondary pleural effusions. Common fungal diseases that may produce pleural effusions are *histoplasmosis, coccidioidomycosis*, and *blastomycosis.*

Pleural Effusion Resulting From Diseases of the Gastrointestinal Tract

Pleural effusion is sometimes associated with diseases of the gastrointestinal tract such as pancreatitis, subphrenic abscess, intrahepatic abscess, esophageal perforation, abdominal operations, and diaphragmatic hernia.

Pleural Effusion Resulting From Collagen Vascular Diseases

Pleural effusion occasionally develops as a complication of collagen vascular diseases. Such diseases include rheumatoid pleuritis, systemic lupus erythematosus, Sjögren's syndrome, familial Mediterranean fever, and Wegener's granulomatosis.

OTHER PATHOLOGIC FLUIDS THAT SEPARATE THE PARIETAL FROM THE VISCERAL PLEURA

In addition to transudate and exudate, other pathologic fluids can separate the parietal pleura from the visceral pleura.

Empyema

The accumulation of pus in the pleural cavity is called *empyema.* Empyema commonly develops as a result of inflammation. Thoracentesis may confirm the diagnosis and determine the specific causative organism. The pus is usually removed by chest tube drainage. Open thoracotomy drainage may occasionally be necessary.

Chylothorax

Chylothorax is the presence of chyle in the pleural cavity. Chyle is a milky liquid produced from the food in the small intestine during digestion. It consists mainly of fat particles in a stable emulsion. Chyle is taken up by fingerlike intestinal lymphatics called *lacteals* and transported by the thoracic duct to the neck. From the thoracic duct the chyle moves into the venous circulation and mixes with blood. The presence of chyle in the pleural cavity is usually caused by trauma to the neck or thorax or by cancer occluding the thoracic duct.

Hemothorax

The presence of blood in the pleural space is known as a *hemothorax.* Most of these are caused by penetrating or blunt chest trauma. An iatrogenic hemothorax may develop from trauma caused by the insertion of a central venous or pulmonary artery catheter.

Blood can gain entrance into the pleural space from trauma to the chest wall, diaphragm, lung, or mediastinum. A hematocrit of the pleural fluid should always be obtained if the pleural fluid looks like blood. A hemothorax is said to be present only when the hematocrit of the pleural fluid is at least 50% that of the peripheral blood.

OVERVIEW

of the Cardiopulmonary Clinical Manifestations Associated with PLEURAL EFFUSION

The following clinical manifestations result from the pathologic mechanisms caused (or activated) by **Atelectasis** (see Figure 9-7)—the major anatomic alteration of the lungs associated with pleural effusion (see Figure 24-1).

CLINICAL DATA OBTAINED AT THE PATIENT'S BEDSIDE

The Physical Examination
Vital Signs

Increased respiratory rate (see page 31 ◆▶)
Several pathophysiologic mechanisms operating simultaneously may lead to an increased ventilatory rate:
- Stimulation of peripheral chemoreceptors (hypoxemia)
- Decreased lung compliance/increased ventilatory rate relationship
- Activation of the deflation receptors
- Activation of the irritant receptors
- Stimulation of J receptors
- Pain/anxiety

Increased heart rate (pulse), cardiac output, and blood pressure (see pages 11 and 99 ◆▶)

Chest Pain/Decreased Chest Expansion (see page 42 ◆▶)

Cyanosis (see page 45 ◆▶)

Cough (Dry, Nonproductive) (see page 47 ◆▶)

Chest Assessment Findings (see page 22 ◆▶)
- Tracheal shift
- Decreased tactile and vocal fremitus
- Dull percussion note
- Diminished breath sounds
- Displaced heart sounds

CLINICAL DATA OBTAINED FROM LABORATORY TESTS AND SPECIAL PROCEDURES

Pulmonary Function Study Findings

Lung Volume and Capacity Findings
(see page 61 ◆▶)

V_T	RV	FRC	TLC
N or ↓	↓	↓	↓
VC	IC	ERV	RV/TLC%
↓	↓	↓	N

Arterial Blood Gases

Small Pleural Effusion
Acute Alveolar Hyperventilation with Hypoxemia (see page 70 ◆▶)

pH	$Paco_2$	HCO_3^-	Pao_2
↑	↓	↓ (Slightly)	↓

Large Pleural Effusion
Acute Ventilatory Failure with Hypoxemia (see page 73 ◆▶)

pH*	$Paco_2$	HCO_3^-*	Pao_2
↓	↑	↑(Slightly)	↓

*When tissue hypoxia is severe enough to produce lactic acid, the pH and HCO_3^- values will be lower than expected for a particular $Paco_2$ level.

Oxygenation Indices (see page 82 ◆▶)

$\dot{Q}_S/\dot{Q}_T$	Do_2†	$\dot{V}o_2$	$C(a-\bar{v})o_2$
↑	↓	Normal	↑(severe)
O_2ER	Svo_2		
↑	↓		

†The Do_2 may be normal in patients who have compensated to the decreased oxygenation status with (1) an increased cardiac output, (2) an increased hemoglobin level, or (3) a combination of both. When the Do_2 is normal, the O_2ER is usually normal.

Hemodynamic Indices (Severe Pleural Effusion)
(see page 99 ◆▶)

CVP	RAP	$\overline{PA}$	PCWP
↑	↑	↑	↓
CO	SV	SVI	CI
↓	↓	↓	↓
RVSWI	LVSWI	PVR	SVR
↑	↓	↑	↓

RADIOLOGIC FINDINGS

Chest Radiograph
- Blunting of the costophrenic angle
- Fluid level on the the affected side (see Figure 23-2)
- Depressed diaphragm

OVERVIEW

of the Cardiopulmonary Clinical Manifestations Associated with
PLEURAL EFFUSION (Continued)

- Mediastinal shift (possibly) to unaffected side
- Atelectasis
- Meniscus sign

The diagnosis of a pleural effusion is generally based on the chest X-ray. A pleural effusion of less than 300 ml usually cannot be seen on an upright chest X-ray film. In moderate pleural effusion (>1000 ml) in the upright position, an increased density usually appears at the costophrenic angle. The fluid first accumulates posteriorly in the most dependent part of the thoracic cavity between the inferior surface of the lower lobe and the diaphragm. As the fluid volume increases, it extends upward around the anterior, lateral, and posterior thoracic walls. Interlobar fissures are sometimes highlighted as a result of fluid filling. On the typical radiograph the lateral costophrenic angle is obliterated, a so-called meniscus sign may develop, and the outline of the diaphragm on the affected side is lost (Figures 23-2

and 23-3). In severe cases the weight of the fluid may cause the diaphragm to become inverted (concave). Clinically, this inversion is seen only in left-sided pleural effusions; the gastric air bubble is pushed downward, and the superior border of the left diaphragmatic leaf is concave. In addition, the mediastinum may be shifted to the unaffected side, and the intercostal spaces may appear widened.

Pleural effusion, atelectasis, and parenchymal infiltrates can obliterate one or both diaphragms. Therefore when a posteroanterior or lateral chest radiograph suggests pleural effusion, additional radiographic studies are generally necessary to document the presence of pleural fluid or other pathology. The lateral decubitus radiograph is recommended because free fluid gravitates to the most dependent part of the pleural space and layers out there (Figure 23-4).

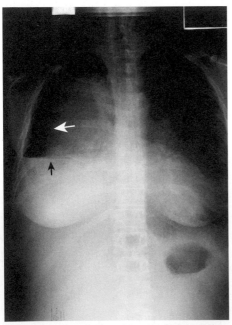

Figure 23–2   Right-sided pleural effusion *(small black arrow)* complicated by a pneumothorax *(large white arrow).*

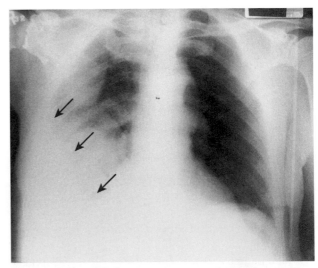

Figure 23–3   Chest radiograph of a patient with a pulmonary abscess in the right lung, extrapleural bleeding *(arrows),* and pleural effusion. (From Rau JL, Jr., Pearce DJ: *Understanding chest radiographs,* Denver, 1984, Multi-Media Publishing.)

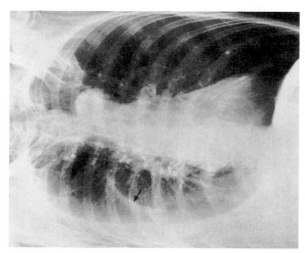

Figure 23–4 Subpulmonic pleural effusion. Right lateral decubitus view. Subdiaphragmatic fluid has run up the lateral chest wall, producing a band of soft tissue density (meniscus sign). The medial curvilinear shadow *(arrow)* indicates fluid in the major fissure.

General Management of Pleural Effusion

The management of each patient with a pleural effusion must be individualized. Questions to be asked include the following: Should a thoracentesis be performed? Can the underlying cause be treated? What is the appropriate antibiotic? Should a chest tube be inserted? When it is determined that a chest tube should be inserted, it is normally placed in the fourth or fifth intercostal space at the midaxillary line. Typically, a #28 to #36 French gauge thoracostomy tube is used for adults, with a smaller size used for children.

An etiologic diagnosis is necessary for the appropriate treatment of a patient with pleural effusion. Examination of the effusion may reveal blood after trauma or surgery, pus in empyema, or milky fluid in chylothorax. The presence of blood in the pleural fluid in the absence of trauma or surgery suggests malignant disease or pulmonary embolization.

When the cause of the pleural effusion is not readily evident, microscopic and chemical examination of pleural fluid may determine whether the effusion is a transudate or an exudate. If the fluid is a transudate, treatment is directed to the underlying problem (e.g., congestive heart failure, cirrhosis, nephrosis). When an exudate is present, a cytologic examination may identify a malignancy. The fluid also may be examined for its biochemical makeup (e.g., protein, sugar, various enzymes) and for the presence of bacteria.

RESPIRATORY CARE TREATMENT PROTOCOLS

Oxygen Therapy Protocol

Oxygen therapy is used to treat hypoxemia, decrease the work of breathing, and decrease myocardial work. The hypoxemia that develops in pleural effusion is mostly caused by the atelectasis and pulmonary shunting associated with the disorder. Hypoxemia caused by capillary shunting is often refractory to oxygen therapy (see Oxygen Therapy Protocol, Protocol 9-1).

Hyperinflation Therapy Protocol

Hyperinflation techniques are often administered to offset the alveolar atelectasis associated with pleural effusions (see Hyperinflation Therapy Protocol, Protocol 9-3).

Mechanical Ventilation Protocol

Because acute ventilatory failure and hypoxemia may be seen in severe pleural effusions, continuous mechanical ventilation may be required to maintain an adequate ventilatory status. Continuous mechanical ventilation is justified when the acute ventilatory failure is thought to be reversible (see Mechanical Ventilation Protocol, Protocol 9-5).

PLEURODESIS

On occasion, a thoracentesis may be performed before a procedure called *pleurodesis*. During this procedure, a chemical or medication (e.g., talc, tetracycline, or bleomycin sulfate) is injected into the chest cavity. The chemical or medication causes an intense inflammatory reaction over the outer surface of the lung and inside of the chest cavity. This procedure is performed to cause the surface of the lung to stick to the chest cavity, thus preventing or reducing recurrent fluid accumulation or pneumothorax.

Case Study: PLEURAL DISEASE

Admitting History

Against her doctor's advice, a 38-year-old Caucasian woman discharged herself from the hospital about 2 months earlier. She had originally been admitted for severe right lower lobe pneumonia. After 5 days of treatment, she became angry because she was not allowed to smoke. She was a longtime, three-pack-per-day smoker. When a nurse found her smoking in her hospital bed while on a 2 L/min oxygen nasal cannula, the nurse quickly confiscated her cigarettes and matches.

The woman became upset. She told her doctor that this was the last straw and that she was going to leave the hospital on her own. Her doctor wanted her to remain so that a thorough follow-up could be performed for what was described as a "spot" on her lower right lung. The woman promised that she would make an appointment at the doctor's office the next week. She then got dressed and left. However, 2 days after she left the hospital, she felt so much better that she decided the spot on her lung was not an issue for concern. The woman told her friends that smoking one pack of cigarettes made her feel better than 5 days' worth of nurses, doctors, and hospitals.

On the day of the present admission, the woman appeared at the doctor's office without an appointment. She told the receptionist that something was very wrong. She thought that she had the flu and that it had been getting progressively worse over the last 4 days. At this time, she could speak in short sentences only and was unable to inhale deeply. Seeing that the woman was in obvious respiratory distress, the nurse interrupted the doctor. Within 5 minutes, the doctor had the woman transported and admitted to the hospital a few blocks away.

Physical Examination

The woman appeared malnourished, exhibited poor personal hygiene, and had yellow tobacco stains around her fingers. She appeared to be in moderate to severe respiratory distress. Her skin was cyanotic, and her shirt was wet from perspiration. She demonstrated an occasional hacking, nonproductive cough. She stated that she could not take a deep breath and that maybe the problem stemmed from that spot on her lung.

Her vital signs were as follows: blood pressure 146/92, heart rate 112 bpm, and respiratory rate 36/min and shallow. She was slightly febrile, with an oral temperature of 37.7° C (99.8° F). Palpation showed that the trachea was shifted slightly to the left. Dull percussion notes were found over the right middle and right lower lobes. Auscultation revealed normal vesicular breath sounds over the left lung fields and upper right lobe. No breath sounds could be heard over the right middle and right lower lobes.

The patient's chest X-ray showed a large, right-sided pleural effusion. The right costophrenic angle demonstrated blunting, the right hemidiaphragm was depressed, and the right middle and lower lung lobes were partially collapsed and showed changes consistent with pneumonia (Figure 23-5). The arterial blood gas values (ABGs) on a 3 L/min oxygen nasal cannula were as follows: pH 7.48, $Paco_2$ 24 mm Hg, HCO_3^- 17 mMol/L, and Pao_2 37 mm Hg. The oxygen

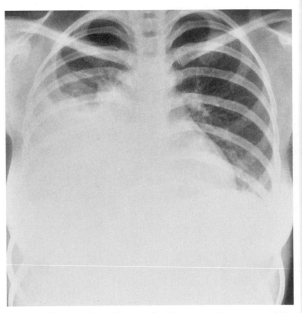

Figure 23–5   Chest X-ray of a 38-year-old woman with pleural disease.

saturation measured by pulse oximetry (Spo$_2$) was 72%. The doctor, assisted by the respiratory therapist, performed a thoracentesis on the patient at the bedside. Slightly more than 2 liters of yellow fluid was withdrawn. The patient then was started on intravenous antibiotics. A portable chest X-ray was ordered, and a respiratory care consult was requested. On the basis of these clinical data, the following SOAP was documented:

Respiratory Assessment and Plan

S "I cannot take a deep breath."

O Malnourished appearance with poor personal hygiene; cyanosis with an occasional hacking, nonproductive cough; vital signs: BP 146/92, HR 112, RR 36 and shallow, T 37.7° C (99.8° F); trachea slightly shifted to the left; dull percussion notes over the right middle and right lower lobes; normal vesicular breath sounds over the left lung fields and right upper lobe; no breath sounds over the right middle and right lower lobes; CXR: large, right-sided pleural effusion, right middle and right lower lobes partially collapsed and consolidated; about 2 L of yellow fluid obtained via thoracentesis; ABGs (on 3 L/min O2 by nasal cannula): pH 7.48 , Paco$_2$ 24, HCO$_3^-$ 17 , Pao$_2$ 37, Spo$_2$ 72 %.

A • Right-sided pneumonia and pleural effusion (CXR)
• Partially collapsed right middle and lower lobes; atelectasis versus pneumonia (CXR)
• Respiratory distress (vital signs, ABGs)
• Acute alveolar hyperventilation with severe hypoxemia (ABGs)
• Metabolic (lactic) acidosis likely (ABGs compared with Pco$_2$-HCO$_3^-$ pH relationship nomogram)

P Begin Hyperinflation Therapy Protocol (incentive spirometry q 2 h) and Oxygen Therapy Protocol (Fio$_2$ = 0.50 per HAFOE mask). Monitor and reevaluate.

• • • • •

3 Hours After Admission

At this time the patient was sitting up in bed. She stated that although she was feeling better, she did not feel great. She still had an occasional dry-sounding, nonproductive cough. Her skin appeared pale and cyanotic. She was no longer perspiring, as she was when she was first admitted. Her vital signs were as follows: blood pressure 135/85, heart rate 100 bpm, respiratory rate 24/min, and temperature normal. Her respiratory efforts, however, no longer appeared shallow. Palpation was not remarkable. Dull percussion notes were found over the right middle and right lower lobes. Normal vesicular breath sounds

were heard over the left lung and upper right lung. Loud bronchial breath sounds were audible over the right middle and right lower lobes.

The patient's chest X-ray showed a small, right-sided pleural effusion. Increased opacity was still present in the right middle and lower lung, consistent with pneumonia. The patient's trachea and mediastinum were in their normal positions. On an Fio$_2$ of 0.50, her ABGs were as follows: pH 7.52, Paco$_2$ 29 mm Hg, HCO$_3^-$ 22 mMol/L, and Pao$_2$ 57 mm Hg. Her Spo$_2$ was 92%. At this time, the following SOAP was charted:

Respiratory Assessment and Plan

S "I'm feeling better but not great yet."

O Cyanotic and pale appearance; occasional dry, nonproductive cough; vital signs: BP 135/85, HR 100, RR 24, T normal; dull percussion notes over right middle and right lower lobes; normal vesicular breath sounds over left lung and over right upper lobe; bronchial breath sounds over right middle and lower lobes; CXR: small right-sided pleural effusion; right middle and right lower lobe consolidation; ABGs: pH 7.52, Paco$_2$ 29, HCO$_3^-$ 22, Pao$_2$ 57; Spo$_2$ 92% on an Fio$_2$ of 0.50.

A • Small right-sided pneumonia and pleural effusion, greatly improved (CXR)
• Atelectasis and consolidation in right middle and lower lung lobes (CXR)
• Continued respiratory distress, but improving (vital signs, ABGs)
• Acute alveolar hyperventilation with moderate hypoxemia, improved (ABGs)

P Up-regulate Hyperinflation Therapy (CPAP mask at 10 cm H$_2$O q 2 h for 15 minutes). Up-regulate Oxygen Therapy per protocol (Fio$_2$ = 0.60 per HAFOE mask). Monitor and reevaluate.

• • • • •

5 Hours After Admission

The patient was situated in a semi-Fowler's position. She appeared relaxed and alert. She stated that she had finally caught her breath. Although she still appeared pale, she did not look cyanotic. No spontaneous cough was observed at this time.

Her vital signs were as follows: blood pressure 128/79, heart rate 88 bpm, respiratory rate 16/min, and temperature normal. Palpation of the chest was unremarkable. Dull percussion notes were found over the right middle and right lower lobes. Normal vesicular breath sounds were heard over the left lung and right upper lobe. Bronchial breath sounds were audible over the right middle and right lower lobes. No current chest X-ray was available. The patient's ABGs on an Fio$_2$ of 0.60 were as follows: pH 7.45,

Paco$_2$ 36 mm Hg, HCO$_3^-$ 24 mMol/L, and Pao$_2$ 77 mm Hg. Her Spo$_2$ was 95%. On the basis of these clinical data, the following SOAP was documented:

Respiratory Assessment and Plan

S "I've finally caught my breath."

O Relaxed, alert appearance, in semi-Fowler's position; paleness but no cyanosis; no spontaneous cough; vital signs: BP 128/79, HR 88, RR 16, T normal; dull percussion notes in right middle and right lower lung lobes; normal vesicular breath sounds over left lung and right upper lobe; bronchial breath sounds over right middle and right lower lobes; ABGs: pH 7.45, Paco$_2$ 36, HCO$_3^-$ 24, Pao$_2$ 77; Spo$_2$ 95%.

A • Small, right-sided pneumonia and pleural effusion, greatly improved (previous CXR)
   • Atelectasis and consolidation in right middle and right lower lung lobes (previous CXR)
   • Normal acid-base status with mild hypoxemia (ABGs)

P Maintain present levels of hyperinflation therapy and oxygen therapy per protocols. Monitor and reevaluate each shift.

Discussion

This case illustrates a patient with pleural effusion, one of the pleural diseases that generally can be improved with appropriate therapy (in this case a 2-liter thoracentesis).

At the end of the **first assessment,** the respiratory care practitioner recognizes that the patient has significant respiratory morbidity. Indeed, the patient has extensive pneumonia and severe hypoxemia, despite alveolar hyperventilation. Understanding that **Atelectasis** is the main pathophysiologic mechanism operating in this case (see Figure 9-7), the practitioner correctly assesses the situation as one that requires careful monitoring and begins oxygen therapy, with a high concentration of oxygen in view of the patient's Pao$_2$. The practitioner recalls that the offending organism(s) is not yet identified and ensures that sputum and thoracentesis fluid cultures are obtained.

A trial of bronchopulmonary hygiene therapy would not be unwarranted in this case, given the patient's cigarette smoking history alone or the degree of severity of the condition. Admittedly, the physical findings in this patient (no wheeze or expiratory prolongation) did not indicate such therapy. Given the patient's history, the respiratory care practitioner also would be interested in the results of the cytologic studies for malignancy in both the sputum and thoracentesis fluid. Frequently, blood gases do not improve immediately after a thoracentesis, despite the fluid removal, because the atelectasis under the pleural effusion takes some time (hours or days) to dissipate. For this reason, hyperinflation therapy after thoracentesis is appropriate.

At the time of the **second assessment,** the patient is beginning to improve, although she has signs of right middle and lower lobe consolidation. Good breath sounds are heard over the left lung and upper right lung, although bronchial breath sounds reflecting consolidation are still noted on the right. The respiratory care practitioner now should be concerned that atelectasis is still present and should increase the hyperinflation therapy with, perhaps, continuous positive airway pressure (CPAP) mask or, possibly, with intensified incentive spirometry or careful use of intermittent positive-pressure breathing (IPPB).

In the **last assessment** the patient continues to do fairly well, although she is far from returning to baseline values. The pneumonitis/atelectasis and mild hypoxemia, which persists despite supplemental oxygen therapy, suggests the need for continued significant (though unchanged) therapy. This case demonstrates that *often in-place therapy does not need to be changed at each assessment.* Indeed, this guide may apply to as many as 50% to 60% of accurately performed seriatim assessments. For pedagogic reasons, this option has not been exercised often in this text. However, this third assessment (in a patient with pleural effusion and underlying atelectasis/pneumonia) is a good case in point.

SELF-ASSESSMENT QUESTIONS

Multiple Choice

1. Which of the following is/are associated with exudative effusion?

   I. Few blood cells
   II. Inflammation
   III. Thin and watery fluid
   IV. Disease of the pleural surfaces

   a. I only
   b. II only
   c. IV only
   d. I and III only
   e. II and IV only

2. Which of the following is probably the most common cause of a transudative pleural effusion?

   a. Pulmonary embolus
   b. Congestive heart failure
   c. Hepatic hydrothorax
   d. Nephrotic syndrome
   e. Peritoneal dialysis

3. A hemothorax is said to be present when the hematocrit of the pleural fluid is at least what percentage of the peripheral blood?

   a. 20
   b. 30
   c. 40
   d. 50
   e. 60

4. Approximately what percentage of patients with pulmonary emboli develop pleural effusion?

   a. 0 to 20
   b. 20 to 30
   c. 30 to 50
   d. 50 to 60
   e. 60 to 80

5. Which of the following is/are associated with pleural effusion?

   I. Increased RV
   II. Decreased FRC
   III. Increased V_T
   IV. Decreased VC

   a. I only
   b. III only
   c. I and III only
   d. II and IV only
   e. II, III, and IV only

True or False

True ☐ False ☐ 1. Chyle in the pleural cavity is commonly caused by trauma to the neck.

True ☐ False ☐ 2. A hyperresonant percussion note is associated with a pleural effusion.

True ☐ False ☐ 3. Left-sided heart failure is more likely to cause a pleural effusion than right-sided heart failure.

True ☐ False ☐ 4. The accumulation of pus in the pleural cavity is called *empyema.*

True ☐ False ☐ 5. Pleural effusion may be caused by a gastrointestinal disorder.

Answers appear in Appendix XI.

CHAPTER 24

Kyphoscoliosis

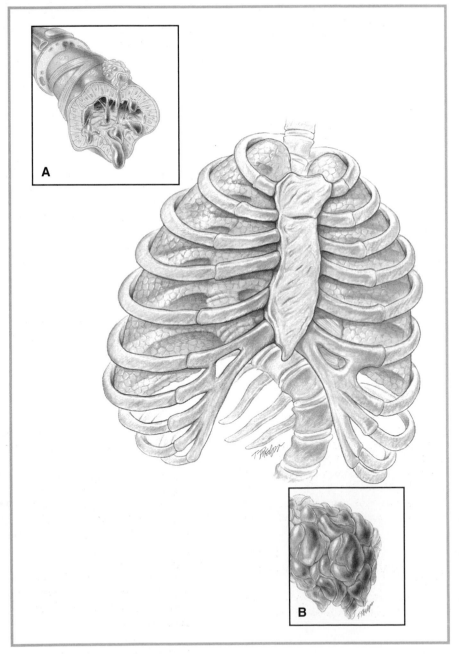

Figure 24–1 Kyphoscoliosis. Posterior and lateral curvature of the spine causing lung compression. Excessive bronchial secretions (**A**) and atelectasis (**B**) are common secondary anatomic alterations of the lungs. See also Plate 16.

Anatomic Alterations of the Lungs

Kyphoscoliosis is a combination of two thoracic deformities that commonly appear together. *Kyphosis* is a posterior curvature of the spine (humpback). In *scoliosis* the spine is curved to one side—typically appearing as an **S** or **C** shape. Its appearance is most obvious in the anterior-posterior plane.

In severe kyphoscoliosis the deformity of the thorax compresses the lungs and restricts alveolar expansion, which in turn causes alveolar hypoventilation and atelectasis. In addition, the patient's ability to cough and mobilize secretions also may be impaired, further causing atelectasis as secretions accumulate throughout the tracheobronchial tree. Because kyphoscoliosis involves both a posterior and lateral curvature of the spine, the thoracic contents generally twist in such a way as to cause a mediastinal shift in the same direction as the lateral curvature of the spine. Severe kyphoscoliosis causes a chronic restrictive lung disorder that makes it more difficult to clear airway secretions. Figure 24-1 illustrates the lung and chest wall abnormalities in a typical case of kyphoscoliosis.

The major pathologic or structural changes of the lungs associated with kyphoscoliosis are as follows:

- Lung restriction and compression as a result of the thoracic deformity
- Mediastinal shift
- Mucus accumulation throughout the tracheobronchial tree
- Atelectasis

Etiology

Kyphoscoliosis affects approximately 2% of the people in the United States—mostly young children who are going through a growing spurt. Kyphoscoliosis rarely develops in the adult—unless it is a worsening condition that started in childhood and was not diagnosed or treated. Kyphoscoliosis may also develop in adults from a degenerative joint condition in the spine. Although the precise cause of kyphoscoliosis is unknown, it is commonly associated with the following conditions:

- Congenital connective tissue and skeletal disorders (e.g., congenital vertebrae defects)
- Hormonal imbalance
- Neuromuscular disorders (e.g., paralytic poliomyelitis, cerebral palsy, spinal muscular atrophy or injury)
- Trauma
- Extraspinal contractures
- Bone infections involving the vertebrae
- Metabolic bone disorders (e.g., rickets, osteoporosis, osteogenesis imperfecta)
- Joint disease
- Tumors

When scoliosis arises without a known cause (about 80% of the cases), it is called *idiopathic kyphoscoliosis*. Depending on the child's age at the time of onset, idiopathic scoliosis is classified as *infantile, juvenile,* or *adolescent.* In *infantile scoliosis* the curvature of the spine develops during the first 3 years of life. In *juvenile scoliosis* the curvature occurs between 4 years and the onset of adolescence. In *adolescent scoliosis* the spine curvature develops after the age of 10. Adolescent scoliosis is the most common. Early signs (i.e., appearing when a child is approximately 8 years of age) of scoliosis include uneven shoulders, prominent shoulder blade or shoulder blades, uneven waist, height, elevated hips, and leaning to one side. Risk factors include the following:

Sex—Girls are 10 times more likely to develop curvature of the spine than boys.

Age—The younger the child is when the diagnosis is first made, the greater the chance of curve progression.

Angle of the curve—The greater the curvature of the spine, the greater the risk that the curve progression will worsen.

Location—In girls with lower back curvature, the curve is less likely to progress.

Height—Taller girls have a greater chance of curve progression.

Spinal problems at birth—Children with scoliosis at birth (congenital scoliosis) may experience a rapid curve progression.

Clinically, scoliosis is commonly defined according to the following factors related to the curvature of the spine:

Shape (Nonstructural and structural scoliosis)—A *nonstructural scoliosis* is a side-to-side curve. This form of scoliosis results from a cause other than the spine itself (e.g., poor posture, leg length discrepancy, pain). A *structural scoliosis* is a curvature of the spine associated with vertebral rotation. A structural scoliosis involves the twisting of the spine and appears in three dimensions.

Location—The curve of the spine may develop in the upper back area (thoracic), the lower back area (lumbar), or between the upper and lower back areas (thoracolumbar).

Direction—The curvature of the spine may bend left or right.

Angle—The angle of the curvature of the spine is determined with a scoliometer by using the vertebra at the apex of the curve as the starting point.

OVERVIEW

of the Cardiopulmonary Clinical Manifestations Associated with KYPHOSCOLIOSIS

The following clinical manifestations result from the pathophysiologic mechanisms caused (or activated) by **Atelectasis** (see Figure 9-7) and **Excessive Airway Secretions** (see Figure 9-11)—the major anatomic alterations of the lungs associated with kyphoscoliosis (see Figure 24-1).

CLINICAL DATA OBTAINED AT THE PATIENT'S BEDSIDE

The Physical Examination

Vital Signs

Increased respiratory rate (see page 31 ◆►)
Several pathophysiologic mechanisms operating simultaneously may lead to an increased ventilatory rate:
- Stimulation of peripheral chemoreceptors (hypoxemia)
- Decreased lung compliance/increased ventilatory rate relationship
- Activation of the deflation receptors
- Activation of the irritant receptors
- Stimulation of the J receptors
- Pain/anxiety

Increased heart rate (pulse), cardiac output, and blood pressure (see pages 11 and 99 ◆►)

Cyanosis (see page 45 ◆►)

Digital Clubbing (see page 46 ◆►)

Peripheral Edema and Venous Distention (see page 47 ◆►)

Because polycythemia and cor pulmonale are associated with kyphoscoliosis, the following may be seen:
- Distended neck veins
- Pitting edema
- Enlarged and tender liver

Cough and Sputum Production (see page 47 ◆►)

Chest Assessment Findings (see page 22 ◆►)
- Obvious thoracic deformity
- Tracheal shift
- Increased tactile and vocal fremitus
- Dull percussion note
- Bronchial breath sounds
- Whispered pectoriloquy
- Crackles, rhonchi, and wheezing

CLINICAL DATA OBTAINED FROM LABORATORY TESTS AND SPECIAL PROCEDURES

Pulmonary Function Study Findings

Expiratory Maneuver Findings (see page 61 ◆►)

FVC	FEV_T	$FEF_{25\%-75\%}$	$FEF_{200-1200}$
↓	N or ↓	N or ↓	N
PEFR	MVV	$FEF_{50\%}$	$FEV_{1\%}$
N	N or ↓	N	N or ↑

Lung Volume and Capacity Findings (see page 62 ◆►)

V_T	RV	FRC	TLC
N or ↓	↓	↓	↓
VC	IC	ERV	RV/TLC%
↓	↓	↓	N

Arterial Blood Gases

Mild to Moderate Kyphoscoliosis
Acute Alveolar Hyperventilation with Hypoxemia (see page 70 ◆►)

pH	$Paco_2$	HCO_3^-	Pao_2
↑	↓	↓ (Slightly)	↓

Severe Kyphoscoliosis
Chronic Ventilatory Failure with Hypoxemia (see page 73 ◆►)

pH	$Paco_2$	HCO_3^-	Pao_2
Normal	↑	↑(Significantly)	↓

Acute Ventilatory Changes Superimposed on Chronic Ventilatory Failure (see page 75 ◆►)
Because acute ventilatory changes are frequently seen in patients with chronic ventilatory failure, the respiratory care practitioner must be familiar with and alert for (1) acute alveolar hyperventilation superimposed on chronic ventilatory failure and (2) acute ventilatory failure superimposed on chronic ventilatory failure.

OVERVIEW

of the Cardiopulmonary Clinical Manifestations Associated with KYPHOSCOLIOSIS (Continued)

Oxygenation Indices (see page 82 ◆▶)

$\dot{Q}_S/\dot{Q}_T$	DO_2*	$\dot{V}O_2$	$C(a-\bar{v})O_2$
↑	↓	Normal	Normal

O_2ER*	$S\bar{v}O_2$		
↑	↓		

*The DO_2 may be normal in patients who have compensated to the decreased oxygenation status with (1) an increased cardiac output, (2) an increased hemoglobin level, or (3) a combination of both. When the DO_2 is normal, the O_2ER is usually normal.

Hemodynamic Indices (Severe Kyphoscoliosis) (see page 99 ◆▶)

CVP	RAP	$\overline{PA}$	PCWP
↑	↑	↑	Normal
CO	SV	SVI	CI
Normal	Normal	Normal	Normal
RVSWI	LVSWI	PVR	SVR
↑	Normal	↑	Normal

LABORATORY FINDINGS

Complete blood cell count (CBC)—Elevated hemoglobin concentration and hematocrit if the patient is chronically hypoxemic

RADIOLOGIC FINDINGS

Chest Radiograph

- Thoracic deformity
- Mediastinal shift
- Increased lung opacity
- Atelectasis in areas of compressed (atelectatic) lungs
- Enlarged heart (cor pulmonale)

The extent of the thoracic deformity in kyphoscoliosis is demonstrated in anteroposterior and lateral radiographs. When present, a mediastinal shift is best shown on an anteroposterior chest radiograph. As the alveoli collapse, the density of the lung increases and is revealed on the chest radiograph as increased opacity. In severe cases, cor pulmonale may be seen (Figure 24-2).

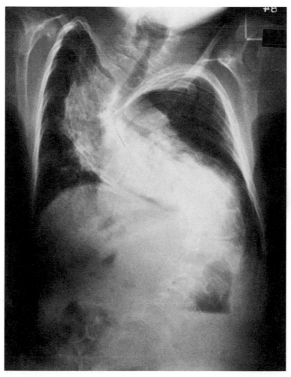

Figure 24–2 Severe kyphoscoliosis in a 14-year-old male patient.

General Management of Scoliosis

In most cases of scoliosis, the degree of abnormal spine curvature is relatively small and requires only observation to ensure that the curve does not worsen. Observation is usually recommended in patients with a spine curvature of less than 20 degrees. In young children who are still growing, observation checkups are usually scheduled in 3- to 6-month intervals. When the curve is determined to be progressing to a more serious degree, treatment may include the following.

BRACES

A brace is recommended for growing children with adolescent idiopathic scoliosis who have a spine curvature of 25 to 45 degrees. Although a brace does not cure scoliosis (or even improve the condition), it has been shown to prevent the curve progression in more than 90% of patients who wear the brace as much as possible, including while they sleep. Today there are a variety of braces available, including the Milwaukee brace, Charleston brace, Boston brace, Wilmington brace, and the thoracolumbosacral orthosis (TLSO). The type of brace is selected according to a number of factors, such as age, the specific characteristics of the curve, and the willingness of the patient to tolerate a specific brace.

For example, the Milwaukee brace is a full-torso brace with a neck ring that serves as a rest for the chin and for the back of the head. This brace has a flat bar in the front and two flat bars in the back. The Milwaukee brace can be used to stabilize a curve anywhere along the spine. A TLSO brace is a closer-fitting brace that is less noticeable under the patient's clothing. The TLSO fits just under the arms and around the rib cage. The TLSO is used primarily to stop the progression of curves that develop below the midpoint of the spine.

SURGERY

Surgery is usually recommended in patients who have curvatures of the spine greater than 40 to 50 degrees. Surgery is usually successful in improving the patient's posture. Surgical procedures include the following.

Posterior Spinal Fusion and Instrumentation

The posterior spinal fusion and instrumentation procedure is the most common. The *fusion* involves placing pieces of bone between two or more vertebrae. The bone sections are taken from the patient's pelvis. Eventually, the bone pieces and the vertebrae fuse together. The *instrumentation* involves the insertion of metal rods, hooks, screws, and wires to prevent the curve from moving for 3 to 12 months and allow the fusion to become solid. In addition, instrumentation applies force to the spine to correct the curvature. Up to 50% improvement of the curvature may occur in patients who elect to have this procedure.

Anterior Spinal Fusion

Occasionally, surgery may involve the anterior portion of the spine. This procedure is performed through the chest cavity and is one of the longest and most complicated orthopedic surgical procedures performed on children.

OTHER APPROACHES

Some physicians may try electrical stimulation of muscles, chiropractic manipulation, and exercise to treat scoliosis. There is no evidence that any of these procedures will stop the progression of spine curvature. Exercise, however, may improve the patient's overall health and well-being.

RESPIRATORY CARE TREATMENT PROTOCOLS

Oxygen Therapy Protocol

Oxygen therapy is used to treat hypoxemia, decrease the work of breathing, and decrease myocardial work. The hypoxemia that develops in kyphoscoliosis is commonly caused by atelectasis and pulmonary shunting. Hypoxemia caused by capillary shunting is often refractory to oxygen therapy. In addition, when the patient demonstrates chronic ventilatory failure during the advanced stages of kyphoscoliosis, caution must be taken not to overoxygenate the patient (see Oxygen Therapy Protocol, Protocol 9-1).

Bronchopulmonary Hygiene Therapy Protocol

A number of bronchial hygiene treatment modalities may be used to enhance the mobilization of the excessive bronchial secretions associated with kyphoscoliosis (see Bronchopulmonary Hygiene Therapy Protocol, Protocol 9-2).

Hyperinflation Therapy Protocol

Hyperinflation modalities are ordered to offset atelectasis (see Hyperinflation Therapy Protocol, Protocol 9-3).

Case Study: KYPHOSCOLIOSIS

Admitting History

A 62-year-old woman began to develop kyphoscoliosis when she was 6 years old. She lived in the mountains of Virginia all her life, first with her parents and later with her two older sisters. Although she wore various types of body braces until she was 17 years old, her disorder was classified as severe by the time she was 15 years old. The doctors, who were few and far between, always told her that she would have to learn to live with her condition the best she could, and as a general rule she did.

She finished high school with no other remarkable physical or personal problems. She was well liked by her classmates and was actively involved in the school newspaper and art club. After graduation she continued to live with her parents for a few more years. At 21 years of age, she moved in with her two older sisters, who were buying a large farmhouse near a small but popular tourist town. All three sisters made various arts and crafts, which they sold at local tourist shops. The woman's physical disability and general health were relatively stable until she was about 40 years old, when she started to experience frequent episodes of dyspnea, coughing, and sputum production. As the years progressed, her baseline condition was marked by increasingly severe dyspnea.

Because the sisters rarely ventured into the city, the woman's medical resources were poor until she was introduced to a social worker at a nearby church. The church had just become part of an outreach program based in a large city nearby. The social worker was charmed by the woman and fascinated by the beauty of the colorful quilts she made.

The social worker, however, also was concerned by the woman's limited ability to move because of her severe chest deformity. In addition, the social worker thought that the woman's cough sounded serious. She noted that the woman appeared grayish-blue, weak, and ill. The sisters told the social worker that their sibling had had a bad "cold" for about 6 months. After much urging, the social worker persuaded the woman to travel, accompanied by her sisters, to the city to see a doctor at a large hospital associated with the church outreach program. The woman was immediately admitted to the hospital. The sisters stayed in a nearby hotel room provided by the hospital.

Physical Examination

The woman appeared to be well nourished and suffering from severe kyphoscoliosis. The lateral curvature of the spine was twisted significantly to the patient's left. In addition, she also demonstrated anterior bending of the thoracic spine. She appeared older than her stated age, and she was in obvious respiratory distress. The patient stated that she was having trouble breathing. Her skin was cyanotic. She had digital clubbing, and her neck veins were distended, especially on the right side. The woman demonstrated a frequent but adequate cough. During each coughing episode she expectorated a moderate amount of thick, yellow sputum.

When the patient generated a strong cough, a large unilateral bulge appeared at the right anterolateral base of her neck, directly posterior to the clavicle. The patient referred to the bulge as her "Dizzy Gillespie pouch." The doctor thought that the bulge was a result of the severe kyphoscoliosis, which had in turn stretched and weakened the suprapleural membrane that normally restricts and contains the parietal pleura at the apex of the lung. Because of the weakening of the suprapleural membrane, any time the woman produced a Valsalva's maneuver for any reason (e.g., for coughing), the increased intrapleural pressure herniated the suprapleural membrane outward. Despite the odd appearance of the bulge, the doctor did not consider it a serious concern at this time.

The patient's vital signs were as follows: blood pressure 160/100, heart rate 90 bpm, respiratory rate 18/min, and oral temperature 36.3° C (97.4° F). Palpation revealed a trachea deviated to the right. Dull percussion notes were produced over both lungs; crackles and rhonchi were heard over them as well. A pulmonary function test (PFT) conducted that morning showed vital capacity (VC), functional residual capacity (FRC), and residual volume (RV) between 45% and 50% of predicted values.

Although the patient's electrolytes were all normal, her hematocrit was 58%, and her hemoglobin level was 18 g/dl. A chest X-ray revealed a severe thoracic and spinous deformity, a mediastinal shift, an enlarged heart with prominent pulmonary artery segments bilaterally, and bilateral infiltrates in the lung bases consistent with pneumonia and atelectasis (Figure 24-3). The patient's arterial blood gas values (ABGs) on room air were as follows: pH 7.52, $Paco_2$ 58 mm Hg, HCO_3^- 42 mMol/L, and Pao_2 49 mm Hg. Her oxygen saturation measured by pulse oximetry (Spo_2) was 78%. The physician requested a respiratory care consult and stated that mechanical ventilation was not an option at this time per the patient's request and his knowledge of the case. On the basis of these clinical data, the following SOAP was documented:

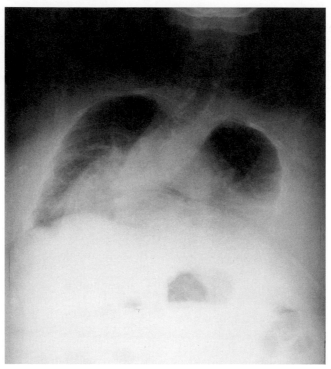

Figure 24–3   Chest X-ray of a 62-year-old female patient with kyphoscoliosis.

Respiratory Assessment and Plan

S "I'm having trouble breathing."

O Well-nourished appearance; severe anterior and left lateral curvature of the spine; cyanosis, digital clubbing, and distended neck veins—especially on the right side; cough: frequent, adequate, and productive of moderate amounts of thick yellow sputum; vital signs: BP 160/100, HR 90, RR 18, T 36.3° C (97.4° F); trachea deviated to the right; both lungs: dull percussion notes, crackles, and rhonchi; PFT: VC, FRC, and RV 45% to 50% of predicted; Hct 58%, Hb 18 g/dl; CXR: severe thoracic and spinous deformity, mediastinal shift, cardiomegaly, and bilateral infiltrates in the lung bases consistent with pneumonia or atelectasis; ABGs (room air): pH 7.52, $Paco_2$ 58, HCO_3^- 42, Pao_2 49; Spo_2 78%

A • Severe kyphoscoliosis (history, CXR, ABGs, physical examination)
 • Increased work of breathing (elevated blood pressure, heart rate, and respiratory rate)
 • Excessive bronchial secretions (sputum, rhonchi)
 • Infection likely (thick, yellow sputum)
 • Good ability to mobilize secretions (strong cough)
 • Atelectasis and consolidation (CXR)

 • Acute alveolar hyperventilation superimposed on chronic ventilatory failure with moderate hypoxemia (ABGs)
 • Possible impending ventilatory failure
 • Cor pulmonale (CXR and physical examination)

P Initiate oxygen therapy protocol (HAFOE at Fio_2 0.28; be careful not to overoxygenate the patient) and bronchopulmonary hygiene therapy protocol (sputum for Gram's stain and culture; C&DB instructions and oral suction prn). Begin hyperinflation therapy protocol (incentive spirometry qid and prn). Begin aerosolized medication protocol (IPPB with aerosolized albuterol 0.5 cc in 1.5 cc 10% acetylcysteine q 4 h). Notify physician of admitting ABGs and possible ventilatory failure. Place mechanical ventilator on standby. When patient is stable, educate about possible future use of noninvasive positive-pressure ventilation (NPPV). Monitor q 1 h × 8 hours, then 23/shift if stable.

• • • • •

10 Hours After Admission

The patient had not improved and was transferred to an intensive care unit. The physician had trouble titrating the cardiac drugs and decided to insert a pulmonary artery catheter, a central venous catheter, and an arterial line. Because of the woman's cardiac problems, several medical students, respiratory therapists, nurses, and doctors were constantly in and out of her room, performing and assisting in various procedures. As a result, working with the patient for any length of time was difficult, and the intensity of respiratory care was less than desirable. Eventually, the patient's cardiac status stabilized, and the physician requested an update on the woman's pulmonary condition.

The respiratory therapist working on the pulmonary consult team found the patient in extreme respiratory distress. She was sitting up in bed, appeared frightened, and stated that she was extremely short of breath. Both of her sisters were in the room; one sister was putting cold towels on the patient's face while the other sister was holding the patient's hands. Both sisters were crying softly.

The woman's skin appeared cyanotic, and perspiration was visible on her face. Her neck veins were still distended. She demonstrated a weak, spontaneous cough. Although no sputum was noted, she sounded congested when she coughed. Dull percussion notes, crackles, and rhonchi were still present throughout both lungs. Her vital signs were as follows: blood pressure 180/120, heart rate 130 bpm, respiratory rate 26/min, and rectal temperature 37.8° C (100° F).

Several of the woman's hemodynamic indices were elevated: CVP, RAP, $\overline{PA}$, RVSWI, and PVR.* All other hemodynamic indices were normal. Her oxygenation indices were as follows: increased $\dot{Q}s/\dot{Q}T$ and O_2ER and decreased Do_2 and $S\overline{v}o_2$. Her $\dot{V}o_2$ and $C(a-\overline{v})o_2$ were normal.† No recent chest X-ray was available. Her ABGs were as follows: pH 7.57, $Paco_2$ 49 mm Hg, HCO_3^- 40 mMol/L, and Pao_2 43 mm Hg. Her Spo_2 was 76%. On the basis of these clinical data, the following SOAP was documented:

Respiratory Assessment and Plan

S Severe dyspnea; "I'm extremely short of breath."

O Extreme respiratory distress; cyanosis and perspiration; distended neck veins; weak, spontaneous cough; sounds of congestion but no sputum produced; bilateral dull percussion

notes, crackles, and rhonchi; vital signs: BP 180/120, HR 130, RR 26, T 37.8° C (100° F); hemodynamics: increased CVP, RAP, $\overline{PA}$, RVSWI, and PVR; all other hemodynamic values, including PCWP, normal; oxygenation indices: increased $\dot{Q}s/\dot{Q}T$, and O_2ER and decreased Do_2 and $S\overline{v}o_2$; $\dot{V}o_2$ and $c(a-\overline{v})o_2$ normal; ABGs; pH 7.57, $Paco_2$ 49, HCO_3^- 40, Pao_2 43; Spo_2 76%

A • Severe kyphoscoliosis (history, physical exam, ABGs, CXR)
   • Increased work of breathing, worsening (increased blood pressure, heart rate, and respiratory rate)
   • Excessive bronchial secretions (rhonchi, congested cough)
   • Atelectasis and consolidation (previous CXR)
   • Acute alveolar hyperventilation superimposed on chronic ventilatory failure with moderate-to-severe hypoxemia (ABGs and history)
   • Continued critically ill status, but chances of avoiding ventilatory failure improving

P Up-regulate oxygen therapy protocol (HAFOE at 0.35). Up-regulate bronchopulmonary hygiene therapy protocol CPT and PD qid). Up-regulate aerosolized medication protocol (increase in IPPB med. nebs. to q 2 h). Contact physician regarding possible ventilatory failure. Discuss therapeutic bronchoscopy with physician. Continue to keep mechanical ventilator on standby. Monitor and reevaluate in 30 minutes

• • • • •

24 Hours After Admission

At this time the respiratory care practitioner found the patient watching the morning news on television with her two sisters. The woman was situated in a semi-Fowler's position eating the last few bites of her breakfast. The patient stated that she felt "so much better" and that "finally I have enough wind to eat some food."

Although her skin still appeared pale and cyanotic, she did not look as bad as she had the day before. On request, she produced a strong cough and expectorated a small amount of white sputum. Her vital signs were as follows: blood pressure 140/85, heart rate 83 bpm, respiratory rate 14/min, and temperature normal. Chest assessment findings demonstrated crackles, rhonchi, and dull percussion notes over both lung fields. The rhonchi were less intense, however, than they had been the day before.

Although the patient's hemodynamic and oxygenation indices were better than they had been the day before, she still had room for improvement. Her hemodynamic parameters, still abnormal, revealed an

---

*CVP, central venous pressure; RAP, right atrial pressure; $\overline{PA}$, mean pulmonary artery pressure; RVSWI, right ventricular stroke work index; PVR, pulmonary vascular resistance.

†$\dot{Q}s/\dot{Q}T$, Cardiac output shunted per total cardiac output; O_2ER, oxygen extraction ratio; Do_2, total oxygen delivery; $S\overline{v}o_2$, mixed venous oxygen saturation;$\dot{V}o_2$, oxygen consumption per unit time; $C(a-\overline{v})o_2$, arterial-mixed venous difference in oxygen content.

elevated CVP, RAP, $\overline{PA}$, RVSWI, and PVR. All other hemodynamic indices were normal. Her oxygenation indices still showed an increased $\dot{Q}s/\dot{Q}T$ and O_2ER and a decreased DO_2 and $S\overline{v}O_2$. Her $\dot{V}O_2$ and $C(a-\overline{v})O_2$ were normal. The patient's chest X-ray taken earlier that morning showed some clearing of the pneumonia and atelectasis described on admission. Her ABGs were as follows: pH 7.45, $Paco_2$ 73 mm Hg, HCO_3^- 48 mMol/L, and PaO_2 68 mm Hg. Her Spo_2 was 93%. On the basis of these clinical data, the following SOAP was recorded:

Respiratory Assessment and Plan

S "I feel so much better. I finally have enough wind to eat some food."

O Pale and cyanotic appearance; cough: strong, small amount of white sputum; vital signs: BP 140/85, HR 83, RR 14, T normal; crackles, rhonchi, and dull percussion notes over both lung fields; rhonchi improving; hemodynamic and oxygenation indices improving, but still an elevated CVP, RAP, $\overline{PA}$, RVSWI, and PVR and still an increased $\dot{Q}s/\dot{Q}T$ and O_2ER and a decreased DO_2 and $S\overline{v}O_2$; CXR: improvement of the bilateral pneumonia and atelectasis; ABGs: pH 7.45, $Paco_2$ 73, HCO_3^- 48, PaO_2 68; Spo_2 93%

A • Generally improved respiratory status (history, CXR, hemodynamic and oxygenation indices, ABG)
   • Significant improvement in problem with excessive bronchial secretions (rhonchi, cough)
   • Improvement in atelectasis and consolidation (CXR)
   • Chronic ventilatory failure with mild hypoxemia (ABGs)
   • Current ABGs likely close to patient's normal (baseline) ABGs

P Down-regulate oxygen therapy, bronchopulmonary hygiene therapy, and aerosolized medication protocols. Continue to monitor and reevaluate (ABGs on reduced FIO_2). Recommend pulmonary rehabilitation and patient and family education (possibly rocking bed, positive expiratory pressure [PEP], or cuirass respiratory ventilation).

Discussion

This case provides an excessive amount of extraneous historical, personal material. This was done to demonstrate, in part, how the respiratory care worker cuts through to the core of the case in the SOAP notes. Care of the patient with symptomatic advanced kyphoscoliosis consists of (1) treatment of the conditions that can complicate it (e.g., bronchitis, pneumonia, atelectasis, pleural effusion) and (2) treatment of the underlying condition itself.

With respect to the issue of long-term ventilatory support, the direct treatment of respiratory pump failure as it occurs in kyphoscoliotic lung disease depends on the patient's willingness to spend the last months or years of life on a ventilator.

Initial evaluation of this patient suggests that infection is present because of the yellow sputum and recent history. The initial chest X-ray also suggests this finding. Clearly respiratory failure is impending, and the therapist's desire to cautiously oxygenate the patient, administer bronchial hygiene and mucolytic aerosols, and to be prepared for ventilator support are all appropriate. The patient's secondary polycythemia and cor pulmonale should improve as overall oxygenation improves, although this improvement may take some time. The patient's hypertension may reflect CO_2 retention, which must be monitored carefully. The digital clubbing and cor pulmonale itself suggest that the hypoxemia is long standing.

At the time of the **second assessment** the patient still demonstrates signs of atelectasis or pneumonia despite vigorous bronchial hygiene therapy. For example, these conditions were verified by the continued observation of the high pulse and respiratory rate, dull percussion notes, acute alveolar hyperventilation, **Atelectasis** on the chest X-ray, and poor response to oxygen therapy (see Figure 9-8).

Atelectasis is often refractory to oxygen therapy, suggesting that therapeutic bronchoscopy might be worthwhile. Although the outlook seems dismal at this point, many clinicians find that vigorous treatment of the complicating factors (in this case hypertension and atelectasis or pneumonia) often carries the day and that the patient does recover, despite early predictions to the contrary.

In the **last assessment**, rehabilitation and family education are appropriately considered. The patient is still retaining CO_2. Indeed, the $Paco_2$ is higher than it was on admission. However, the reader should know that the high $Paco_2$ is close to the patient's normal level. In fact, according to the pH (normal but on the alkalotic side of normal) the patient's usual $Paco_2$ is most likely somewhat higher than this last assessment value.

Comparison with baseline values would be appropriate at this time, and consideration of cuirass ventilation, a rocking bed, or NIPPV to assist nocturnal ventilation may be in order. Oxygenation easily can be assessed by oximetry at home. This case is an excellent example of the value of hemodynamic monitoring (specifically the normal PCWP) in differentiating left-sided from right-sided cardiac failure.

SELF-ASSESSMENT QUESTIONS

Multiple Choice

1. What kind of curvature of the spine is manifested in kyphosis?

   a. Posterior
   b. Anterior
   c. Lateral
   d. Medial
   e. Posterior and lateral

2. Kyphoscoliosis affects approximately what percentage of the U.S. population?

   a. 2
   b. 5
   c. 10
   d. 15
   e. 20

3. Which of the following is/are associated with kyphoscoliosis?

   I. Increased FRC
   II. Decreased V_T
   III. Increased TLC
   IV. Decreased RV

   a. I only
   b. IV only
   c. II and IV only
   d. III and IV only
   e. II, III, and IV only

4. Which of the following are associated with kyphoscoliosis?

   I. Bronchial breath sounds
   II. Hyperresonant percussion note
   III. Whispered pectoriloquy
   IV. Diminished breath sounds

   a. I and III only
   b. II and IV only
   c. III and IV only
   d. II, III, and IV only
   e. I, II, and III only

5. During the advanced stages of kyphoscoliosis, the patient commonly demonstrates which of the following arterial blood gas values?

   I. Increased HCO_3^-
   II. Decreased pH
   III. Increased Pa_{CO_2}
   IV. Normal pH
   V. Decreased HCO_3^-

   a. I only
   b. II only
   c. III and IV only
   d. II and V only
   e. I, III, and IV only

True or False

True ☐ False ☐ 1. When kyphoscoliosis arises without a known cause, it is called *idiopathic kyphoscoliosis.*

True ☐ False ☐ 2. Kyphoscoliosis is classified as an obstructive lung disorder.

True ☐ False ☐ 3. Girls are 10 times more likely to develop curvature of the spine than boys.

True ☐ False ☐ 4. The anatomic alterations of the lungs associated with kyphoscoliosis cause a shuntlike effect.

True ☐ False ☐ 5. Kyphoscoliosis causes the patient's PEFR to increase.

Answers appear in Appendix XI.

PART VII

Environmental Lung Diseases

CHAPTER 25

Pneumoconiosis

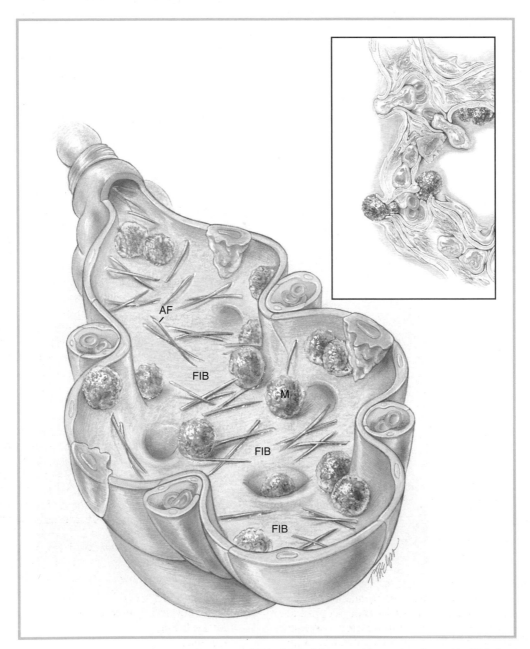

Figure 25–1   Pneumoconiosis, illustrated here in a case of asbestosis (close-up of one alveolar unit). *AF,* Asbestos fiber; *FIB,* fibrosis; *M,* macrophage. *Inset,* Cross-section showing fibrotic thickening of the alveolus, a common secondary anatomic alteration of the lungs. See also Plate 17.

Anatomic Alterations of the Lungs

Pneumoconiosis is a general term used to describe diseases of the lungs that are caused by the chronic inhalation of inorganic dusts and particulate matter, usually of occupational or environmental origin (e.g., coal dust, asbestos, silica; Figure 25-1). When inorganic dusts or particulate matter are inhaled, the smaller particles stick to, and become imbedded in, the moist surfaces of the respiratory bronchioles, alveolar ducts, and alveoli.

The initial lung response is inflammation and phagocytosis of the particles by alveolar macrophages. The macrophages engulf and carry the particles to the terminal bronchioles from where they are normally propelled out of the lungs by the mucociliary escalator. Some particles are carried to the lymphatic vessels and then to the lymph nodes, primarily the nodes around the hilum. During excessive exposure, however, the mucociliary system becomes overwhelmed, which results in the accumulation of particles on its surface. When this happens, the dust particles become enmeshed in a network of collagen and fibrin, and the lungs become fibrotic and stiffen (lung compliance decreases). Characteristic of pneumoconioses is the fact that the pulmonary fibrosis may continue despite the cessation of dust exposure.

Some dust particles (e.g., silica) have a toxic effect on the macrophages that ingest them. The macrophages disintegrate and release substances that activate successive waves of macrophages. When the newly recruited macrophages engulf the liberated dust particles, they in turn disintegrate. Some particles have the ability to penetrate the interstitial space (e.g., asbestos, coal dust, silica). As the disease progresses, the alveoli and adjacent pulmonary capillaries are destroyed and replaced by fibrous, cystlike structures. The cysts are commonly about 1.0 cm in diameter and produce a honeycomb appearance on gross examination. In severe cases, and particularly in asbestosis, fibrotic thickening and calcification of the pleura often produce fibrocalcific pleural plaques. This pathologic process frequently extends into—or involves—the diaphragm. Some environmental irritants, most notably asbestos, also may be carcinogenic.

In general, the pneumoconioses produce a restrictive pulmonary disease. However, because the inorganic dusts and particulate matter also can accumulate in the small airways, chronic inflammation, swelling, and bronchial obstruction frequently develop. When this condition is present, clinical manifestations of airway obstruction are seen. The patient with pneumoconiosis therefore may demonstrate a restrictive disorder, an obstructive disorder, or a combination of both.

The major pathologic or structural changes associated with pneumoconiosis are as follows:

- Destruction of the alveoli and adjacent pulmonary capillaries
- Fibrotic thickening of the respiratory bronchioles, alveolar ducts, and alveoli
- Cystlike structures (honeycomb appearance)
- Fibrocalcific pleural plaques (particularly in asbestosis)
- Airway obstruction caused by inflammation and excessive bronchial secretions
- Bronchospasm
- Bronchogenic carcinoma
- Mesothelioma (in asbestosis)

Etiology

The etiologic determinants for the development of pneumoconiosis include (1) the size of the inhaled particle (only particles between 0.3 and 0.5 μm are likely to reach the alveoli), (2) its chemical nature, (3) its concentration, (4) the length of exposure, and (5) the individual's susceptibility to specific inorganic dusts or particulate matter. Clinically, the diagnosis of a specific cause of a pneumoconiosis may be difficult. In general, the diagnosis is based on the history of the individual, X-ray films, pulmonary function studies, and, in some cases, lung biopsy.

Some of the major causes of pneumoconiosis are covered in the following paragraphs.

ASBESTOSIS

Exposure to asbestos may cause asbestosis. Asbestos fibers are a mixture of fibrous minerals composed of hydrous silicates of magnesium, sodium, and iron in various proportions. There are two primary types: the amphiboles (crocidolite, amosite, and anthophyllite) and chrysotile (most commonly used in industry). Asbestos fibers typically range between 50 and 100 μ in length and are about 0.5 μm in diameter. The chrysotiles have the longest and strongest fibers.

Industrial areas and commercial products associated with asbestos fibers include the following:

- Acoustic products
- Automobile undercoating
- Brake lining
- Cements
- Clutch casings
- Floor tiles
- Fire-fighting suits

- Fireproof paints
- Insulation
- Roofing materials
- Ropes
- Steam pipe material

Asbestos fibers can be seen by microscope within the thickened septa as brown or orange batonlike structures. The fibers characteristically stain for iron with Perls' stain. The pathologic process may affect only one lung, a lobe, or a segment of a lobe. The lower lobes are most commonly affected (see Figure 25-2). Pleural calcification is common and diagnostic in patients with an asbestos exposure history (see Figure 25-3).

COAL WORKER'S PNEUMOCONIOSIS

The deposition and accumulation of large amounts of coal dust cause what is known as *coal worker's pneumoconiosis (CWP)*. CWP also is known as *coal miner's lung, black lung, black phthisis,* and *miner's phthisis.* Miners who use cutting machines at the coal face have the greatest exposure, but even relatively minor exposures may result in the disease. Indeed, cases have been reported in which coal miners' wives develop the disease, presumably from shaking the dust from their husbands' work clothes.

Simple CWP is characterized by the presence of pinpoint nodules called *coal macules (black spots)* throughout the lungs. The coal macules often develop around the first- and second-generation respiratory bronchioles and cause the adjacent alveoli to retract. This condition is called *focal emphysema.*

Complicated CWP or progressive massive fibrosis (PMF) is characterized by areas of fibrotic nodules greater than 1 cm. The fibrotic nodules generally appear in the peripheral regions of upper lobes and extend toward the hilum with growth. The nodules are composed of dense collagenous tissue with black pigmentation. Coal dust by itself is chemically inert. The fibrotic changes in CWP are usually caused by silica.

SILICOSIS

Silicosis (also called *grinder's disease* or *quartz silicosis*) is caused by the chronic inhalation of crystalline, free silica or silicon dioxide particles. Silica is the main component of more than 95% of the rocks of the earth. It is found in sandstone, quartz (beach sand is mostly quartz), flint, granite, many hard rocks, and some clays.

Simple silicosis is characterized by small rounded nodules scattered throughout the lungs. No single nodule is greater than 9 mm. Patients with simple silicosis are usually symptom free.

Complicated silicosis is characterized by nodules that coalesce and form large masses of fibrous tissues, usually in the upper lobes and perihilar regions. In severe cases the fibrotic regions may undergo tissue necrosis and cavitate.

Occupations in which an individual may be exposed to silica include the following:

- Tunneling
- Hard-rock mining
- Sandblasting
- Quarrying
- Stonecutting
- Foundry work
- Ceramics work
- Abrasives work
- Brick making
- Paint making
- Polishing
- Stone drilling
- Well drilling

BERYLLIOSIS

Beryllium is a steel-gray, lightweight metal found in certain plastics and ceramics, rocket fuels, and X-ray tubes. As a raw ore, beryllium is not hazardous. When it is processed into the pure metal or one of its salts, however, it may cause a tissue reaction when inhaled or implanted into the skin. The acute inhalation of beryllium fumes or particles may cause a toxic or allergic pneumonitis sometimes accompanied by rhinitis, pharyngitis, and tracheobronchitis. The more complex form of berylliosis is characterized by the development of granulomas and a diffuse interstitial inflammatory reaction.

OTHER FORMS OF PNEUMOCONIOSIS

Additional causes of pneumoconiosis include the following:

Aluminum
- Ammunition workers
Baritosis (barium)
- Barite millers and miners
- Ceramics workers
Kaolinosis (clay)
- Brick makers and potters
- Ceramics workers
Siderosis (iron)
- Welders
Talcosis (certain talcs)
- Ceramics workers
- Papermakers
- Plastics and rubber workers

OVERVIEW
of the Cardiopulmonary Clinical Manifestations Associated with PNEUMOCONIOSIS

The following clinical manifestations result from the pathophysiologic mechanisms caused (or activated) by an **Increased Alveolar-Capillary Membrane Thickness** (see Figure 9-9), **Bronchospasm** (see Figure 9-10), and **Excessive Bronchial Secretions** (see Figure 9-11)—the major anatomic alterations of the lungs associated with pneumoconiosis (see Figure 25-1).

CLINICAL DATA OBTAINED AT THE PATIENT'S BEDSIDE

The Physical Examination
Vital Signs

Increased respiratory rate (see page 31 ◆►)
Several pathophysiologic mechanisms operating simultaneously may lead to an increased ventilatory rate:
- Stimulation of peripheral chemoreceptors (hypoxemia)
- Decreased lung compliance/increased ventilatory rate relationship
- Stimulation of the J receptors
- Pain/anxiety

Increased heart rate (pulse), cardiac output, and blood pressure
(see pages 11 and 99 ◆►).

Cyanosis (see page 45 ◆►)

Digital Clubbing (see page 46 ◆►)

Peripheral Edema and Venous Distention
(see page 47 ◆►)

Because polycythemia and cor pulmonale are associated with pneumoconiosis, the following may be seen:
- Distended neck veins
- Pitting edema
- Enlarged and tender liver

Cough and Sputum Production
(see page 47 ◆►)

Chest Assessment Findings
(see page 22 ◆►)
- Increased tactile and vocal fremitus
- Dull percussion note
- Bronchial breath sounds
- Crackles, rhonchi, and wheezing
- Pleural friction rub
- Whispered pectoriloquy

CLINICAL DATA OBTAINED FROM LABORATORY TESTS AND SPECIAL PROCEDURES

Pulmonary Function Study Findings
Expiratory Maneuver Findings (see page 61 ◆►)

FVC	FEV_T	$FEF_{25\%-75\%}$	$FEF_{200-1200}$
↓	↓	↓	↓
PEFR	MVV	$FEF_{50\%}$	$FEV_{1\%}$
↓	↓	↓	normal/↓

Lung Volume and Capacity Findings
(see page 62 ◆►)

V_T	RV	FRC	TLC
↓	↓	↓	↓
VC	IC	ERV	RV/TLC ratio
↓	↓	↓	normal/↓

Decreased Diffusion Capacity (DL_{CO})
(see page 67 ◆►)

Arterial Blood Gases
Mild to Moderate Pneumoconiosis
Acute Alveolar Hyperventilation with Hypoxemia
(see page 70 ◆►)

pH	$Paco_2$	HCO_3	PaO_2
↑	↓	↓ (Slightly)	↓

Severe Pneumoconiosis with Extensive Fibrosis
Chronic Ventilatory Failure with Hypoxemia
(see page 73 ◆►)

pH	$Paco_2$	HCO_3^-	Pao_2
Normal	↑	↑(Significantly)	↓

Acute Ventilatory Changes Superimposed on Chronic Ventilatory Failure (see page 75 ◆►)
Because acute ventilatory changes frequently are seen in patients with chronic ventilatory failure, the respiratory care practitioner must be familiar with and alert for (1) acute alveolar hyperventilation superimposed on chronic ventilatory failure and (2) acute ventilatory failure superimposed on chronic ventilatory failure.

OVERVIEW

of the Cardiopulmonary Clinical Manifestations Associated with
PNEUMOCONIOSIS (Continued)

Oxygenation Indices (see page 82 ◆▶)

$\dot{Q}_s/\dot{Q}_T$	DO_2*	$\dot{V}O_2$	$C(a-\bar{v})O_2$
↑	↓	Normal	Normal

O_2ER	$S\bar{v}O_2$		
↑	↓		

*The DO_2 may be normal in patients who have compensated to the decreased oxygenation status with (1) an increased cardiac output, (2) an increased hemoglobin level, or (3) a combination of both. When the DO_2 is normal, the O_2ER is usually normal.

Hemodynamic Indices (Severe Pneumoconiosis) (see page 99 ◆▶)

CVP	RAP	$\overline{PA}$	PCWP
↑	↑	↑	Normal
CO	SV	SVI	CI
Normal	Normal	Normal	Normal
RVSWI	LVSWI	PVR	SVR
↑	Normal	↑	Normal

LABORATORY FINDINGS

Complete blood cell count (CBC)—Elevated hemoglobin concentration and hematocrit if the patient is chronically hypoxemic

RADIOLOGIC FINDINGS

Chest Radiograph

- Small rounded opacities scattered throughout the lung
- Irregularly shaped opacities
- Irregular cardiac and diaphragmatic borders
- Pleural plaques
- Honeycomb appearance

Because of the inflammation, tissue thickening, fibrosis, calcification, and pleural plaques, the density of the lungs on the X-ray progressively increases. The increased lung density resists X-ray penetration and is revealed on X-ray films as increased opacity (i.e., whiter in appearance).

Patients with simple silicosis often show small rounded opacities scattered throughout the lungs. In complicated silicosis, huge densities are often seen in the upper lung fields. The hilar region may be elevated, and the lower lobes may show emphysematous changes. Another characteristic feature in a small percentage of patients with silicosis is the appearance of eggshell-like calcifications around the hilar region.

In patients with CWP the rounded opacities scattered throughout the lung are smaller and less well defined than those seen in silicosis. In general, however, the radiographic appearance of silicosis and CWP is quite similar. When large opacities are present (greater than 1 cm), complicated CWP is diagnosed. Cavity formation also may be seen on the chest X-ray.

In patients with asbestosis, the opacity is frequently described as a clouding or as having a "ground-glass" appearance and is particularly apparent in the lower lung lobes (Figure 25-2). When substantial calcifications and pleural plaques are present in the pleural space, irregularly shaped opacities are often seen. Calcified pleural plaques also may be seen on the superior border of the diaphragm (Figure 25-3). The inflammatory response elicited by the asbestos fibers also may produce a fuzziness and irregularity of the cardiac and diaphragmatic borders. Pleural effusion may be present in patients with asbestosis.

Finally, because several of the pneumoconioses are capable of causing cavity formation and cystlike structures, a honeycomb pattern may be seen.

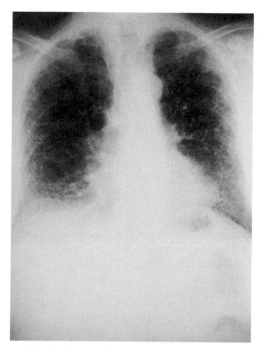

Figure 25–2   Chest X-ray of a patient with asbestosis.

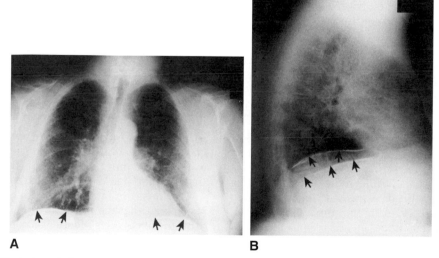

A   **B**

Figure 25–3   Calcified pleural plaques on the superior border of the diaphragm *(arrows)* in a patient with asbestosis. Thickening of the pleural margins also is seen along the lower lateral borders of the chest. **A,** Anteroposterior view. **B,** Lateral view.

General Management of Pneumoconiosis

Control of occupational diseases is the responsibility of the worker, management, the community health department, and the state and federal governments. Prevention is the key. It involves education in protective measures, management cooperation in supplying proper equipment and conditions, inspection and testing services provided by management and by the government, adequate medical and first aid services at the work site, adequate hospitalization insurance and compensation, and research to improve safety.

After the disease is established, it has no effective cure. Of course, individuals who demonstrate suspicious clinical manifestations should be removed from any environment in which they are exposed to inorganic dusts and particulate matter. The long-term prognosis of workers who develop pneumoconiosis is poor. Treatment is directed toward symptoms of the disease.

RESPIRATORY CARE TREATMENT PROTOCOLS

Oxygen Therapy Protocol

Oxygen therapy is used to treat hypoxemia, decrease the work of breathing, and decrease myocardial work. Because of the hypoxemia associated with pneumoconiosis, supplemental oxygen may be required. The hypoxemia that develops in pneumoconiosis is most commonly caused by the alveolar thickening, fibrosis, and capillary shunting associated with the disorder. Hypoxemia caused by capillary shunting is often refractory to oxygen therapy. In addition, when the patient demonstrates chronic ventilatory failure during the advanced stages of a pneumoconiosis disorder, caution must be taken not to overoxygenate the patient (see Oxygen Therapy Protocol, Protocol 9-1).

Bronchopulmonary Hygiene Therapy Protocol

Because of the excessive mucus production and accumulation associated with pneumoconiosis, a number of bronchial hygiene treatment modalities may be used to enhance the mobilization of bronchial secretions (see Bronchopulmonary Hygiene Therapy Protocol, Protocol 9-2).

Aerosolized Medication Protocol

Both sympathomimetic and parasympatholytic agents are commonly used to offset bronchial smooth muscle constriction (see Aerosolized Medication Protocol, Protocol 9-4), especially if concomitant chronic obstructive pulmonary disease is present.

Mechanical Ventilation Protocol

Mechanical ventilation may be needed to provide and support alveolar gas exchange and eventually return the patient to spontaneous breathing (e.g., when an acute pneumonia complicates the patient's condition). Because acute ventilatory failure superimposed on chronic ventilatory failure is often seen in patients with severe pneumoconiosis disorders, continuous mechanical ventilation may sometimes be required. Continuous mechanical ventilation is justified when the acute ventilatory failure is thought to be reversible (see Mechanical Ventilation Protocol, Protocol 9-5).

Case Study: PNEUMOCONIOSIS

Admitting History

A 72-year-old man is well known to the treating hospital staff members, having received care there for more than 12 years. While in the U.S. Navy during World War II, he worked on the East Coast in the ship construction industry. After his discharge in 1945, he returned to his home in Mississippi for about 6 months; he then moved to Detroit, Michigan, and worked for an automobile manufacturer. His primary job for the next 20 years was undercoating automobiles.

In the early 1970s the man was transferred to a nearby automotive plant, where he worked on an assembly line fastening bumpers and chrome trim to cars. He was popular with his fellow workers and considered a hard worker by the management. When he retired in 1980, he was one of four supervisors in charge of the chrome trim assembly line.

Although the man smoked two packs a day for more than 40 years, his health was essentially unremarkable until about 4 years before he retired. At that time he started to experience periods of coughing, dyspnea, and weakness. A complete examination provided by the company concluded that the man had moderate pneumoconiosis.

On the basis of the man's work history, the doctor speculated that the pneumoconiosis was caused by asbestos fibers. This theory was confirmed later with a Perls' stain of sputum, and the diagnosis of asbestosis was noted in the patient's chart. Just before the man retired, his pulmonary function tests (PFTs) showed a mild-to-moderate combined restrictive and obstructive disorder.

Although the man was able to enjoy a couple of relatively good years of retirement with his wife, his health declined rapidly thereafter. His cough and dyspnea quickly became a daily problem. Despite his deteriorating health, the man continued to smoke. When he was 68 years old, he was hospitalized for 8 days to treat pneumonia and severe respiratory distress. When he was discharged at that time, his PFTs still showed a moderate-to-severe restrictive and obstructive disorder. He started using oxygen at home regularly.

Approximately 10 months before the current admission, the man was hospitalized for congestive heart failure. He was treated aggressively and sent home within 5 days. At the time of discharge, his PFT results showed that he had a worsening restrictive and obstructive respiratory disorder. His arterial blood gas values (ABGs) on 2 L/min oxygen by nasal cannula were as follows: pH 7.38, $Paco_2$ 86 mm Hg, HCO_3^- 46 mmol/L, and Pao_2 63 mm Hg.

Approximately 3 hours before the current admission, the man awoke from an afternoon nap extremely short of breath. His wife stated that he coughed almost continuously and had difficulty speaking. She measured his oral temperature, which read 38° C (100° F). Concerned, she drove her husband to the hospital emergency room.

Physical Examination

As the man was wheeled into the emergency room, he appeared nervous, weak, and in obvious respiratory distress. He was on 1.5 L/min oxygen by nasal cannula, which was connected to an E-tank that was attached to the wheelchair. His skin felt damp and clammy to the touch. He appeared pale and cyanotic. His neck veins were distended, and his fingers and toes were clubbed. He demonstrated a frequent but weak cough productive of a moderate amount of thick, whitish-yellow secretions. He had peripheral edema (3+) of the ankles and feet. He said this was the worst his breathing had ever been.

The patient's vital signs were as follows: blood pressure 180/96, heart rate 108 bpm, respiratory rate 32/min, and oral temperature 38.3° C (100.8° F). Palpation of the chest was negative. Percussion produced bilateral dull notes in the lung bases. Wheezing, rhonchi, and crackles were auscultated throughout both lungs. A pleural friction rub could be heard over the right middle lobe between the sixth and seventh ribs, between the anterior axillary line and midaxillary line.

The patient's lower lobes had a diffuse, "ground-glass" appearance on the chest X-ray. Irregularly shaped opacities in the right and left lower pleural spaces were identified by the radiologist as calcified pleural plaques. A possible infiltrate consistent with pneumonia also was visible in the right middle lobes. In addition, the chest X-ray suggested that the right side of the heart was moderately enlarged (Figure 25-4). His ABGs on a 1.5 L/min oxygen nasal cannula were as follows: pH 7.56, $Paco_2$ 51 mm Hg, HCO_3^- 38 mMol/L, and Pao_2 47 mm Hg.

The physician started the patient on intravenous (IV) furosemide (Lasix) to treat the man's cor pulmonale and began administering an antibiotic to treat suspected pneumonia. A respiratory care practitioner was called to obtain a sputum culture, perform a respiratory care evaluation, and outline further respiratory therapy. The physician said that she did not want to commit the patient to a ventilator unless absolutely necessary. On the basis of this information, the following SOAP was recorded:

Respiratory Assessment and Plan

S "This is the worst my breathing has ever been."
O Vital signs: BP 180/96, HR 108, RR 32, T 38.3° C (100.8° F); weak appearance; skin: cyanotic,

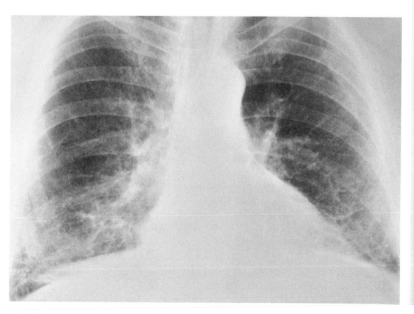

Figure 25–4 Chest X-ray of a 72-year-old man with pneumoconiosis.

damp, and clammy; distended neck veins and digital clubbing; cough: frequent, weak, moderate amount of thick, whitish yellow secretions; peripheral edema (3+) of ankles and feet. Bilateral dull percussion notes in lung bases. Over both lungs: wheezing, rhonchi, and crackles; pleural friction rub over right middle lobe between sixth and seventh ribs, between anterior axillary line and midaxillary line; CXR: "ground-glass" appearance in lower lobes; calcified pleural plaques in right and left lower pleural spaces; consolidation in right middle lung lobe; right heart enlargement; ABGs (1.5 L/min O_2 by nasal cannula): pH 7.56, $Paco_2$ 51, HCO_3^- 38, Pao_2 47.

A
- Respiratory distress (general appearance, vital signs, ABGs)
- Pulmonary fibrosis (history, diagnosis of asbestosis, CXR)
- Alveolar consolidation in right middle lobe (CXR)
- Pleurisy (asbestosis or pneumonitis) in area of right middle lobe (pleural friction rub)
- Excessive bronchial secretions (rhonchi, sputum production)
- Chest infection likely (yellow sputum)
- Bronchospasm (wheezing)
- Wheezing possibly caused by bronchial secretions
- Acute alveolar hyperventilation superimposed on chronic ventilatory failure with moderate-to-severe hypoxemia (history, ABGs)
- Possible impending ventilatory failure (ABGs)

P Begin Oxygen Therapy Protocol (HAFOE at F_{IO_2} 0.28) and Aerosolized Medication Protocol (2 cc premixed albuterol qid), followed by Bronchopulmonary Hygiene Therapy Protocol (C&DB q 4 h; obtaining sputum for Gram's stain and culture). Initiate Hyperinflation Therapy Protocol (incentive spirometry followed by C&DB). Monitor with alarming pulse oximeter set at 85% Spo_2.

• • • • •

The Next Morning

Throughout the night the patient's condition remained unstable. He continued to cough frequently but could not expectorate secretions adequately on his own. When the therapist assisted the patient during coughing episodes, a moderate amount of thick, white and yellow sputum was produced. Even though he was conscious, alert, and able to follow simple directions, he did not answer any of the respiratory care practitioner's specific questions about his breathing.

His skin was cold and damp to the touch, and he appeared short of breath. His color was improved, but he still appeared pale and cyanotic. His neck veins were still distended, although not so severely as they had been on admission, and edema of his ankles and feet could still be seen. The patient's vital signs were as follows: blood pressure 192/108, heart rate 113 bpm, respiratory rate 34/min, and oral temperature 38° C (100.4° F). Palpation of the chest was negative.

Dull percussion notes were elicited over the lung bases. Wheezing, rhonchi, and crackles continued to be auscultated throughout both lungs. A pleural friction rub could still be heard over the right middle lung between the sixth and seventh ribs, between the anterior axillary line and midaxillary line. No recent chest X-ray was available. His ABGs were as follows: pH 7.57, $Paco_2$ 47 mm Hg, HCO_3^- 36 mMol/L, and Pao_2 40 mm Hg. His oxygen saturation measured by pulse oximetry (Spo_2) was 77%. On the basis of these clinical data, the following SOAP was documented:

Respiratory Assessment and Plan

S N/A (patient too dyspneic to reply)

O Condition unstable; cough: frequent, weak, productive of thick, white and yellow secretions; skin: cyanotic, pale, cool, and damp; distended neck veins and peripheral edema, but improving; vital signs: BP 192/108, HR 113, RR 34, T 38° C (100.4° F); dull percussion notes over both lung bases; wheezing, rhonchi, and crackles throughout both lungs; pleural friction rub over right middle lobe between sixth and seventh ribs, between anterior axillary line and midaxillary line; ABGs: pH 7.57, $Paco_2$ 47, HCO_3^- 36, Pao_2 40; Spo_2 77%.

A
- Continued respiratory distress (general appearance, vital signs, ABGs)
- Pulmonary fibrosis in lower lobes (history, diagnosis of asbestosis, recent CXR)
- Alveolar consolidation in right middle lobe (CXR, pneumonia)
- Pleurisy or pneumonia that has extended into pleural space over right middle lobe (pleural friction rub)
- Excessive bronchial secretions (rhonchi, sputum production)
- Infection likely (yellow sputum)
- Bronchospasm (wheezing)
- Wheezing not improving in response to bronchodilator treatment
- Wheezing possibly caused by bronchial secretions
- Acute alveolar hyperventilation superimposed on chronic ventilatory failure with severe hypoxemia, worsening (history, ABGs)
- Impending ventilatory failure (ABGs)

P Up-regulate oxygen therapy per protocol (HAFOE at F_{IO_2} 0.40). Continue Bronchopulmonary Hygiene Therapy and Aerosolized Medication Protocols (adding intensive nasotracheal suctioning q 2 h and 2 cc acetylcysteine to the premix albuterol). Continue Hyperinflation Therapy Protocol (continuing to coach and monitor incentive spirometry; if FVC falls below 15 cc/kg, substituting IPPB with previously discussed aerosolized medications while awake). Continue to monitor closely.

• • • • •

20 Hours Later

At 6.15 AM the alarm on the patient's cardiac monitor sounded. The electrocardiogram (ECG) strip showed several premature ventricular contractions followed by ventricular flutter and fibrillation. The head nurse called for a code blue. Cardiopulmonary resuscitation was started immediately. Because of the severe hypotension (blood pressure 80/50), epinephrine and dopamine were administered through the patient's intravenous line. Approximately 12 minutes into the code, the patient exhibited a normal sinus rhythm. Spontaneous respiration was absent.

The patient was intubated, transferred to the intensive care unit (ICU), and placed on a mechanical ventilator. The initial ventilator settings were in assist control mode as follows: 12 breaths per minute, F_{IO_2} 1.0, pressure support 14 cm H_2O, and 10 cm H_2O positive end-expiratory pressure (PEEP). His cardiopulmonary status remained unstable. Premature ventricular contractions were frequently seen on the ECG monitor. A pulmonary artery catheter and arterial line were inserted.

The patient's skin was pale, cyanotic, and clammy. His neck veins were still distended, and his ankles and feet were swollen. Vital signs were as follows: blood pressure 135/90, heart rate 84 bpm, and rectal temperature 38.3° C (100.8° F). Palpation of the chest wall was negative. Dull percussion notes were noted over the lung bases. Wheezing, rhonchi, and crackles continued to be auscultated throughout both lungs. Thick, greenish-yellow sputum was frequently suctioned from the patient's endotracheal tube.

A pleural friction rub still could be heard over the right middle lung lobe between the sixth and seventh ribs, between the anterior axillary line and midaxillary line. A chest X-ray had been taken but had not yet been interpreted by the radiologist. The patient's hemodynamic indices were as follows: elevated central venous pressure (CVP), right atrial pressure (RAP), mean pulmonary artery pressure ($\overline{PA}$), right ventricular stroke work index (RVSWI), and pulmonary vascular resistance (PVR). All other hemodynamic values were normal. His ABGs were as follows: pH 7.53, $Paco_2$ 56 mm Hg, HCO_3^- 38 mMol/L, and Pao_2 246 mm Hg. His Spo_2 was 98%. At this time, the following SOAP note was charted:

Respiratory Assessment and Plan

S N/A (patient intubated on ventilator)

O Vital signs: BP 135/90 on vasopressors, HR 84, T 38.3° C (100.8° F); frequent premature ventricular contractions; skin: pale, cyanotic, and clammy; distended neck veins; peripheral edema of ankles and feet; dull percussion notes over lung bases; wheezing, rhonchi, and crackles throughout both lungs; thick, greenish-yellow sputum frequently suctioned; pleural friction rub over right middle lung lobe between sixth and seventh ribs and between anterior axillary line and midaxillary line; hemodynamic indices: elevated CVP, RAP, $\overline{PA}$, RVSWI, and PVR; ABGs: pH 7.53, $Paco_2$ 56, HCO_3^- 38, Pao_2 246, Spo_2 98%.

A
- Pulmonary fibrosis, lower lung lobes (history, diagnosis of asbestosis, recent CXR)
- Alveolar consolidation, right middle lobe (recent CXR showing pneumonia)
- Pneumonia possibly extended into pleural space over right middle lobe (pleural friction rub)
- Excessive bronchial secretions (rhonchi, sputum production)
- Infection likely (greenish-yellow sputum, possible new organism)
- Bronchospasm possible (wheezing)
- Wheezing not improving in response to bronchodilator treatment
- Wheezing possibly caused by bronchial secretions
- Acute alveolar hyperventilation superimposed on chronic ventilatory failure and overly corrected hypoxemia (ABGs)
- Overventilation (mechanical) and overoxygenation

P Down-regulate Oxygen Therapy Protocol (reduction of F_{IO_2} to 0.50). Down-regulate Mechanical Ventilation Protocol (decreasing tidal volume). Continue Bronchopulmonary Hygiene Therapy and Aerosolized Medication per protocol. Continue Hyperinflation Therapy Protocol (depending on mean airway pressure). Continue to closely monitor and reevaluate.

Discussion

The admitting history reveals that the patient had been diagnosed with moderate pneumoconiosis (probable asbestosis) and that he has been a heavy smoker for more than 40 years. Not surprisingly, pulmonary function tests in the past had shown mild-to-moderate combined obstructive and restrictive pulmonary disorders.

Significant new findings are the history suggesting congestive heart failure and the arterial blood gases on his discharge from the hospital 10 months before this admission, which demonstrated chronic ventilatory failure. The patient's recent fever and cough before his emergency room admission suggest an infectious cause for his symptoms. His cyanosis, neck-vein distention, and digital clubbing suggest chronic hypoxemia. The sputum purulence confirms that infection may indeed be present and that the assessing therapist's desire to obtain a sputum culture is appropriate. The pleural rub demonstrated by this patient could be related to his asbestosis or to a pneumonic infiltrate extending to the pleural surface.

In the **initial assessment** the patient's severe hypertension and his fever should be noted. Both deserve vigorous therapy if his pulmonary function is to improve at all. The patient's severe hypoxemia reflects **Alveolar-Capillary Membrane Thickening** (see Figure 9-9), **Bronchospasm** (see Figure 9-10), and **Excessive Bronchial Secretions** (see Figure 9-11). The latter is possibly treatable, and therapy is appropriately directed to reduction of intrapulmonary shunting. Note that the pulmonary capillary wedge pressure (PCWP) was not measured in the first assessments. Such measurements may have identified an element of left ventricular failure in this hypertensive patient as well. The patient is hyperventilating with respect to his earlier outpatient blood gases. This assessment should record the patient's underlying pulmonary conditions (chronic pulmonary fibrosis, bronchitis, and congestive heart failure) but should really zero in on the treatable issues, specifically the pulmonary infection, as suggested by the sputum and chest X-ray film.

At the time of the **second evaluation,** the patient's hypoxemia has worsened despite oxygen therapy. If not already being used, Venturi oxygen mask (HAFOE) therapy is indicated here, and additional mucolytics and endobronchial suctioning also may be indicated. The trial of hyperinflation therapy would have to be made carefully, given the patient's known airway obstruction. The physician may have ordered a trial of diuretic therapy to reduce the fluid retention. The therapist's opinion that the wheezing might have been caused by bronchial secretions, rather than by out-and-out bronchospasm, quite possibly is correct. However, the distinction is academic because both aerosolized medication therapy and mucolytics should be used in this setting.

The **last assessment** reveals ventricular arrhythmias. The change in the patient's sputum color from thick and white to greenish-yellow suggests superinfection with another organism, and reculture of the sputum is appropriate. The patient is hyperoxygenated, and the F_{IO_2} should be reduced appropriately. Ventilator parameters should be adjusted to provide good pulmonary expansion while avoiding high mean airway pressures.

Despite all that was done for this patient, he died as a result of left-sided congestive heart failure and pneumonia complicating his pulmonary asbestosis.

SELF-ASSESSMENT QUESTIONS

Multiple Choice

1. The length of asbestos fibers commonly ranges between which of the following?

   a. 5 and 10 μ
   b. 10 and 20 μ
   c. 15 and 25 μ
   d. 25 and 50 μ
   e. 50 and 100 μ

2. Which of the following expiratory maneuver findings is/are associated with the pneumoconioses?

      I. Increased MVV
     II. Decreased FEV_T
    III. Increased PEFR
    IV. Decreased FVC

   a. II only
   b. III only
   c. I and III only
   d. II and IV only
   e. I, III, and IV only

3. Which of the following oxygenation indices is/are associated with the pneumoconioses?
      I. Decreased $C(a-\bar{v})o_2$
     II. Increased O_2ER
    III. Decreased $S\bar{v}o_2$
    IV. Increased $\dot{V}o_2$

   a. I only
   b. III only
   c. II and III only
   d. I and IV only
   e. II, III, and IV only

4. The fibrotic changes that develop in coal worker's pneumoconiosis usually result from which of the following?

   a. Barium
   b. Silica
   c. Iron
   d. Coal dust
   e. Clay

5. Which of the following is/are associated with the pneumoconioses?

      I. Pleural friction rub
     II. Dull percussion note
    III. Cor pulmonale
    IV. Elevated $\overline{PA}$

   a. I and II only
   b. II and IV only
   c. III and IV only
   d. II, III, and IV only
   e. I, II, III, and IV

Fill in the Blanks

The five major etiologic determinants for the development of the pneumoconioses are the following:

1. _____
   _____

2. _____
   _____

3. _____
   _____

4. _____
   _____

5. _____
   _____

Answers appear in Appendix XI.

PART VIII

Neoplastic Disease

CHAPTER 26

Cancer of the Lung

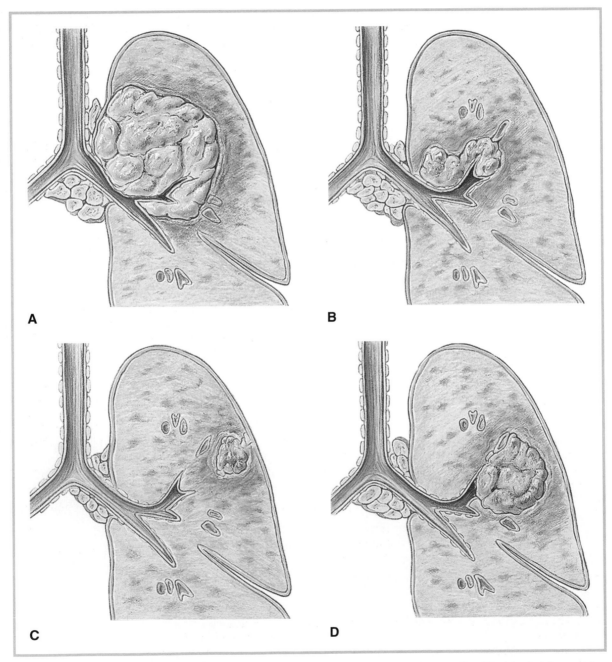

Figure 26–1 Cancer of the lung. **A,** Squamous (epidermoid) cell carcinoma. **B,** Small-cell (oat-cell) carcinoma. **C,** Adenocarcinoma. **D,** Large-cell carcinoma. See also Plate 18.

Anatomic Alterations of the Lungs

Cancer is a general term that refers to abnormal new tissue growth characterized by the progressive, uncontrolled multiplication of cells. This abnormal growth of new cells is called a *neoplasm* or *tumor*. A tumor may be localized or invasive, benign or malignant.

Benign tumors do not endanger life unless they interfere with the normal functions of other organs or affect a vital organ. They grow slowly and push aside normal tissue but do not invade it. They are usually encapsulated, well-demarcated growths. They are not invasive or metastatic; that is, tumor cells do not travel by way of the bloodstream or lymphatics and invade or form secondary tumors in other organs.

Malignant tumors are composed of embryonic, primitive, or poorly differentiated cells. They grow in a disorganized manner and so rapidly that nutrition of the cells becomes a problem. For this reason, necrosis, ulceration, and cavity formation are commonly associated with malignant tumors. They also invade surrounding tissues and may be metastatic.

Although malignant changes may develop in any portion of the lung, they most commonly originate in the mucosa of the tracheobronchial tree. Lung cancer arises from the epithelium of the tracheobronchial tree. Thus a tumor that originates in the bronchial mucosa is called *bronchogenic carcinoma*. The terms *lung cancer* and *bronchogenic carcinoma* are used interchangeably.

As a tumor enlarges, the surrounding bronchial airways and alveoli become irritated, inflamed, and swollen. The adjacent alveoli may fill with fluid and become consolidated or collapse. In addition, as the tumor protrudes into the tracheobronchial tree, excessive mucus production and airway obstruction develop. As the surrounding blood vessels erode, blood enters the tracheobronchial tree. Peripheral tumors also may invade the pleural space and impinge on the mediastinum, chest wall, ribs, or diaphragm. A secondary pleural effusion is often seen in lung cancer. A pleural effusion further compresses the lung and causes atelectasis.

The major pathologic or structural changes associated with bronchogenic carcinoma are as follows:

- Inflammation, swelling, and destruction of the bronchial airways and alveoli
- Excessive mucus production
- Tracheobronchial mucus accumulation and plugging
- Airway obstruction (either from blood, from mucus accumulation, or from a tumor projecting into a bronchus)
- Atelectasis
- Alveolar consolidation
- Cavity formation
- Pleural effusion (when a tumor invades the parietal pleura and mediastinum)

Etiology

Lung cancer is the leading cause of cancer deaths in the United States. More than 160,000 new cases of lung cancer are reported in the United States annually—about 90,000 in males and about 70,000 in females. Although lung cancer accounts for about 13% of all cancers in both men and women, it is responsible for about 31% of all cancer deaths in men and about 25% of all cancers in women. The mortality rate for lung cancer in men recently has leveled off. In women, however, the mortality rate is still rising—primarily because of the increased rate of cigarette smoking among women. Among women, the lung cancer death rate is now higher than the death rate of any other cancer—including breast cancer. Death from lung cancer generally begins when patients are between 35 and 44 years of age. A sharp increase in lung cancer deaths is seen among patients between 45 and 55 years of age. The incidence of lung cancer death progressively increases to 74 years of age and then levels off and decreases in extremely old individuals.

Cigarette smoking is the most common cause of lung cancer. Heavy smokers are about 25% more likely to develop lung cancer than nonsmokers. It is estimated that cigarette smoke contains more than 4000 different chemicals, many of which have proved to be carcinogens. Passive, or second-hand, smoking is associated with as much as a 30% increase in the risk for lung cancer. A genetic predisposition toward developing lung cancer also plays a role in the incidence of lung cancer.

Environmental or occupational risk factors for lung cancer include the following:

- Benzopyrene and radon particles associated with uranium mining
- Radiation and nuclear fallout
- Polycyclic aromatic hydrocarbons and arsenicals
- Asbestos fibers
- Diesel exhaust
- Nitrogen mustard gases
- Nickel
- Silica
- Vinyl chloride
- Chlormethyl methyl ether
- Air pollution
- Coal and iron mining

TYPES OF CANCERS

There are four major types of bronchogenic tumors: (1) squamous (epidermoid) cell carcinoma, (2) adenocarcinoma (including bronchioalveolar cell carcinoma) (3) large-cell carcinoma, and (4) small-cell (oat-cell) carcinoma (Figure 26-1). For therapeutic reasons, these bronchogenic tumors are commonly divided into the following two groups:

- Small-cell lung cancer
  - Small-cell (or oat-cell carcinoma)

- Non–small-cell cancer
  - Squamous cell carcinoma
  - Adenocarcinoma
  - Large-cell carcinoma

Each group grows and spreads in different way. For example, small-cell lung cancer spreads aggressively and responds best to chemotherapy and radiation therapy. It occurs almost exclusively in smokers and accounts for about 25% of all lung cancers in the United States. Non–small-cell lung cancer is more common and accounts for about 75% of all lung cancers in America. When confined to a small area and identified early, this type of cancer often can be removed surgically. Table 26-1 provides a general characteristics of these cancer cell types, including evaluation and treatment. A more in-depth description of each cancer cell type follows.

SMALL-CELL LUNG CANCER

Small-Cell (Oat-Cell) Carcinoma

Small-cell carcinoma arises from the Kulchitsky (or K-type) cells in the bronchial epithelium; it is commonly found near the hilar region. Because the tumor cells often are compressed into an oval shape, this form of cancer is commonly referred to as *oat-cell carcinoma.* Cell size ranges from 6 to 8 µm. Small-cell carcinoma accounts for 20% to 25% of all bronchogenic carcinomas. The tumor grows quite rapidly (a doubling time of about 30 days) and

metastasizes early. Small-cell carcinoma has the strongest correlation with cigarette smoking and is associated with the worst prognosis. Staging for small-cell carcinoma is divided into only two categories: limited disease (20% to 30%) or extensive disease (70% to 80%). Mean survival time for untreated small-cell carcinoma is about 1 to 3 months. When treated, about 10% of the patients are alive 2 years after completing treatment (see Figure 26-1, *A*).

NON–SMALL-CELL LUNG CANCER

Squamous (Epidermoid) Cell Carcinoma

Squamous cell carcinoma is the most common type of lung cancer in men (about 30% to 50% of the cases). It is commonly located near the hilar region, projecting into the large bronchi. Squamous cell tumors may be seen to project into the bronchi during bronchoscopy. The tumor originates from the basal cells of the bronchial epithelium and grows through the epithelium before invading the surrounding tissues. The tumor has a slow growth rate (a doubling time of about 100 days) and a late metastatic tendency (mostly to hilar lymph nodes). In about one third of the cases, squamous cell carcinoma originates in the periphery. Because of the location in the central bronchi, obstructive manifestations are often nonspecific and include a nonproductive cough and hemoptysis. Pneumonia and atelectasis are often secondary complications of squamous cell carcinoma. Cavity formation with or without an air-fluid interface is seen in 10% to 20% of the cases (see Figure 26-1, *B*).

Adenocarcinoma (Including Bronchioalveolar Cell Carcinoma)

Adenocarcinoma arises from the mucus glands of the tracheobronchial tree. In fact, the glandular configuration and the mucus production caused by this type of cancer are the pathologic features that distinguish

TABLE 26–1	General Characteristics of Lung Cancer Types, Growth Rate, and Metastasis	
Cell Type	**Growth Rate**	**Metastasis**
Non–small-cell cancer		
Squamous cell carcinoma	Slow	Late; usually to hilar lymph nodes
Adenocarcinoma	Moderate	Early
Large-cell carcinoma	Rapid	Early and widespread
Small-cell (oat-cell) carcinoma	Very rapid	Very early; to mediastinum or distally in lung

adenocarcinoma from the other types of bronchogenic carcinoma. Adenocarcinoma is the most common type of lung cancer in women and in people who do not smoke. Adenocarcinoma tumors are usually smaller than 4 cm and are most commonly found in the peripheral regions of the lung parenchyma. The growth rate is moderate (a doubling time of about 180 days), and the metastatic tendency is early. Secondary cavity formation and pleural effusion are common (see Figure 26-1, *C*).

Bronchioloalveolar cell carcinoma is included under the category of adenocarcinoma. These tumors typically arise from the terminal bronchioles and alveoli. They have a slow growth rate, and their metastasis pattern is unpredictable.

Large-Cell Carcinoma (Undifferentiated)

Large-cell carcinoma accounts for about 10% to 15% of all bronchogenic carcinoma cases. Because this tumor has lost all evidence of differentiation, it is commonly referred to as *undifferentiated large-cell anaplastic cancer.* Although these tumors commonly arise peripherally, they may also be found centrally—often distorting the trachea and large airways. Large-cell carcinoma has a rapid growth rate and early and widespread metastasis. Common secondary complications include chest wall pain, pleural effusion, pneumonia, hemoptysis, and cavity formation (see Figure 26-1, *D*).

SCREENING AND DIAGNOSIS

A routine chest X-ray is the most common screening test used to identify an abnormal mass or nodule in a patient's lung. A computed tomography (CT) scan and positron emission tomography (PET) scans are also frequently used to reveal extremely small lesions and determine whether the cancer has spread to other areas. A definitive diagnosis, however, can be made only by viewing a tissue sample (biopsy) under a microscope. Common procedures used to obtain a tissue biopsy include bronchoscopy, mediastinoscopy, transbronchial needle biopsy or an open-lung biopsy, sputum cytology, thoracentesis, and video thoracoscopy (see Chapter 7).

STAGING OF LUNG CANCER

Staging is the process of classifying information about cancer. The system describes the cancer cell type, the size of the tumor, the level of lymph node involvement, and the extent to which the cancer has spread. The patient's prognosis and treatment depend, to a large extent, on the staging results. The system most often used for the staging of lung cancer is the *TNM classification* (Table 26-2). *T* represents the extent of the *primary tumor*, *N* denotes the *lymph node* involvement, and *M* indicates the *extent of metastasis.* On the basis of the TNM findings, roman numerals are used to identify stages, with 0 being the least advanced and IV the most advanced. Figure 26-2 provides five representative illustrations of the staging of lung cancer by the TNM classification system. A general overview and description of the staging process for non–small-cell lung cancer and small-cell lung cancer follows*:

NON–SMALL-CELL LUNG CANCER

Non–small-cell lung cancer is staged according to the size of the tumor, the level of lymph node involvement, and the extent to which the cancer has spread. The stages for non–small-cell lung cancer include the following:

Stage 0: The cancer is limited to the lining of the bronchial airways. There is no involvement of the lung tissue or distant metastasis. Stage 0 cancers usually are found during bronchoscopy. When found and treated early, cancers at this stage can often be cured. (TisNOMO)

Stage I: The tumor is less than 3 cm and is located in lobar or distal airways. There is no lung tissue involvement or distant metastasis. (T1NOMO)

Stage II: In this stage the cancer has invaded neighboring lymph nodes or spread to the chest wall. There is no distant metastasis. (T1N1MO)

Stage III A: The tumor is any size. The tumor is in the main bronchus, or the tumor is accompanied by atelectasis or obstructive pneumonitis of the entire lung. Local invasion involves chest wall, diaphragm, mediastinal, pleural, or parietal pericardium. There is the presence of metastasis to ipsilateral peribronchial or ipsilateral hilar lymph nodes or both. There is no distant metastasis. (T3N1MO)

Stage III B: The cancer has spread locally to areas such as the mediastinum, heart, great vessels, trachea, esophagus, vertebral body, or carina; or presence of malignant pleural/pericardial effusion—all within the chest. There may be involvement of any of the lymph node groups. There is no distant metastasis. (T4, any N, MO)

---

*Note: Not all the subcategories for each stage are provided in this overview. See Table 26-2 for all the stages and their respective definitions.

TABLE 26–2 1997 Revised International System for Staging Lung Cancer

Symbol	Definition
Primary Tumor (T)	
T0	No evidence of tumor
Tx	Tumor that cannot be assessed or is not apparently radiologically or bronchoscopically (malignant cells in bronchopulmonary secretions)
Tis	Carcinoma in situ
T1	Tumor with the following characteristics:
a	Size: ≤3 cm
b	Airway location: in lobar bronchus or distal airways
c	Local invasion: none, surrounded by lung or visceral pleura
T2	Tumor with any of the following characteristics:
a	Size: >3 cm
b	Airway location: tumor in the main bronchus (within 2 cm of the carina) or tumor with atelectasis involvement of the main bronchus (distance to the carina is 2 cm or more) or presence of atelectasis or obstructive pneumonitis that extends to hilar region but does not involve the entire lung
c	Local invasion: involvement of the visceral pleura
T3	Tumor with the following location or invasion:
a	Size: any
b	Airway location: tumor in the main bronchus (within 2 cm of the carina) or tumor with atelectasis or obstructive pneumonitis of the entire lung
c	Local invasion: invasion of chest wall (including superior sulcus tumors), diaphragm, mediastinal pleura, or parietal pericardium
T4	Tumor with the following location or invasion:
a	Size: any
b	Airway location: satellite tumor nodule(s) within the ipsilateral primary-tumor lobe of the lung
c	Local invasion: invasion of the mediastinum, heart, great vessels, trachea, esophagus, vertebral body, or carina; or presence of malignant pleural/pericardial effusion
Lymph Nodes (N)	
Nx	Regional lymph nodes cannot be assessed
N0	Absence of regional lymph node involvement
N1	Presence of metastasis to ipsilateral peribronchial or ipsilateral hilar lymph nodes or both (including direct extension to intrapulmonary nodes)
N2	Presence of metastasis to ipsilateral mediastinal or subcarinal lymph nodes or both
N3	Presence of metastasis to any of the following lymph node groups: contralateral mediastinal, contralateral hilar, ipsilateral or contralateral scalene, or supraclavicular
Distant Metastasis (M)	
Mx	Metastasis cannot be assessed
M0	Absence of distant metastasis
M1	Presence of distant metastasis (separate metastatic tumor nodule[s] in the ipsilateral nonprimary-tumor lobe[s] of the lung also are grouped as M1)
Stage Grouping— TNM Subsets	
Stage 0	TisN0M0
Stage IA	T1N0M0
Stage IB	T2N0M0
Stage IIA	T1N1M0
Stage IIB	T2N1N0; T3N0M0
Stage IIIA	T3N1M0; T(1-3)N2M0
Stage IIIB	T4, any N, M0; any T, N3M0
Stage IV	Any T; any N; M1

From Mountain CF: Revisions in the international system for staging lung cancer. *Chest* 111(6):1710, 1997.

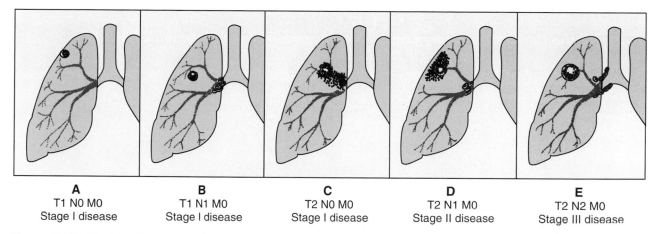

A	B	C	D	E
T1 N0 M0	T1 N1 M0	T2 N0 M0	T2 N1 M0	T2 N2 M0
Stage I disease	Stage I disease	Stage I disease	Stage II disease	Stage III disease

Figure 26–2   Staging of lung cancer by the TNM classification system. (From McCance KL, Huether SE: *Pathophysiology: The biologic basis for disease in adults and children*, ed 4, St. Louis, 2002, Mosby.)

Stage IV: The cancer is of any size, involves any of the lymph node groups, and has spread to other parts of the body, such as the liver, bones, or brain. (any T; any N; M1)

SMALL-CELL LUNG CANCER

Small-cell lung cancer is staged differently than non–small-cell cancer. Roman numerals are not used to identify the stages. Small-cell lung cancer is usually classified as either limited or extensive:

Limited: The cancer is confined to only one lung and to its neighboring lymph nodes.

Extensive: The cancer has spread beyond one lung and nearby lymph nodes. It may have invaded both lungs, more remote lymph nodes, or other organs.

OVERVIEW

of the Cardiopulmonary Clinical Manifestations Associated with CANCER OF THE LUNG

The following clinical manifestations result from the pathologic mechanisms caused (or activated) by **Atelectasis** (see Figure 9-7), **Alveolar Consolidation** (see Figure 9-8), and **Excessive Bronchial Secretions** (see Figure 9-11)—the major anatomic alterations of the lungs associated with cancer of the lung (see Figure 26-1).

CLINICAL DATA OBTAINED AT THE PATIENT'S BEDSIDE

The Physical Examination
Vital Signs

Increased respiratory rate (see page 31 ◆▷)
Several pathophysiologic mechanisms operating simultaneously may lead to an increased ventilatory rate:
- Stimulation of peripheral chemoreceptors (hypoxemia)
- Decreased lung compliance/increased ventilatory rate relationship
- Stimulation of the J receptors
- Pain/anxiety

Increased heart rate (pulse), cardiac output, and blood pressure (see pages 11 and 99 ◆▷)

Cyanosis (see page 45 ◆▷)

Cough, Sputum Production, and Hemoptysis (see page 47 ◆▷)

Chest Assessment Findings (see page 22 ◆▷)
- Crackles, rhonchi, and wheezing

CLINICAL DATA OBTAINED FROM LABORATORY TESTS AND SPECIAL PROCEDURES

Pulmonary Function Study Findings
Expiratory Maneuver Findings (see page 61 ◆▷)

FVC	FEV_T	$FEF_{25\%-75\%}$	$FEF_{200-1200}$
↓	N or ↓	N or ↓	N
PEFR	MVV	$FEF_{50\%}$	$FEV_{1\%}$
N	N or ↓	N	N or ↑

OVERVIEW

of the Cardiopulmonary Clinical Manifestations Associated with CANCER OF THE LUNG (Continued)

Lung Volume and Capacity Findings
(see page 62 ◆►)

V_T	RV	FRC	TLC
N or ↓	↓	↓	↓
VC	IC	ERV	RV/TLC%
↓	↓	↓	N

Arterial Blood Gases

Localized (e.g., lobar) Lung Cancer
Acute Alveolar Hyperventilation with Hypoxemia
(see page 70 ◆►)

pH	$Paco_2$	HCO_3^-	Pao_2
↑	↓	↓(Slightly)	↓

Extensive or Widespread Lung Cancer
Acute Ventilatory Failure with Hypoxemia
(see page 73 ◆►)

pH	Pao_2	HCO_3^-*	Pao_2
↓	↑	↑(Slightly)	↓

*When tissue hypoxia is severe enough to produce lactic acid, the pH and HCO_3^- values will be lower than expected for a particular $Paco_2$ level.

Oxygenation Indices (see page 82 ◆►)

$\dot{Q}_S/\dot{Q}_T$	Do_2†	$\dot{V}o_2$	$C(a-\bar{v})o_2$
↑	↓	Normal	Normal
O_2ER	$S\bar{v}o_2$		
↑	↓		

†The Do_2 may be normal in patients who have compensated to the decreased oxygenation status with (1) an increased cardiac output, (2) an increased hemoglobin level, or (3) a combination of both. When the Do_2 is normal, the O_2ER is usually normal.

Hemodynamic Indices (when hypoxemia and acidemia are present, or when a tumor invades the mediastinum and compresses the superior vena cava)
(see page 99 ◆►)

CVP	RAP	$\bar{PA}$	PCWP
↑	↑	↓	↓
CO	SV	SVI	CI
↓	↓	↓	↓
RVSWI	LVSWI	PVR	SVR
↑	↓	↑	Normal

RADIOLOGIC FINDINGS

Chest Radiograph
- Small oval or coin lesion
- Large irregular mass
- Alveolar consolidation
- Atelectasis
- Pleural effusion (see Chapter 23)
- Involvement of the mediastinum or diaphragm

A routine chest X-ray often provides the first indication or suspicion of lung cancer. Depending on how long the tumor has been growing, the chest X-ray may show a small radiodense nodule (called a *coin lesion*) or a large irregular radiodense mass. Unfortunately, by the time a tumor is identified radiographically, regardless of its size, it is usually in the invasive stage and thus difficult to treat. Another common X-ray presentation of lung cancer is that of volume loss involving a single lobe or an individual segment within a lobe.

Because there are four major forms of lung cancer, chest X-ray findings are variable. In general, squamous cell and small-cell carcinoma usually appear as a white mass near the hilar region; adenocarcinoma appears in the peripheral portions of the lung; and large-cell carcinoma may appear in either the peripheral or the central portion of the lung. Figure 26-3 is a representative example of a bronchogenic carcinoma in the right upper lobe and a coin lesion in the left lung field. Common secondary chest X-ray findings caused by bronchial obstruction include alveolar consolidation, atelectasis, pleural effusion, and mediastinal or diaphragmatic involvement. The X-ray appearance of cavity formation within a bronchogenic carcinoma is similar regardless of the type of cancer.

Clinically, a PET scan is an excellent test to rule out a possible cancerous area identified on either a chest X-ray or a CT scan. For example, Figure 8-12 shows a chest radiograph that identifies two suspicious findings—one small nodule in the right upper lung lobe and a larger density in the left lower lung lobe, just behind the heart. Figure 8-13 shows two CT scans that also identify the two suspicious findings and their precise location. Figures 8-14, 8-15, and 8-16 show PET scans that all confirm a "hot spot" (likely cancer) in the lower left lobe. However, the PET scan shown in Figure 8-17 confirms that the nodule in the right upper lobe is benign (i.e., no "hot spot" is noted).

Finally, the PET/CT image provides an image of excellent quality and high sensitivity and specificity in detecting malignant lesions in the chest. Figure 8-18 shows a CT/PET scan alongside a CT scan and a PET scan—all the images show the same malignant nodule in the right upper lung lobe.

OVERVIEW

of the Cardiopulmonary Clinical Manifestations Associated with CANCER OF THE LUNG (Continued)

Bronchoscopy Findings

• Bronchial tumor or mass lesion

The fiberoptic bronchoscope provides direct visualization of a bronchial tumor for further inspection, biopsy, and assessment of the extent of the disease (Figure 26-4).

COMMON NONRESPIRATORY CLINICAL MANIFESTATIONS

• Hoarseness
• Difficulty in swallowing
• Superior vena cava syndrome (distention of the neck veins and neck and facial edema)
• Weakness
• Electrolyte abnormalities

When a bronchogenic tumor invades the mediastinum, it may involve the left recurrent laryngeal nerve, the esophagus, or the superior vena cava. When the tumor involves the left recurrent laryngeal nerve, the patient's voice becomes hoarse. When the tumor compresses the esophagus, swallowing may become difficult. When a tumor invades the mediastinum and compresses the superior vena cava, blood return to the heart from the head and upper part of the body may be interrupted. When obstruction occurs, the symptoms include an increased ventilatory rate and cough, which is greatly aggravated by recumbency. Clinically, this condition is called *superior vena cava syndrome.*

GENERAL COMMENTS

The clinical manifestations associated with lung cancer may be caused by local effects, tumor extensions into the mediastinum, paraneoplastic endocrine syndromes, or tumor metastases. The most common local symptoms are cough, chest pain, dyspnea, and hemoptysis. Less common symptoms include superior vena cava syndrome, hoarseness resulting from vocal cord paralysis, wheezing, shoulder and upper back pain, and Horner's syndrome (constriction of the pupil and enophthalmos) related to an apical (Pancoast) tumor. Symptoms of metastatic lung cancer include bone pain and central nervous system symptoms such as headache, seizures, or symptoms mimicking a cerebrovascular accident (CVA). Asymptomatic axillary and supraclavicular lymph node metastasis also may be present. Deep venous thrombophlebitis is present at the time of diagnosis in 5% to 10% of patients with lung cancer.

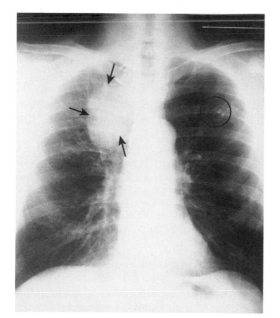

Figure 26–3 Posteroanterior chest radiograph showing a large mass in the right upper lobe *(arrows)*. Note the nodular density in the left lung field *(circle)*. (From Rau JL, Jr., Pearce DJ: *Understanding chest radiographs,* Denver, 1984, Multi-Media Publishing.)

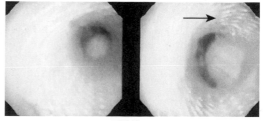

Figure 26–4 Bronchoscopic view of a tumor protruding into the right mainstem bronchus. A wire stent is in place to help hold the airway open.

General Management of Cancer of the Lung

The treatment of lung cancer depends on the patient's overall health, the type of cancer, the size of the tumor, and the location.

Small-Cell Lung Cancer

Because most small-cell lung cancers have spread outside of the lungs by the time they are discovered, surgery is usually not a treatment option. The most effective treatment option is chemotherapy, either alone or in combination with radiation therapy.

CHEMOTHERAPY

Chemotherapy uses powerful drugs to destroy cancer cells. For small-cell lung cancer, chemotherapy is used to slow the growth of the tumor, prevent the tumor from spreading further, or relieve symptoms (palliative care). A combination of drugs is usually administered in a series of treatments over a few weeks or months. Breaks are provided between treatment sessions to allow the body to recover. Unfortunately, because the drugs can damage healthy cells along with the cancer cells, serious side effects are common. Fast-growing cells are especially likely to be affected (e.g., cells in the digestive tract, bone marrow, and hair). In addition, the patient may experience nausea and vomiting, dizziness, fatigue, and increased risk of infection. Chemotherapeutic agents include paclitaxel (Taxol), carboplatin (Paraplatin), vinorelbine tartrate (Navelbine) gemcitabine hydrochloride (Gemzar), docetaxel (Taxotere), and combinations of the above with cisplatin (Platinol).

RADIATION THERAPY

Radiation therapy uses X-rays to kill the cancer cells. It is used in about 50% of all cancer cases, either alone or in combination with other forms of treatment. The patient may receive radiation therapy from outside the body (external radiation) or from radioactive substances that are placed inside needles, seeds, or catheters and inserted into or near the tumor (internal radiation). The type of radiation therapy the patient receives depends on the type and stage of the cancer being treated. The patient may receive radiation therapy before, during, or after chemotherapy.

The goal of treatment is to kill cancer cells without hurting normal tissue cells. Side effects of radiation therapy include redness, swelling, sloughing of skin at the point the radiation enters the patient's body, and an increased risk of infection. In addition, the patient may experience nausea, vomiting, change of taste, fatigue, and malaise. Because small-cell lung cancer often spreads to the brain, brain radiation therapy may be given to prevent cancer from invading that part of the body. Brain radiation therapy can cause short-term memory loss, fatigue, and nausea.

COMFORT (SUPPORTIVE) CARE

Radiation therapy and chemotherapy may not be tolerated when the patient has extensive small-cell lung cancer and is in poor health. The patient may choose to receive only comfort or palliative care, which means treating the symptoms of the cancer rather than the cancer itself.

Non–Small-Cell Lung Cancer

Surgery is usually the treatment of choice for early-stage non–small-cell lung cancer. Depending on the severity and extent of the tumor, surgery may include the removal of only the portion of the lung that contains the tumor (wedge resection), one lobe (lobectomy), or the entire lung (pneumonectomy).

TREATMENT ACCORDING TO STAGES—A GENERAL OVERVIEW

Stage I and Stage II

Surgical resection is the principal form of treatment for patients with Stage I or Stage II lung cancer. Radiation therapy often follows surgical resection to reduce the rate of tumor regrowth in the area of the original tumor. When the patient is medically unable to withstand a surgical resection procedure, radiation therapy alone may be used to treat the tumor.

Stage III

Stage III is commonly divided into the following three groups:

1. Patients with obvious Stage III disease who show enlarged lymph nodes on chest X-ray or CT scan.

   Treatment options: These patients are not considered good candidates for surgery. They may benefit from a combination of both radiation and chemotherapy (either concurrent or sequential).

2. Patients with normal-appearing but cancerous mediastinal lymph nodes that are identified during mediastinoscopy.

Treatment options: Surgery may be an option for these patients. Initially, the patient usually undergoes a preoperative radiation or chemotherapy (either concurrent or sequential). If this therapy is successful, a follow-up surgical resection of any remaining tumor may be helpful.

3. Classic Stage III B patients with tumors of any size and cancerous lymph nodes within the mediastinum and/or the carina (tracheal ridge), hilum, upper ribs, or upper collarbone region.

   Treatment options: Surgery is not an option for these patients. A combination treatment plan with chemo-radiotherapy (either concurrent or sequential) may be administered to patients who have noncancerous effusion (fluid that is free of cancer cells). Unfortunately, the survival rate for these patients is only as long as Stage IV (about 8 months), in spite of aggressive therapy.

Stage IV (or Recurrent Lung Cancer)

Patients with Stage IV, or recurrent, lung cancer have the option of chemotherapy alone or no therapy with comfort care. Research indicates that treatment can improve overall survival compared with comfort care only. Chemotherapy also may help to relieve symptoms in patients who experience significant symptoms from their disease.

RESPIRATORY CARE TREATMENT PROTOCOLS

Oxygen Therapy Protocol

Oxygen therapy is used to treat hypoxemia, decrease the work of breathing, and decrease myocardial work. Because hypoxemia is associated with lung cancer, supplemental oxygen may be required. However, capillary shunting is common because of the alveolar compression and consolidation often produced by lung cancer. Hypoxemia caused by capillary shunting often is refractory to oxygen therapy (see Oxygen Therapy Protocol, Protocol 9-1).

Bronchopulmonary Hygiene Therapy Protocol

Because of the excessive mucus production and accumulation associated with lung cancer, a number of bronchial hygiene treatment modalities may be used to enhance the mobilization of bronchial secretions (see Bronchopulmonary Hygiene Therapy Protocol, Protocol 9-2).

Hyperinflation Therapy Protocol

Hyperinflation techniques are used to offset (at least temporarily) the alveolar compression and consolidation associated with lung cancer (see Hyperinflation Therapy Protocol, Protocol 9-3).

Aerosolized Medication Protocol

Aerosolized bronchodilators and mucolytics often are indicated, particularly when chronic obstructive pulmonary disease (COPD) co-exists, as it does in more than 75% of all cases of lung cancer (see Aerosolized Medication Protocol, Protocol 9-4).

BRONCHOSCOPY

In addition to its role in diagnosis and staging, bronchoscopy is used to treat lung cancer as part of photodynamic therapy, laser therapy, brachytherapy, and the placement of airway stents (see Figure 26-4). These techniques require the assistance of respiratory care practitioners but are not discussed in any depth here.

Case Study: CANCER OF THE LUNGS

Admitting History

A 66-year-old retired man lives with his wife in a small, two-bedroom ranch house in Peoria, Illinois, during the summer months. During the rest of the year, they live in a 22-foot trailer in a retirement park just outside Las Vegas, Nevada. The trailer park is located conveniently on the casinos' shuttle-bus route; a bus comes by at the top of every hour.

Both the man and his wife are described by their children as addicted gamblers. They gamble almost every day of the year. During the summer months, they play keno and blackjack on the Par-A-Dice Riverboat Casino, which is docked along the shores of the Illinois River in downtown East Peoria. While in Las Vegas, they play bingo, blackjack, and the slot machines at several different casinos. They dress in matching warm-up suits, ride the bus to one of the casinos, and gamble until 10 or 11 PM every day.

Their children, adults with their own families, homes, and jobs in the Peoria area, are concerned about their parents' gambling. They have tried to no avail to get their parents to see a compulsive-gambling therapist, who actually is provided by the Par-A-Dice Riverboat Casino.

Their children's concern is justified. Their parents are always gambling on a shoestring budget.

Although they still own their trailer and small home in Peoria, within the last 2 years they have gambled away most of their life savings, which included stocks, bonds, and mutual funds. Because they let their health insurance premium lapse, their policy recently was cancelled. They still receive a small monthly pension check, however, and some Social Security income.

Before he retired, the man worked for 17 years as a boiler tender for Methodist Hospital in Peoria. He also was a part-time firefighter. For more than 52 years, he smoked between two and a half and three packs of unfiltered cigarettes daily. While in Las Vegas about 3 months earlier, the man began experiencing periods of dyspnea, coughing, and weakness. His cough was productive of small amounts of clear secretions. Also around this time, his wife first noticed that his voice sounded hoarse.

Although he missed several days of gambling and remained in bed because of weakness, he did not seek medical attention. He hates doctors and thought that he suffered merely from a bad cold and the flu. When he returned to Peoria for the summer, however, the children became concerned and insisted that he see a doctor. Despite the man's lack of health insurance, two medical students from the University of Illinois, who were working as a team, ordered a full diagnostic workup.

A pulmonary function test (PFT) showed that the man had a restrictive and obstructive pulmonary disorder. CT scanning revealed several masses, ranging from 2 to 5 cm in diameter, in the right and left mediastinum in the hilar regions. The masses, especially on the right side, also could be seen clearly on the posteroanterior chest radiograph (Figure 26-5). Both the CT scan and the chest X-ray showed an increased opacity consistent with atelectasis of the medial basal segments of the left lower lobe as well.

A fiberoptic bronchoscopic examination was conducted by the pulmonary physician, with the assistance of a respiratory care practitioner trained in special procedures. It showed several large, protruding bronchial masses in the second- and third-generation bronchi of the right lung and the second-, third-, and fourth-generation bronchi of the left lung. During the bronchoscopy, several mucus plugs were suctioned. Biopsy of three of the larger tumors was positive for squamous cell bronchogenic carcinoma, and the man was admitted to the hospital.

The physician told the patient that he had cancer and that his prognosis was poor. Treatment, at best, would be palliative. The patient asked what the odds were on his life expectancy. The physician stated that the patient had only about a 50% chance of living longer than 6 to 8 weeks. Surgery was out of the question. In the interim, however, the physician promised to do what was possible to make the man comfortable. The physician outlined a treatment plan of radiation therapy and chemotherapy and requested a respiratory care consult.

Physical Examination

The respiratory care practitioner reviewed the admitting history information in the patient's chart and found the man sitting up in bed in obvious respiratory distress. He appeared weak. His skin was cyanotic, and his face, arms, and chest were damp with perspiration. Wheezing was audible with the

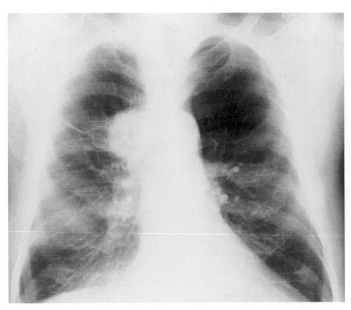

Figure 26–5   Chest X-ray of a 66-year-old man with cancer of the lungs.

aid of a stethoscope. He stated in a hoarse voice that he had coughed up a cup of sputum since breakfast 2 hours earlier. He demonstrated a weak cough every few minutes or so. His cough was productive of large amounts of blood-streaked sputum. The viscosity of the sputum was thin. After each coughing episode, he stated that he wanted a cigarette and then laughed.

His vital signs were as follows: blood pressure 155/85, heart rate 90 bpm, respiratory rate 22/min, and temperature normal. Palpation was unremarkable. Percussion produced dull notes over the left lower lobe. On auscultation, rhonchi, wheezing, and crackles could be heard throughout both lung fields. His arterial blood gas values (ABGs) on a 2 L/min oxygen nasal cannula were as follows: pH 7.51, $Paco_2$ 29 mm Hg, HCO_3^- 22 mMol/L, and Pao_2 66 mm Hg. His oxygen saturation measured by pulse oximetry (Spo_2) was 92%. On the basis of these clinical data, the following SOAP was documented:

Respiratory Assessment and Plan

S "I've coughed up a cup of sputum since breakfast."

O Vital signs: BP 155/85, HR 90, RR 22, T normal; perspiring and weak and cyanotic appearance; voice hoarse-sounding; weak cough; large amounts of blood-streaked sputum; dull percussion notes over left lower lobe; rhonchi, wheezing, and crackles throughout both lung fields; recent PFT: restrictive and obstructive pulmonary disorder; CT scan and CXR: 2- to 5-cm masses in right and left mediastinum in hilar regions and atelectasis of left lower lobe. Bronchoscopy: protruding tumors in both left and right large airways, mucus plugging. Biopsy: squamous cell bronchogenic carcinoma. ABGs (2 L/min O_2 by nasal cannula): pH 7.51, $Paco_2$ 29, HCO_3^- 22, Pao_2 66; Spo_2 92%

A • Bronchogenic carcinoma (CT scan and biopsy)
   • Respiratory distress (vital signs, ABGs)
   • Excessive bloody bronchial secretions (sputum, rhonchi)
   • Mucus plugging (bronchoscopy)
   • Poor ability to mobilize secretions (weak cough)
   • Atelectasis of left lower lobe (CXR)
   • Acute alveolar hyperventilation with mild hypoxemia (ABGs)

P Initiate Oxygen Therapy Protocol (4 L nasal cannula and titration by oximetry). Also begin Aerosolized Medication Protocol (0.5 cc albuterol in 2 cc 10% acetylcysteine q 6 h), followed by Bronchopulmonary Hygiene Therapy Protocol (C&DB). Begin Hyperinflation Therapy Protocol (incentive spirometry q 2 h and prn). Closely monitor and reevaluate.

• • • • •

3 Days After Admission

A respiratory care practitioner evaluated the patient during morning rounds. After reviewing the patient's chart, the practitioner went to the patient's bedside and discovered that the man was not tolerating the chemotherapy well. He had been vomiting intermittently for the past 10 hours and was still in obvious respiratory distress. He appeared cyanotic and tired, and his hospital gown was wet from perspiration. His cough was still weak and productive of large amounts of moderately thick, clear, and white sputum. He stated in a hoarse voice that he still was not breathing very well.

His vital signs were as follows: blood pressure 166/90, heart rate 95 bpm, respiratory rate 28/min, and temperature normal. Dull percussion notes were elicited over both the right and left lower lobes. Rhonchi, wheezing, and crackles were auscultated throughout both lung fields. His ABGs were as follows: pH 7.55, $Paco_2$ 25 mm Hg, HCO_3^- 20 mMol/L, and Pao_2 53 mm Hg. His Spo_2 was 88%. On the basis of these clinical data, the following SOAP was documented:

Respiratory Assessment and Plan

S "I'm still not breathing very well."

O Vital signs: BP 166/90, HR 95, RR 28, T normal; vomiting over past 10 hours; cyanosis, tiredness, and dampness from perspiration; cough: weak and productive of moderately thick, clear, and white sputum; dull percussion notes over both right and left lower lobes; rhonchi, wheezing, and crackles over both lung fields; ABGs: pH 7.55, $Paco_2$ 25, HCO_3^- 20, Pao_2 53, Spo_2 88%

A • Bronchogenic carcinoma (previous CT scan and biopsy)
   • Trouble tolerating chemotherapy well (excessive vomiting)
   • Continued respiratory distress
   • Excessive bronchial secretions (sputum, rhonchi)
   • Mucus plugging still likely (previous bronchoscopy, secretions becoming thicker)
   • Poor ability to mobilize secretions (weak cough)
   • Atelectasis of left lower lobes; atelectasis likely in right lower lobe now (CXR, dull percussion notes)
   • Acute alveolar hyperventilation with moderate hypoxemia, worsening (ABGs)
   • Possible impending ventilatory failure

P Up-regulate Oxygen Therapy Protocol (oxygen mask). Up-regulate Aerosolized Medication Protocol (increasing treatment frequency to q 3 h). Up-regulate Bronchopulmonary Hygiene Therapy Protocol (CPT and PD q 3 h).

Up-regulate Hyperinflation Therapy Protocol (changing incentive spirometry to IPPB). Contact physician about possible ventilatory failure. Discuss therapeutic bronchoscopy. Closely monitor and reevaluate.

• • • • •

16 Days After Admission

Although the physician's original intention and hope was to discharge the patient soon, stabilizing the man for any length of time proved difficult. Over the next 2 weeks, the patient had continued to be nauseated on a daily basis. He did, however, have occasional periods of relief during which he could breathe, but he generally was in respiratory distress.

On this day the respiratory therapist observed and collected the following clinical data:

The patient was lying in bed in the supine position. His eyes were closed, and he was unresponsive to the therapist's questions. The patient was in obvious respiratory distress. He appeared pale, cyanotic, and diaphoretic. No cough was observed at this time, but rhonchi easily could be heard from across the patient's room. The nurse in the patient's room stated that the doctor had called the rhonchi a "death rattle" earlier. The patient's vital signs were as follows: blood pressure 170/105, heart rate 110 bpm, respiratory rate 12/min and shallow, and rectal temperature normal. Percussion was not performed. Rhonchi, wheezing, and crackles were heard throughout both lung fields. His ABGs were as follows: pH 7.28, $Paco_2$ 63 mm Hg, HCO_3^- 27 mmol/L, and Pao_2 66 mm Hg. His Spo_2 was 90%. At this time, the following SOAP was recorded:

Respiratory Assessment and Plan

S   N/A (patient comatose)
O   Unresponsive; pale, cyanotic, and perspiring appearance; no cough noted; rhonchi heard without stethoscope; vital signs: BP 170/105, HR 110, RR 12 and shallow, T normal; rhonchi, wheezing, and crackles over both lung fields; ABGs: pH 7.28, $Paco_2$ 63, HCO_3^- 27, Pao_2 66; Spo_2 90%
A   • Bronchogenic carcinoma (previous CT scan and biopsy)
   • Excessive bronchial secretions (rhonchi)
   • Mucus plugging still likely (previous bronchoscopy, rhonchi)
   • Poor ability to mobilize secretions (no cough)
   • Atelectasis (history)
   • Acute ventilatory failure with moderate hypoxemia (ABGs)
P   Contact physician about acute ventilatory failure, and discuss code status. Up-regulate oxygen therapy, bronchopulmonary hygiene therapy, and aerosolized medication therapy per respective protocols. Monitor and reevaluate.

Discussion

This case demonstrates the few specific treatments that a respiratory care practitioner can bring to the care of patients with lung cancer. Specifically, it illustrates that most of the patients have concomitant obstructive pulmonary disease with a need for good bronchial hygiene therapy. The patient's comfort must be kept in mind at all times.

The **first assessment** was performed soon after bronchoscopy and diagnosis. The patient's blood-stained sputum may reflect the primary tumor or, more likely, bleeding from the bronchoscopy sites. The practitioner must monitor this sputum as the day goes along. No improvement in the patient's wheezing can be expected if an endobronchial tumor is the cause, but it may improve if obstructive pulmonary disease (from cigarette smoking) is the causative factor.

The rhonchi, wheezing, and crackles indicate the need for vigorous bronchial hygiene therapy. The **Atelectasis** in the left lower lobe suggests that a trial of careful hyperinflation therapy is in order (see Figure 9-7). The ABGs drawn on 2 L/min O_2 show moderate hypoxemia, despite alveolar hyperventilation. A trial of oxygen by Venturi mask (or nonrebreathing mask) would be helpful. The patient's anxiety may be alleviated with appropriate treatment of the hypoxemia.

The **second assessment** reveals that the patient may have developed atelectasis in both the right and left lower lobes (where the tumor masses were noted previously). This case may present a setting in which therapeutic bronchoscopy or laser-assisted endobronchial resection of the tumor masses may be helpful. The patient continued to be hypoxemic, despite alveolar hyperventilation. A higher Fio_2 (through a Venturi oxygen mask) might be indicated. Vigorous suctioning should be done. Ordering at least one cycle of ventilator support for such a patient would not be surprising, given that the patient just recently received radiation and chemotherapy. His wishes in this respect should be checked against his living will or durable power of attorney for health care, if such a document exists.

The **last assessment** indicates that the patient did not elect aggressive therapy and that he was now slipping into acute ventilatory failure. All health-care personnel have agreed that the patient is close to death. The practitioner may be excused for not suggesting the use of chest physical therapy and postural drainage at this time, because of the patient's wishes. *Aerosolized morphine* is now being used to relieve dyspnea in terminally ill cancer patients. If, however, aggressive therapy were still in order, formal evaluation and treatment of superimposed atelectasis or pneumonia, or both, would be in order.

SELF-ASSESSMENT QUESTIONS

Multiple Choice

1. Which of the following is the most common form of bronchogenic carcinoma?

   a. Squamous cell carcinoma
   b. Oat-cell carcinoma
   c. Large-cell carcinoma
   d. Adenocarcinoma
   e. Small-cell carcinoma

2. Which of the following arises from the mucus glands of the tracheobronchial tree?

   a. Small-cell carcinoma
   b. Adenocarcinoma
   c. Squamous cell carcinoma
   d. Oat-cell carcinoma
   e. Large-cell carcinoma

3. Which of the following carcinoma has the strongest correlation with cigarette smoking?

   a. Adenocarcinoma
   b. Small-cell carcinoma
   c. Large-cell carcinoma
   d. Squamous cell carcinoma

4. Which of the following has the fastest growth (doubling) rate?

   a. Large-cell carcinoma
   b. Small-cell carcinoma
   c. Adenocarcinoma
   d. Squamous cell carcinoma
   e. Epidermoid carcinoma

5. Which of the following is associated with bronchogenic carcinoma?

   I. Alveolar consolidation
   II. Pleural effusion
   III. Alveolar hyperinflation
   IV. Atelectasis

   a. III only
   b. II and III only
   c. I and IV only
   d. II and III only
   e. I, II, and IV only

True or False

True ☐ False ☐ 1. Necrosis, ulceration, and cavitation are commonly associated with malignant tumors.

True ☐ False ☐ 2. It is estimated that about 85% of lung cancer cases are caused by cigarette smoking.

True ☐ False ☐ 3. Small-cell carcinoma arises from the Kulchitsky's cells in the bronchial epithelium.

True ☐ False ☐ 4. Benign tumors are metastatic.

True ☐ False ☐ 5. Adenocarcinoma is most commonly found in the peripheral portion of the lung parenchyma.

Answers appear in Appendix XI.

PART IX

Diffuse Alveolar Disease

CHAPTER 27

Acute Respiratory Distress Syndrome

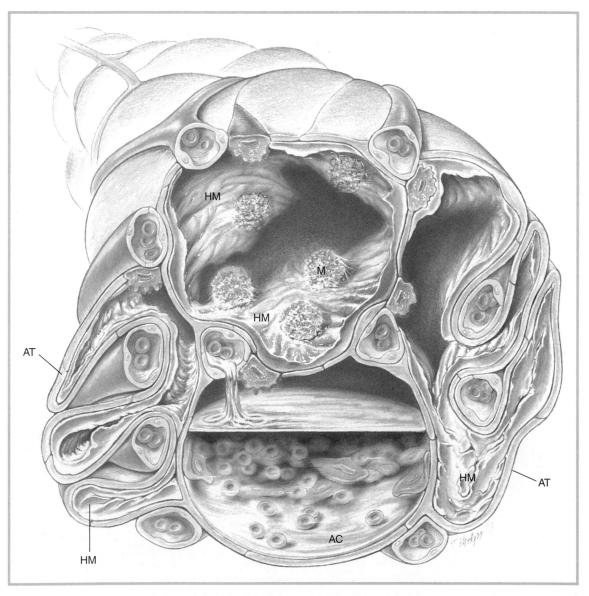

Figure 27–1   Cross-sectional view of alveoli in adult respiratory distress syndrome. *HM,* Hyaline membrane; *AT,* atelectasis; *AC,* alveolar consolidation; *M,* macrophage. See also Plate 19.

Anatomic Alterations of the Lungs

The lungs of patients affected by acute respiratory distress syndrome (ARDS) undergo similar anatomic changes, regardless of the etiology of the disease. In response to injury the pulmonary capillaries become engorged, and the permeability of the alveolar-capillary membrane increases. Interstitial and intra-alveolar edema and hemorrhage ensue, as well as scattered areas of hemorrhagic alveolar consolidation. These processes result in a decrease in alveolar surfactant and in alveolar collapse, or atelectasis.

As the disease progresses, the intra-alveolar walls become lined with a thick, rippled hyaline membrane identical to the hyaline membrane seen in newborns with infant respiratory distress syndrome (hyaline membrane disease). The membrane contains fibrin and cellular debris. In prolonged cases there is hyperplasia and swelling of the type II cells. Fibrin and exudate develop and lead to intra-alveolar fibrosis.

In gross appearance the lungs of patients with ARDS are heavy and "red," "beefy," or "liver-like." The anatomic alterations that develop in ARDS create a restrictive lung disorder (Figure 27-1).

The major pathologic or structural changes associated with ARDS are as follows:

- Interstitial and intra-alveolar edema and hemorrhage
- Alveolar consolidation
- Intra-alveolar hyaline membrane
- Pulmonary surfactant deficiency or abnormality
- Atelectasis

Historically, ARDS was first referred to as the "shock lung syndrome" when the disease was first identified in combat casualties during World War II. Since that time, the disease has appeared in the medical literature under many different names, all based on the etiology believed to be responsible for the disease. In 1967 the disease was first described as a specific entity, and the term *adult respiratory distress syndrome* was suggested. This term is predominantly used today. In alphabetical order, some of the other names that have appeared in the medical journals to identify ARDS are as follows:

- Adult hyaline membrane disease
- Adult respiratory distress syndrome
- Capillary leak syndrome
- Congestion atelectasis
- Da Nang lung (because of the high incidence of ARDS associated with casualties in the Vietnam War)
- Hemorrhagic pulmonary edema
- Noncardiac pulmonary edema
- Oxygen pneumonitis
- Oxygen toxicity
- Postnontraumatic pulmonary insufficiency
- Postperfusion lung
- Postpump lung
- Posttraumatic pulmonary insufficiency
- Shock lung syndrome
- Stiff lung syndrome
- Wet lung
- White lung syndrome

Etiology

A multitude of etiologic factors may produce ARDS. In alphabetical order, some of the better-known causes follow:

- Aspiration (e.g., of gastric contents or water in near-drowning episodes)
- Central nervous system (CNS) disease (particularly when complicated by increased intracranial pressure)
- Cardiopulmonary bypass (especially when the bypass is prolonged)
- Congestive heart failure (leads to increased alveolar fluid leakage)
- Disseminated intravascular coagulation (seen in patients with shock; it is a condition of paradoxical simultaneous clotting and bleeding that produces microthrombi in the lungs)
- Drug overdose (e.g., heroin, barbiturates, morphine, methadone)
- Fat or air emboli (the fat emboli act as a source of harmful vasoactive material, including fatty acids and serotonin)
- Fluid overload (which promotes alveolar fluid leakage)
- Infections (bacterial, viral, fungal, parasitic, mycoplasmal)
- Inhalation of toxins and irritants (e.g., chlorine gas, nitrogen dioxide, smoke, ozone; oxygen also may be included in this category of irritants)
- Immunologic reaction (e.g., allergic alveolar reaction to inhaled material or Goodpasture's syndrome)
- Massive blood transfusion (in stored blood the quantity of aggregated white blood cells [WBCs], red blood cells [RBCs], platelets, and fibrin increases; these blood components may in turn occlude or damage small blood vessels)
- Nonthoracic trauma
- Oxygen toxicity (e.g., when patients are treated with an excessive oxygen concentration—usually greater than 60%—for a prolonged period)

- Pulmonary ischemia (resulting from shock and hypoperfusion; may cause tissue necrosis, vascular damage, and capillary leakage)
- Radiation-induced lung injury
- Shock (e.g., hypovolemia)

- Systemic reactions to processes initiated outside the lungs (e.g., reactions caused by hemorrhagic pancreatitis, burns, complicated abdominal surgery, septicemia)
- Thoracic trauma (direct contusion to the lungs)
- Uremia

OVERVIEW
of the Cardiopulmonary Clinical Manifestations Associated with ACUTE RESPIRATORY DISTRESS SYNDROME

The following clinical manifestations result from the pathologic mechanisms caused (or activated) by **Atelectasis** (see Figure 9-7), **Alveolar Consolidation** (see Figure 9-8), and **Increased Alveolar-Capillary Membrane Thickness** (see Figure 9-9)—the major anatomic alterations of the lungs associated with ARDS (see Figure 27-1).

CLINICAL DATA OBTAINED AT THE PATIENT'S BEDSIDE

The Physical Examination

Vital Signs

Increased respiratory rate (see page 31 ◆)
Several pathophysiologic mechanisms operating simultaneously may lead to an increased ventilatory rate:

- Stimulation of peripheral chemoreceptors (hypoxemia)
- Decreased lung compliance/increased ventilatory rate relationship
- Stimulation of J receptors
- Anxiety

Increased heart rate (pulse), cardiac output, and blood pressure (see pages 11 and 99 ◆)

Substernal/Intercostal Retractions
(see page 43 ◆)

Cyanosis (see page 45 ◆)

Chest Assessment Findings (see page 22 ◆)

- Dull percussion note
- Bronchial breath sounds
- Crackles

CLINICAL DATA OBTAINED FROM LABORATORY TESTS AND SPECIAL PROCEDURES

Pulmonary Function Study Findings
Expiratory Maneuver Findings (see page 61 ◆)

FVC	FEV_T	$FEF_{25\%-75\%}$	$FEF_{200-1200}$
↓	N or ↓	N or ↓	N
PEFR	MVV	$FEF_{50\%}$	$FEV_{1\%}$
N	N or ↓	N	N or ↑

Lung Volume and Capacity Findings
(see page 62 ◆)

V_T	RV	FRC	TLC
N or ↓	↓	↓	↓
VC	IC	ERV	RV/TLC%
↓	↓	↓	N

Decreased Diffusion Capacity (D_{LCO})
(see page 67 ◆)

Arterial Blood Gases

Mild to Moderate ARDS
Acute Alveolar Hyperventilation with Hypoxemia (see page 70 ◆)

pH	$Paco_2$	HCO_3^-	Pao_2
↑	↓	↓ (Slightly)	↓

Severe ARDS
Acute Ventilatory Failure with Hypoxemia (see page 73 ◆)

pH	$Paco_2$	HCO_3^-*	Pao_2
↓	↑	↑(Slightly)	↓

*When tissue hypoxia is severe enough to produce lactic acid, the pH and HCO_3^- values will be lower than expected for a particular $Paco_2$ level.

Oxygenation Indices (see page 82 ◆)

$\dot{Q}_S/\dot{Q}_T$	Do_2†	$\dot{V}o_2$	$C(a-\bar{v})o_2$
↑	↓	Normal	Normal
O_2ER	$S\bar{v}o_2$		
↑	↓		

†The Do_2 may be normal in patients who have compensated to the decreased oxygenation status with an increased cardiac output. When the Do_2 is normal, the O_2ER is usually normal.

OVERVIEW
of the Cardiopulmonary Clinical Manifestations Associated with
ACUTE RESPIRATORY DISTRESS SYNDROME (Continued)

Hemodynamic Indices (severe)
(see page 99 ◆▷)

CVP	RAP	$\overline{PA}$	PCWP
↑	↑	↑	↑
CO	SV	SVI	CI
↓	↓	↓	↓
RVSWI	LVSWI	PVR	SVR
↑	↓	↑	↑

RADIOLOGIC FINDINGS

Chest Radiograph

- Increased opacity

The structural changes that develop in ARDS increase the radiodensity of the lungs. The increased lung density resists X-ray penetration and is revealed on the radiograph as increased opacity (i.e., whiter in appearance). Therefore the more severe the ARDS, the denser the lungs become and the whiter the radiograph (Figure 27-2). Ultimately, the lungs may have a "ground-glass" appearance.

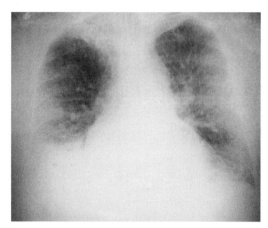

Figure 27–2 Chest X-ray of a patient with moderately severe ARDS.

General Management of ARDS

RESPIRATORY CARE TREATMENT PROTOCOLS

Oxygen Therapy Protocol

Oxygen therapy is used to treat hypoxemia, decrease the work of breathing, and decrease myocardial work. Because of the hypoxemia associated with ARDS, supplemental oxygen often is required. The hypoxemia that develops in ARDS most commonly is caused by widespread alveolar consolidation, atelectasis, and capillary shunting. Hypoxemia caused by capillary shunting often is refractory to oxygen therapy (see Oxygen Therapy Protocol, Protocol 9-1).

Hyperinflation Therapy Protocol

Hyperinflation measures commonly are administered to offset the alveolar consolidation and atelectasis associated with ARDS (see Hyperinflation Therapy Protocol, Protocol 9-3).

Mechanical Ventilation Protocol

Mechanical ventilation may be needed to provide and support alveolar gas exchange and eventually return the patient to spontaneous breathing. Continuous mechanical ventilation is justified when the acute ventilatory failure is thought to be reversible.

Today, the ventilation strategy for most patients with ARDS entails *low tidal volumes* and *high respiratory rates.* The initial tidal volume is usually set at 4 to 8 ml/kg, compared with 12 to 15 ml/kg for patients who do not have ARDS. Ventilatory rates as high as 35 breaths/min may be needed to maintain an adequate minute volume. Positive end-expiratory pressure (PEEP) and continuous positive airway pressure (CPAP) are used with small tidal volumes to reduce atelectasis. The therapeutic goal of low-tidal volume ventilation is to (1) decrease high transpulmonary pressures, (2) reduce overdistention of the lungs, and (3) decrease barotrauma. The patient's Pa_{CO_2} often is allowed to increase (permissive hypercapnia) as a tradeoff to protect the lungs from high airway pressures. In most cases, an increased ventilatory rate adequately offsets the decreased tidal volume used in the management of ARDS. The Pa_{CO_2}, however, should not be permitted to increase to the point of severe acidosis (e.g., a pH below 7.2; see Mechanical Ventilation Protocol, Protocol 9-5).

MEDICATIONS AND PROCEDURES COMMONLY PRESCRIBED BY THE PHYSICIAN

Antibiotics

Antibiotics are commonly administered in an effort to treat secondary bacterial infections (see Appendix II).

Diuretic Agents

Diuretic agents frequently, but often to no effect, are ordered for patients with ARDS in an attempt to reduce interstitial edema (see Appendix II).

Corticosteroids

Although the exact mode of action of corticosteroids is not known, they have been shown to be somewhat effective in treating patients with ARDS. Corticosteroids are used to suppress inflammation and edema (see Appendix II).

Case Study: ACUTE RESPIRATORY DISTRESS SYNDROME

Admitting History and Physical Examination

This comatose 47-year-old woman was admitted to the emergency department of a small community hospital. Her husband found her lying in bed with an empty bottle of "sleeping pills" on the bedside table and a "goodbye note" on the desk blaming her husband's infidelity for her suicide attempt.

In the emergency department she was found to be in a moderately deep coma, responding to deep painful stimulation but otherwise nonresponsive. She was of average size and, according to the husband, had previously been in good health. She did not smoke or drink and was taking no other medication. Her blood pressure and pulse were within normal limits, but her respirations were shallow and noisy.

The emergency department physician decided to lavage her stomach. During the introduction of the nasogastric tube, the patient vomited and aspirated liquid gastric contents. At this time it was decided to transfer her by ambulance to a tertiary care medical center about 30 miles away. The pH of the gastric contents was not determined.

On arrival at the medical center, the patient was comatose but responsive to mild painful stimulation. Her weight was 60 kg and her rectal temperature was 101.5° F. Her blood pressure was 100/60, heart rate 114/min, and respirations 28/min. On auscultation, there were scattered crackles on the right side.

A chest X-ray showed bilateral moderate fluffy infiltrates, mostly on the right side. Blood gases on 5 Lpm O_2 were pH 7.51, Pa_{CO_2} 29, HCO_3^- 22, and Pa_{O_2} 52. At this time the respiratory care practitioner recorded the following SOAP note:

Respiratory Assessment and Plan

S   N/A

O   Patient is comatose. BP 100/60; HR 114; RR 28, T 101.5°; bilateral crackles; CXR: bilateral infiltrates, worse on right side; ABG on 5 LPM O_2: pH 7.51, Pa_{CO_2} 29, HCO_3^- 22, and Pa_{O_2} 52.

A   • Sedative drug overdose with coma (history)
   • Acute alveolar hyperventilation with moderate hypoxemia (ABG)
   • Impending ventilatory failure
   • Aspiration pneumonitis without previous history of pulmonary disease (history and X-ray)

P   Confer with physician. Oxygen therapy per protocol: 100% O_2 via nonrebreathing mask. Plan intubation and ventilatory support according to protocol. Arterial line placement. Continuous oximetry. Repeat ABG 1 hour after intubation and prn.

The patient was admitted to the intensive care unit, intubated, and mechanically ventilated with these settings: V_T 300 ml, IMV 12 bpm, $F_{I_{O_2}}$ 0.4, and 110 cm H_2O of PEEP. An arterial line was placed in her left radial artery, and an intravenous infusion was started with lactated Ringer's solution. An hour later, blood gases were as follows: pH 7.43, $Paco_2$ 36, HCO_3^- 23, and Pao_2 40.

• • • • •

Over the next 72 hours, the patient's oxygenation status continued to deteriorate in spite of an increased Fio_2, PEEP, and pressure-controlled mechanical ventilation. When the arterial oxygen tension did not improve appreciably on an Fio_2 of 0.75 and a PEEP of 20 cm H_2O, a Swan-Ganz catheter was placed in the pulmonary artery. In view of the PEEP, the pressure readings were difficult to interpret. A mean pulmonary artery pressure of 27 mm Hg, however, did suggest increased pulmonary vascular resistance.

A chest X-ray confirmed good position of the endotracheal tube and revealed ARDS with extensive, diffuse infiltrates and atelectasis, worse on the right side. Arterial blood gases on an Fio_2 of 1.0, +25 cm H_2O of PEEP, V_T of 500, and IMV of 16 were pH 7.41, $Paco_2$ 41, HCO_3^- 24, and Pao_2 38. Her spontaneous respiratory rate was 40/min (between the mechanically ventilated breaths), and there were crackles, wheezes, and rhonchi in all lung fields. Moderate to large amounts of purulent sputum frequently were suctioned from the endotracheal tube. Her blood pressure was 90/60, and her heart rate was 130/min. Her temperature was 100.2° F. At this time, the respiratory care practitioner charted the following SOAP note:

Respiratory Assessment and Plan

S N/A (patient comatose)

O Patient remains comatose. BP 90/60, HR 130, RR 40, T 100.2° F. Bilateral crackles, rhonchi, and wheezes. ABGs on Fio_2 1.0 and +25 PEEP: pH 7.41, $Paco_2$ 41, HCO_3^- 24, and Pao_2 38. CXR: ARDS with bilateral infiltrates and atelectasis, worse on the right side. Purulent sputum. PA pressure (mean) 27 mm Hg.

A • Severe and worsening hypoxemia (ABG)
• Persistent coma (physical exam)
• Aspiration pneumonitis progressing to ARDS with bilateral infiltrates and atelectasis (X-ray)

• Increasing airway secretions with infection (crackles, rhonchi, and purulent sputum)

P Call physician to discuss worsening Pao_2 and reconfirm PEEP upper limit. Bronchopulmonary Hygiene Therapy and Aerosolized Medication Protocols (add 2 ml 10% acetylcysteine to 0.5 ml albuterol and aerosolize q 2 h. Suction prn). Gram's stain and culture sputum. Closely monitor and reevaluate.

Because it was apparent that current management would not be successful, the physician decided to alert the **Extracorporeal Membrane Oxygenation** (ECMO) team and place the patient on extracorporeal membrane oxygenation. This was done, and the patient was maintained on ECMO for 13 hours, when she developed ventricular tachycardia followed by ventricular fibrillation. Attempts to reestablish normal cardiac function were not successful, and the patient was pronounced dead 45 minutes later.

Discussion

This was possibly a preventable death. Gastric lavage *never* should be performed on an unconscious patient unless the airway is first protected with a cuffed endotracheal tube. This is one of the very few categorical imperatives in pulmonary medicine. The following three etiologic factors known to produce ARDS may have been operative in this patient: drug overdose, aspiration of gastric contents, and breathing an excessive Fio_2 for a long period (very unlikely). As time progressed, the patient's lungs became stiffer and physiologically nonfunctional as a result of the anatomic alterations associated with ARDS.

Her crackles, rhonchi, refractory hypoxemia, and X-ray findings all reflected the pathophysiologic changes seen in patients with **Atelectasis** (see Figure 9-7) and/or **Increased Alveolar-Capillary Membrane Thickening** (see Figure 9-9). Hyperinflation therapy in the form of PEEP was used with mechanical ventilation right from the start.

Increasing the Fio_2 and PEEP, adding bronchodilator and mucolytic aerosols, and, finally, going to ECMO to manage this case were clearly indicated and appropriate—but not enough in the final analysis.

SELF-ASSESSMENT QUESTIONS

Multiple Choice

1. In response to injury, the lungs of an ARDS patient undergo which of the following changes?

   I. Atelectasis
   II. Decreased alveolar-capillary membrane permeability
   III. Interstitial and intra-alveolar edema
   IV. Hemorrhagic alveolar consolidation

   a. I and III only
   b. II and IV only
   c. I, II, and IV only
   d. I, III, and IV only
   e. I, II, III, and IV

2. Historically, ARDS was first referred to as which of the following?

   a. Oxygen toxicity
   b. Shock lung syndrome
   c. Adult hyaline membrane disease
   d. Congestion atelectasis
   e. White lung

3. What is the generic name of Lasix?

   a. Furosemide
   b. Spironolactone
   c. Aldactone
   d. Thiazide
   e. Hydrochlorothiazide

4. During the early stages of ARDS, the patient commonly demonstrates which of the following arterial blood gas values?

   I. Decreased pH
   II. Increased $Paco_2$
   III. Decreased HCO_3^-
   IV. Normal Pao_2

   a. II only
   b. III only
   c. II and III only
   d. III and IV only
   e. I and II only

5. Which of the following oxygenation indices is/are associated with ARDS?

   I. Increased $\dot{V}o_2$
   II. Decreased Do_2
   III. Increased $S\bar{v}o_2$
   IV. Decreased $\dot{Q}s/\dot{Q}t$

   a. I only
   b. II only
   c. III only
   d. II and III only
   e. I, III, and IV only

True or False

True ☐ False ☐ **1.** The hyaline membrane that develops in ARDS is identical to the hyaline membrane seen in newborns with infant respiratory distress syndrome.

True ☐ False ☐ **2.** The lung compliance of patients with ARDS is very high.

True ☐ False ☐ **3.** Bronchial breath sounds are associated with ARDS.

True ☐ False ☐ **4.** The RV is increased in patients with ARDS.

True ☐ False ☐ **5.** Chest X-ray findings in ARDS reveal a decreased opacity.

Answers appear in Appendix XI.

PART X

Chronic Noninfectious Parenchymal Disease

CHAPTER 28

Chronic Interstitial Lung Diseases

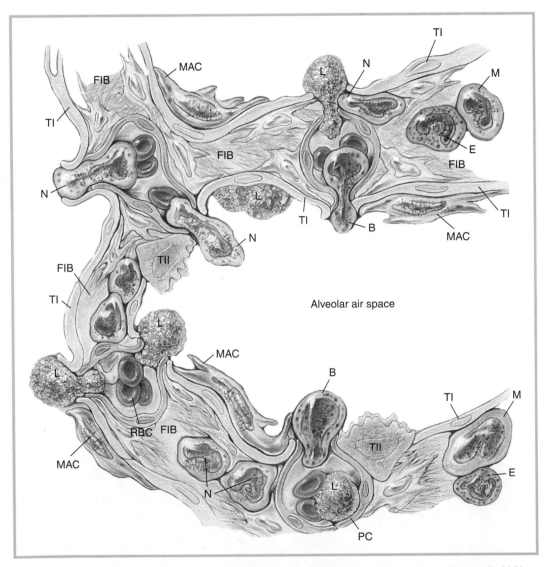

Figure 28–1 Chronic interstitial lung disease. Cross-sectional microscopic view of alveolar-capillary unit. *N*, Neutrophil; *E*, eosinophil; *B*, basophil; *M*, monocyte; *MAC*, macrophage; *L*, lymphocyte; *FIB*, fibroblast (fibrosis); *TI*, type I alveolar cell; *TII*, type II alveolar cell; *RBC*, red blood cell; *PC*, pulmonary capillary. See also Plate 20.

Anatomic Alterations of the Lungs

Interstitial lung diseases comprise a large group of pulmonary disorders that are all associated with pulmonary inflammatory changes. Often, the term *interstitial lung disorder* is made more specific by using a name closely related to the etiology or specific pathology associated with the disease. For example, farmer's lung (caused by inhalation of moldy hay) and pulmonary alveolar proteinosis (so named because of the proteinlike material that fills the alveoli) are both considered interstitial lung disorders, and both manifest the same basic pulmonary pathophysiology. The anatomic alterations may involve the bronchi, alveolar walls, and adjacent alveolar spaces. In severe cases, the extensive inflammation leads to fibrosis, granulomas, honeycombing, and cavitation.

During the acute stage of any interstitial lung disease, the general inflammatory condition is characterized by edema and the infiltration of a variety of white blood cells (e.g., neutrophils, eosinophils, basophils, monocytes, macrophages, and lymphocytes) in the alveolar walls and interstitial spaces (Figure 28-1). Bronchial inflammation and bronchial smooth muscle constriction also may be present.

During the chronic stage the general inflammatory response is characterized by the infiltration of numerous white blood cells (especially monocytes, macrophages, and lymphocytes) and some fibroblasts in the alveolar walls and interstitial spaces. Airway hyperactivity may be present. This stage may be followed by further interstitial thickening, fibrosis, granulomas, and, in some cases, honeycombing and cavity formation. Pleural effusion also may be present. In the chronic stages the basic pathologic features of interstitial fibrosis are identical in any interstitial lung disorder (so-called end-stage pulmonary fibrosis).

In general, the interstitial lung disorders produce a restrictive pattern in pulmonary function testing. However, because inflammation and smooth muscle constriction also can develop in the small airways, the clinical manifestations associated with an obstructive disorder may also be seen. Therefore the patient with interstitial lung disease may demonstrate a restrictive disorder, an obstructive disorder, or a combination of both.

Although a fully satisfactory classification system is not available, the interstitial lung disorders are commonly divided into two broad groups according to whether the alveolar inflammation and fibrosis are associated with the presence or absence of granuloma. The term *granuloma* is an imprecise description applied to (1) any small nodular, delimited aggregation of mononuclear inflammatory cells or (2) a similar collection of modified macrophages resembling epithelial cells, usually surrounded by a rim of lymphocytes. Granuloma formation represents a chronic inflammatory response initiated by various infective and noninfective agents.

The major pathologic or structural changes associated with chronic interstitial lung diseases are as follows:

* Fibrotic thickening of the respiratory bronchioles, alveolar ducts, and alveoli
* Granulomas
* Destruction of the alveoli and adjacent pulmonary capillaries
* Honeycombing and cavity formation
* Airway obstruction caused by inflammation and bronchial constriction

Etiology

More than 140 different disease processes are known to produce an interstitial lung disorder, and the list continues to grow. In this group of disease entities, however, no specific etiologic agent can be identified in more than 65% of the cases, in spite of the fact that a specific name may be attached to a particular disease entity. Box 28-1 lists some of the more common interstitial lung disorders. A discussion of the more common interstitial lung diseases follows.

INTERSTITIAL INFLAMMATION WITH GRANULOMA FORMATION

Extrinsic Allergic Alveolitis

Extrinsic allergic alveolitis (also called *hypersensitivity pneumonitis*) is an immunologically mediated inflammation of the lungs caused by the inhalation of a variety of offending agents (antigens) such as pollen, animal dander, organic dusts, and spores of certain molds. Table 28-1 lists a variety of offending agents known to cause extrinsic allergic alveolitis. The term *extrinsic allergic alveolitis* is often renamed according to the specific agent known to cause the disorder. For example, extrinsic allergic alveolitis caused by inhalation of moldy hay is called *farmer's lung*.

To understand the clinical and pathophysiologic features of extrinsic allergic alveolitis, a basic understanding of the hypersensitivity reaction is required (Table 28-2). There are four types of allergic or hypersensitivity reactions; three are mediated by humoral antibodies, and one is mediated by T cells. It appears that the Type III hypersensitivity reaction is the underlying cause for most of the pathologic changes associated with extrinsic allergic alveolitis. The diagnosis of

BOX 28–1

Common Interstitial Lung Disorders

Interstitial Inflammation with Granuloma Formation

Extrinsic allergic alveolitis (hypersensitivity pneumonitis)
Sarcoidosis
Eosinophilic granuloma (histiocytosis X)
Pulmonary vasculitides
  Wegener's granulomatosis
  Churg-Strauss syndrome
  Lymphomatoid granulomatosis

Interstitial Inflammation without Granuloma Formation

Idiopathic pulmonary fibrosis
Drug-induced interstitial lung disease
Radiation-induced interstitial lung disease
Irritant gases
Collagen vascular diseases
  Rheumatoid arthritis
  Systemic lupus erythematosus
  Polymyositis-dermatomyositis
  Progressive systemic sclerosis
  Sjögren's syndrome

Miscellaneous Diffuse Interstitial Lung Diseases

Goodpasture's syndrome
Idiopathic pulmonary hemosiderosis
Chronic eosinophilic pneumonia
Bronchiolitis obliterans with organizing pneumonia
Lymphangioleiomyomatosis
Alveolar proteinosis

TABLE 28–1 Antigens, Their Source, and the Disease Entities that Can Produce Hypersensitivity Pneumonitis

Disease	Source of Antigen	Antigens
Air-conditioning and humidifier lung	Fungi in air conditioners and humidifiers	Thermophilic actinomycetes
Aspergillosis	Ubiquitous	*Aspergillus fumigatus, A. flavus, A. niger, A. nidulans*
Bagassosis (sugar cane workers)	Moldy bagasse	*Thermoactinomyces vulgaris*
Bird breeder's lung	Pigeon, parrot, hen droppings	Avian proteins
Byssinosis	Cotton, flax, hemp workers	Unknown
Farmer's lung	Moldy hay	*Micropolyspora faeni, T. vulgaris*
Malt worker's lung	Moldy barley, malt dust	*A. clavatus, A. fumigatus*
Maple-bark pneumonitis	Moldy maple bark	*Coniosporium corticale*
Mushroom worker's lung	Mushroom compost	*M. faeni, T. vulgaris*
"New Guinea" lung	Moldy thatch dust	Thatch of huts
Pituitary snuff-taker's lung	Heterologous pituitary powder	Heterologous antigen of pituitary snuff
Sisal worker's lung	Unknown	Unknown
Suberosis	Moldy oak bark, cork dust	*Penicillium*
Wheat weevil disease	Infested wheat flour	*Sitophilus granarius*

extrinsic allergic alveolitis generally depends on an occupational history and, subsequently, is confirmed with blood tests (antibody measurements) or skin testing.

Sarcoidosis

Sarcoidosis is a multisystem granulomatous disease of unknown etiology. It may affect any part of the body but most frequently involves the lung, lymph nodes, liver, spleen, skin, eyes, and small bones of the hands and feet. The lung is the most frequently affected organ, with manifestations generally including interstitial lung disease, enlargement of the mediastinal lymph nodes, or a combination of both. One of the clinical hallmarks of sarcoidosis is an increase in all three major immunoglobulins (IgM, IgG, and IgA).

The incidence of sarcoidosis varies from one country to another and even in different regions of the same country. For example, Sweden, Northern Ireland, Denmark, and Germany have a high prevalence, whereas neighboring countries such as Finland have a relatively low prevalence. In the United States the incidence is about 10 cases per 100,000. The disease is more common among African-Americans and appears most frequently in patients between 10 and 40 years of age, with the highest incidence between 20 and 30 years of age. Women are affected more than men, especially among African-Americans.

TABLE 28–2 Hypersensitivity or Allergic Reaction

Group	Reaction	Pulmonary Pathology	Examples
TYPE I: anaphylaxis	When first exposed to a certain antigen, the lymphoid cells from specific IgE antibodies in turn bond to the surface of the mast cells. Subsequent exposure to the same antigen creates an antigen-antibody reaction on the surface of the mast cell, which causes the mast cell to degranulate and release chemical mediators such as histamine, leukotrienes [formerly called slow reacting substance of anaphylaxis (SRS-A)], eosinophilic chemotactic factor of anaphylaxis (ECFA), neutrophil chemotactic factor (NCF), prostaglandins, and platelet-activating factor (PAF).	The release of chemical mediators causing smooth muscle constriction of the bronchi, dilation of blood vessels, increased capillary permeability, infiltration of eosinophils, and tissue edema	Bronchial asthma, allergic rhinitis, and eczema
TYPE II: cytotoxic	When certain antigens are introduced into the body, they may bond to the surface of red blood cells, leukocytes, or platelets. When this happens, antibodies are formed to destroy the antigens attached to the cells. The disease that develops depends on the blood cell to which the antigen is attached. For example, when antibodies attack the antigen attached to red blood cells, hemolysis, jaundice, and anemia develop. When antibodies attack the leukocytes, increased susceptibility to infection ensues. When antiplatelet antibodies are formed, the results may be thrombocytopenia and hemorrhagic manifestations. Unlike the Type I reaction, only one exposure to the antigen is necessary in the Type II reaction.	Cellular and tissue inflammation	Goodpasture's syndrome, blood transfusion, pericillin therapy (occasionally)
TYPE III: immune complex–mediated hypersensitivity	When an offending soluble or particulate antigen is introduced into the body (e.g., inhaled into the lungs) antibodies are formed. The antibodies, in turn, attach themselves to the capillaries at the spot where the antigen entered the body. The next exposure to the offending antigen elicits immune complexes that lead to the destruction of endothelial cells by the individual's own immunologic defense system.	Damage to the endothelial lining, deposition of fibrin in the wall of the blood vessel, microthrombosis, local ischemia, necrosis of the vessel walls, and granuloma formation	Extrinsic allergic alveolitis (hypersensitivity pneumonitis)
TYPE IV: cell-mediated reactions	The Type IV reaction is mediated by T lymphocytes and involves the same basic mechanism related to the protective response to the T cells. The reaction takes 24 to 48 hours to develop and is therefore called *delayed hypersensitivity*.	Infiltration of macrophages and lymphocytes with possible granuloma formation, caseation, and necrosis	Tuberculosis, poison ivy, poison oak, contact dermatitis, and eczema; possibly sarcoidosis and Wegener's granulomatosis

The initial diagnosis of sarcoidosis usually is based on the clinical presentation, followed by confirmation with a chest radiograph and histologic evidence obtained by biopsy.

Eosinophilic Granuloma

Eosinophilic granuloma (also called *histiocytosis X*) is characterized by numerous small interstitial granulomas scattered throughout the lungs. Often their location is just below the visceral pleura of the lungs, causing what is known as a "reverse bat-wing" appearance on the chest X-ray. The interstitial granulomas are composed of moderately large, pale histiocytes (also called *histiocytosis X cells*), which are the hallmark of this disorder. Histiocytic cells are a particular type of macrophage having unique rodlike structures called *X bodies* within their cytoplasm that can be seen by electron microscopy. In addition to histiocytes, there is an infiltration by eosinophils, lymphocytes, and alveolar macrophages. Eosinophilic granuloma is a disorder of unknown etiology. It most commonly appears in smokers and ex-smokers between 20 and 40 years of age, and males are slightly more often affected than females.

THE PULMONARY VASCULITIDES

The pulmonary vasculitides (also called *granulomatous vasculitides*) consist of a heterogeneous group of pulmonary disorders characterized by inflammation and destruction of the pulmonary vessels. The major disorders in this category include Wegener's granulomatosis, Churg-Strauss syndrome, and lymphomatoid granulomatosis.

Wegener's Granulomatosis

Wegener's granulomatosis is a multisystem disorder characterized by (1) a necrotizing, granulomatous vasculitis; (2) focal and segmental glomerulonephritis; and (3) variable degrees of systemic vasculitis of the small veins and arteries. In the lungs, numerous 1- to 9-cm-diameter nodules are commonly seen in the upper lobes, and cavity formation is often associated with the larger lesions.

Wegener's granulomatosis is considered an aggressive and fatal disorder, although the prognosis has significantly improved with the recent availability of cytotoxic agents (e.g., cyclophosphamide). This disorder most commonly is seen in males older than 50 years of age. Diagnosis is confirmed by an open lung biopsy. Histologic examination reveals lesions with marked central necrosis. The area surrounding the necrotizing lesion consists of inflammatory white blood cells (WBCs) with some fibroblasts. Inflammatory cell infiltrate and necrotizing vasculitis are seen in the adjacent blood vessels.

Churg-Strauss Syndrome

Churg-Strauss syndrome is a necrotizing vasculitis that predominantly involves the small vessels of the lungs. The granulomatous lesions are characterized by a heavy infiltrate of eosinophils, central necrosis, and peripheral eosinophilia. Cavity formation is rare in this disorder. Clinically, symptoms of asthma usually precede the onset of vasculitis. In recent years, rapid tapering of oral steroids with substitution of leukotriene inhibitors such as montelukast (Singulair) and zafirlukast (Accolate) has been associated with deaths from fulminant Churg-Strauss syndrome reactions. Neurologic disorders such as mononeuritis multiplex, a simultaneous disease of several peripheral nerves, are frequently associated with this disorder. Diagnosis is usually confirmed with an open lung biopsy, and the disease is often rapidly fatal.

Lymphomatoid Granulomatosis

Lymphomatoid granulomatosis is a rare necrotizing vasculitis that primarily involves the lungs, although neurologic and cutaneous lesions sometimes are seen. The lesions are usually in the lower lobes, and cavities develop in more than one third of the cases. Pleural effusion is common.

Although the clinical presentation is similar to that of Wegener's granulomatosis, there are some distinct differences. For example, more mature lymphoreticular cells are involved in the formation of the granulomatous lesions and no glomerulonephritis is seen. Histologically, the lesions simulate malignant lymphoma. This disorder most commonly is seen in males between 50 and 70 years of age. Diagnosis is confirmed by open lung biopsy.

INTERSTITIAL INFLAMMATION WITHOUT GRANULOMA FORMATION

Idiopathic Pulmonary Fibrosis

Idiopathic pulmonary fibrosis (IPF) is a progressive inflammatory disease with varying degrees of fibrosis and, in severe cases, honeycombing. The precise etiology is unknown. Although *IPF* is the most frequent term used for this disorder, numerous other names appear in the literature, such as *acute interstitial fibrosis of the lung, cryptogenic fibrosing alveolitis, Hamman-Rich syndrome, honeycomb lung, interstitial fibrosis,* and *interstitial pneumonitis.*

IPF commonly is separated into the following two major disease entities according to the predominant histologic appearance: desquamative interstitial pneumonia (DIP) and usual interstitial pneumonia (UIP). In DIP the most prominent features are hyperplasia and desquamation of the alveolar Type II cells. The alveolar spaces are packed with macrophages, and there is an even distribution of the interstitial mononuclear infiltrate.

In UIP the most prominent features are interstitial and alveolar wall thickening caused by chronic inflammatory cells and fibrosis. In severe cases, fibrotic connective tissue replaces the alveolar walls, the alveolar architecture becomes distorted, and eventually honeycombing develops. When honeycombing is present, the inflammatory infiltrate is significantly reduced. The prognosis for patients with DIP is significantly better than that for patients with UIP.

Some experts believe that DIP and UIP are two distinct interstitial lung disease entities. Others, however, believe that DIP and UIP are different stages of the same disease process. This disorder most commonly seen is seen in males between 40 and 70 years of age. Diagnosis generally is confirmed by an open lung biopsy. Most patients diagnosed with IPF have a more chronic progressive course, and death usually occurs in 4 to 10 years. Death usually is the result of progressive acute ventilatory failure, complicated by pulmonary infection.

Drug-Induced Interstitial Lung Disease

As the list of pharmacologic agents continues to grow, so does the list of possible side effects. Unfortunately, the lungs are major target organs affected by these side effects. Although it is impossible to discuss in detail the various lung-related side effects of every drug, it is possible to describe some of the general concerns related to drug-induced lung disease and list some of the pharmacologic agents that may be responsible.

The chemotherapeutic or cytotoxic agents (anticancer agents) are by far the largest group of agents associated with interstitial lung disease. Bleomycin, mitomycin, busulfan, cyclophosphamide, methotrexate, and carmustine (BCNU) are the major offenders. Nitrofurantoin (an antibacterial drug used in the treatment of urinary tract infections) also is associated with interstitial lung disease. Gold and penicillamine for the treatment of rheumatoid arthritis also have been shown to cause interstitial lung disease. The diagnosis may be difficult in these cases because the underlying disease (rheumatoid arthritis) itself also is a possible cause of diffuse parenchymal disease.

The excessive administration of oxygen (oxygen toxicity) also is known to cause diffuse pulmonary injury and fibrosis (see Chapter 27). As a general rule, the risk of these drugs causing an interstitial lung disorder is directly related to the dosage. Drug-induced interstitial disease may be seen as early as 1 month to as late as several years after exposure to these agents.

The precise etiology of drug-induced interstitial lung disease is not known. Diagnosis is confirmed by an open lung biopsy. When interstitial fibrosis is found with no infectious organisms, a drug-induced interstitial process must be suspected.

Radiation-Induced Interstitial Lung Disease

Radiation therapy for tumors of the breast, lung, or thorax is a potential cause of interstitial lung disease. Radiation-induced lung disease commonly is divided into the following two major phases: the acute, or early, pneumonitic phase and the late fibrotic phase. Acute pneumonitis rarely is seen in patients who receive a total radiation dose of less than 3500 rads. On the other hand, doses in excess of 6000 rads over 6 weeks almost always cause interstitial lung disease in and near the radiated areas.

The acute pneumonitic phase develops approximately 2 to 3 months after exposure. Chronic radiation fibrosis is seen in all patients who develop acute pneumonitis. The late phase of fibrosis may develop (1) immediately after the development of acute pneumonitis, (2) without an acute pneumonitic period, or (3) after a symptom-free latent period. When fibrosis does develop, it generally does so between 6 and 12 months after radiation exposure. Pleural effusion often is associated with the late fibrotic phase.

The precise cause of radiation-induced lung disease is not known. The establishment of a diagnosis is similar to that for drug-induced interstitial disease (i.e., by obtaining a history of recent radiation therapy and confirming the diagnosis with an open lung biopsy).

Irritant Gases

The inhalation of irritant gases may cause an acute chemical pneumonitis and, in severe cases, interstitial lung disease. Most exposures occur in an industrial setting. Table 28-3 lists some of the more common irritant gases and the industrial settings where they may be found.

COLLAGEN VASCULAR DISEASES

The collagen vascular diseases (also called *connective tissue disorders*) include rheumatoid arthritis, systemic lupus erythematosus, progressive systemic

TABLE 28–3 Common Irritant Gases Associated with Interstitial Lung Disease

Gas	Industrial Setting
Chlorine	Chemical and plastic industries
	Water disinfection
Ammonia	Commercial refrigeration
	Smelting of sulfide ores
Ozone	Welding
	Manufacture of bleaches and peroxides
Nitrogen dioxide	May be liberated after exposure of nitric acid to air
Phosgene	Used in the production of aniline dyes

sclerosis (scleroderma), polymyositis-dermatomyositis, and Sjögren's syndrome. All of these disorders are multisystem inflammatory diseases that are immunologically mediated. The organ systems that may be involved vary with each disease, but all may affect the lungs.

Rheumatoid Arthritis

Rheumatoid arthritis primarily is an inflammatory joint disease. It may, however, involve the lungs in the form of (1) pleurisy, with or without effusion; (2) interstitial pneumonitis; (3) necrobiotic nodules, with or without cavities; (4) Caplan's syndrome; and (5) pulmonary hypertension secondary to pulmonary vasculitis.

Pleurisy with or without effusion is the most common pulmonary complication associated with rheumatoid arthritis. When present, the effusion is generally unilateral (often on the right side). Men appear to develop rheumatoid pleural complications more often than women. Rheumatoid interstitial pneumonitis is characterized by alveolar wall fibrosis, interstitial and intra-alveolar mononuclear cell infiltration, and lymphoid nodules. In severe cases, extensive fibrosing alveolitis and honeycombing may develop. Rheumatoid interstitial pneumonitis is also more common in male patients. Necrobiotic nodules are characterized by the gradual degeneration and swelling of lung tissue.

The pulmonary nodules generally appear as well-circumscribed masses that often progress to cavitation. The nodules usually develop in the periphery of the lungs and are more common in men. Histologically, the pulmonary nodules are identical to the subcutaneous nodules that develop in rheumatoid arthritis.

Caplan's syndrome (also called *rheumatoid pneumoconiosis*) is a progressive pulmonary fibrosis of the lung commonly seen in coal miners.

Caplan's syndrome is characterized by rounded densities in the lung periphery that often undergo cavity formation and, in some cases, calcification. Pulmonary hypertension is a common secondary complication caused by the progression of fibrosing alveolitis and pulmonary vasculitis.

Systemic Lupus Erythematosus

Systemic lupus erythematosus (SLE) is a multisystem disorder that mainly involves the joints and skin. It also may cause serious problems in numerous other organs, including the kidneys, lungs, nervous system, and heart. Involvement of the lungs appears in about 50% to 70% of the cases. Pulmonary manifestations are characterized by (1) pleurisy with or without effusion, (2) atelectasis, (3) diffuse infiltrates and pneumonitis, (4) diffuse interstitial lung disease, (5) uremic pulmonary edema, (6) diaphragmatic dysfunction, and (7) infections.

Pleurisy with or without effusion is the most common pulmonary complication of SLE. The effusions usually are exudates with high protein concentration and are frequently bilateral. Atelectasis commonly develops in response to the pleurisy, effusion, and diaphragmatic elevation associated with SLE. Diffuse noninfectious pulmonary infiltrates and pneumonitis are common. In severe cases, chronic interstitial pneumonitis may develop. Because SLE frequently impairs the renal system, uremic pulmonary edema may occur. Recently, SLE has been found to be associated with diaphragmatic dysfunction and reduced lung volume. Some research suggests that a diffuse myopathy affecting the diaphragm is the source of this problem. Approximately 50% of the cases have a complicating pulmonary infection.

Polymyositis-Dermatomyositis

Polymyositis is a diffuse inflammatory disorder of the striated muscles that primarily weakens the limbs, neck, and pharynx. *Dermatomyositis* is the term used when an erythematous skin rash accompanies the muscle weakness. Pulmonary involvement develops in response to (1) recurrent episodes of aspiration pneumonia caused by esophageal weakness and atrophy, (2) hypostatic pneumonia secondary to a weakened diaphragm, and (3) drug-induced interstitial pneumonitis.

Polymyositis-dermatomyositis is seen more often in women than men, at about a 2:1 ratio. The disease occurs primarily in two age groups: before the age of 10 and between 40 and 50 years of age. In about 40% of the patients, the pulmonary manifestations are seen 1 to 24 months before the striated muscle or skin shows signs of symptoms.

Progressive Systemic Sclerosis

Progressive systemic sclerosis (also called *scleroderma*) is a disorder that primarily involves the skin and the small blood vessels. Other affected organ systems include the pulmonary vasculature, esophagus, gastrointestinal tract, heart, lungs, and kidneys. The esophagus is the organ most often affected. Progressive systemic sclerosis of the lung appears in the form of interstitial lung disease and fibrosis. Of all the collagen vascular disorders, progressive systemic sclerosis is the one in which pulmonary involvement is most severe and most likely to cause significant scarring of the lung parenchyma.

The pulmonary complications include diffuse interstitial fibrosis, severe pulmonary hypertension, pleural disease, and aspiration pneumonitis (secondary to esophageal involvement). Progressive systemic sclerosis also may involve the small pulmonary blood vessels and appears to be independent of the fibrotic process involving the alveolar walls. The disease most commonly is seen in women between 30 and 50 years of age.

Sjögren's Syndrome

Sjögren's syndrome is a lymphocytic infiltration that primarily involves the salivary and lacrimal glands and is manifested by dry mucous membranes, usually of the mouth and eyes. Pulmonary involvement also frequently occurs in Sjögren's syndrome and includes (1) pleurisy with or without effusion, (2) interstitial fibrosis that is indistinguishable from that of other collagen vascular disorders, and (3) infiltration of lymphocytes of the tracheobronchial tree mucous glands, which in turn causes atrophy of the mucous glands, mucus plugging, atelectasis, and secondary infections. Sjögren's syndrome occurs most often in women (90%) and is commonly associated with rheumatoid arthritis (50% of patients with Sjögren's syndrome).

MISCELLANEOUS DIFFUSE INTERSTITIAL LUNG DISEASES

Goodpasture's Syndrome

Goodpasture's syndrome is a disease of unknown etiology that involves two organ systems—the lungs and the kidneys. In the lungs, there are recurrent episodes of pulmonary hemorrhage and, in some cases, pulmonary fibrosis—presumably as a consequence of the bleeding episodes. In the kidneys, there is a glomerulonephritis characterized by the infiltration of antibodies within the glomerular basement membrane. These circulating antibodies function against the patient's own glomerular basement membrane (GBM). They are commonly abbreviated as anti-GBM antibodies. It is believed that the anti-GBM antibodies cross-react with the basement membrane of the alveolar wall and that their deposition in the kidneys and lungs is responsible for producing the pathophysiologic processes of the disease.

Goodpasture's syndrome usually is seen in young adults. The average survival period after diagnosis is about 15 weeks. About 50% of the patients die from massive pulmonary hemorrhage, and about 50% die from chronic renal failure. An interesting feature of Goodpasture's syndrome is that the patient frequently demonstrates an increased DL_{CO}, which is in direct contrast to most interstitial lung disorders. The increased carbon monoxide uptake commonly seen in this disorder is thought to be caused by the increased amount of retained blood in the pulmonary tissue.

Idiopathic Pulmonary Hemosiderosis

Idiopathic pulmonary hemosiderosis is a disease entity of unknown etiology that is characterized by recurrent episodes of pulmonary hemorrhage similar to that seen in Goodpasture's syndrome. Histologic examination reveals an alveolar hemorrhage with hemosiderin-laden macrophages and hyperplasia of the alveolar epithelium. Unlike Goodpasture's syndrome, however, there is no evidence of circulating anti-GBM antibodies attacking the alveolar or glomerular basement membranes, and this disorder is not associated with renal disease.

Idiopathic pulmonary hemosiderosis most often is seen in children. As in Goodpasture's syndrome, patients commonly demonstrate an increased DL_{CO}, which is in direct contrast to most interstitial lung disorders. Again, the increased uptake of carbon monoxide is thought to be caused by the increased amount of blood retained in the lungs.

Chronic Eosinophilic Pneumonia

Chronic eosinophilic pneumonia is characterized by infiltration of eosinophils and, to a lesser extent, macrophages into the alveolar and interstitial spaces. Clinically, a unique feature of this disorder often is seen on the chest radiograph, consisting of a peripheral distribution of pulmonary infiltrates. This radiographic pattern is commonly referred to as a *photographic negative of pulmonary edema*. This is because of the dense peripheral infiltration, with the sparing of the perihilar areas, seen in chronic eosinophilic pneumonia, compared with the central pulmonary infiltration with the sparing of the lung periphery seen in pulmonary edema. An increased number of eosinophils also is commonly seen in the peripheral blood. Histologic diagnosis is made by means of an open lung biopsy.

Bronchiolitis Obliterans with Organizing Pneumonia

Bronchiolitis obliterans with organizing pneumonia, more commonly known by the acronym *BOOP*, is characterized by connective tissue plugs in the small airways (hence the term *bronchiolitis obliterans*) and mononuclear cell infiltration of the surrounding parenchyma (hence the term *organizing pneumonia*). Although the majority of BOOP cases have no identifiable cause and therefore are considered idiopathic, BOOP has been associated with connective tissue disease, toxic gas inhalation, and infection. The chest radiograph commonly shows patchy infiltrates of alveolar rather than interstitial involvement.

Lymphangioleiomyomatosis

Lymphangioleiomyomatosis (LAM) is a rare disease of the smooth muscles of the lungs affecting women of childbearing age. It is characterized by the proliferation of nodules composed of atypical smooth muscles along the lymphatics of the lung, thorax, and abdomen. Common clinical features associated with LAM are recurrent pneumothorax, hemoptysis, and chylothorax. The diagnosis of LAM is confirmed with an open lung biopsy. The prognosis is poor; the disease slowly progresses over 2 to 10 years, ending in death resulting from ventilatory failure.

Alveolar Proteinosis

Alveolar proteinosis is a disorder of unknown etiology. It is characterized by the filling of the alveoli with an amorphous proteinaceous material. The material is a lipoprotein similar to the pulmonary surfactant produced by the Type II cells. In addition, the alveolar macrophages generally are dysfunctional in this disorder. The disease most commonly is seen in adults between 20 and 50 years of age. Men are affected twice as often as women. The chest radiograph typically reveals bilateral infiltrates that are most prominent in the perihilar regions (butterfly pattern). It is often indistinguishable from pulmonary edema but does not produce cardiac enlargement. Air bronchograms commonly are seen. The diagnosis of alveolar proteinosis is confirmed by transbronchial or open lung biopsy.

OVERVIEW
of the Cardiopulmonary Clinical Manifestations Associated with CHRONIC INTERSTITIAL LUNG DISEASES

The following clinical manifestations result from the pathophysiologic mechanisms caused (or activated) by an **Increased Alveolar-Capillary Membrane Thickness** (see Figure 9-9) and **Bronchospasm** (see Figure 9-10)—the major anatomic alterations of the lungs associated with chronic interstitial lung disease (see Figure 28-1).

CLINICAL DATA OBTAINED AT THE PATIENT'S BEDSIDE

The Physical Examination
Vital Signs

Increased respiratory rate (see page 31 ◆▶)
Several pathophysiologic mechanisms operating simultaneously may lead to an increased ventilatory rate:
- Stimulation of peripheral chemoreceptors (hypoxemia)
- Decreased lung compliance/increased ventilatory rate relationship
- Stimulation of the J receptors
- Pain/anxiety

Increased heart rate (pulse), cardiac output, and blood pressure (see pages 11 and 99 ◆▶)

Cyanosis (see page 45 ◆▶)

Digital Clubbing (see page 46 ◆▶)

Peripheral Edema and Venous Distention (see page 47)

Because polycythemia and cor pulmonale are associated with chronic interstitial lung disease, the following may be seen:
- Distended neck veins
- Pitting edema
- Enlarged and tender liver

Nonproductive Cough (see page 47)

Chest Assessment Findings (see page 22 ◆▶)
- Increased tactile and vocal fremitus
- Dull percussion note
- Bronchial breath sounds
- Crackles, rhonchi, and wheezing
- Pleural friction rub
- Whispered pectoriloquy

OVERVIEW

of the Cardiopulmonary Clinical Manifestations Associated with
CHRONIC INTERSTITIAL LUNG DISEASES (Continued)

CLINICAL DATA OBTAINED FROM LABORATORY TESTS AND SPECIAL PROCEDURES

Pulmonary Function Study Findings

Expiratory Maneuver Findings
(see pages 61 and 62 ◆)

FVC	FEV_T	$FEF_{25\%-75\%}$	$FEF_{200-1200}$
↓	N or ↓	N or ↓	N or ↓
PEFR	MVV	$FEF_{50\%}$	$FEV_{1\%}$
N or ↓	N or ↓	N or ↓	N or ↓

Lung Volume and Capacity Findings
(see pages 62 and 66 ◆)

V_T	RV	FRC	TLC
N or ↓	↓	↓	N or ↓
VC	IC	ERV	RV/TLC%
↓	N or ↓	N or ↓	N or ↑

Decreased Diffusion Capacity (see page 67 ◆)
There is an exception to the expected decreased diffusion capacity in the following two interstitial lung diseases: Goodpasture's syndrome and idiopathic pulmonary hemosiderosis. The DLco is often elevated in response to the increased amount of blood retained in the alveolar spaces that is associated with these two disorders.

Arterial Blood Gases

Mild to Moderate Chronic Interstitial Lung Disease
Acute Alveolar Hyperventilation with Hypoxemia (see page 70 ◆)

pH	$Paco_2$	HCO_3^-	Pao_2
↑	↓	↓(Slightly)	↓

Severe Chronic Interstitial Lung Disease
Chronic Ventilatory Failure with Hypoxemia (see page 73 ◆)

pH	$Paco_2$	HCO_3^-	Pao_2
Normal	↑	↑(Significantly)	↓

Acute Ventilatory Changes Superimposed on Chronic Ventilatory Failure (see page 75 ◆)
Because acute ventilatory changes frequently are seen in patients with chronic ventilatory failure, the respiratory care practitioner must be familiar with and alert for (1) acute alveolar hyperventilation superimposed on chronic ventilatory failure and (2) acute ventilatory failure superimposed on chronic ventilatory failure.

Oxygenation Indices (see page 82 ◆)

$\dot{Q}s/\dot{Q}_T$	Do_2*	Vo_2	$C(a-\bar{v})O_2$
↑	↓	Normal	Normal
O_2ER*	$S\bar{v}o_2$		
↑	↓		

*The Do_2 may be normal in patients who have compensated to the decreased oxygenation status with (1) an increased cardiac output, (2) an increased hemoglobin level, or (3) a combination of both. When the Do_2 is normal, the O_2ER is usually normal.

Hemodynamic Indices (Severe)
(see page 99)

CVP	RAP	$\overline{PA}$	PCWP
↑	↑	↑	Normal
CO	SV	SVI	CI
Normal	Normal	Normal	Normal
RVSWI	LVSWI	PVR	SVR
↑	Normal	↑	Normal

LABORATORY FINDINGS

Complete blood count—Elevated hemoglobin concentration and hematocrit

RADIOLOGIC FINDINGS (VARY ACCORDING TO THE ETIOLOGY)

Chest Radiograph
- Bilateral infiltrates
- Granulomas
- Cavity formation
- Honeycombing
- Air bronchograms
- Pleural effusion (see Chapter 23)

Bilateral diffuse interstitial infiltrates and nodular densities in the lower lung lobes generally are seen on the radiographs of affected patients. Cavity formation commonly is associated with Wegener's granulomatosis, lymphomatoid granulomatosis, and rheumatoid arthritis (Figure 28-2). Pleural effusion commonly is seen in patients with lymphomatoid granulomatosis, rheumatoid arthritis, systemic lupus erythematosus, and progressive systemic sclerosis (Figure 28-3). A honeycomb or reticulonodular pattern also may be seen in patients with chronic interstitial lung disease (Figure 28-4).

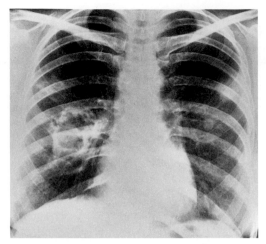

Figure 28–2 Wegener's granulomatosis. Numerous nodules with a large (6 cm) cavitary lesion adjacent to the right hilus. Its walls are thick and irregular. (Courtesy Dr. GJ Hunger, London. From Armstrong P et al: *Imaging of diseases of the chest,* ed 2, St. Louis, 1995, Mosby.)

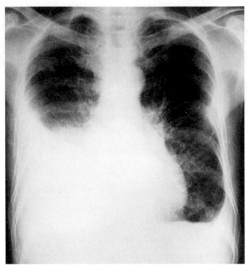

Figure 28–3 Pleural effusion in rheumatoid disease. Bilateral pleural effusions are present with mild changes of fibrosing alveolitis. The effusions were painless, and the one on the right had been present, more or less unchanged, for 5 months. (From Armstrong P et al: *Imaging of diseases of the chest,* ed 2, St. Louis, 1995, Mosby.)

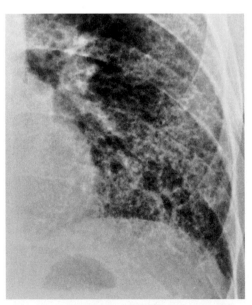

Figure 28–4 Reticulonodular pattern in a chest X-ray of a patient with interstitial pulmonary fibrosis resulting from scleroderma. (From Armstrong P et al: *Imaging of diseases of the chest,* ed 2, St. Louis, 1995, Mosby.)

General Management of Chronic Interstitial Lung Diseases

RESPIRATORY CARE TREATMENT PROTOCOLS

Oxygen Therapy Protocol

Oxygen therapy is used to treat hypoxemia, decrease the work of breathing, and decrease myocardial work. Because of the hypoxemia associated with interstitial lung diseases, supplemental oxygen often is required. The hypoxemia that develops in an interstitial lung disorder most commonly is caused by the alveolar thickening, fibrosis, and capillary shunting associated with the disorder. Hypoxemia caused by capillary shunting often is refractory to oxygen therapy. In addition, when the patient demonstrates chronic ventilatory failure during the advanced stages of an interstitial lung disorder, caution must be taken not to overoxygenate the patient (see Oxygen Therapy Protocol, Protocol 9-1).

Aerosolized Medication Protocol

Both sympathomimetic and parasympatholytic agents commonly are used to offset bronchial smooth muscle constriction (see Aerosolized Medication Protocol, Protocol 9-4).

Mechanical Ventilation Protocol

Mechanical ventilation may be needed to provide and support alveolar gas exchange and eventually return the patient to spontaneous breathing. Because acute ventilatory failure superimposed on chronic ventilatory failure often is seen in patients with severe interstitial lung disease, continuous mechanical ventilation often is required. Continuous mechanical ventilation is justified when the acute ventilatory failure is thought to be reversible (see Mechanical Ventilation Protocol, Protocol 9-5).

MEDICATIONS AND PROCEDURES COMMONLY PRESCRIBED BY THE PHYSICIAN

The management of interstitial lung disorders is directed at the inflammation associated with the various disorders.

Corticosteroids

Corticosteroids are commonly administered with reasonably good results, but the benefit varies remarkably from one patient to another (see Appendix II).

Other Agents

In patients with Wegener's granulomatosis, the prognosis has dramatically improved since the development of cytotoxic agents (e.g., cyclophosphamide).

OTHER TREATMENTS

Plasmapheresis

Treatment of Goodpasture's syndrome is directed at reducing the circulating anti-GBM antibodies that attack the patient's glomerular basement membrane. Plasmapheresis, which directly removes the anti-GBM antibodies from the circulation, has been of some benefit.

Case Study: CHRONIC INTERSTITIAL LUNG DISEASES

Admitting History

A 56-year-old African-American woman visited the health maintenance organization (HMO) clinic associated with her job because of shortness of breath and an ongoing dry, hacking cough. Before this visit, she seldom saw a physician because she always perceived herself to be in perfect health. As a child, she was rarely ill and saw her doctor only for immunizations and preschool physicals.

The woman, a well-known editor at a prestigious publishing house, said that she had "little time" in her busy life to go through the "hassle" that her HMO required of her to make an appointment with a physician. Her last experience with the HMO system was frustrating. She especially did not approve of the physician assigned to see her.

On this day, her worst fears were confirmed. For almost 5 hours, she was shuffled from one waiting room to another and asked to fill out forms, provide blood samples, and submit to pulmonary function tests (PFT). During this visit the closest person to a physician she saw was a young physician's assistant (PA), who slowly took a thorough history. As the PA was closing her interview with the patient, the physician entered the room. The patient sarcastically stated, "You mean I'm finally going to see a real doctor?"

Physical Examination

On observation the patient appeared to be a stunning, well-nourished woman who looked much younger than her stated years. Her clothing was impeccable, and her jewelry was simple but elegant.

The woman stated that she had made an appointment because of her recent inability to participate in aerobic exercise classes at work. She said that her shortness of breath, which had worsened progressively over the past several weeks, was accompanied by a dry, hacking cough. She said that her cough was especially annoying. It awakened her from sleep at night. At first, she said, she had tried to cut down on her aerobics classes, but recently she had been unable to tolerate them at all. She said that she had never smoked.

As she talked, the woman frequently demonstrated pursed-lip breathing. Her cough was frequent, dry, and nonproductive and was obviously annoying to her. She demonstrated a moderate degree of digital clubbing, and her nail beds were cyanotic. She also demonstrated a mild degree of peripheral edema, and her neck veins were slightly distended. Her liver was enlarged and tender.

The woman's vital signs were as follows: blood pressure 145/90, heart rate 96 bpm, respiratory rate 28/min, and temperature 98.5° F. On auscultation, bronchial breath sounds and crackles could be heard bilaterally. Over the lung bases, tactile and vocal fremitus were notable. Rare wheezes were heard intermittently. Percussion was unremarkable.

Her PFT obtained a few hours earlier showed both a restrictive and an obstructive lung disorder, and the pulmonary carbon monoxide diffusion capacity (D_{LCO}) was 50% of the value predicted. Her chest X-ray revealed bilateral diffuse interstitial infiltrates and nodular densities in the lower lung lobes.

Air bronchograms also were visible. Her heart was enlarged, suggesting right ventricular hypertrophy (Figure 28-5). Her laboratory work showed an increase in immunoglobulin M (IgM), immunoglobulin G (IgG), and immunoglobulin A (IgA) antibodies. Her arterial blood gas values (ABGs) on room air were as follows: pH 7.53, $Paco_2$ 29 mm Hg, HCO_3^- 21 mmol/L, and Pao_2 61 mm Hg. At this point the physician elected to admit the woman to the hospital. The physician also requested a respiratory care consultation and scheduled a transbronchial lung biopsy. On the basis of these data, the following SOAP was written:

Respiratory Assessment and Plan

S "I had to stop taking my aerobic class because of shortness of breath."

O Vital signs: BP 145/90, HR 96, RR 28, T normal; cyanosis, digital clubbing; frequent, dry, nonproductive cough; peripheral edema, distended neck veins, and enlarged and tender liver; pursed-lip breathing; bilateral bronchial breath sounds and crackles; tactile and vocal fremitus over lung bases; PFTs: moderate restrictive and obstructive disorder; 50% reduction in D_{LCO}; CXR: bilateral diffuse interstitial infiltrates and nodular densities in lower lung lobes, air bronchograms, right ventricular cardiomegaly; ABGs (room air): pH 7.53, $Paco_2$ 29, HCO_3^- 21, Pao_2 61

A • Moderate respiratory distress (history, vital signs, ABGs)

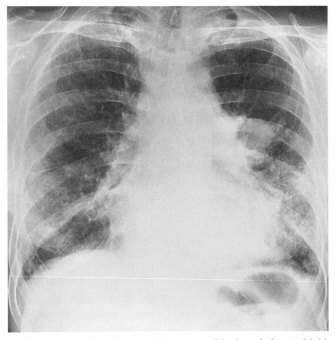

Figure 28-5   Chest X-ray of a 56-year-old woman with chronic interstitial lung disease.

- Bilateral interstitial infiltrates (CXR) with combined obstructive and restrictive elements (PFTs)
- Bronchial obstruction, possibly bronchospasm (PFT)
- Cor pulmonale (CXR)
- Acute alveolar hyperventilation with mild-to-moderate hypoxemia (ABGs)

P Begin pulse oximetry. Initiate Oxygen Therapy per protocol (2 L/min by nasal cannula) and trial period of Hyperinflation Therapy Protocol (incentive spirometry). Begin trial of Aerosolized Medication Protocol (salmeterol 2 puffs MDI bid). Monitor and reevaluate (e.g., per shift)

• • • • •

2 Days After Admission

The respiratory care practitioner found the patient sitting up in bed editing a manuscript. She complained to the therapist that she had a lot of work to do and that she was getting tired of being in the hospital. Despite her verbal comments, she appeared weak, fatigued, and in obvious respiratory distress. She still had a frequent, dry cough. She often demonstrated pursed-lip breathing as she talked, and her nail beds were still cyanotic.

Her vital signs were as follows: blood pressure 142/91, heart rate 90 bpm, respiratory rate 22/min, and temperature normal. On auscultation, bronchial breath sounds and crackles were audible bilaterally. The histology report regarding the transbronchial lung biopsy established a diagnosis of sarcoidosis, after which she was started on oral corticosteroids (prednisone, 40 mg/day).

A morning chest X-ray showed unchanged bilateral diffuse interstitial infiltrates and nodular densities in the lower lung lobes. Air bronchograms also were visible. A gallium lung scan indicated moderate pulmonary activity. Evidence of cor pulmonale was still present. The patient's peak expiratory flow rate (PEFR) both before and after bronchodilator therapy was 280 L/min. Her ABGs were as follows: pH 7.48, $Paco_2$ 32 mm Hg, HCO_3^- 23 mmol/L, and Pao_2 67 mm Hg. The woman's oxygen saturation measured by pulse oximetry (Spo_2) was 94%. At this time, the following SOAP was charted:

Respiratory Assessment and Plan

S "I'm getting tired of being in the hospital."
O Appearance weak and tired; cough: frequent, dry; pursed-lip breathing and cyanotic nail beds; vital signs: BP 142/91, HR 90, RR 22, T normal; bilateral bronchial breath sounds and crackles; PEFR: 280 before and after bronchodilator therapy; CXR: bilateral diffuse

interstitial infiltrates and nodular densities in lower lobes and air bronchograms; right ventricular cardiomegaly; histology report: sarcoidosis; gallium scan positive; ABGs: pH 7.48, $Paco_2$ 32, HCO_3^- 23, Pao_2 67; Spo_2 94%

A
- Moderate respiratory distress (general observation, vital signs, ABGs)
- Bilateral interstitial infiltrates (CXR)
- Active sarcoidosis (histology report, CXR, gallium scan)
- Bronchial obstruction (PEFR), probably from sarcoidosis—without reversibility from bronchodilator
- Acute alveolar hyperventilation with mild hypoxemia (ABGs)

P Continue oxygenation therapy per protocol. Discontinue hyperinflation and bronchodilator therapies per protocols. (With the confirmation of sarcoidosis, the effectiveness of hyperinflation and bronchodilator therapy is questionable.) Continue to monitor and reevaluate. Ensure that pulmonary rehabilitation and home care personnel see patient.

• • • • •

3 Days Later

The physician requested a repeat respiratory care evaluation and recommendations regarding the patient's discharge. The respiratory care practitioner noted that the patient was not in as much respiratory distress on her present oxygen setting. Although she appeared comfortable, she still had a frequent dry, hacking cough and demonstrated pursed-lip breathing as she talked. She stated that she felt much better. Her nail beds no longer appeared cyanotic.

Her vital signs were as follows: blood pressure 133/86, heart rate 86 bpm, respiratory rate 15/min, and temperature normal. On auscultation, bronchial breath sounds were heard bilaterally. A morning chest X-ray showed no change in the bilateral diffuse interstitial infiltrates and nodular densities. Air bronchograms again were seen. Her ABGs on supplemental oxygen at 3 L/min per nasal cannula were as follows: pH 7.44, $Paco_2$ 36 mm Hg, HCO_3^- 23 mmol/L, and Pao_2 84 mm Hg. The patient's Spo_2 was 95%. She desaturated to 80% on oxygen with walking exercise. On the basis of these clinical data, the following SOAP was documented:

Respiratory Assessment and Plan

S "I feel much better."
O No longer in respiratory distress (on present O_2 setting); cough: frequent, dry, and hacking; pursed-lip breathing and cyanosis; vital signs: BP 133/86, HR 86, RR 15, T normal;

bronchial breath sounds bilaterally; CXR: bilateral diffuse interstitial infiltrates and nodular densities; air bronchograms also seen; ABGs (on 3 lpm by nasal cannula): pH 7.44, $Paco_2$ 36, HCO_3^- 23, Pao_2 84; Spo_2 95% at rest; desaturates significantly with exercise.

A • Bilateral interstitial infiltrates (CXR)
  • Sarcoidosis (histology report)
  • Bronchial obstruction (PEFR)
  • Normal acid-base status with corrected hypoxemia (ABGs)
  • Overall clinical improvement

P Recommend home care oxygen therapy per protocol. Check pneumococcal and influenza vaccine status.

Discussion

Respiratory care of the patient with chronic interstitial lung disease involves the provision of adequate oxygenation, reversal or prevention of atelectasis, and treatment of any obstructive component that may be present. At least three interstitial lung diseases have a definite obstructive component: sarcoidosis, cystic fibrosis, and eosinophilic granuloma (histiocytosis X).

The **first assessment** suggests that hypoxemia and cor pulmonale may be complicating the patient's course early in the disease. Her dyspnea, tachypnea, tachycardia, and nonrefractory hypoxemia are consistent with **Increased Alveolar-Capillary Thickening** (see Figure 9-9). Interestingly, some airway obstruction is picked up on pulmonary function testing, suggesting that a somewhat atypical clinical scenario—airway obstruction and possible **Bronchospasm,** or at least airway obstruction—also may be present in this case (see Figure 9-10). Oxygen therapy certainly

is indicated. While the workup is proceeding, not much more can be done to treat her illness. This patient was undiagnosed when she came to the clinic, and the effects of corticosteroid therapy would take some time before they would be felt.

In the **second assessment** a gallium scan indicates that the patient has cytoactive sarcoidosis, for which corticosteroid therapy might be helpful. The patient is modestly hypoxic, and oxygen therapy should be up-regulated. Neither wheezing nor crackles has improved, even on a rapid-acting bronchodilator. Thus hyperinflation and bronchodilator therapy might safely be discontinued. These therapies were instituted only on a trial basis.

At the time of the **third assessment,** with continued improvement in oxygenation with appropriate oxygen therapy, all that remains is to prepare for discharge of this patient on a simple program of supplemental oxygen therapy, as indicated. This patient should be recognized by this time as having chronic lung disease, no matter what her symptom status. Only time will tell how much of her interstitial disease will be helped by oral corticosteroids.

This patient is at the age at which both pneumococcal vaccine and influenza vaccine should be given. The pneumococcal vaccine can be given at any time of the year and should be repeated every 2 to 5 years in patients with chronic lung disease. Influenza vaccine should be given yearly during the Fall months. A note should be added to the patient's chart that this action has been recommended.

That this patient presented with cor pulmonale suggests that a significant amount of parenchymal lung damage already exists and that supplemental oxygen therapy may be needed for a long time, if not for the remainder of her lifetime.

SELF-ASSESSMENT QUESTIONS

Multiple Choice

1. Which of the following is another name for extrinsic allergic alveolitis?

   a. Sarcoidosis
   b. Hypersensitivity pneumonitis
   c. Alveolar proteinosis
   d. Idiopathic pulmonary hemosiderosis
   e. Chronic eosinophilic pneumonia

2. Which of the following allergic reactions appears to be the underlying cause for most of the pathologic changes associated with extrinsic allergic alveolitis?

   a. Type I: Anaphylaxis
   b. Type II: Cytotoxic
   c. Type III: Immune complex–mediated hypersensitivity
   d. Type IV: Cell-mediated reactions
   e. None of the above

3. Which of the following is/are associated with interstitial inflammation accompanied by granuloma formation?

   I. Rheumatoid arthritis
   II. Extrinsic allergic alveolitis
   III. Sarcoidosis
   IV. Churg-Strauss syndrome

   a. I only
   b. II only
   c. III and IV only
   d. II and III only
   e. II, III, and IV only

4. What is another common name for eosinophilic granuloma?

   a. Histiocytosis X
   b. Wegener's granulomatosis
   c. Goodpasture's syndrome
   d. Polymyositis-dermatomyositis
   e. Alveolar proteinosis

5. Which of the following is/are considered pulmonary vasculitides?

   I. Rheumatoid arthritis
   II. Wegener's granulomatosis
   III. Lymphomatoid granulomatosis
   IV. Churg-Strauss syndrome

   a. I only
   b. III only
   c. II, III, and IV only
   d. I, II, and III only
   e. I, II, III, and IV

6. Which of the following disorders is associated with desquamative interstitial pneumonia and usual interstitial pneumonia?

   a. Idiopathic pulmonary fibrosis
   b. Eosinophilic granuloma
   c. Rheumatoid arthritis
   d. Sarcoidosis
   e. Goodpasture's syndrome

7. Which of the following is/are collagen vascular diseases?

   I. Histiocytosis X
   II. Rheumatoid arthritis
   III. Sjögren's syndrome
   IV. Alveolar proteinosis

   a. I only
   b. III only
   c. II and IV only
   d. I and IV only
   e. II and III only

8. Which of the following pulmonary function study findings is/are associated with chronic interstitial lung disease?

   I. Increased FRC
   II. Decreased FEV_T
   III. Increased RV
   IV. Decreased FVC

   a. I only
   b. III only
   c. II and IV only
   d. III and IV only
   e. II, III, and IV only

9. Which of the following hemodynamic indices is/
   are associated with advanced or severe
   interstitial lung disease?

   I. Increased CVP
   II. Decreased PCWP
   III. Increased $\overline{PA}$
   IV. Decreased RAP

   a. I only
   b. IV only
   c. I and III only
   d. II and IV only
   e. I, III, and IV only

10. A pleural effusion is commonly associated with
   which of the following chronic interstitial lung
   diseases?

   I. Systemic lupus erythematosus
   II. Rheumatoid arthritis
   III. Lymphomatoid granulomatosis
   IV. Goodpasture's syndrome

   a. I only
   b. III only
   c. II and IV only
   d. III and IV only
   e. I, II, and III only

Answers appear in Appendix XI.

PART XI

Neurologic Disorders and Sleep Apnea

CHAPTER 29

Guillain-Barré Syndrome

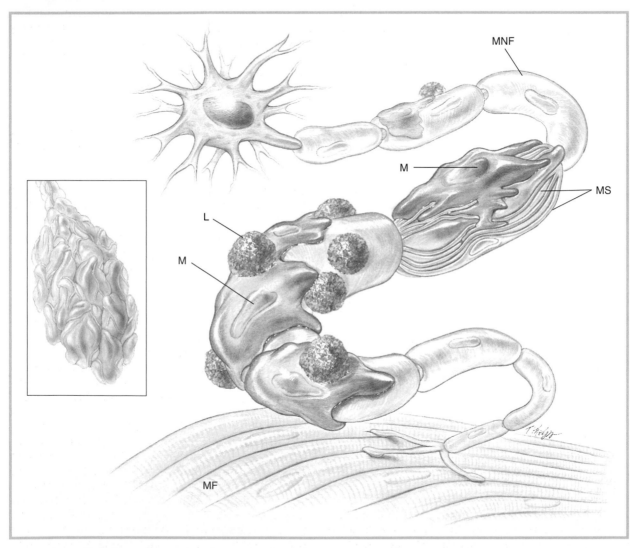

Figure 29–1 Guillain-Barré syndrome. Lymphocytes and macrophages attacking and stripping away the myelin sheath of a peripheral nerve. *MNF,* Myelinated nerve fiber; *L,* lymphocyte; *M,* macrophage; *MS,* myelin sheath (cross-sectional view; note the macrophage attacking the myelin sheath); *MF,* muscle fiber. *Inset,* Atelectasis, a common secondary anatomic alteration of the lungs. See also Plate 21.

Anatomic Alterations of the Lungs Associated with Guillain-Barré Syndrome

Guillain-Barré syndrome is a relatively rare disorder of the peripheral nervous system in which flaccid paralysis of the skeletal muscles and loss of reflexes develop in a previously healthy patient. In severe cases, paralysis of the diaphragm and ventilatory failure can develop. Clinically, this is a medical emergency. If the ventilatory failure is not properly managed, mucus accumulation with airway obstruction, alveolar consolidation, and atelectasis may develop.

Paralysis of the skeletal muscles develops in response to various pathologic changes in the peripheral nerves. Microscopically, the nerves show demyelination, inflammation, and edema. As the anatomic alterations of the peripheral nerves intensify, the ability of the neurons to transmit impulses to the muscles decreases, and eventually paralysis ensues (Figure 29-1).

Other names found in the literature for Guillain-Barré syndrome are as follows:

- Landry-Guillain-Barré-Strohl syndrome
- Acute idiopathic polyneuritis
- Postinfectious polyneuritis
- Landry's paralysis
- Acute postinfectious polyneuropathy
- Acute polyradiculitis
- Polyradiculoneuropathy

The major pathologic or structural changes of the lungs associated with the ventilatory failure that may accompany Guillain-Barré syndrome are as follows:

- Mucus accumulation
- Airway obstruction
- Alveolar consolidation
- Atelectasis

Etiology

The annual incidence of Guillain-Barré syndrome is 1 to 2 per 100,000 people in the United States. The mortality rate is 4% to 6%, and the morbidity rate (permanent disabling weakness, imbalance, or sensory loss) is between 5% and 10%. Although the condition is uncommon in early childhood, it may occur in all age groups and in either gender. A greater incidence has been noted among people 45 years of age and older, among male subjects, and among Caucasians (the condition is 50% to 60% more common in Caucasians). There is no obvious seasonal clustering of cases.

The precise cause of Guillain-Barré syndrome is not known. It is probably an immune disorder that causes inflammation and deterioration of the patient's peripheral nervous system. Studies of serial serum samples have shown high antibody titers during the early stages of the disorder. Elevated levels of specific antibodies include IgM and complement-activating antibodies against isolated human peripheral nerve myelin, or anti-PNM antibodies. Studies have shown that serum antibody titers fall rapidly during the recovery period.

Lymphocytes and macrophages appear to attack and strip off the myelin sheath of the peripheral nerves and leave swelling and fragmentation of the neural axon (see Figure 29-1). It is believed that the myelin sheath covering the peripheral nerves (or the myelin-producing Schwann cell) is the actual target of the immune attack.

The onset of Guillain-Barré syndrome frequently occurs 1 to 4 weeks after a febrile episode such as an upper respiratory or gastrointestinal illness. Numerous viruses and some bacterial agents have been implicated as precursors to Guillain-Barré syndrome. Infectious mononucleosis, for example, has been associated with as many as 25% of the cases. Other possible infective agents include parainfluenza 2, vaccinia, variola, measles, mumps, hepatitis A and B viruses, *Mycoplasma pneumoniae*, *Salmonella typhi*, and *Chlamydia psittaci*. Although the significance of the association is controversial, during the nationwide immunization campaign in the United States in 1976, more than 40 million adults were vaccinated with swine influenza vaccine, and more than 500 cases of Guillain-Barré syndrome were reported among the vaccinated individuals, with 25 deaths.

If diagnosed early, patients with Guillain-Barré syndrome have an excellent prognosis. The diagnosis typically is based on the patient's clinical history. Significant signs include paresthesias, paralysis, cerebrospinal fluid (CSF) findings, and abnormal electromyography (EMG) results. When Guillain-Barré syndrome is present, the CSF has an unusually high protein level (500 mg/dl) with a normal cell count. An EMG helps to establish the diagnosis and the extent of neurologic involvement. The EMG measures the electrical activity of a muscle in response to nerve stimulation. It also measures the nature and speed of electrical conduction along a nerve. Functional spontaneous recovery is expected in about 85% to 95% of the cases, although approximately 40% may have some minor residual symptoms.

Common Noncardiopulmonary Manifestations

- Progressive ascending paralysis of the skeletal muscles

- Tingling sensation and numbness (distal paresthesia)
- Loss of deep tendon reflexes
- Sensory nerve impairment
- Peripheral facial weakness
- Decreased gag reflex
- Decreased ability to swallow

The early symptoms of Guillain-Barré syndrome include fever, malaise, nausea, and prostration, with a subsequent tingling sensation and numbness in the extremities (distal paresthesia). The feet and lower portions of the legs usually are affected first. The tingling and numbness are followed by skeletal muscle paralysis and the loss of deep tendon reflexes.

The muscle paralysis then moves upward (ascending paralysis) to the arms, neck, and pharyngeal and facial muscles (cranial nerves IX and X). The muscle weakness and paralysis commonly develop during a single day, although they may develop over several days. Paralysis generally peaks in fewer than 10 days. Sensory nerve impairment also may be present. The patient's gag reflex generally is decreased or absent, and swallowing is usually difficult (dysphagia). Therefore the management of oral secretions is often a problem.

Although Guillain-Barré syndrome is typically an ascending paralysis (i.e., moving from the lower portions of the legs and body upward), muscle paralysis may affect the facial and arm muscles first and then move downward. Although the weakness is commonly symmetric, a single arm or leg may be involved before paralysis spreads. The paralysis also may affect all four limbs simultaneously. Progression of the paralysis may stop at any point. After the paralysis reaches its maximum, it usually remains unchanged for a few days or weeks. Improvement generally begins spontaneously and continues for weeks or, in rare cases, months.

OVERVIEW
of the Cardiopulmonary Clinical Manifestations Associated with
GUILLAIN-BARRÉ SYNDROME

The following clinical manifestations result from the pathologic mechanisms caused (or activated) by **Atelectasis** (see Figure 9-7), **Alveolar Consolidation** (see Figure 9-8), and **Excessive Bronchial Secretions** (see Figure 9-11)—the major anatomic alterations of the lungs associated with Guillain-Barré syndrome (when ventilatory failure is not properly managed) (see Figure 29-1).

CLINICAL DATA OBTAINED AT THE PATIENT'S BEDSIDE

The Physical Examination
Cyanosis (see page 45 ◆▶)

Chest Assessment Findings
  (see page 22 ◆▶)
- Diminished breath sounds
- Crackles and rhonchi

Autonomic Nervous System Dysfunctions
- Heart rate and rhythm abnormalities
- Blood pressure abnormalities

Autonomic nervous system dysfunction develops in approximately 50% of all cases. The autonomic dysfunction involves the overreaction or underreaction of the sympathetic or parasympathetic nervous system. Clinically, the patient may manifest various cardiac arrhythmias, such as sinus tachycardia (the most common), bradycardia, ventricular tachycardia, atrial flutter, atrial fibrillation, and asystole. Hypertension and hypotension also may be seen. Although the loss of bowel and bladder sphincter control is uncommon, transient sphincter paralysis may occur during the evolution of symptoms. The autonomic involvement may be transient or may persist throughout the duration of the disorder.

CLINICAL DATA OBTAINED FROM LABORATORY TESTS AND SPECIAL PROCEDURES

Pulmonary Function Study Findings
Expiratory Maneuver Findings (see page 61 ◆▶)

FVC	FEV$_T$	FEF$_{25\%-75\%}$	FEF$_{200-1200}$
↓	↓	↓	↓
PEFR	MVV	FEF$_{50\%}$	FEV$_{1\%}$
↓	↓	↓	↓

Lung Volume and Capacity Findings
  (see page 62 ◆▶)

V$_T$	RV	FRC	TLC
↓	↓	↓	↓
VC	IC	ERV	RV/TLC%
↓	↓	↓	N

OVERVIEW
of the Cardiopulmonary Clinical Manifestations Associated with
GUILLAIN-BARRÉ SYNDROME (Continued)

Arterial Blood Gases
Acute Ventilatory Failure with Hypoxemia
(see page 73 ◆▶)

pH	$Paco_2$	HCO_3^-*	Pao_2
↓	↑	↑(Slightly)	↓

*When tissue hypoxia is severe enough to produce lactic acid, the pH and HCO_3^- values will be lower than expected for a particular $Paco_2$ level.

Oxygenation Indices (see page 82 ◆▶)

$\dot{Q}_S/\dot{Q}_T$	Do_2†	$\dot{V}o_2$	$C(a-\bar{v})o_2$
↑	↓	Normal	Normal
O_2ER	$S\bar{v}o_2$		
↑	↓		

†The Do_2 may be normal in patients who have compensated to the decreased oxygenation status with an increased cardiac output. When the Do_2 is normal, the O_2ER is usually normal.

RADIOLOGIC FINDINGS

Chest Radiograph
- Normal
- Increased opacity (when atelectasis is present)

If the ventilatory failure associated with Guillain-Barré syndrome is properly managed, the chest X-ray should be normal. If the bronchopulmonary hygiene and ventilatory failure is improperly managed, however, alveolar consolidation from secondary pneumonia and atelectasis may occur from excess secretion accumulation in the tracheobronchial tree. This increases the density of the lung segments affected.

General Management of Guillain-Barré Syndrome

Guillain-Barré syndrome is a potential medical emergency that must be monitored closely after the diagnosis has been made. The primary treatment should be directed at stabilization of vital signs and supportive care for the patient. Initially, such patients should be managed in an intensive care unit. Frequent measurements of the patient's vital capacity, blood pressure, oxygen saturation, and arterial blood gases should be performed. Mechanical ventilation should be initiated when the clinical data demonstrate impending or acute ventilatory failure. Bronchopulmonary Hygiene and Hyperinflation Therapy Protocols should be instituted to prevent mucus accumulation, airway obstruction, alveolar consolidation, and atelectasis.

As in any patient who is paralyzed, the risk of thromboembolism increases. Because of this danger, the patient commonly receives subcutaneously administered heparin, elastic stockings, and passive range-of-motion exercises (every 3 to 4 hours) for all extremities. To prevent skin breakdown, the patient should be turned frequently. A rotary bed or Stryker frame may be required. Urinary catheterization is required in paralyzed patients. Blood pressure disturbances and cardiac arrhythmias require immediate attention.

For example, nitroprusside (Nipride) or phentolamine (Regitine) are commonly administered during severe hypertensive episodes. Episodes of bradycardia are commonly treated with atropine.

PLASMAPHERESIS

In severe cases, *plasmapheresis* (also known as *plasma exchange*) has been shown effective in decreasing the morbidity and shortening the clinical course of Guillain-Barré syndrome. Plasmapheresis entails the removal of damaged antibodies from the patient's blood plasma, followed by the retransfusion of the blood cells. Type-specific fresh frozen plasma or albumin generally is used to replace the withdrawn plasma. It is believed that plasmapheresis removes the antibodies from the plasma that contribute to the immune system attack on the peripheral nerves. This procedure has been shown to reduce antibody titers during the early stages of the disorder.

As a general rule, a fairly conservative plasmapheresis regimen is performed. In the normal-sized adult, a total of five exchanges of 3 L each over 8 to 10 days is usually adequate. Studies have shown that plasmapheresis within the first 7 days of the onset of neurologic symptoms significantly decreases the number of days that the patient requires mechanical ventilation. It is recommended, however, that only severely affected patients with worsening symptoms receive plasmapheresis. Patients with mild symptoms or symptoms that have improved or ceased to worsen should not undergo plasmapheresis.

INFUSION OF IMMUNOGLOBULIN

The infusion of high doses of immunoglobulin (containing healthy antibodies) from blood donors can block the damaging antibodies. However, combining both the plasma exchange therapy and the infusion of immunoglobulin offers no benefit. In other words, the mixing of treatments or administering of one form of therapy after the other is no more effective than either treatment alone.

CORTICOSTEROIDS

Corticosteroids have been found to be ineffective in the treatment of Guillain-Barré syndrome. In fact, the administration of oral or intravenous corticosteroids may actually prolong the patient's recovery time.

RESPIRATORY CARE TREATMENT PROTOCOLS

Oxygen Therapy Protocol

Oxygen therapy is used to treat hypoxemia, decrease the work of breathing, and decrease myocardial work. Because of the hypoxemia that may develop in Guillain-Barré syndrome, supplemental oxygen may be required. However, because of the alveolar consolidation and atelectasis associated with Guillain-Barré syndrome, capillary shunting may be present. Hypoxemia caused by capillary shunting or alveolar hypoventilation is refractory to oxygen therapy (see Oxygen Therapy Protocol, Protocol 9-1).

Bronchopulmonary Hygiene Therapy Protocol

Because of the excessive mucus production and accumulation associated with Guillain-Barré syndrome, a number of bronchopulmonary hygiene treatment modalities may be used to enhance the mobilization of bronchial secretions (see Bronchopulmonary Hygiene Therapy Protocol, Protocol 9-2).

Hyperinflation Therapy Protocol

Hyperinflation measures are commonly administered to offset the alveolar consolidation and atelectasis associated with Guillain-Barré syndrome (see Hyperinflation Therapy Protocol, Protocol 9-3).

Mechanical Ventilation Protocol

Mechanical ventilation may be necessary to provide and support alveolar gas exchange and eventually return the patient to spontaneous breathing. Because acute ventilatory failure is often seen in patients with severe Guillain-Barré syndrome, continuous mechanical ventilation is often required. Continuous mechanical ventilation is justified when the acute ventilatory failure is thought to be reversible (see Mechanical Ventilation Protocol, Protocol 9-5).

PHYSICAL THERAPY/REHABILITATION

Physical therapy usually begins long before the patient recovers from the effects of Guillain-Barré syndrome—often while the patient is still being mechanically ventilated. In long-term cases, for example, the patient's arms and legs will be manually moved on a regular basis to keep the muscles flexible and strong. After recovery, the patient frequently requires physical therapy to regain full strength and normal mobility. Hydrotherapy (whirlpool therapy) is commonly used to relieve pain and facilitate limb movement. Full recovery may require as little as a few weeks or as long as a few years. Approximately 30% of the patients will still experience residual weakness after 3 years. Approximately 3% may experience a relapse, with muscle weakness and a tingling sensation, many years after the initial illness.

Case Study: GUILLAIN-BARRÉ SYNDROME

Admitting History/Physical Examination

A 48-year-old career U.S. Navy physician visited the hospital base clinic because of the acute onset of severe muscle weakness. He had joined the Navy immediately after medical school. Throughout his time in the service, he had the opportunity to pursue his passion—competitive water-ski jumping. For many years he was the first-place winner at most tournaments, including the nationals held yearly. For almost 25 years, he progressed through the age divisions, always remaining the top seed, always capturing the highest title.

The man was in outstanding physical condition. He was an avid runner and weight lifter, and during the off season he often traveled to a warm climate to practice his water-ski jumping. He never smoked and was never hospitalized. He had an occasional "cold," for which he was treated by his peers. About 2 years ago, he began to focus all his attention on his 19-year-old son, who was quickly following in his father's footsteps, having just captured the Men's 1 division in collegiate ice hockey.

The man stated that he had felt good until 2 weeks before his admission, at which time he experienced a flulike syndrome for 3 days. About 10 days after returning to work, he noticed a tingling sensation in his feet during his morning patient rounds. By dinner time that same day, the tingling sensation had radiated from his feet to about the level of his knees. Thinking that he was tired from being on his feet all day, he went to bed early that evening. The next morning, however, his legs were completely numb, although he could still move them. Alarmed, he asked his son to drive him to the clinic. After examining him, his doctor (a personal friend) admitted him for a diagnostic workup and observation.

Over the next 3 days, the laboratory results showed that the patient's cerebrospinal fluid had an elevated protein concentration with a normal cell count. The electrodiagnostic studies showed a progressive ascending paralysis of the man's arms and legs. He began to have difficulty eating and swallowing his food. The respiratory care practitioners, who were monitoring his vital capacity, pulse oximetry, and arterial blood gas values (ABGs), reported a progressive deterioration in all the values. A diagnosis of Guillain-Barré syndrome was recorded in the patient's chart.

When the man's ABGs reached pH 7.29, $Paco_2$ 53 mm Hg, HCO_3^- 23 mMol/L, and Pao_2 86 mm Hg (on a 2 L/min oxygen nasal cannula), the respiratory therapist called the attending physician and reported his assessment of acute ventilatory failure. The doctor transferred the patient to the intensive care unit (ICU), intubated him, and placed him on a mechanical ventilator. The initial ventilator settings were as follows: intermittent mechanical ventilation (IMV) mode, 12 breaths per minute, tidal volume 0.85 L, and Fio_2 0.40.

Approximately 15 minutes after the patient was committed to the ventilator, he appeared comfortable. No spontaneous breaths were noted between the 12 intermittent mandatory ventilations. His vital signs were as follows: blood pressure 126/82 and heart rate 68 bpm. He was afebrile. A portable chest X-ray revealed that the endotracheal tube was in a good position and the lungs were adequately aerated. Normal vesicular breath sounds were auscultated over both lung fields. His ABGs were as follows: pH 7.51, $Paco_2$ 29 mm Hg, HCO_3^- 22 mMol/L, and Pao_2 204 mm Hg. His oxygen saturation measured by pulse oximetry (Spo_2)

was 98%. On the basis of these clinical data, the following SOAP was documented:

Respiratory Assessment and Plan

S N/A (intubated on ventilator)
O Vital signs: BP 126/82, HR 68, RR 12 (controlled); afebrile; no spontaneous breaths; CXR: normal; normal breath sounds; ABGs (on $Fio2 = 0.40$): pH 7.51, $Paco_2$ 29, HCO_3^- 22, Pao_2 204; Spo_2 98%
A • Acute alveolar hyperventilation with excessive oxygenation (ABGs)
  • Excessive alveolar ventilation (increased pH and decreased $Paco_2$)
  • Fio_2 too high (ABGs)
P Adjust mechanical ventilator settings (decreasing tidal volume and Fio_2) according to protocol. Monitor closely and reevaluate.

• • • • •

3 Days After Admission

The patient's cardiopulmonary status so far had been unremarkable. No improvement was seen in his muscular paralysis. No changes had been made in his ventilator settings over the past 48 hours. His skin color appeared good. Palpation and percussion of the chest were unremarkable. On auscultation, however, crackles and rhonchi could be heard over both lung fields.

Moderate amounts of thick, whitish, clear secretions were being suctioned from the patient's endotracheal tube regularly. His vital signs were as follows: blood pressure 124/83, heart rate 74 bpm, and rectal temperature 37.7° C (99.8° F). A recent portable chest X-ray revealed no significant pathologic process. His ABGs were as follows: pH 7.44, $Paco_2$ 35 mm Hg, HCO_3^- 24 mMol/L, and Pao_2 98 mm Hg. His Spo_2 was 97%. On the basis of these clinical data, the following SOAP was documented:

Respiratory Assessment and Plan

S N/A
O Skin color good; crackles and rhonchi over both lung fields; moderate amount of whitish, clear secretions being suctioned regularly; vital signs: BP 124/83, HR 74, T 37.7° C (99.8° F); CXR: unremarkable; ABGs: pH 7.44, $Paco_2$ 35, HCO_3^- 24, and Pao_2 98; Spo_2 97%
A • Normal acid-base and oxygenation status on present ventilator settings (ABGs)
  • Excessive sputum accumulation; possible progression to mucus plugging and atelectasis (crackles, rhonchi, whitish and clear secretions)
P Begin bronchopulmonary hygiene therapy per protocol (vigorous tracheal suctioning and

obtaining of sputum stain and culture).
Begin Hyperinflation Therapy Protocol (10 cm
H_2O positive end-expiratory pressure [PEEP]
to offset any early development of atelectasis).
Monitor and reevaluate (4 × per shift).

• • • • •

5 Days After Admission

The patient remained alert and comfortable, except
for the ET tube. His muscular paralysis remained
unchanged. His skin color appeared good, and no
remarkable information was noted during palpation
and percussion. Although crackles and rhonchi could
still be heard over both lung fields, they were not as
intense as they had been 48 hours earlier. A small
amount of clear secretions was suctioned from the
patient's endotracheal tube. His vital signs were as
follows: blood pressure 118/79, heart rate 68 bpm,
and temperature normal. A recent portable chest
X-ray appeared normal. His ABGs were as follows:
pH 7.42, $Paco_2$ 37 mm Hg, HCO_3^- 24 mMol/L, and Pao_2
97 mm Hg. His Spo_2 was 97%. The sputum culture
was unremarkable. On the basis of these clinical data,
the following SOAP note was recorded:

Respiratory Assessment and Plan

S   N/A
O   Skin color good; crackles and rhonchi over both
lung fields improving; small amount of clear
secretions suctioned; vital signs: BP 118/79,
HR 68, T normal; no spontaneous respirations;
CXR: normal; ABGs: pH 7.42, $Paco_2$ 37,
HCO_3^- 24, Pao_2 97; Spo_2 97%
A • Normal acid-base and oxygenation status on
present ventilator settings (ABGs)
 • Respiratory muscle pump insufficiency
(no spontaneous respirations)
 • Secretion control improving (crackles,
rhonchi, clear secretions)
P   Continue Ventilator Management Protocol.
Continue Bronchopulmonary Hygiene Therapy
protocol. Continue Hyperinflation Therapy
Protocol. Monitor and reevaluate (forced
expiratory volume in 1 second [FEV_1],
negative inspiratory force [NIF] 2 × per shift).

Discussion

Guillain-Barré syndrome is a neuromuscular paralysis that ensues after infection from a neurotropic
virus. This patient has a classic history of ascending
paralysis and paresthesias and the diagnostic finding
of albuminocytologic dissociation in the spinal fluid.
In this setting, serial forced vital capacity (FVC)
maneuvers must be charted. Once respiratory failure
supervenes, intubation and respiratory support on a
ventilator become necessary.

By the time of the **first assessment,** early CO_2
retention is present, and, given the clinical setting,
the patient is appropriately intubated. The initial
blood gases show hyperoxia and hyperventilation.
An appropriate response would be to adjust the ventilator settings by reducing the tidal volume or frequency (or both) and the Fio_2. At the time of this
assessment, the patient exhibits no evidence of
airway obstruction or secretions. Therefore bronchial hygiene therapy is not indicated. Indeed, all
that needs to be done is to ensure adequate ventilation and oxygenation on the ventilator.

However, 3 days later, at the time of the **second
assessment,** crackles and rhonchi are heard over all
lung fields, and the time has come to begin vigorous
bronchial hygiene therapy with suctioning and possibly even therapy with mucolytic agents. Because of
the risk of **Atelectasis,** hyperinflation therapy, in the
form of PEEP on the ventilator, is indicated (see
Figure 9-7). The sputum should be cultured to see
whether any infectious organisms are present.

At the time of the **final assessment** (2 days later),
the evidence for airway secretions is lessened because
the rhonchi no longer can be heard over the lung
fields, and the small amount of sputum suctioned
appears clear. At this point, down-regulation of bronchial hygiene therapy is indicated.

Serial FVC, forced expiratory volume in 1 second
(FEV_1), or negative inspiratory force (NIF) measurements should continue to be made until the patient
is ready to be extubated, thereafter for at least several days. Indeed, extubation occurred about 3 weeks
after the initiation of mechanical ventilation. The
patient recovered without incident and returned to
his active lifestyle within a year.

SELF-ASSESSMENT QUESTIONS

Multiple Choice

1. In Guillain-Barré syndrome, which of the following pathologic changes develop in the peripheral nerves?

    I. Inflammation
    II. Increased ability to transmit nerve impulses
    III. Demyelination
    IV. Edema

    a. I and IV only
    b. II and III only
    c. III and IV only
    d. II, III, and IV only
    e. I, III, and IV only

2. Which of the following is associated with Guillain-Barré syndrome?

    I. Alveolar consolidation
    II. Mucus accumulation
    III. Alveolar hyperinflation
    IV. Atelectasis

    a. I only
    b. I and II only
    c. III and IV only
    d. I, II, and IV only
    e. II, III, and IV only

3. Guillain-Barré syndrome is more common in:

    I. People older than 45 years of age
    II. Blacks than in whites
    III. Males than in females
    IV. Early childhood

    a. I only
    b. IV only
    c. I and III only
    d. III and IV only
    e. II and III only

4. Which of the following are possible precursors to Guillain-Barré syndrome?

    I. Mumps
    II. Swine influenza vaccine
    III. Infectious mononucleosis
    IV. Measles

    a. I and III only
    b. II and IV only
    c. III and IV only
    d. II, III, and IV only
    e. I, II, III, and IV

5. Spontaneous recovery from Guillain-Barré syndrome is expected in approximately what percentage of cases?

    a. 45 to 55
    b. 55 to 65
    c. 65 to 75
    d. 75 to 85
    e. 85 to 95

True or False

True ☐ False ☐ **1.** In Guillain-Barré syndrome a tingling sensation and numbness usually begin in the feet and lower portions of the legs.

True ☐ False ☐ **2.** Guillain-Barré syndrome is called a *descending paralysis.*

True ☐ False ☐ **3.** Paralysis in Guillain-Barré syndrome usually takes approximately 12 weeks to peak.

True ☐ False ☐ **4.** Hypertension and hypotension may be associated with Guillain-Barré syndrome.

True ☐ False ☐ **5.** Plasmapheresis has been shown to reduce the antibody titers during the early stages of Guillain-Barré syndrome.

Answers appear in Appendix XI.

CHAPTER 30

Myasthenia Gravis

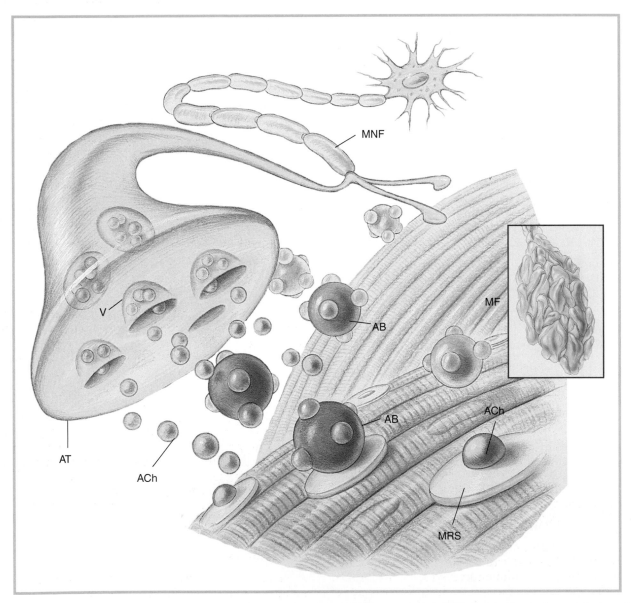

Figure 30–1 Myasthenia gravis, a disorder of the neuromuscular junction that interferes with the chemical transmission of acetylcholine. *MNF,* Myelinated nerve fiber; *AT,* axonal terminal; *V,* vesicle; *ACh,* acetylcholine; *MF,* muscle fiber; *MRS,* muscle receptor site; *AB,* antibody. Note that the antibodies have a physical structure similar to that of ACh, which permits them to connect to (and block ACh from) the muscle receptor sites. *Inset,* Atelectasis, a common secondary anatomic alteration of the lungs. See also Plate 22.

Anatomic Alterations of the Lungs Associated with Myasthenia Gravis

Myasthenia gravis is a chronic disorder of the neuromuscular junction that interferes with the chemical transmission of acetylcholine (ACh) between the axonal terminal and the receptor sites of voluntary muscles (Figure 30-1). It is characterized by fatigue and weakness, with improvement following rest. Because the disorder affects only the myoneural (motor) junction, sensory function is not lost.

The abnormal weakness may be confined to an isolated group of muscles (e.g., the drooping of one or both eyelids), or it may manifest as a generalized weakness that in severe cases includes the diaphragm. When the diaphragm is involved, ventilatory failure can develop. If the ventilatory failure is not properly managed, mucus accumulation with airway obstruction, alveolar consolidation, and atelectasis may develop.

The major pathologic or structural changes of the lungs associated with the ventilatory failure that may accompany myasthenia gravis are as follows:

- Mucus accumulation
- Airway obstruction
- Alveolar consolidation
- Atelectasis

Etiology

The cause of myasthenia gravis appears to be related to circulating antibodies of the autoimmune system (anti-ACh receptor antibodies). It is believed that the antibodies disrupt the chemical transmission of ACh at the neuromuscular junction by (1) blocking the ACh from the receptor sites of the muscular cell, (2) accelerating the breakdown of ACh, and (3) destroying the receptor sites (see Figure 30-1). Although the specific events that activate the formation of the antibodies remain unclear, the thymus gland is almost always abnormal; it is generally presumed that the antibodies arise within the thymus or in related tissue.

According to estimates, myasthenia gravis affects between 20,000 and 70,000 people in the United States annually. It is most common in young women and older men. The disease usually has a peak age of onset in females between 15 and 35 years, compared with 40 to 70 years in males. The clinical manifestations associated with myasthenia gravis are often provoked by emotional upset, physical stress, exposure to extreme temperature changes, febrile illness, and pregnancy. Death caused by myasthenia gravis is possible, especially during the first few years after onset. After the disease has been in progress for 10 years, however, death from myasthenia gravis is rare.

SCREENING AND DIAGNOSIS

The diagnosis of myasthenia gravis is based on (1) the clinical history, (2) neurologic examination, (3) electromyography, (4) blood analysis, (5) edrophonium test, and (6) computed tomography or magnetic resonance imaging.

Clinical History

Signs and symptoms of myasthenia gravis include facial muscle weakness (including drooping eyelids); double vision; difficulty in breathing, talking, chewing or swallowing; muscle weakness in arms and legs; and fatigue brought on by repetitive motions.

Neurologic Examination

Neurologic tests may include the evaluation of reflexes, muscle strength, muscle tone, senses of touch and sight, gait, posture, coordination, balance, and mental abilities.

Electromyography

Electromyography usually is performed to confirm the diagnosis of myasthenia gravis, identify the specific muscles involved, and determine the degree of fatigability. Electromyography entails the repetitive stimulation of a nerve, such as the ulnar nerve, with the simultaneous recording of the muscle response. Clinically, the degree of fatigability often is evaluated by having the patient use certain muscles for a sustained period. For example, the patient may be instructed to gaze upward for an extended period, blink continuously, hold both arms outstretched as long as possible, or count aloud as long as possible in one breath (normal is about 50). A dynamometer sometimes is used to measure the force of repetitive muscle contractions.

Blood Analysis

A blood test may reveal the presence of acetylcholine receptor antibodies. About 75% of patients with myasthenia gravis have an elevated level of these antibodies.

Edrophonium Test

The diagnosis usually is confirmed with the injection of edrophonium (Tensilon). Tensilon, a short-acting drug, blocks cholinesterase from breaking down ACh after it has been released from the terminal axon. This action increases the myoneural concentration of ACh, which in turn offsets the influx of antibodies at the neuromuscular junction. When muscular weakness is caused by myasthenia gravis, a dramatic transitory improvement in muscle function (lasting about 10 minutes) is seen after the administration of Tensilon.

Computed Tomography or Magnetic Resonance Imaging

A computed tomography (CT) scan or magnetic resonance imaging (MRI) may be used to identify an abnormal thymus gland or the presence of a thymoma.

Common Noncardiopulmonary Manifestations

WEAKNESS OF STRIATED MUSCLES

- Eye muscles
  - Drooping of the upper eyelids (ptosis)
- Extraocular muscles
  - Double vision (diplopia)
- Muscles of the lower portion of the face
  - Speech impairment
- Chewing and swallowing muscles (dysphagia)
- Skeletal muscles of the arms and legs

The onset of myasthenia gravis is usually gradual. Ptosis followed by diplopia caused by weakness of the external ocular muscles are usually the first symptoms. Weakness of the extraocular muscles is usually asymmetric and may progress to complete external paralysis in one or both eyes (ocular myasthenia). For some patients, these may be the only symptoms.

In many patients, however, the disease progresses to a generalized skeletal muscle disorder. In such patients the lower facial and neck muscles are almost always affected. The orbicularis oris is usually weak, which causes a vertical snarl when the patient attempts to smile. Chewing and swallowing become difficult as the muscles of the jaw, soft palate, and pharynx weaken. The patient also may regurgitate food and fluid through the nose when swallowing. Muscle fatigue in the pharyngeal area represents a significant danger because food and fluids may be aspirated. During periods of muscle fatigue the patient's ability to articulate frequently deteriorates, and the voice is usually high and nasal in quality. Weakness of the neck muscles commonly causes the patient's head to fall forward unless it is supported. Clinically, the patient is often seen to support the chin with one hand to either hold the head up or assist in speaking.

As the disorder becomes more generalized, weakness develops in the arms and legs. The muscle weakness is usually more pronounced in the proximal parts of the extremities. The patient has difficulty in climbing stairs, lifting objects, maintaining balance, and walking. In severe cases, the weakness of the upper limbs may be such that the hand cannot be lifted to the mouth. Muscle atrophy or pain is rare. Tendon reflexes almost always remain intact.

Clinical manifestations during the early stages of the disorder are often elusive. The patient may (1) demonstrate normal health for weeks or months at a time, (2) show signs of weakness only late in the day or evening, or (3) develop a sudden and transient generalized weakness that includes the diaphragm. Ventilatory failure is always a sinister possibility.

If the ventilatory failure associated with myasthenia gravis is properly managed, the chest X-ray findings should be normal. If it is improperly managed, however, alveolar consolidation and atelectasis develop from the accumulation of excess secretions in the tracheobronchial tree.

OVERVIEW
of the Cardiopulmonary Clinical Manifestations Associated with MYASTHENIA GRAVIS

The following clinical manifestations result from the pathologic mechanisms caused (or activated) by **Atelectasis** (see Figure 9-7), **Alveolar Consolidation** (see Figure 9-8), and **Excessive Bronchial Secretions** (see Figure 9-11)—the major anatomic alterations of the lungs associated with myasthenia gravis (when ventilatory failure is not properly managed) (see Figure 30-1).

CLINICAL DATA OBTAINED AT THE PATIENT'S BEDSIDE

The Physical Examination

Cyanosis (see page 45 ◆►)

Chest Assessment Findings (see page 22 ◆►)

- Diminished breath sounds
- Crackles and rhonchi

OVERVIEW

of the Cardiopulmonary Clinical Manifestations Associated with MYASTHENIA GRAVIS (Continued)

CLINICAL DATA OBTAINED FROM LABORATORY TESTS AND SPECIAL PROCEDURES

Pulmonary Function Study Findings

Expiratory Maneuver Findings (see page 61 ◆)

FVC	FEV_T	$FEF_{25\%-75\%}$	$FEF_{200-1200}$
↓	↓	↓	↓
PEFR	MVV	$FEF_{50\%}$	$FEV_{1\%}$
↓	↓	↓	↓

Lung Volume and Capacity Findings
(see page 62 ◆)

V_T	RV	FRC	TLC
↓	↓	↓	↓
VC	IC	ERV	RV/TLC%
↓	↓	↓	N

Arterial Blood Gases

Acute Ventilatory Failure with Hypoxemia
(see page 73 ◆)

pH	Pa_{CO_2}	HCO_3^-*	Pa_{O_2}
↓	↑	↑(Slightly)	↓

*When tissue hypoxia is severe enough to produce lactic acid, the pH and HCO_3^- values will be lower than expected for a particular Pa_{CO_2} level.

Oxygenation Indices (see page 82 ◆)

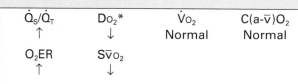

$\dot{Q}_S/\dot{Q}_T$	DO_2*	$\dot{V}O_2$	$C(a-\bar{v})O_2$
↑	↓	Normal	Normal
O_2ER	$S\bar{v}O_2$		
↑	↓		

*The DO_2 may be normal in patients who have compensated to the decreased oxygenation status with an increased cardiac output. When the DO_2 is normal, the O_2ER is usually normal.

RADIOLOGIC FINDINGS

Chest Radiograph
- Normal
- Increased opacity (when atelectasis or consolidation is present)

General Management of Myasthenia Gravis

In the past, many patients with myasthenia gravis died within the first few years of the disease. Today, a number of therapeutic measures provide most patients with marked relief of symptoms and allow them to live a normal life. Because ventilatory failure is possible, patients with myasthenia gravis should be monitored closely during critical periods. Frequent measurements of the patient's vital capacity, blood pressure, oxygen saturation, and arterial blood gases should be performed. Mechanical ventilation should be initiated when the patient's clinical data demonstrate impending or acute ventilatory failure. Bronchopulmonary Hygiene and Hyperinflation Therapy Protocols should be instituted to prevent mucus accumulation, airway obstruction, alveolar consolidation, and atelectasis.

During a myasthenic crisis, the treatment modalities described in the following paragraphs also may be used.

CHOLINESTERASE INHIBITORS

Cholinesterase inhibitors that enhance the action of ACh are used to treat myasthenia gravis. The most popular agents are edrophonium chloride (Tensilon), neostigmine (Prostigmin), and pyridostigmine (Regonol, Mestinon). These agents inhibit the function of cholinesterase. This action increases the concentration of ACh to compete with the circulating anti-ACh antibodies, which interfere with the ability of ACh to stimulate the muscle receptors. Although the anticholinesterase drugs are effective in mild cases of myasthenia gravis, they are not completely effective in severe cases.

IMMUNOSUPPRESSANTS

Corticosteroids (e.g., prednisone) and similar agents, such as cyclophosphamide (Cytoxan, Neosar) and azathioprine (Imuran), are used to suppress the immune system. These agents usually are used for more severe cases. The patient's strength often improves strikingly with steroids. Patients receiving long-term steroid therapy, however, frequently develop serious complications such as diabetes, cataracts, gastrointestinal bleeding, infections, aseptic necrosis of the bone, osteoporosis, myopathies, and psychoses.

Adrenocorticotropic Hormone Therapy

The administration of adrenocorticotropic hormone (ACTH) has proved useful in severely ill patients with myasthenia gravis. A disadvantage to this therapy, however, is that patients tend to worsen before improving. Paradoxically, patients who demonstrate the greatest initial weakness often show the most improvement later.

THYMECTOMY

Although controversial, thymectomy has been helpful in many patients with myasthenia gravis, especially young adult females. The thymus gland in the myasthenic patient frequently appears to be the source of anti-ACh receptor antibodies. In some patients, muscle strength improves soon after surgery, whereas in others improvement takes months or years.

Plasmapheresis

This blood plasma exchange procedure is used to "filter" the blood of acetylcholine receptor antibodies by replacing the patient's plasma with a donor's plasma. Plasmapheresis can be a life-saving intervention in the treatment of myasthenia gravis. However, it is time-consuming and associated with many side effects, such as low blood pressure, infection, and blood clots.

RESPIRATORY CARE TREATMENT PROTOCOLS

Oxygen Therapy Protocol

Oxygen therapy is used to treat hypoxemia, decrease the work of breathing, and decrease myocardial work. Because of the hypoxemia that may develop in myasthenia gravis, supplemental oxygen may be required. However, because of the alveolar consolidation and atelectasis associated with myasthenia gravis, capillary shunting may be present. Hypoxemia caused by capillary shunting is refractory to oxygen therapy (see Oxygen Therapy Protocol, Protocol 9-1).

Bronchopulmonary Hygiene Therapy Protocol

Because of the excessive mucus production and accumulation associated with myasthenia gravis, a number of bronchial hygiene treatment modalities may be used to enhance the mobilization of bronchial secretions (see Bronchopulmonary Hygiene Therapy Protocol, Protocol 9-2).

Hyperinflation Therapy Protocol

Hyperinflation measures are commonly administered to offset the alveolar consolidation and atelectasis associated with myasthenia gravis (see Hyperinflation Therapy Protocol, Protocol 9-3).

Mechanical Ventilation Protocol

Mechanical ventilation may be needed to provide and support alveolar gas exchange and eventually return the patient to spontaneous breathing. Because acute ventilatory failure is often seen in patients with severe myasthenia gravis, continuous mechanical ventilation is often required. Continuous mechanical ventilation is justified when the acute ventilatory failure is thought to be reversible (see Mechanical Ventilation Protocol, Protocol 9-5).

Case Study: MYASTHENIA GRAVIS

Admitting History

A 35-year-old Spanish-American woman is a schoolteacher with a 3-year-old son and an unemployed husband who is still "finding his real place in life." The woman is a high achiever. She recently received her doctoral degree in education, but she has continued to work in the classroom with the grade-school children she loves so much. She was named Teacher of the Year in the large city where she lives. Her colleagues at school consider her a nonstop worker. She has never smoked.

At home, she is always on the move. She has just finished remodeling her kitchen and two bathrooms. She also does her own backyard landscaping on the weekends, a job she particularly enjoys. She reads and plays with her son whenever they have time together. Although she enjoys cooking (a skill she learned from her mother), she does not like to shop for groceries. Fortunately, this is a chore that her husband enjoys.

Three weeks before the current admission, the woman noticed that her eyes "felt tired." She began to experience slight double vision. Thinking that she was working too hard, she slowed down a bit and went to bed earlier for about a week. However, she progressively felt weaker. Her legs quickly became tired, and she began having trouble chewing her food. Concerned, the woman finally went to see her doctor. After reviewing the woman's recent history and performing a careful physical examination, the physician admitted her to the hospital for further evaluation and treatment.

Over the next 48 hours, the woman's physical status declined progressively. After the administration of edrophonium (Tensilon), her muscle strength increased significantly for about 10 minutes. Electromyography disclosed extensive muscle involvement and a high degree of fatigability in all the affected muscles. A diagnosis of myasthenia gravis was recorded in the patient's chart.

The woman began to choke and aspirate food during meals, and a nasogastric feeding tube was inserted. Her speech became more and more slurred. Her upper eyelids drooped, and she was unable to hold her head off her pillow on request. The respiratory therapists who monitored her vital capacity, pulse oximetry, and arterial blood gas values (ABGs) reported a progressive worsening in all parameters.

When the woman's ABGs were pH 7.32, $Paco_2$ 51 mm Hg, HCO_3^- 23 mMol/L, and Pao_2 59 mm Hg (on room air), the respiratory therapist called the physician and reported an assessment of acute ventilatory failure. The doctor had the patient transferred to the intensive care unit, intubated, and placed on a mechanical ventilator. The initial ventilator settings were as follows: intermittent mechanical ventilation (IMV) mode, 10 breaths per minute, tidal volume 0.8 L, and Fio_2 0.5, and positive end-expiratory pressure (PEEP) of 7 cm H_2O.

Approximately 25 minutes after the patient was placed on the ventilator, she appeared stable. No spontaneous ventilations were seen. Her vital signs were as follows: blood pressure 132/86, heart rate 90 bpm, and rectal temperature 38° C (100.5° F). A portable chest X-ray had been ordered but not yet taken. Normal vesicular breath sounds were auscultated over the right lung, and diminished-to-absent breath sounds were auscultated over the left lung. On an Fio_2 of 0.5, her ABGs were as follows: pH 7.28, $Paco_2$ 64 mm Hg, HCO_3^- 26 mMol/L, and Pao_2 52 mm Hg.

Her oxygen saturation measured by pulse oximetry (Spo_2) was 80%. On the basis of these clinical data, the following SOAP was recorded:

Respiratory Assessment and Plan

S   N/A (patient intubated)

O   No spontaneous ventilations; vital signs: BP 132/86, HR 90, RR 10 (controlled), T 38° C (100.5° F); normal breath sounds over right lung; diminished-to-absent breath sounds over left lung; ABGs (on Fio_2 = 0.50): pH 7.28, $Paco_2$ 64, HCO_3^- 26, Pao_2 52; Spo_2 80%

A   • Possible aspiration pneumonia (observed aspiration of food)
   • Endotracheal tube possibly placed in right main stem bronchi (diminished-to-absent breath sounds over left lung, ABGs)
     • Acute ventilatory failure with moderate hypoxemia (ABGs)
     • Condition likely caused by misplacement of endotracheal tube

P   Notify physician stat. Check CXR. Pull endotracheal tube back, if necessary. Monitor and reevaluate immediately.

• • • • •

45 Minutes Later

After the patient's endotracheal tube was pulled back 4 cm, normal vesicular breath sounds could be auscultated over both lungs. The chest X-ray confirmed that the endotracheal tube was in a good position above the carina and that both lungs were adequately aerated.

Her vital signs were as follows: blood pressure 123/75, heart rate 74 bpm, and temperature normal. The ventilator settings were readjusted, and repeat ABGs were as follows: pH 7.53, $Paco_2$ 27 mm Hg, HCO_3^- 22 mMol/L, and Pao_2 176 mm Hg. Her Spo_2 was 98%. On the basis of these clinical data, the following SOAP was written:

Respiratory Assessment and Plan

S   N/A (patient intubated on ventilator)

O   Vital signs: BP 123/75, HR 74, T normal; normal bronchovesicular breath sounds over both lung fields; CXR: endotracheal tube in good position; lungs adequately ventilated; ABGs: pH 7.53, $Paco_2$ 27, HCO_3^- 22, Pao_2 176; Spo_2 98%

A   • Acute ventilator-induced alveolar hyperventilation (respiratory alkalosis) with overly corrected hypoxemia (ABGs)

P   Adjust present mechanical ventilation setting per protocol (decreasing tidal volume). Down-regulate oxygen therapy per protocol. Monitor and reevaluate.

• • • • •

3 Days After Admission

No changes in the patient's ventilator settings were necessary over the previous 48 hours. No improvement was seen in her muscular paralysis. The woman appeared pale, and her vital signs were as follows: blood pressure 146/88, heart rate 92 bpm, and temperature 37.9° C (100.2° F). Large amounts of thick, yellowish sputum were being suctioned from her endotracheal tube approximately every 30 minutes.

Rhonchi were auscultated over both lung fields. A sputum sample was obtained and sent to the laboratory to be cultured. A portable chest X-ray showed a new infiltrate in the right lower lobe consistent with pneumonia or atelectasis. The ABGs were as follows: pH 7.28, $Paco_2$ 36 mm Hg, HCO_3^- 17 mMol/L, and Pao_2 41 mm Hg. Her Spo_2 was 69%. On the basis of these clinical data, the following SOAP was recorded:

Respiratory Assessment and Plan

S   N/A

O   No improvement seen in muscular paralysis; skin: pale; vital signs: BP 146/88, HR 92, T 37.9° C (100.2° F); large amounts of thick, yellowish sputum; rhonchi over both lung fields; CXR: pneumonia and atelectasis in right lower lobe; ABGs: pH 7.28, $Paco_2$ 36, HCO_3^- 17, Pao_2 41; Spo_2 69%

A   • Excessive bronchial secretions (rhonchi, sputum)
  • Infection likely (yellow sputum, fever, CXR: pneumonia)
  • Metabolic acidosis with moderate-to-severe hypoxemia (ABGs)
  • Condition likely caused by lactic acid (ABGs)

P   Up-regulate Bronchopulmonary Hygiene Therapy Protocol (med. neb. with 0.5 cc L-albuterol in 2 cc 10% acetylcysteine q 4 h; therapist to suction patient frequently; sputum culture check in 24 and 48 hours). Perform Hyperinflation Therapy Protocol (adding 10 cm H_2O PEEP to ventilator settings). Up-regulate Oxygen Therapy Protocol. Monitor closely and reevaluate (checking ABGs in 30 minutes).

Discussion

As with the patient with Guillain-Barré syndrome, this case of myasthenia gravis provides another chance to discuss ventilatory pump failure secondary to neuromuscular disease. The presentation of this patient with diplopia, dysphagia, and progressive muscle weakness is classic for this condition. The positive Tensilon test noted in the history was necessary for a final diagnosis. Also important to note is that aspiration of gastric contents is not uncommon in these cases.

In the **first assessment** the therapist should recognize that this case is more than simple respiratory pump failure. The reader sees that the patient was intubated recently and that breath sounds no longer are present in the entire left lung (inadvertent right main stem bronchus intubation). A history of aspiration is also noted. The reader should confirm the impression with a chest X-ray and (very quickly) pull the endotracheal tube back and recheck its new placement with another X-ray. At this point, oxygenating the patient is of primary importance. Increasing the F_{IO_2} to between 0.80 and 1.0 is appropriate. Any attempt to wean the patient at this early junction should not proceed.

The **second assessment** should reflect that the patient is improving and is now hyperventilated and hyperoxygenated on the current ventilator settings. The therapist should adjust the ventilator therapy accordingly and begin the process of longitudinal evaluation of forced vital capacity, forced expiratory volume in 1 second, and negative inspiratory force that is appropriate for this condition if weaning is to be accomplished successfully.

The **final assessment** suggests that the patient has taken another turn for the worse. The sputum is now purulent, rhonchi are heard over both lung fields, and a right lower lobe pneumonia or atelectasis has developed. The patient now has an uncompensated metabolic acidemia that requires evaluation.

The therapist should have anticipated this development, obtained appropriate cultures, and if not done before, prophylactically started bronchopulmonary hygiene and aerosolized medication therapies with frequent suctioning, percussion, postural drainage, and possibly mucolytics. The metabolic acidemia is out of proportion to the patient's condition as described. The reader may wish to review other possible causes of metabolic acidemia at this time (e.g., diabetic ketoacidosis, renal failure).

Unfortunately the patient's pulmonary condition progressively deteriorated, and she died 3 weeks later.

SELF-ASSESSMENT QUESTIONS

True or False

True ☐ False ☐ **1.** Alveolar hyperinflation is associated with myasthenia gravis.

True ☐ False ☐ **2.** The cause of myasthenia gravis appears to be related to circulating antibodies that disrupt the transmission of acetylcholine.

True ☐ False ☐ **3.** Myasthenia gravis is more common in men than in women.

True ☐ False ☐ **4.** Tensilon is used to confirm the diagnosis of myasthenia gravis because of its ability to block cholinesterase.

True ☐ False ☐ **5.** The onset of myasthenia gravis is usually sudden.

True ☐ False ☐ **6.** In myasthenia gravis the extremity muscles (arms and legs) are usually the first to weaken.

True ☐ False ☐ **7.** Neostigmine is used to treat patients with myasthenia gravis.

True ☐ False ☐ **8.** A thymectomy may be beneficial in young adult females with myasthenia gravis.

True ☐ False ☐ **9.** In males the incidence of myasthenia gravis is greatest between 15 and 35 years of age.

True ☐ False ☐ **10.** After the disease has been present for 10 years, death from myasthenia gravis is rare.

Answers appear in Appendix XI.

CHAPTER 31

Sleep Apnea

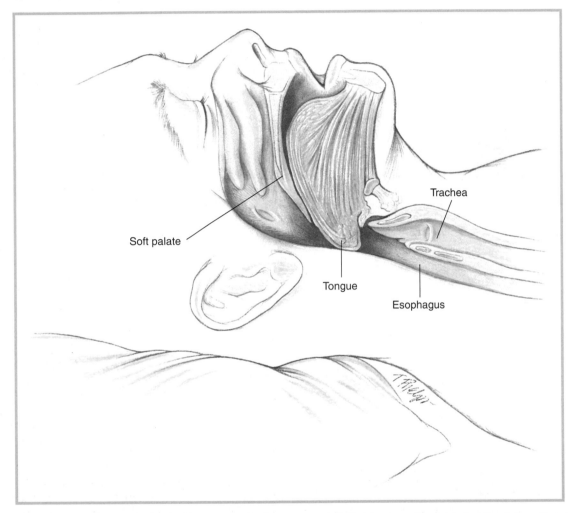

Figure 31–1 Obstructive sleep apnea. When the genioglossus muscle fails to oppose the force that tends to collapse the airway passage during inspiration, the tongue moves into the oropharyngeal area and obstructs the airway. See also Plate 23.

Despite the fact that the clinical characteristics of sleep apnea have been described in the literature for centuries, it was not until the late 1970s and early 1980s that this disorder became generally acknowledged by the medical community. Before this time, it was assumed that individuals who breathed normally while awake also did so during sleep. It also was assumed that patients with lung disorders were not likely to develop more severe respiratory problems when asleep than when awake. Both of these assumptions are now recognized as incorrect.

Stages of Sleep and Characteristic Cardiopulmonary Patterns

During sleep the normal individual slips in and out of two major sleep stages: non–rapid eye movement (non-REM) sleep (also called *quiet* or *slow-wave sleep*) and rapid eye movement (REM) sleep (also called *active* or *dreaming sleep*). Each stage is associated with characteristic electroencephalographic (EEG), behavioral, and breathing patterns.

NON-REM SLEEP

Non-REM sleep usually begins immediately after an individual dozes off. This phase consists of four separate stages, each progressing into a deeper sleep. During stages 1 and 2 the ventilatory rate and tidal volume continually increase and decrease, and brief periods of apnea may be seen. The EEG tracing shows increased slow-wave activity (slow-wave sleep) and loss of alpha rhythm. Cheyne-Stokes respiration also is commonly seen in older male adults during non-REM sleep, especially at high altitudes.

During stages 3 and 4, ventilation becomes slow and regular. Minute ventilation is commonly 1 to 2 L/min less than during the quiet wakeful state. Typically, the Pa_{CO_2} levels are higher (4 to 8 mm Hg), the Pa_{O_2} levels are lower (3 to 10 mm Hg), and the pH is lower (0.03 to 0.05 units) during stages 3 and 4.

Normally, non-REM sleep lasts for 60 to 90 minutes. Although an individual typically moves in and out of all four stages during non-REM sleep, most of the time is spent in stage 2. An individual may move into REM sleep at any time directly from any of the four non-REM sleep stages, although the lighter stages (1 and 2) are commonly the levels of sleep just before REM sleep.

REM SLEEP

During REM sleep a burst of fast alpha rhythms occurs in the EEG tracing. During this period the ventilatory rate becomes rapid and shallow. Sleep-related hypoventilation and apnea frequently are demonstrated during this period. Apneic periods occur in normal adults as often as five times per hour. These apneas may last 15 to 20 seconds without producing any discernible effects. In the normal infant, apneas are shorter (approximately 10 seconds in length), although even these may be cause for concern. A marked reduction in both the hypoxic ventilatory response and the hypercapnic ventilatory response occurs during REM sleep. The heart rate also becomes irregular, and the eyes move rapidly. Dreaming occurs mainly during REM sleep, and profound atonia (paralysis) of movement occurs. The skeletal muscle paralysis primarily affects the arms, legs, and intercostal and upper airway muscles. The activity of the diaphragm is maintained.

The muscle paralysis that occurs during REM sleep can affect an individual's ventilation in two major ways. First, because the muscle tone of the intercostal muscles is low during this period, the negative intrapleural pressure generated by the diaphragm often causes a paradoxical motion of the rib cage. In other words, during inspiration the tissues between the ribs move inward, and during expiration the tissues bulge outward. This paradoxical motion of the rib cage causes the functional residual capacity to decrease. During the wakeful state the intercostal muscle tone tends to stiffen the tissue between the ribs. Second, the loss of muscle tone in the upper airway involves muscles that normally contract during each inspiration and hold the upper airway open. These muscles include the posterior muscles of the pharynx, the genioglossus (which normally causes the tongue to protrude), and the posterior cricoarytenoid (the major abductor of the vocal cords). *The loss of muscle tone in the upper airway may result in airway obstruction.* The negative pharyngeal pressure produced when the diaphragm contracts during inspiration tends to bring the vocal cords together, collapse the pharyngeal wall, and suck the tongue back into the oropharyngeal cavity.

REM sleep periods last between 5 and 40 minutes and recur approximately every 60 to 90 minutes. The REM sleep periods lengthen and become more frequent toward the end of a night's sleep. REM sleep constitutes about 20% to 25% of the total sleep time. Most studies show that it is more difficult to awaken a subject during REM sleep.

Types of Sleep Apnea

Apnea is defined as the cessation of breathing for a period of 10 seconds or longer. Sleep apnea is diagnosed in patients who have more than five episodes of apnea per hour that may occur in either or both non-REM and REM sleep, over a 6-hour period. Generally, the episodes of apnea per hour are more frequent and severe during REM sleep and in the supine body position. They last more than 10 seconds and occasionally may exceed 100 seconds in length. Some patients have as many as 500 periods of apnea per night. Sleep apnea may occur in all age groups; in infants, it may play an important role in sudden infant death syndrome (SIDS).

OBSTRUCTIVE SLEEP APNEA

Obstructive sleep apnea is the sleep disorder most commonly encountered in the clinical setting. It is caused by an anatomic obstruction of the upper airway in the presence of continued ventilatory effort (Figure 31-1). During periods of obstruction, patients commonly appear quiet and still, as though they are holding their breath, followed by increasingly desperate efforts to inhale. Often the apneic episode ends only after an intense struggle. A snorting sound called "fricative breathing" may be heard at the end of the apneic periods. In severe cases, the patient may suddenly awaken, sit upright in bed, and gasp for air. Patients with obstructive sleep apnea usually demonstrate perfectly normal and regular breathing patterns during the wakeful period. Obstructive sleep apnea is seen more often in male subjects than in female subjects (by an 8:1 ratio), and it is especially common in middle-aged men. Approximately 1% to 4% of the adult male population appear to be be affected. It is commonly seen in obese persons who have short necks, a combination that may significantly narrow the pharyngeal airway. In men, a neck diameter of more than 17 inches is suspect; in women, a neck diameter greater than 16 inches predisposes a subject to the condition. In fact, a large number of patients with obstructive sleep apnea demonstrate the pickwickian syndrome (named after a character in Charles Dickens's *The Posthumous Papers of the Pickwick Club*, published in 1837). Dickens's description of Joe, the fat boy who snored and had excessive daytime sleepiness, included many of the classic features of what is now recognized as the sleep apnea syndrome. However, many patients with sleep apnea are not obese, and therefore clinical suspicion should not be limited to this group.

Some clinical disorders associated with obstructive sleep apnea are as follows:

- Obesity (hypoventilation syndrome)
- Anatomic narrowing of upper airway (nasopharyngeal narrowing)
  - Excessive pharyngeal tissue
  - Enlarged tonsils or adenoids
  - Deviated nasal septum, or allergic rhinitis, causing obligate mouth breathing
  - Laryngeal stenosis or vocal cord dysfunction
  - Laryngeal web
  - Pharyngeal neoplasms
  - Micrognathia and/or retrognathia
  - Macroglossia
  - Goiter
- Hypothyroidism
- Testosterone administration
- Myotonic dystrophy
- Shy-Drager syndrome
- Down syndrome

The general clinical manifestations of obstructive sleep apnea can be summarized as follows:

- Chronic loud snoring
- Hypertension
- Morning headaches
- Systemic hypertension
- Congestive heart failure
- Nausea
- Dry mouth on awakening
- Intellectual and personality changes (short-term memory loss, loss of executive function)
- Depression
- Sexual impotence
- Nocturnal enuresis
- Excessive daytime sleepiness (hypersomnolence)
- Automobile accidents or job malperformance related to sleepiness
- Pulmonary hypertension and/or cor pulmonale (rarely)

Polysomnographic monitoring demonstrates the following in obstructive sleep apnea:

- Apnea-related oxygen desaturation (4% or greater drop in Spo_2)
- More than five obstructive apneas of more than 10 seconds per hour of sleep, and one or more of the following:
  - Frequent arousals from the apneas, premature ventricular contractions (PVCs), other serious cardiac arrhythmias, including:
    - Profound bradycardia and/or asystole
    - Shortened sleep latency with or without a mean sleep latency test (MSLT) demonstrating a mean sleep latency of less than 10 minutes

CENTRAL SLEEP APNEA

Central sleep apnea occurs when the respiratory centers of the medulla fail to send signals to the respiratory muscles. It is characterized by cessation of airflow at the nose and mouth along with cessation of inspiratory efforts (absence of diaphragmatic excursions), as opposed to obstructive sleep apnea, which is characterized by the presence of heightened inspiratory efforts during apneic periods.

Central sleep apnea is associated with cardiovascular, metabolic, or central nervous system disorders. As previously mentioned, a small number of brief central apneas normally occur with the onset of sleep or the onset of REM sleep. Central sleep apnea, however, is diagnosed when the frequency of the apnea episodes is excessive (more than 30 in a 6-hour period).

Clinical disorders associated with central sleep apnea include the following:

- Congestive heart failure (Cheyne-Stokes respiration)
- Metabolic alkalosis
- Idiopathic (hypoventilation syndrome)
- Encephalitis
- Brain stem neoplasm
- Brain stem infarction
- Bulbar poliomyelitis
- Cervical cordotomy
- Spinal surgery
- Hypothyroidism

The general noncardiopulmonary clinical manifestations of central sleep apnea can be summarized as follows:

- Tendency for the patient to be of normal weight
- Mild snoring
- Insomnia
- Although not as common as in obstructive apnea, some of the following may occur:
  - Daytime fatigue
  - Depression
  - Sexual dysfunction

MIXED SLEEP APNEA

Mixed sleep apnea is a combination of obstructive and central sleep apneas. It usually begins as central apnea followed by the onset of ventilatory effort without airflow (obstructive apnea). Clinically, patients with predominantly mixed apnea are classified (and treated) as having obstructive sleep apnea.

Figure 31-2 illustrates the patterns of airflow, respiratory effort (reflected through the esophageal pressure), and arterial oxygen saturation in central, obstructive, and mixed apneas.

Diagnosis

The diagnosis of sleep apnea begins with a careful history from the patient, especially noting the presence of snoring, sleep disturbance, and persistent daytime sleepiness. This is followed by a careful examination of the upper airway and perhaps by pulmonary function studies to determine whether upper airway obstruction is present.

The patient's blood is evaluated for the presence of polycythemia, reduced thyroid function, and bicarbonate retention. Arterial blood gas values are obtained to determine resting, wakeful oxygenation and acid-base status. When possible, a carboxyhemoglobin level should be obtained. A chest X-ray, electrocardiogram (ECG), and echocardiogram are helpful in evaluating the presence of pulmonary hypertension, the state of right and left ventricular compensation, and the presence of any other cardiopulmonary disease.

The diagnosis and type of sleep apnea are confirmed with polysomnographic sleep studies, which include (1) an EEG and electro-oculogram (EOG) to identify the sleep stages; (2) use of a monitoring device for airflow in and out of the patient's lungs; (3) an ECG to identify cardiac arrhythmias; (4) impedance pneumography, intercostal electromyography, or esophageal manometry to monitor the patient's ventilatory rate and effort; and (5) ear oximetry or transcutaneous oxygen monitoring to detect changes in oxygen saturation.

Patients diagnosed as having predominantly central sleep apnea are evaluated carefully for lesions

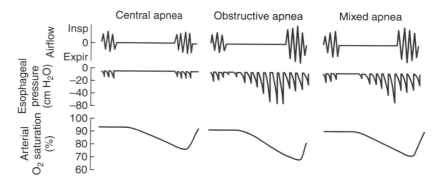

Figure 31–2 Patterns of airflow, respiratory efforts (reflected through the esophageal pressure), and arterial oxygen saturation produced by central, obstructive, and mixed apneas.

involving the brain stem. Patients diagnosed as having obstructive sleep apnea may undergo a computed tomographic (CT) evaluation or a cephalometric head X-ray of the upper airway to determine the site (or sites) and severity of the pharyngeal narrowing.

The steps typically involved in diagnosing sleep apnea can be summarized as follows:

- History
- Examination of the neck and upper airway structures, heart and lungs
- Spirometry (flow-volume loops in the erect and supine positions) to assess for extrathoracic airway obstruction and "chatter" (sawtooth pattern)
- Arterial blood gas analysis
- Hemoglobin and carboxyhemoglobin levels
- Nocturnal recording oximetry
- Thyroid function
- Chest radiograph
- ECG
- Polysomnographic (sleep) study
- Computed axial tomographic (CAT) scan of the upper airway (obstructive apnea) or cephalometric head X-ray (in selected patients)

OVERVIEW
of the Cardiopulmonary Clinical Manifestations Associated with SLEEP APNEA

CLINICAL DATA OBTAINED AT THE PATIENT'S BEDSIDE

The Physical Examination
Cyanosis (see page 45 ◆▶)

CLINICAL DATA OBTAINED FROM LABORATORY TESTS AND SPECIAL PROCEDURES

Pulmonary Function Study Findings
Lung Volume and Capacity Findings
(see page 62 ◆▶)

V_T	RV	FRC	TLC
↓	↓	↓	↓
VC	IC	ERV	RV/TLC%
↓	↓	↓	N

Obviously, pulmonary function cannot easily be studied during sleep. However, patients with obstructive sleep apnea commonly demonstrate a sawtooth pattern on maximal inspiratory and expiratory flow-volume loops. Also characteristic of obstructive sleep apnea is a ratio of expiratory-to-inspiratory flow rates at 50% of the vital capacity ($FEF_{50\%}/FIF_{50\%}$) that exceeds 1.0 in the absence of obstructive pulmonary disease.

In addition, because the muscle tone of the intercostal muscles is low during periods of REM-related apneas, the negative intrapleural pressure generated by the diaphragm often causes a paradoxical motion of the rib cage—that is, during inspiration the tissue between the ribs moves inward, and during expiration the tissue bulges outward. This paradoxical motion of the rib cage may cause the VC, RV, FRC, and TLC to decrease further. This pathologic condition further contributes to the nocturnal hypoxemia seen in patients with sleep apnea syndrome.

Arterial Blood Gases
Severe Sleep Apnea
Chronic Ventilatory Failure with Hypoxemia
(see page 73 ◆▶)

pH	$Paco_2$	HCO_3^-	Pao_2
Normal	↑	↑(Significantly)	↓

Acute Ventilatory Changes Superimposed on Chronic Ventilatory Failure (see page 75 ◆▶)
Because acute ventilatory changes frequently are seen in patients with chronic ventilatory failure, the respiratory care practitioner must be familiar with and alert for (1) acute alveolar hyperventilation superimposed on chronic ventilatory failure and (2) acute ventilatory failure superimposed on chronic ventilatory failure.

Oxygenation Indices (see page 82 ◆▶)

$\dot{Q}_S/\dot{Q}_T$	Do_2*	$\dot{V}o_2$	$C(a-\bar{v})O_2$
↑	↓	Normal	Normal
O_2ER	$S\bar{v}o_2$		
↑	↓		

*The Do_2 may be normal in patients who have compensated to the decreased oxygenation status with (1) an increased cardiac output, (2) an increased hemoglobin level, or (3) a combination of both. When the Do_2 is normal, the O_2ER is usually normal.

OVERVIEW
of the Cardiopulmonary Clinical Manifestations Associated with
SLEEP APNEA (Continued)

Hemodynamic Indices (Severe Sleep Apnea)
(see page 99 ◆)

CVP	RAP	$\overline{PA}$	PCWP
↑	↑	↑	↑
CO	SV	SVI	CI
↓	↓	↓	↓
RVSWI	LVSWI	PVR	SVR
↑	↑	↑	↑

During periods of apnea the heart rate decreases then increases after the termination of apnea. It is believed that the carotid body peripheral chemoreceptors are responsible for this response—that is, when ventilation is kept constant or is absent (e.g., during an apneic episode), hypoxic stimulation of the carotid body peripheral chemoreceptors slows the cardiac rate. Therefore it follows that when the lungs are unable to expand (e.g., during periods of obstructive apnea), the depressive effect of the carotid bodies on the heart rate predominates. The increased heart rate noted when ventilation resumes is activated by the excitation of the pulmonary stretch receptors.

Although changes in cardiac output during periods of apnea have been difficult to study, several studies have reported a reduction in cardiac output (about 30%) during periods of apnea, followed by an increase (10% to 15% above controls) after the termination of apnea. Both pulmonary and systemic arterial blood pressures increase in response to the nocturnal oxygen desaturation that develops during periods of sleep apnea. The magnitude of the pulmonary hypertension is related to the severity of the alveolar hypoxia and hypercapnic acidosis. Repetition of these transient episodes of pulmonary hypertension many times a night every night for years may contribute to the development of the right ventricular hypertrophy, cor pulmonale, and eventual cardiac decompensation seen in such patients.

Episodic systemic vasoconstriction secondary to sympathetic adrenergic neural activity is believed to be responsible for the elevation in systemic blood pressure that is commonly seen during apneas. Sleep apnea is now recognized as one of the most frequent and correctable causes of systemic hypertension.

RADIOLOGIC FINDINGS

Chest Radiograph
- Right- or left-sided heart failure

Because of the pulmonary hypertension and polycythemia associated with persistent periods of apnea, right- and/or left-sided heart failure may develop. This condition may be identified on a chest X-ray and may help in diagnosis.

CARDIAC ARRHYTHMIAS

- Sinus arrhythmia
- Sinus bradycardia
- Sinus pauses
- Atrioventricular block (second degree)
- Premature ventricular contractions
- Ventricular tachycardia

In severe cases of sleep apnea, sudden arrhythmia-related death is always possible. Periods of apnea commonly are associated with sinus arrhythmia, sinus bradycardia, and sinus pauses (greater than 2 seconds). The extent of sinus bradycardia is directly related to the severity of the oxygen desaturation. Obstructive apneas usually are associated with the greatest degrees of cardiac slowing. To a lesser extent, atrioventricular heart block (second degree), premature ventricular contractions, and ventricular tachycardia are seen. Apnea-related ventricular tachycardia is viewed as a life-threatening event.

General Management of Sleep Apnea

Over the past few years, it has become apparent that many pathologic conditions are associated with sleep apnea, including hypoxemia, fragmented sleep, cardiac arrhythmias, and neurologic disorders. In general, the prognosis is more favorable for obstructive and mixed apneas than for central sleep apnea.

WEIGHT REDUCTION

Many patients with obstructive sleep apnea are overweight, and although the excess weight alone is not the cause of the apnea, weight reduction clearly leads to a reduction in apnea severity. The precise reason is not known. Because weight reduction may take months and because maintaining weight loss is often difficult, weight reduction as a single form of therapy often fails.

SLEEP POSTURE

It is generally believed that most obstructive apnea is more severe in the supine position and, in fact, may be present only in this position (positional sleep apnea). Apnea and daytime hypersomnolence have significantly improved in some patients who have been instructed to sleep on their sides and avoid the supine posture. Others may benefit from sleeping in a head-up position (e.g., in a lounge chair). The effect of this change in sleeping habits can be documented by recording oximetry in the supine and lateral decubitus positions.

OXYGEN THERAPY

Because of the hypoxemia-related cardiopulmonary complications of apnea (arrhythmias and pulmonary hypertension), oxygen therapy is sometimes used to offset or minimize the oxygen desaturation, particularly in central sleep apnea (see Oxygen Therapy Protocol, Protocol 9-1). Usually, no improvement in sleep fragmentation or hypersomnolence occurs with supplemental oxygen.

DRUG THERAPY

Drugs used to treat central sleep apnea include REM inhibitors such as protriptyline (Vivactil). Acetazolamide (Diamox) is a carbonic anhydrase inhibitor that causes a bicarbonate diuresis and mild metabolic acidosis, which in turn stimulates respiration. It occasionally is also helpful in cases of central sleep apnea.

Protriptyline Hydrochloride

The most frequent and severe episodes of apnea occur during REM sleep in patients with obstructive sleep apnea. Protriptyline hydrochloride, which is a tricyclic antidepressant, causes a marked decrease in REM sleep. When the amount of REM sleep is decreased, the incidence of REM apneic episodes also is decreased. Some patients demonstrate improved upper airway muscle tone during REM and non-REM sleep when protriptyline hydrochloride is administered. A reduction in daytime hypersomnolence also may be seen. Protriptyline hydrochloride is not usually helpful in obstructive sleep apnea.

SURGERY

Some non-obese patients with obstructive sleep apnea benefit from surgical correction or bypass of the anatomic defect or obstruction that is responsible for the apneic episodes. The procedures described in the following paragraphs are presently available.

Uvulopalatopharyngoplasty

Uvulopalatopharyngoplasty (UPPP) is the surgical procedure most commonly used to treat snoring and sleep apnea. During this surgery, the soft palate tissue is shortened by removing the posterior third, including the uvula. The pillars of the palatoglossal arch and the palatopharyngeal arch are tied together, and the tonsils are removed if they are still present. As much excess lateral posterior wall tissue is removed as possible. UPPP is effective in a proportion of cases, especially in patients who are not obese. The success of this type of surgery is between 30% and 50%.

Laser-Assisted Uvulopalatoplasty

Laser-assisted uvulopalatoplasty (LAUP) is performed to eliminate snoring. This surgical procedure entails using a laser to remove tissue from the back of the throat. Although a LAUP is often helpful in the elimination of snoring, it has not proved effective in treating sleep apnea.

Nasal Surgery

Nasal surgery may be performed to remove polyps or straighten a deviated nasal septum.

Tracheostomy

Tracheal intubation with or without tracheostomy is often the treatment of choice in emergency situations and in patients who do not respond satisfactorily to drug therapy or other treatment interventions.

Mandibular Advancement

Approximately 6% of patients with obstructive sleep apnea have a mandibular malformation. For example, patients who have obstructive sleep apnea because of retrognathia or mandibular micrognathia may benefit from surgical mandibular advancement.

MECHANICAL VENTILATION

Continuous Positive Airway Pressure

As previously mentioned, the cause of many obstructive sleep apneas is related to (1) an anatomic configuration of the pharynx and (2) the decreased muscle tone that normally develops in the pharynx during REM sleep. When patients with obstructive sleep apnea inhale, the pharyngeal muscles and surrounding tissues are sucked inward in response to the negative airway pressure generated by the contracting diaphragm. Nocturnal continuous positive airway pressure (CPAP) is useful in preventing the collapse of the hypotonic airway and is the standard treatment for most cases of obstructive sleep apnea (Figure 31-3). CPAP is not indicated in pure central sleep apnea.

Continuous Mechanical Ventilation

Intubation and continuous mechanical ventilation may be used for short-term therapy when acute ventilatory failure develops in central or obstructive sleep apnea.

Negative-Pressure Ventilation

In patients with central sleep apnea, the noninvasive approach of negative-pressure ventilation without an endotracheal tube may be useful. For example, a negative-pressure cuirass, which is applied to the patient's chest and upper portion of the abdomen, may effectively control ventilation throughout the night. A negative-pressure cuirass is convenient for home use. Negative-pressure ventilation is contraindicated in obstructive sleep apnea.

PHRENIC NERVE PACEMAKER

The implantation of an external phrenic nerve pacemaker may be useful in patients with central sleep apnea resulting from the absence of a signal from the central nervous system to the diaphragm by way of the phrenic nerve. This procedure, however, has not received wide application.

MEDICAL DEVICES

Oral appliances that optimally position the tongue and jaw are the most successful alternatives to surgery and CPAP by mask or "nasal pillows." Recent studies suggest that when oral appliances are carefully selected and applied, a 50% reduction in the number of apneas can be expected in 70% of patients. The devices are best used in patients with mild-to-moderate obstructive sleep apnea. Follow-up polysomnography is mandatory to ensure the effectiveness of the device.

Neck Collar

A small number of patients have used a collar (similar to those used to stabilize cervical fractures) to increase the diameter of the airway and reduce the apnea. The therapeutic success of this procedure is questionable.

OTHER THERAPEUTIC APPROACHES

Regardless of the type of sleep apnea, the patient should be advised to avoid drugs that depress the central nervous system. For example, alcohol and sedatives have been shown to increase the severity and frequency of sleep apnea. All obese patients with sleep apnea should be encouraged to lose weight.

Table 31-1 summarizes the major therapy modalities described above for obstructive and central apnea and their effectiveness.

Figure 31–3 **A,** Normal airway. **B,** Obstructed airway during sleep. **C,** Nasal CPAP generates a positive pressure and holds the airway open during sleep.

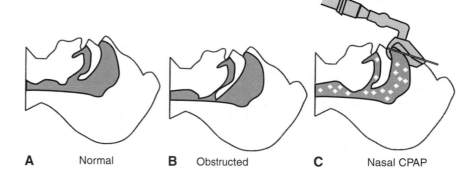

| **A** Normal | **B** Obstructed | **C** Nasal CPAP |

TABLE 31–1 Therapy Modalities for Sleep Apnea

Therapy	Type of Apnea	
	Obstructive	Central
Oxygen therapy	Therapeutic	Therapeutic
Carbonic anhydrase inhibitor drugs		
Acetazolamide	Contraindicated	Indicated
REM inhibitor drugs		
Protriptyline hydrochloride	Therapeutic	Not indicated
Surgical		
Tracheostomy	Therapeutic (100%)	Not indicated
Palatopharyngoplasty	Therapeutic	Not indicated
Mandibular advancement	Therapeutic	Not indicated
Mechanical ventilation		
Continuous positive airway pressure	Therapeutic	Not indicated
Mechanical ventilation	Short-term	Short-term
Negative-pressure ventilation	Contrainidicated	Therapeutic
Endotracheal tube at night	Short-term	Not indicated
Phrenic nerve pacemaker	Not indicated	Experimental
Medical devices	Experimental	Not indicated

Case Study: OBSTRUCTIVE SLEEP APNEA

Admitting History

A 55-year-old Caucasian man had been in the U.S. Marine Corps for more than 25 years when he retired with honors at 46 years of age with the rank of sergeant. He completed tours in Vietnam, Grenada, and Beirut. His last assignment was in Iraq and Kuwait during Operation Desert Storm. During his military career, he received several medals, including a Purple Heart for a leg wound that he incurred in Vietnam when he pulled a fellow marine to safety. During his last 3 years in the service, he was assigned to a desk job, working with new recruits as they progressed through various stages of boot camp.

Although it was not mandatory that he retire, he felt that it was time. He had gained a great deal of weight over the years, and his ability to meet the physical challenge of being a Marine had become progressively more difficult. In addition, when he was doing paperwork at his office, he was aware that he was catnapping while on the job. He knew that if he had observed a fellow Marine doing the same, he would have been quick to issue a severe reprimand. In view of these developments, the man regretfully retired from the service.

For a few years after he retired, he continued to work for the Marines as a volunteer at a local recruitment office. At first he enjoyed this job a great deal. He often found that his military experiences enhanced his ability to talk in a meaningful way to new recruits. Over the past few years, however, working had become progressively more difficult for him, and his attendance was increasingly sporadic. He was often tardy for work. He told the other recruitment volunteers that he was always tired and was experiencing severe morning headaches. His co-workers frequently found him irritable and quick to anger.

The man was having trouble at home, too. Several months before this admission, his wife began sleeping in a room vacated by their daughter, who had recently married. She said that she no longer could sleep with her husband because of his loud snoring and constant thrashing in bed. About this time, the man became clinically depressed and sexually impotent. Despite much discussion and encouragement from his wife, he did not seek medical advice until a few hours before this admission, when he became extremely short of breath. His wife drove him to the local emergency room, where he was evaluated.

Physical Examination

On observation the man appeared to be in severe respiratory distress. He was obese, weighing more than 160 kg (355 lb), and was perspiring profusely. His skin appeared cyanotic, and his neck veins were distended. He had edema (4+) of his feet and legs extending to midcalf. His blood pressure was 194/118, heart rate was 78 bpm, respiratory rate was 22/min, and temperature was normal. Although the man was in obvious discomfort, he stated that he was breathing OK. His wife quickly piped up, "There's that damn Marine coming out again!"

The man's breath sounds were normal but diminished. The diminished breath sounds were believed to be due primarily to the patient's obesity. Palpation of the chest was unremarkable, and percussion was unreliable because of the obesity. A chest X-ray showed cardiomegaly; the lungs appeared unremarkable. To treat presumed cor pulmonale, the physician immediately started the patient on diuretics. His awake arterial blood gas values (ABGs) on room air were as follows: pH 7.54, $Paco_2$ 58 mm Hg, HCO_3^- 48 mmol/L, and Pao_2 52 mm Hg. His oxygen saturation measured by pulse oximetry (Spo_2) was 87%.

Because of the patient's history and present clinical manifestations, the respiratory therapist on duty suspected that the man suffered from obstructive sleep apnea. The therapist suggested this possibility to the emergency room physician, who requested a polysomnographic study. The physician asked the respiratory therapist to document her assessment. The following SOAP was charted:

Respiratory Assessment and Plan

S "I'm breathing OK."

O Weight: 160 kg (355 lb); skin: flushed and cyanotic; distended neck veins and edema of feet and legs (4+) to midcalf; vital signs: BP 194/118, HR 78, RR 22, T normal; oropharyngeal exam typical for obstructive sleep apnea; diminished breath sounds, likely due to obesity; CXR: cor pulmonale; lungs appear normal; ABGs (on room air): pH 7.54, $Paco_2$ 48, HCO_3^- 48, Pao_2 52; Spo_2 87%

A • Obstructive sleep apnea likely (history, cor pulmonale, ABGs, physical appearance)
   • Acute alveolar hyperventilation superimposed on chronic ventilatory failure with moderate hypoxemia (ABGs)
   • Impending ventilatory failure

P Initiate oxygen therapy per protocol. If obstructive sleep apnea is confirmed, start continuous positive airway pressure (CPAP) calibration study. Monitor and reevaluate (vital signs, ECG and Spo_2 q. h).

• • • • •

Over the Next 72 Hours

The diagnosis of severe obstructive sleep apnea was quickly established. Along with the patient's classic history of obstructive sleep apnea, the polysomnogram documented more than 325 periods of obstructive apnea in the study night. The continuous positive airway pressure (CPAP) titration study indicated that 12 cm H_2O CPAP was required to effectively treat the apneic syndrome. In addition to the patient's short, muscular neck and extreme obesity, an oropharyngeal examination revealed a small mouth and large tongue for his body size. The free margin of the soft palate hung low in the oropharynx, nearly obliterating the view behind it. The uvula was widened (4+) and elongated; the tonsillar pillars were widened (3+). Air entry through the nares was reduced bilaterally. The patient's hemocrit was 51% and hemoglobin level was 17 g/dl.

A complete pulmonary function test (PFT) showed that the man had a severe restrictive disorder. In addition, a saw-toothed pattern was seen in the maximal inspiratory and expiratory flow-volume loops. A chest X-ray obtained on the patient's second day of hospitalization showed reduction in heart size, and the lungs were clear. A brisk diuresis was in process. The patient stated that he was breathing much better.

On inspection the patient no longer appeared short of breath. Although he still appeared flushed, he did not look as cyanotic as he had on admission. His neck veins were no longer distended, and the peripheral edema of his legs and feet had improved. His breath sounds were clear but diminished. His room air ABGs were as follows: pH 7.38, $Paco_2$ 82 mm Hg, HCO_3^- 44 mmol/L, and Pao_2 66 mm Hg. His Spo_2 was 91%. The physician again called for a respiratory care evaluation. On the basis of these clinical data, the following SOAP was recorded:

Respiratory Assessment and Plan

S "I'm breathing much better."

O Recent diagnosis: obstructive sleep apnea— more than 325 periods of obstructive apnea documented during sleep study; short muscular neck; narrow upper airway; obesity; Hct. 51%; Hb 17 g/dl; PFTs: severe restrictive disorder; saw-tooth pattern seen on maximal inspiratory and expiratory flow-volume loops; no longer appearing short of breath; cyanotic appearance but improved; clear but diminished breath sounds; ABGs (on room air): pH 7.38, $Paco_2$ 82, HCO_3^- 44, Pao_2 66; Spo_2 91%

A • Obstructive sleep apnea confirmed (history, polysomnographic study, ABGs)
   • Chronic ventilatory failure with mild hypoxemia

P Continue oxygen therapy per protocol. Request CPAP calibration study. Ensure that patient sleeps in the head-up position and refrains from sleeping on his back. Monitor and reevaluate.

Discussion

Although the diagnosis of obstructive sleep apnea is made most frequently in the outpatient setting, recent experience has shown that it often may be diagnosed in the course of an acute hospitalization. In the present case, although the patient was first seen in the emergency room, it soon became clear that he was ill enough to be admitted, and his workup proceeded from there.

In the **first assessment** the therapist must perform a careful examination of the patient's nasopharynx and oropharynx, as well as his chest. The typical upper airway anatomy of obstructive sleep apnea is visible. While the patient's polysomnogram and CPAP titration study are in progress, the therapist appropriately ensures the patient's oxygenation (probably by use of a Venturi oxygen mask) to prevent alveolar hypoventilation. In a patient with as classic a case as this, a split night study (half standard polysomnography, half CPAP titration) may be in order. Autotitrating CPAP may be helpful in this setting.

The patient's neck vein distention, polycythemia, cardiomegaly, and peripheral edema all suggest cor pulmonale. This condition will improve once the patient's overall hypoventilation is treated. Many physicians would go ahead and give the patient a bicarbonate-losing diuretic, watching for worsening of metabolic acidosis while this step is being done. The therapist (in this first assessment) correctly analyzes the situation as being potentially hazardous, and this assessment includes impending ventilatory failure, which is a real possibility.

After the **second assessment** the diagnosis has been made. Pulmonary function tests have shown upper airway obstruction and a restrictive disorder. The therapist ensures that a chest X-ray is taken to rule out any other significant pulmonary condition. None is found. The patient's Pa_{CO_2}, however, has worsened, and the therapist must make some choices regarding treatment. The therapist elects to have the patient refrain from sleeping on his back and to sleep in the head-up position instead. In addition, the physician would likely ask for a nutrition consultation at this time because the patient needs to begin a drastic weight-loss program.

At the end of this case the patient still is not markedly improved and awaits the benefits of continuous positive airway pressure (CPAP) therapy. Indeed, the CPAP therapy was eventually helpful. The patient had a 9-kg (20-lb) diuresis during the first week of its use, and good oxygenation was achieved with 10 cm H_2O CPAP pressure.

A diagnosis of obstructive sleep apnea often can complicate other primary respiratory disorders, such as chronic obstructive pulmonary disease (COPD), pneumonia, atelectasis, or chest wall deformity. In these settings the care is more complicated and, if anything, should be even more data-driven, with careful examination of all subjective and objective data.

Patients with obstructive sleep apnea have a significant risk of cardiovascular and central nervous system morbidity and mortality (myocardial infarctions, arrhythmias, hypertension, and cerebrovascular accidents). Psychiatric effects such as depression, sleep-related job malperformance, and daytime motor vehicle accidents also are seen. Current evidence suggests that such patients need not experience these effects if the sleep disorder–related breathing problem is treated effectively. Compliance with CPAP therapy is important but difficult to measure. Improvement in daytime somnolence is one surrogate for more direct measurements of compliance, such as recording of oximetry in the patient's home. Close clinical monitoring is important if good therapeutic outcomes are to be achieved consistently.

Note: The field of sleep-disordered breathing holds much promise for the respiratory therapist trained in polysomnographic studies. Nasal CPAP therapy should come naturally to him or her, as should recognition of untoward cardiovascular events. The difficult part is that of EEG pattern recognition, which is now being taught as an "add-on" in some respiratory care training programs.

SELF-ASSESSMENT QUESTIONS

Multiple Choice

1. What is another name for non–rapid eye movement (non-REM) sleep?

    I. Slow-wave sleep
    II. Active sleep
    III. Dreaming sleep
    IV. Quiet sleep

   a. I only
   b. III only
   c. IV only
   d. I and IV only
   e. II and III only

2. During non-REM sleep, ventilation becomes slow and regular during which stage(s)?

    I. Stage 1
    II. Stage 2
    III. Stage 3
    IV. Stage 4

   a. II only
   b. III only
   c. I and II only
   d. II and III only
   e. III and IV only

3. The pickwickian syndrome is associated with which of the following?

    I. Central sleep apnea
    II. Obesity
    III. Loud snoring
    IV. Obstructive sleep apnea
    V. Absence of diaphragmatic excursion

   a. I only
   b. IV only
   c. I and V only
   d. IV and V only
   e. II, III, and IV only

4. During periods of apnea, the patient commonly demonstrates which of the following?

    I. Systemic hypotension
    II. Decreased cardiac output
    III. Increased heart rate
    IV. Pulmonary hypertension

   a. I and III only
   b. II and IV only
   c. III and IV only
   d. I, II, and III only
   e. II, III, and IV only

5. Periods of severe sleep apnea are commonly associated with which of the following?

    I. Ventricular tachycardia
    II. Sinus bradycardia
    III. Premature ventricular contraction
    IV. Sinus arrhythmia

   a. I and IV only
   b. II and III only
   c. III and IV only
   d. II, III, and IV only
   e. I, II, III, and IV

6. During REM sleep, there is paralysis of the:

    I. Arm muscles
    II. Upper airway muscles
    III. Leg muscles
    IV. Intercostal muscles
    V. Diaphragm

   a. IV only
   b. V only
   c. IV and V only
   d. I, II, III, and IV only
   e. I, II, III, IV, and V

7. Normally, REM sleep constitutes about what percentage of the total sleep time?

   a. 5 to 10
   b. 10 to 20
   c. 20 to 25
   d. 25 to 30
   e. 35 to 40

8. Which of the following therapy modalities are therapeutic for obstructive apnea?

    I. Phrenic pacemaker
    II. CPAP
    III. Theophylline
    IV. Negative-pressure ventilation

   a. I only
   b. II only
   c. III and IV only
   d. I and IV only
   e. I, II, III, and IV

9. Which of the following therapy modalities are therapeutic for central sleep apnea?

    I. Negative-pressure ventilation
    II. CPAP
    III. Tracheostomy
    IV. Endotracheal tube at night

a. I only
b. II only
c. III only
d. II and III only
e. II, III, and IV only

10. How long do normal periods of apnea during REM sleep last?

a. 0 to 5 seconds
b. 5 to 10 seconds
c. 10 to 15 seconds
d. 15 to 20 seconds
e. 30 to 40 seconds

Answers appear in Appendix XI.

PART XII

Newborn and Early Childhood Respiratory Disorders

Clinical Manifestations Common with Newborn and Early Childhood Respiratory Disorders

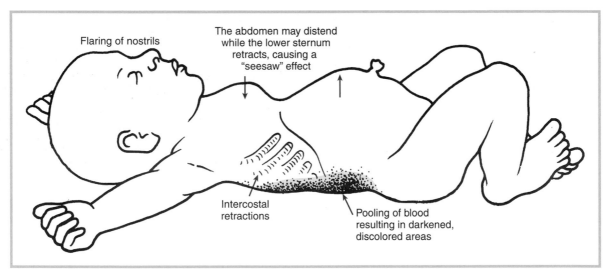

Flaring of nostrils

The abdomen may distend while the lower sternum retracts, causing a "seesaw" effect

Intercostal retractions

Pooling of blood resulting in darkened, discolored areas

Figure 32–1 Clinical manifestations associated with increased negative intrapleural pressure during inspiration in infants, exaggerated in infants with IRDS.

Respiratory disorders are the leading causes of admission to the neonatal intensive care unit (NICU). Essential to the understanding of respiratory distress at any age, but especially in the newborn, is the axiom "Oxygen is the primary nutrient of the human body." The clinical manifestations presented by a baby in early respiratory distress include lethargy, cyanosis, increased respiratory rate, nasal flaring, expiratory grunting, intercostal retractions, substernal retraction, tachycardia, increased blood pressure, and acute alveolar hyperventilation with hypoxemia. The late, ominous manifestations include a decreased respiratory rate, gasping respirations, apnea, bradycardia, decreased blood pressure, and acute ventilatory failure with both CO_2 retention and hypoxemia.

Although many of the pathophysiologic mechanisms and clinical manifestations presented by the newborn with a respiratory disorder are identical to those seen in the older child or adult (see Part I, Chapters 1 through 10), some of the pathophysiologic mechanisms and clinical manifestations are unique to the newborn. The more important clinical manifestations associated with neonatal respiratory disorders and the primary pathophysiologic mechanisms responsible for these clinical manifestations are outlined in this chapter.

Clinical Manifestations Associated with Increased Negative Intrapleural Pressures During Inspiration

The thorax of the newborn infant is quite flexible— that is, the compliance of the infant's thorax is high. This flexibility is a result of the large amount of cartilage found in the skeletal structure of newborns. Because of the structural alterations associated with many newborn respiratory disorders, however, the compliance of the infant's *lungs* is low. In an effort to offset the decreased lung compliance, the infant must generate high negative intrapleural pressures

Clinical Manifestations Associated with Increased Negative Intrapleural Pressures During Inspiration

- Intercostal retractions
- Substernal retraction/abdominal distention ("seesaw") movement
- Cyanosis of the dependent portions of the thoracic and abdominal areas

during inspiration. This condition causes the following (Figure 32-1):

- The soft tissues between the ribs retract during inspiration.
- The substernal area retracts and the abdominal area protrudes in a seesaw fashion during inspiration. The substernal retraction is caused by high negative intrapleural pressure, and the abdominal distention is caused by the contraction (depression) of the diaphragm during inspiration.
- The blood vessels in the more dependent portions of the thoracic and abdominal areas dilate and pool blood, causing these areas to appear cyanotic.

FLARING NOSTRILS (OR NASAL FLARING)

Flaring nostrils frequently are observed in infants in respiratory distress. This clinical manifestation probably is a facial reflex to facilitate the movement of gas into the tracheobronchial tree. The dilator naris, which originates from the maxilla and inserts into the ala of the nose, is the muscle responsible for this movement. When activated, the dilator naris pulls the alae laterally and widens the nasal aperture, providing a larger orifice for gas to enter during inspiration (Figure 32-2).

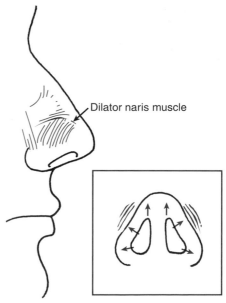

Dilator naris muscle

Figure 32–2 The dilator naris muscles cause the nostrils to dilate during a stressful inspiration.

EXPIRATORY GRUNTING

An audible expiratory grunt frequently is heard in infants with respiratory problems. Depending on the listener's auditory perception, the expiratory grunt may sound like an expiratory cry. It often is first detected on auscultation. The expiratory grunt is a natural physiologic mechanism that generates high positive pressures in the alveoli, which, at least in part, counteracts the hypoventilation associated with the disorder (e.g., infant respiratory distress syndrome). In short, as the gas pressure in the alveoli increases, the infant's PAo$_2$ increases. During exhalation the infant's epiglottis covers the glottis, which causes the intrapulmonary air pressure to increase. When the epiglottis abruptly opens, gas rushes past the infant's vocal cords and produces an expiratory grunt or cry.

 APNEA OF PREMATURITY

Periodic breathing frequently is seen in the newborn and is described as cycles of short pauses in respiration followed by an increased breathing rate. What is called *apnea of prematurity* also is a common form of apnea in the newborn. It is defined as a cessation of breathing effort that is longer than 20 seconds or any respiratory pause that is long enough to cause

bradycardia, cyanosis, or both to appear in a baby of less than 37 weeks' gestation. About 75% of premature babies weighing less than 1250 g suffer from severe apnea. More than 25% of infants weighing more than 1500 g manifest severe apnea. In general, the younger the infant, the greater the number of apneic episodes that may occur.

Premature infants are believed to be susceptible to apneic episodes because of immature functioning of the chemoreceptors, receptors in the airways, and central nervous system. Rapid eye movement (REM) sleep also is thought to play an important role in causing sleep apnea. Box 32-1 lists factors that trigger apneic episodes.

 PERSISTENT PULMONARY HYPERTENSION OF THE NEWBORN

Persistent pulmonary hypertension of the newborn (PPHN) commonly is seen in infants with an underlying respiratory disorder such as *meconium aspiration syndrome* (MAS), *transient tachypnea of the newborn* (TTN), *infant respiratory distress syndrome* (IRDS), *pulmonary air leak syndromes*, and *diaphragmatic hernia*. Box 32-2 lists disorders commonly associated with PPHN.

PPHN is caused in part by reflex pulmonary vasoconstriction that can be activated by myriad

---

BOX 32–1

Factors that Trigger Apnea in the Premature Infant

Control of Ventilation
REM sleep
Decreased hypoxia and hypercapnia response
Ondine's curse (idiopathic alveolar hypoventilation)

Reflex Stimulation
Suctioning of the nasopharynx and trachea
Laryngeal stimulation
Bowel movements (vagal response)
Hiccups

Environmental Conditions
Ambient temperature changes

Neurologic Disorders
Seizures
Intracranial hemorrhage
Meningitis

Drug Depression
Sedatives
Analgesics
Prostaglandins

Respiratory Diseases
Infant respiratory distress syndrome
Pneumonia
Transient tachypnea of the newborn
Meconium aspiration syndrome
Bronchopulmonary dysplasia
Diaphragmatic hernia

Cardiac Disorders
Patent ductus arteriosus
Congestive heart failure
Right to left intracardiac shunting

Systemic Processes
Hypothermia
Hypoglycemia
Hyponatremia
Hypocalcemia
Sepsis (group B *Streptococcus*)

Body Position
Head flexion

Anatomic Abnormalities
Micrognathia
Choanal atresia
Microglossia

BOX 32–2

Factors Associated with Persistent Pulmonary Hypertension of the Newborn (PPHN)

Maternal Factors
Diabetes
Cesarean section
Hypoxia

Cardiovascular Factors
Systemic hypotension
Congenital heart disease
Shock

Hematologic Factors
Increased hematocrit
Septicemia
Maternal-fetal blood loss
  Abruptio placentae
  Placenta previa
Acute blood loss

Respiratory Diseases
Meconium aspiration syndrome (MAS)
Transient tachypnea of the newborn (TTN)

Infant respiratory distress syndrome (IRDS)
Pneumonia
Pulmonary air leak syndromes
Diaphragmatic hernia

Fetal Factors
Intrauterine stress
Hypoxia
Decreased pH
Placental vascular abnormalities

Other Factors
Central nervous system disorders
Hypoglycemia
Hypocalcemia
Neuromuscular disease

---

stimuli, including alveolar hypoxia, hypercapnia, and decreased pH. As a result of the high pulmonary vascular resistance, right-to-left shunting develops—that is, nonoxygenated blood bypasses the infant's lungs via the ductus arteriosus and foramen ovale (see fetal circulation pathways; Figure 32-3).

After birth, approximately 80% of the pulmonary vascular resistance (PVR) normally decreases within the first 24 hours in response to (1) increased Pa_{O_2} and pH; (2) lung expansion; and (3) release of vasoactive substances, including prostaglandins, bradykinin, and endothelium-derived relaxing factor (ERF). In infants with PPHN, however, the PVR stays high because of pulmonary vascular hyperreactivity to irritating stimuli. Clinically, PPHN usually appears within the first 12 hours of life with cyanosis, tachypnea, intercostal retractions, nasal flaring, and grunting. Arterial blood gases typically show what is termed *shunt physiology:* a low Pa_{O_2} that is refractory to oxygen therapy. Cardiomegaly may develop as a result of the increased right ventricular afterload caused by the increased PVR.

◆ ARTERIAL BLOOD GASES

Acute alveolar hyperventilation with hypoxemia and acute ventilatory failure with hypoxemia commonly are seen in newborn babies with pulmonary disorders. However, the pathophysiologic mechanisms responsible for the infant's low arterial oxygen level (Pa_{O_2}) are often different from those seen in adults.

This is especially true for newborn infants who have MAS, TTN, IRDS, pulmonary air leak syndromes, respiratory syncytial virus infections, and/or diaphragmatic hernia.

There are three major mechanisms responsible for the decreased Pa_{O_2} observed in the disorders of the newborn just mentioned: (1) pulmonary shunting and venous admixture, (2) PPHN, and (3) infant fatigue. During the early or mild stages of the disorder, the infant commonly hyperventilates, causing the Pa_{CO_2} to decrease and the pH to increase. During the advanced or late stages of the disorder, the infant often goes into acute ventilatory failure. When this occurs, there is a progressive increase in the Pa_{CO_2}, a secondary increase in the HCO_3^-, and a decrease in the pH. The decreased pH also may result from the decreased Pa_{O_2} and the metabolic acidosis that results from anaerobic metabolism and lactic acid accumulation. If this is the case, the calculated HCO_3^- reading and pH will be lower than expected for a particular Pa_{CO_2} level.

Assessment of the Newborn

As already discussed in Chapter 10, good assessment skills include (1) the systematic collection of clinical data, (2) the evaluation of the data, and (3) the formulation of an appropriate treatment plan. As with the older child or adult, the newborn with respiratory disease must be evaluated frequently. To enhance this

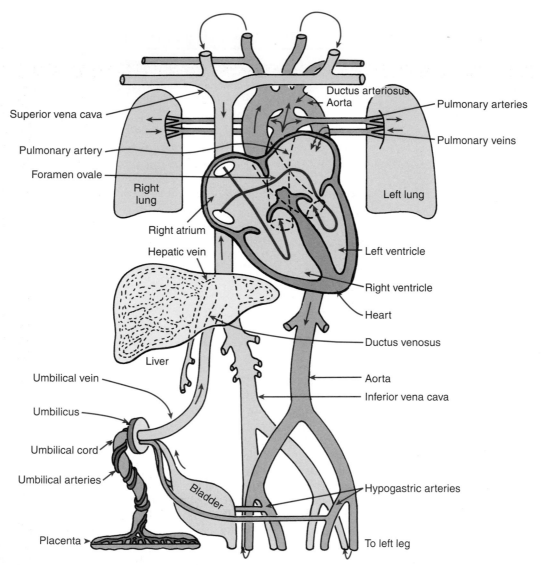

Figure 32-3 Fetal circulation.

process, Figure 32-4 illustrates objective data, assessments, and treatment plans commonly associated with newborn respiratory disorders. Another common assessment tool for the newborn is the Apgar score.

APGAR SCORE

The Apgar score is a rating system for the rapid identification of infants requiring immediate intervention or transfer to an NICU. The Apgar evaluation is performed 1 minute after birth and again 5 minutes later. It is based on a rating of five factors that reflect

the infant's ability to adjust to extrauterine life. As shown in Figure 32-5, the infant's heart rate, respiratory effort, muscle tone, reflex irritability, and color are scored from a low value of 0 to a normal value of 2. The five scores are combined and the totals at 1 minute and 5 minutes are recorded. For example, Apgar 8/10 is a score of 8 at 1 minute and 10 at 5 minutes.

A score of 0 to 3 represents severe distress, a score of 4 to 6 indicates moderate distress, and a score of 7 to 10 represents an absence of difficulty in adjusting to extrauterine life. The 5-minute score is normally higher than the 1-minute score. A low 1-minute score

A — NEONATAL RESPIRATORY CARE POCKET CARD

Clinical manifestations that commonly develop in response to respiratory disease

History	Objective Data — Inspection	Auscultation	ABGs/Pulse Oximetry	Chest Radiograph	ASSESSMENT — Common Causes of Clinical Indicators	Plan
Prematurity, maternal diabetes, C-section, multiple births, sibling with RDS	• Retractions • Nasal flaring • Paradoxical (see-saw) respirations • Cyanosis or pallor	• Expiratory grunting • Poor air entry • May have crackles	↓PO2/SpO2 while on ↑FIO2 (Note: premature infants need PCO2 in 60-80 range) Avoid SpO2 >95%	Reticulogranular, ground glass appearance with air bronchograms	RESPIRATORY DISTRESS SYNDROME (RDS) • Surfactant deficiency • Atelectasis	• Oxygen therapy • Hyperinflation therapy (CPAP/PEEP) • Mechanical ventilation • Surfactant administration
Prematurity, history of RDS, mechanical ventilation	• Decreased chest movement	• Diminished or distant breath sounds	Further ↓PO2/SpO2 while on ↑FIO2	Small cystic areas with possibly flattened diaphragms	PULMONARY INTERSTITIAL EMPHYSEMA (PIE) • Airtrapping	• Oxygen therapy • Decrease ventilator pressures • Permissive hypercapnia • Possibly high frequency ventilation and/or selective mainstem intubation • Monitor for barotrauma
Low birth weight, RDS, prolonged mechanical ventilation, supplemental oxygen, slow growth	• Cyanosis if off O2 • Barrel chest	• Wheezes • Crackles • Rhonchi	↑PCO2 with normal pH, ↓PO2/SpO2	Cystic pattern	BRONCHOPULMONARY DYSPLASIA (BPD) • Airtrapping • Bronchospasm	• Oxygen therapy • Bronchodilator therapy • Bronchial hygiene therapy • Permissive hypercapnia • Fluid management • Increased calorie intake
Usually full term, possibly C-section, perinatal complications	• Tachypnea • Retractions	• Crackles	↓PCO2; ↓PO2/SpO2	Perihilar streaking with enlarged cardiac silhouette	TRANSIENT TACHYPNEA OF THE NEWBORN • Airway fluid	• Oxygen therapy
Stress and/or asphyxia in utero, meconium noted in amniotic fluid, usually full term to post term	• Dyspnea • Meconium-stained umbilical cord or fingernails	• Crackles • Rhonchi	↓PCO2 (May increase as patient fatigues), ↓PO2/SpO2	Hyperaeration	MECONIUM ASPIRATION SYNDROME (MAS) • Airway secretions • Airtrapping	• Suction oropharynx and trachea before delivery • Oxygen therapy • Bronchial hygiene therapy • Possible hyperventilation (to further ↓PCO2 and ↑pH) if hypertension likely • May need to consider ECMO, HFV, etc. • Monitor for barotrauma
Possible underlying problem with meconium aspiration, congenital heart disease, or perinatal asphyxia. Minimal ↑PO2 with 100%O2 challenge	• Persistent cyanosis disproportionate to degree of pulmonary disease on CXR • Tachypnea	• Corresponds to underlying cardiopulmonary disorder	Fluctuations in PO2/SpO2	Normal to mild pulmonary parenchymal disease	PERSISTENT PULMONARY HYPERTENSION OF THE NEWBORN (PPHN) • Pulmonary vasoconstriction • Reopening of fetal circulation pathways	• Oxygen therapy • Mechanical ventilation • Treat underlying cause • May need to consider ECMO, HFV, nitric oxide, etc.
May have normal pregnancy and delivery (full term); may have dusky, cyanotic episodes. Minimal ↑PO2 with 100% O2 challenge.	• May be normal in appearance if Left→Right shunt present • Cyanotic if Right→Left shunt present	• Heart murmur may be present	PO2 may vary widely depending on heart lesion: low with Right→Left shunt; more normal with Left→Right	May have irregular heart shape ie., boot or egg) depending on lesion	CONGENITAL HEART DISEASE • Pulmonary shunting	• Evaluation to identify problem • Cardiac catheterization • Surgery; pre and post-op supportive care
Problems with breathing; difficulty with eating and breathing (e.g., dusky with feeding), noisy breathing	• Varies with lesion • Respiratory distress, drooling, gastric distension	• Varies with lesion	Usually ↓PCO2 and ↓PO2, extent of which varies with lesion	Normal to highly irregular, depending on lesion	CONGENITAL ANOMALIES of the respiratory system • Airway obstruction	• Evaluation to identify problem • Radiographic procedures/operative procedures to diagnose and treat • Pre and post-op supportive care

ISBN: 0-9659350-4-3 by Terry DesJardins, MEd, RRT and Patricia Beck Koff, MEd, RRT. © Simon & Kolz Publishing 1998. All rights reserved. To order: 319-557-5846

Continued

Figure 32-4 Common neonatal clinical manifestations (objective data), assessments, and treatment plans. (See bottom of parts A and B of this figure for complete source information.)

		Objective Data Clinical manifestations that commonly develop in response to respiratory disease				**ASSESSMENT**	**Plan**
History	**Inspection**	**Auscultation**	**ABGs/ Pulse Oximetry**	**Chest Radiograph**		**COMMON CAUSES OF CLINICAL INDICATORS**	
Infant or young child (usually newborn–3y.o.), upper respiratory infection, barking cough	• Tachypnea • Retractions • Nasal flaring • May have cyanosis	• Barking cough • Stridor	↓PCO₂ and ↓PO₂/SpO₂	Subglottic edema on neck radiograph–steeple sign		LARYNGOTRACHEOBRONCHITIS (CROUP) (typically parainfluenza viruses, occasionally bacterial in origin) • Laryngeal edema	• Oxygen therapy • Cool mist • Racemic epinephrine • Steroids
Toddler or school age child (usually 2y.o. or >), acute onset of fever and respiratory distress	• Stridor • Dyspnea • Drooling • May have cyanosis	• Stridor	↓PCO₂ and ↓PO₂/SpO₂	Epiglottis appears as large, round, soft tissue density on neck radiograph–thumb sign		EPIGLOTTITIS (H. Influenza Type B; vaccine available) • Edema	• Emergency attention • Oxygen therapy • Intubation in OR or tracheostomy in OR • Antibiotics
Upper respiratory infection, apnea (newborn–2y.o. or older child with chronic cardiopulmonary condition)	• Tachypnea, retractions, nasal flaring, nasal secretions • Cyanosis if severe	• Wheezes • Rhonchi	↓PO₂/SpO₂	May vary from normal to streaky infiltrates or hyperaeration		BRONCHIOLITIS (typically RSV organism) • Airway secretions • Bronchospasm	• Supportive • Oxygen therapy • Mist hood/tent • Bronchial hygiene therapy • Trial of bronchodilator therapy • Mechanical ventilation rare • Possible ribavirin via SPAG if critically ill)
Upper respiratory infection, late onset of fever, may c/o earache	• Tachypnea, retractions, nasal flaring, nasal secretions • Cyanosis if severe	• Crackles • Wheezes • Bronchial sounds	↓PO₂/SpO₂	Infiltrates and/or consolidation		PNEUMONIA • Consolidation • Airway secretions	• Supportive as above if viral • Antibiotics if bacterial with supportive care also provided
Wheezing, family history of asthma/allergies, frequent respiratory infections, or chronic unexplained cough	• Accessory muscle use • Decreased chest excursion • Pursed-lip breathing	• Wheezes, • Prolonged expiration • Crackles	↑PCO₂ (increasing PCO₂ is an ominous sign), ↓PO₂/SpO₂	May be normal or show hyperaeration		ASTHMA (most common chronic disease in childhood; see Expert Guidelines ref. below) • Inflammation • Reversible airway obstruction/bronchospasm	(See Expert Guidelines ref. below) • Plan varies with severity • Inhaled B-2 agonists, steroids, anticholinergics, mast cell stabilizers, leukotriene modifiers, PEF or FEV₁ assessments, oxygen therapy, possible mechanical ventilation • Discharge teaching of med use, peakflow self-monitoring, and school management plan
Meconium ileus at birth, excessive thick respiratory secretions, frequent respiratory infections, failure to thrive	• Accessory muscle use • Barrel chest • Clubbed fingertips	• Rhonchi • Wheezes • Crackles	May have↓PO₂/SpO₂	Hyperaeration, peribronchial thickening, bronchiectasis, increased AP diameter		CYSTIC FIBROSIS (one of the most common hereditary disorders) • Excessive secretions • Airtrapping	• Bronchial hygiene therapy (postural drainage and percussion, PEP mask therapy, mucolytics) • Bronchodilators • Antibiotics if indicated • Oxygen therapy • Nutritional support • May need to consider lung transplant
Previously healthy, acute onset of choking, coughing. Occasionally chronic unexplained cough	• Drooling • Stridor • May have cyanosis	• Asymmetrical breath sounds • Wheezes	May be normal, May have↓PO₂/SpO₂	Asymmetrical expansion of chest with forced expiratory film		FOREIGN BODY OBSTRUCTION • Airway obstruction	Rigid bronchoscopy with anesthesia, followed by bronchial hygiene therapy and bronchodilator therapy
Presence of underlying disorder such as shock, sepsis, near drowning, aspiration	• Dyspnea • Tachypnea progressing to cyanosis • Irritability	• Crackles • Rhonchi • Bronchial sounds	↓PCO₂ (PCO₂ increases as disease progresses), ↓PO₂/SpO₂, which continues to worsen despite treatment	Normal early in course, progressively shows fluffy infiltrates and patchy, nodular densities		ADULT RESPIRATORY DISTRESS SYNDROME (ARDS) • Increased alveolar-capillary membrane • Atelectasis • Consolidation	• Oxygen therapy • Hyperinflation therapy (CPAP) • Mechanical ventilation • May need to consider HFV, ECMO • Monitor for barotrauma

PEDIATRIC RESPIRATORY CARE POCKET CARD

B

References: Hay, Current Pediatric Diagnosis and Treatment, 12th Ed. (N.Y. Appleton & Lange, 1995) and Koff, et al., Neonatal and Pediatric Respiratory Care, 2nd Ed. (St. Louis: Mosby, 1993), Excerpt from Expert Panel Report II: Guidelines for the Diagnosis and Management of Asthma, Respir. Care 1997; 42(5):499

Figure 32-4 Cont'd. (See page 433 for legend.)

	0	1	2	1 Minute	5 Minute
Heart rate	Absent	Slow, irregular	More than 100 beats per minute		
Respiratory effort	Apnea	Irregular, slow, shallow, gasping	Strong cry		
Muscle tone	Flaccid/limp	Some flexion of extremities	Well flexed		
Reflex irritability	None-no response to stimulus	Grimace (withdraws)	Crying		
Skin color	Pale blue (shock)	Blue hands and feet, body pink	Pink all over		

Figure 32-5 Apgar score interpretation (add the points in the 1-minute and 5-minute columns): 0-3 = severe distress; 4-6 = moderate distress; 7-10 = mild to no distress.

requires immediate intervention, including the administration of oxygen and oral and nasal suctioning. A baby with a low score that remains low after 5 minutes requires expert care, which may include transfer to the NICU, continuous positive airway pressure (CPAP), umbilical catheterization, and mechanical ventilation. In the newborn who is lethargic, apneic, pale, blue, and bradycardic at birth, assessments to verify that resuscitation efforts are being done correctly and effectively typically follow this order: First, the heart rate returns to normal. This is followed by spontaneous respiratory movements and improved color. The last assessment to be made is that of the baby's tone and reflex irritability.

SELF-ASSESSMENT QUESTIONS

Multiple Choice

1. Which of the following trigger apneic episodes?

   I. Hypoglycemia
   II. Nasotracheal suctioning
   III. Head flexion
   IV. MAS

   a. I only
   b. IV only
   c. II and III only
   d. II, III, and IV only
   e. I, II, III, and IV

2. Clinically, PPHN usually presents within the first:

   a. 3 hours of life
   b. 6 hours of life
   c. 12 hours of life
   d. 24 hours of life
   e. 48 hours of life

3. When resuscitation of the newborn is being done correctly, which of the following begins to improve first?

   a. Tone
   b. Heart rate
   c. Reflex irritability
   d. Respiratory movements
   e. Color

4. Which of the following is associated with PPHN?

   I. Hypoglycemia
   II. Decreased pH
   III. Hypercalcemia
   IV. Systemic hypotension

   a. I only
   b. III only
   c. II and IV only
   d. I, II, and IV only
   e. I, II, III, and IV

5. The Apgar evaluation is performed 1 minute after birth, and again:

   a. 3 minutes after birth
   b. 5 minutes after birth
   c. 10 minutes after birth
   d. 15 minutes after birth
   e. 20 minutes after birth

True or False

True ☐ False ☐ **1.** The compliance of the newborn infant's thorax is low.

True ☐ False ☐ **2.** About 75% of premature babies weighing less than 1250 g suffer from severe apnea.

True ☐ False ☐ **3.** An Apgar score between 4 and 6 indicates mild to no distress.

True ☐ False ☐ **4.** PPHN can be activated by a variety of stimuli, including hypoxia.

True ☐ False ☐ **5.** Flaring nostrils in the newborn is probably a facial reflex to facilitate the movement of gas into the tracheobronchial tree.

Answers appear in Appendix XI.

CHAPTER 33

Meconium Aspiration Syndrome

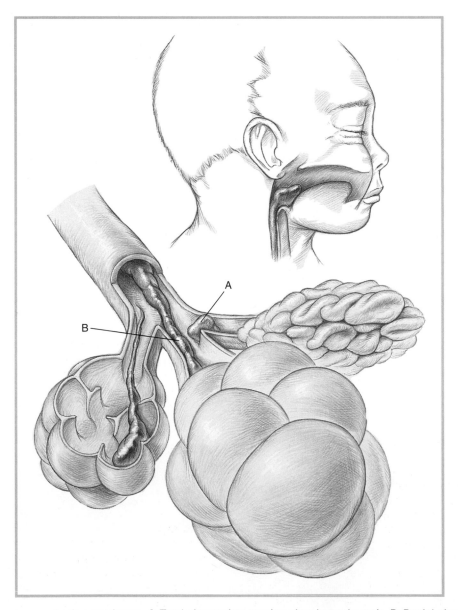

Figure 33–1 Meconium aspiration syndrome. **A,** Total obstruction causing alveolar atelectasis. **B,** Partial obstruction causing air trapping and alveolar hyperinflation. See also Plate 24.

Anatomic Alterations of the Lungs

During normal intrauterine fetal development, the infant periodically demonstrates normal rapid, shallow respiratory chest movements. This normal action moves amniotic fluid in and out of the oropharynx while the glottis remains closed. During periods of fetal hypoxemia, however, the infant may demonstrate very deep, gasping inspiratory movements that may force the contents of the naso-oropharynx to pass through the glottis into the airways. The aspiration of minimal amounts of clear amniotic fluid usually is not associated with serious anatomic or functional problems of the lungs. During fetal hypoxemia, however, the aspirate may contain a mix of fetal stool (meconium) and amniotic fluid—hence the phrase *meconium aspiration syndrome (MAS)*.

MAS is a clinical entity seen primarily in full-term or post-term infants who have had some degree of hypoxemia either prenatally or during the birth process. When the fetus experiences in-utero hypoxia, the intestinal response is vasoconstriction, increased gastrointestinal peristalsis, anal sphincter relaxation, and passage of meconium into the amniotic fluid. Meconium is the material that collects in the intestine of the fetus and forms the first stools of the newborn. It is thick and sticky, highly viscous, and usually green to black in color. Meconium is a heterogeneous mixture of intestinal tract secretions, amniotic fluid, pulmonary fetal fluid, and intrauterine debris such as epithelial cells, mucus, lanugo, blood, and vernix.

Aspiration of meconium leads to one or more of the following complications. *First,* the physical presence of the meconium results in upper airway obstruction at birth because the high viscosity of the meconium prevents it from penetrating past the glottis. Shortly after birth (within 1 hour), and especially if gasping inspirations are present, clumps of meconium rapidly migrate past the glottis and penetrate the smaller airways (Figure 33-1). In cases of severe intrauterine hypoxemia, however, meconium may already be present in the distal airways at birth.

The thick, tenacious meconium can partially or totally obstruct the airways. Airways that are partially obstructed cause a "ball-valve" effect. This condition in turn leads to air trapping and alveolar hyperinflation. Excessive hyperinflation commonly leads to alveolar rupture and air leak syndromes (see Chapter 36) such as pneumomediastinum or pneumothorax. Totally obstructed airways lead to alveolar shrinkage and atelectasis. This combination of areas of overexpanded alveoli adjacent to areas of atelectasis creates both an increased functional residual capacity (FRC) and a decrease in air flow during exhalation.

The *second* chain of events that can develop from MAS is a chemical pneumonitis, which is characterized by an acute inflammatory reaction and edema of the bronchial mucosa and alveolar epithelium. This reaction commonly leads to excessive bronchial secretions and alveolar consolidation. Meconium commonly promotes the growth of bacteria, which in turn augments the development of alveolar pneumonitis and consolidation. Meconium aspiration also interferes with alveolar protein B, decreasing pulmonary surfactant production. In this way, infant respiratory distress syndrome (IRDS) also may complicate MAS (see Chapter 35).

Third, as a consequence of the hypoxemia associated with MAS, infants with the condition often develop hypoxia-induced pulmonary arterial vasoconstriction and vasospasm, which causes a state of pulmonary hypertension. This results in blood shunting from right to left through the ductus arteriosus and the foramen ovale; intrapulmonary shunts occasionally are seen also. As a consequence, the blood flow is diverted away from the lungs (pulmonary hypoperfusion), which worsens the hypoxemia. Clinically, this condition is referred to as *persistent pulmonary hypertension of the neonate* (PPHN; previously called *persistent fetal circulation [PFC]*).

The major pathologic or structural changes associated with MAS are as follows:

- Physical presence of the meconium leading to:
  Partially obstructed airways, air trapping, and alveolar hyperinflation
  Pulmonary air leak syndromes (pneumomediastinum or pneumothorax)
  Totally obstructed airways and absorption atelectasis
- Edema of the bronchial mucosa and alveolar epithelium
- Excessive bronchial secretions
- Alveolar consolidation
- Hypoxia-induced pulmonary vasospasm and vasoconstriction:
  Pulmonary hypertension
  Right-to-left shunting
  Worsening hypoxia
  Pulmonary hypoperfusion

Etiology

Meconium-stained amniotic fluid occurs in about 8% to 10% of all births. About 5% of these infants acquire MAS. About 30% of the infants with MAS require mechanical ventilation. Approximately 11% of the infants with MAS will develop a pneumothorax and about 4% will die. As discussed earlier, the fetal passage of meconium is caused by fetal hypoxemia and stress, which in turn causes a vagal response that relaxes anal sphincter tone and allows meconium to move into the amniotic fluid.

MAS rarely is seen in infants younger than 36 weeks' gestation because the release of meconium requires strong peristalsis and sphincter tone, which usually are not present among preterm infants. Thus, the post-term infant (infants older than 42 weeks' gestation) is especially at risk for MAS, because both strong peristalsis and sphincter tone are present in babies of this age. Other infants who are at high risk for MAS are those who are small for gestational age, those who are delivered in the breech position, and those whose mothers are toxemic, hypertensive, or obese.

OVERVIEW
of the Cardiopulmonary Clinical Manifestations Associated with
MECONIUM ASPIRATION SYNDROME

The following clinical manifestations result from the pathologic mechanisms caused (or activated) by **Atelectasis** (see Figure 9-7), **Alveolar Consolidation** (see Figure 9-8), and **Excessive Bronchial Secretions** (see Figure 9-11)—the major anatomic alterations of the lungs associated with meconium aspiration syndrome (see Figure 33-1).

CLINICAL DATA OBTAINED AT THE PATIENT'S BEDSIDE

The Physical Examination

Vital Signs

Increased respiratory rate (see page 31 ◆►)
Normally, a newborn infant's respiratory rate is about 40 to 60 breaths per minute. In MAS the respiratory rate generally is well over 60 breaths per minute. Several pathophysiologic mechanisms operating simultaneously may lead to an increased ventilatory rate:
- Stimulation of the peripheral chemoreceptors (hypoxemia)
- Decreased lung compliance/increased ventilatory rate relationship
- Stimulation of the central chemoreceptors

Increased heart rate (pulse), cardiac output, and blood pressure (see pages 11 and 99 ◆►)

Apnea (see page 430 ◆►)

Clinical Manifestations Associated with Increased Negative Intrapleural Pressure During Inspiration (see page 429 ◆►)
- Intercostal retractions
- Substernal retraction/abdominal distention (see-saw movement)
- Cyanosis of the dependent portion of the thoracic and abdominal areas
- Flaring nostrils

Chest Assessment Findings (see page 22 ◆►)
- Wheezes
- Rhonchi
- Crackles

Expiratory Grunting (see page 430 ◆►)
Cyanosis (see page 45 ◆►)
Common General Appearance Clinical Manifestations
- Meconium stains on the fingernails, toenails, and umbilical cord, and wrinkles and creases in the skin
- Barrel chest (when airways are partially obstructed)

CLINICAL DATA OBTAINED FROM LABORATORY TESTS AND SPECIAL PROCEDURES

Pulmonary Function Study Findings (extrapolated data for instruction purposes)

Expiratory Maneuver Findings (see page 61 ◆►)

FVC	FEV$_T$	FEF$_{25\%-75\%}$	FEF$_{200-1200}$
↓	N or ↓	N or ↓	N
PEFR	MVV	FEF$_{50\%}$	FEV$_{1\%}$
N	N or ↓	N	N or ↑

Lung Volume and Capacity Findings (see page 62 ◆►)

V$_T$	RV*	FRC*	TLC
N or ↓	↓	↓	↓
VC	IC	ERV	RV/TLC%
↓	↓	↓	N

*↑ When airways are partially obstructed.

Arterial Blood Gases

Mild to Moderate Meconium Aspiration Syndrome
Acute Alveolar Hyperventilation with Hypoxemia (see page 70 ◆►)

pH	Paco$_2$	HCO$_3^-$	Pao$_2$
↑	↓	↓ (Slightly)	↓

OVERVIEW

of the Cardiopulmonary Clinical Manifestations Associated with MECONIUM ASPIRATION SYNDROME (Continued)

Advanced Meconium Aspiration Syndrome

Acute Ventilatory Failure with Hypoxemia (see page 73 ◆▶)

pH*	$Paco_2$	HCO_3^-*	Pao_2
↓	↑	↑(Slightly)	↓

*When tissue hypoxia is severe enough to produce lactic acid, the pH and HCO_3^- values will be lower than expected for a particular $Paco_2$ level.

Oxygenation Indices (see page 82 ◆▶)

$\dot{Q}_s/\dot{Q}_T$	Do_2†	$\dot{V}o_2$	$C(a-\bar{v})o_2$
↑	↓	Normal	Normal
O_2ER	$S\bar{v}o_2$		
↑	↓		

†The Do_2 may be normal in patients who have compensated to the decreased oxygenation status with an increased cardiac output. When the Do_2 is normal, the O_2ER is usually normal.

RADIOLOGIC FINDINGS

Chest Radiograph

The chest X-ray may show focal or generalized problem areas. When significant partial airway obstruction, air trapping, and alveolar hyperinflation are present, the chest X-ray appears hyperlucent and the diaphragms may be depressed. The practitioner should be alert for the sudden development of a pneumothorax or pneumomediastinum in infants with MAS (Figure 33-2). When alveolar atelectasis and consolidation are present, the chest X-ray shows irregular densities throughout the lungs. Although the chest X-ray picture clearly is different from that seen in IRDS, it is difficult to differentiate the X-ray appearance of MAS from that of pneumonia (Figure 33-3).

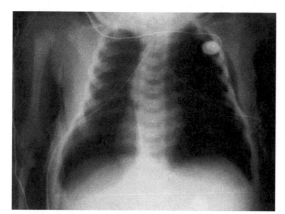

Figure 33–2 Meconium aspiration with bilateral pneumothorax.

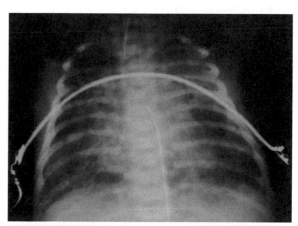

Figure 33–3 Classic meconium aspiration. Bilateral infiltrates associated with meconium aspiration. Well-expanded lungs.

General Management of MAS

The respiratory care practitioner should be proactive whenever an infant is at risk for meconium aspiration. When amniotic fluid is found to be stained with meconium or particulate, the nasopharynx and oral pharynx should be suctioned thoroughly as the head appears (during delivery, if possible). Immediately after delivery, the infant should be intubated and the upper airways should be suctioned until all the meconium has been cleared. This measure should be routine for all infants born through particulate meconium, even if meconium is not visualized in the oropharynx. *Positive-pressure ventilation should not be administered until a thorough suctioning of the upper airways has been completed,* because any particulate meconium remaining in the upper airways likely will be forced into the lower airways in response to positive-pressure ventilation.

After the infant is stabilized and has been transported to the neonatal intensive care unit, vigorous bronchial hygiene (e.g., postural drainage, percussion, suctioning) of the airways should be performed per protocol. Appropriate oxygen therapy should be administered per protocol; in severe cases, mechanical ventilation may be necessary. As already mentioned, however, mechanical ventilation should be avoided or applied cautiously to prevent the possibility of dislodging unseen particulate meconium and pushing it further down the infant's airways. In addition, a high incidence of pneumothorax is associated with MAS. If some mechanical ventilation is necessary, an inspiration/expiration ratio that permits a long exhalation time (to allow gas enough time to flow past partially obstructed airways) should be used. Finally, the infant should be monitored closely for possible superimposed infection. Antibiotics may be indicated and steroids may be required to offset the inflammatory response in chemical pneumonitis. Pulmonary surfactant is often administered when MAS is complicated by IRDS (see Chapter 35)

Case Study: MAS

Admitting History and Physical Examination

This 38-week-gestation newborn male infant was delivered by emergency cesarean section because of sudden maternal vaginal hemorrhage. The mother was a primigravida Caucasian 19-year-old with a history of no prenatal care. She was a heavy smoker and had an uncertain history of recreational psychopharmaceutical drug use during pregnancy. Rupture of membranes was believed to have occurred about 18 hours before delivery.

At delivery, the infant was found to have the umbilical cord wound around his neck once, moderately tightly. He was covered with meconium. He was limp and blue and did not show any spontaneous movement or respiratory effort when he was handed to the neonatologist, who was heading the resuscitation team of one registered nurse and a registered respiratory therapist. While receiving 100% free-flow oxygen to the oral and nasal area, the infant was dried and warmed. With the aid of a laryngoscope, several clumps of meconium were suctioned from the infant's oral and pharyngeal areas. On two separate passes below the vocal cords, no meconium was visualized or suctioned.

In spite of these efforts, the infant demonstrated no spontaneous respirations, and his heart rate was less than 60/min. Because of this, manual ventilation could no longer be avoided. At this time, the respiratory therapist started to ventilate the infant with a bag-valve-mask resuscitation bag, at an Fio_2 of 1.0 and a respiratory rate of 30/min. The nurse started chest compressions at about 90 per minute, with a rhythm of 3 compressions to one breath. Bilateral crackles and rhonchi were auscultated.

At 1 minute, the Apgar score was 1 for the heart rate. By the third minute, the baby's heart rate was 80/min. The infant was gasping occasionally and demonstrated some central pinkness. Although compressions were stopped, bagging continued at 40 breaths per minute. At the fifth minute, the Apgar score was 6 (heart rate 2, respirations 1, tone 1, reflex irritability 0, and color 2). The neonatologist decided at this time to intubate the baby with a 3.5-mm endotracheal tube. The respiratory therapist taped the tube at the 8.5-cm mark at the lip after careful auscultation confirmed the position. The baby was transferred to the neonatal intensive care unit (NICU) and placed on a ventilator. Initial ventilator settings were respiratory rate 40, inspiratory time (IT) 0.35 sec, Fio_2 100%, positive inspiratory pressure (PIP) 25, positive end-expiratory pressure (PEEP) 5, and flow 8 Lpm. A chest X-ray was ordered. At this time, the respiratory therapist documented the following in the infant's chart:

Respiratory Assessment and Plan

S   N/A

O   Apneic at birth, hypoactive, cyanotic, covered with meconium. 1 minute Apgar 1, 5 minute Apgar 6.

Bilateral crackles and rhonchi. Meconium suctioned from oral and pharyngeal areas.

A • Possible MAS (meconium in airway)
 • Airway secretions (meconium?) (crackles and rhonchi)
 • Probable asphyxic episode. Likely combined respiratory and metabolic acidosis (history, cyanosis)

P Mechanical Ventilation Protocol in combination with Oxygen Therapy and Hyperinflation Therapy Protocol (RR 40, F_{IO_2} 100%, PIP 25, flow 8 Lpm, and PEEP 5). Bronchopulmonary Hygiene Protocol (suction prn & CPT qid). Assist physician with surfactant administration. Monitor closely (oximetry, vital signs, watch for signs of acute air leak, pulmonary hemorrhage).

• • • • •

Over the next hour, an umbilical artery catheter (UAC) was inserted; it showed a pH of 7.19, $Paco_2$ 37, HCO_3^- 14, Pao_2 87, and Spo_2 94%. Although the infant's skin was now completely pink, bilateral crackles and rhonchi were still present. The chest X-ray revealed hyperinflation in both the right and left lungs. There was whiteout of the right upper and middle lobes, most likely caused by atelectasis. Clumps of white patches of atelectasis (resembling small popcorn balls) were seen throughout the remainder of the lungs. The endotracheal tube tip was at the clavicle level, and the UAC tip was appropriately positioned at T-8. The following SOAP note was recorded at this time:

Respiratory Assessment and Plan

S N/A
O Pink skin. Bilateral crackles and rhonchi. Atelectasis in the right upper and middle lobes. Air trapping right and left lower lobes. ABGs: pH 7.19, $Paco_2$ 37, HCO_3^- 14, Pao_2 87, and Spo_2 94 (on F_{IO_2} 1.0)

A • Airway secretions (crackles and rhonchi)
 • Atelectasis (chest X-ray)
 • Uncompensated metabolic acidosis (ABG)

P Continue Mechanical Ventilation Protocol in combination with Oxygen Therapy and Hyperinflation Therapy Protocols (RR 40, F_{IO_2} 100%, PIP 30 cm H_2O, and PEEP 5 cm H_2O). Continue Bronchopulmonary Hygiene Protocol (suction prn & CPT qid). Monitor closely (vital signs, watch for signs of acute air leak, pulmonary hemorrhage).

The neonatologist administered sodium bicarbonate to correct the baby's metabolic acidosis. The baby progressively improved over the next 4 days. On the fifth day, the baby was off the ventilator; on the seventh, he was discharged from the hospital. The mother was scheduled to see Social Services on a weekly basis.

Discussion

Inspection—the first step in the assessment process—was of the utmost importance in this case. The umbilical cord wrapped around the infant's neck, the presence of meconium, the blue skin, and the absence of spontaneous respirations all were important clinical indicators demonstrating the severity of the baby's condition. Paramount in this case is the fact that the baby was not manually ventilated—in spite of the fact that the baby had no spontaneous respirations—until after several clumps of meconium were suctioned from the infant's oral and laryngeal areas. Great care must be taken not to blow any meconium, blood, or amniotic fluid deeper down the tracheobronchial tree. The neonatal team must always be alert for the presence of a ball-valve meconium obstruction and the possibility of a pneumothorax. A ball-valve obstruction was verified in this case by the identification of alveolar hyperinflation on the chest X-ray. Fortunately, a pneumothorax did not develop.

As with adult subjects, several of the clinical manifestations in this case can be traced back through the "clinical scenarios" associated with **Atelectasis** (see Figure 9-7) and **Excessive Bronchial Secretions** (see Figure 9-11). For example, the increased lung density caused by the atelectasis was revealed on the chest X-ray, and the crackles and rhonchi were produced by the excessive airway secretions recorded in the second SOAP. Although it was not used in this case, high-frequency oscillatory ventilation or jet ventilation is often used with these babies. Either ventilator management approach appears to benefit the patient equally. The therapeutic effect of these ventilator techniques is that they ventilate by air streams that flow down the center of the airways while gas leaving the lungs moves along the peripheral walls of the airways, thus moving meconium and secretions out of the lungs.

These babies are very sensitive to external stimuli. Great caution should be taken not to overstimulate them. They should be suctioned only as needed. When suctioning is necessary, the respiratory therapist should not prolong the suctioning process but should get in and out of the infant's trachea as fast as possible. Often, these babies are given eye patches and earplugs to decrease external sensory stimulation. Occasionally, they will be paralyzed to minimize their reactions to stimuli and resistance to ventilation.

SELF-ASSESSMENT QUESTIONS

Multiple Choice

1. When the fetus experiences in utero hypoxia, which of the following occur?

    I. Vasoconstriction
    II. Inspiratory gasping
    III. Sphincter constriction
    IV. Increased intestinal peristalsis

  a. I only
  b. II only
  c. I, II, and IV only
  d. II, III, and IV only
  e. I, II, III, and IV

2. Aspiration of meconium may lead to which of the following?

    I. Ball-valve effect
    II. Atelectasis
    III. Total airway obstruction
    IV. Alveolar hyperinflation
    V. Chemical pneumonitis

  a. I only
  b. II only
  c. I, II, and IV only
  d. II, III, and IV only
  e. I, II, III, and IV

3. Meconium-stained amniotic fluid is seen in approximately what percentage of all births?

  a. 1
  b. 3
  c. 10
  d. 15
  e. 20

4. Which of the following clinical manifestations are associated with meconium aspiration syndrome?

    I. Apnea
    II. Intercostal retractions
    III. Barrel chest
    IV. Expiratory grunting

  a. I only
  b. II only
  c. I, II, and IV only
  d. II, III, and IV only
  e. I, II, III, and IV

5. Meconium aspiration decreases pulmonary surfactant production because it interferes with which alveolar protein?

  a. Protein A
  b. Protein B
  c. Protein C
  d. Protein D
  e. Protein E

Complete the Following

During the advanced stages of meconium aspiration syndrome, the infant's:
1. RV _____ decreases _____ increases _____ remains the same
2. VC _____ decreases _____ increases _____ remains the same
3. pH _____ decreases _____ increases _____ remains the same
4. FRC _____ decreases _____ increases _____ remains the same
5. Pa_{CO_2} _____ decreases _____ increases _____ remains the same

Answers appear in Appendix XI.

CHAPTER 34

Transient Tachypnea of the Newborn

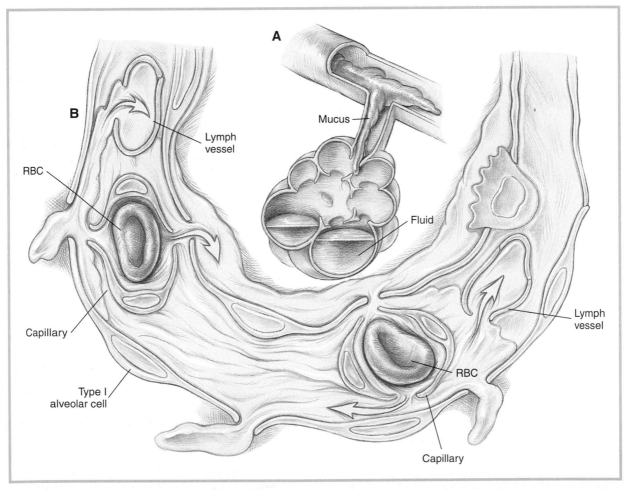

Figure 34–1 Transient tachypnea of the newborn. **A,** Excessive bronchial secretions and pulmonary capillary congestion. **B,** Cross-section of alveolus with interstitial edema. See also Plate 25.

Anatomic Alterations of the Lungs

Transient tachypnea of the newborn (TTN) also is called *type II respiratory distress syndrome* or *"wet lung" syndrome*. Initially (i.e., within the first 24 to 48 hours after birth), TTN produces clinical symptoms similar to those associated with the early stages of infant respiratory distress syndrome (see Chapter 35). Because the swallowing and cough efforts of infants with this disorder commonly are depressed, the clearance of bronchial secretions is compromised, resulting in the accumulation of bronchial secretions. This condition often leads to air trapping and alveolar hyperinflation. In addition, there is a delay in the infant's pulmonary fluid absorption by the lymphatic system and pulmonary capillaries. It is thought that this condition results, in part, from the infant's hypoxemia and inadequate inspiratory effort, producing a delayed changeover to adult circulatory anatomy and physiology. As a consequence of the hypoxemia, these babies often develop hypoxia-induced pulmonary arterial vasoconstriction and vasospasm, causing a state of pulmonary hypertension.

This condition results in blood shunting from right to left through the ductus arteriosus and the foramen ovale; intrapulmonary shunts may also occur occasionally. As a consequence, the blood flow is diverted away from the lungs (pulmonary hypoperfusion), which worsens the hypoxemia. Clinically, this condition is referred to as *persistent pulmonary hypertension of the neonate* ([PPHN]; previously called *persistent fetal circulation [PFC]*). As this condition worsens, the infant develops pulmonary capillary congestion, interstitial edema, decreased lung compliance, decreased tidal volume, and increased dead space (Figure 34-1). As a general rule, however, the abnormal anatomic alterations of the lungs associated with TTN usually begin to resolve in about 24 to 48 hours after birth.

The major pathologic or structural changes associated with TTN are as follows:

- Excessive bronchial secretions and incomplete absorption of pulmonary fetal fluid
- Air trapping and alveolar hyperinflation
- Pulmonary capillary congestion
- Interstitial edema
- Hypoxia-induced pulmonary vasospasm and vasoconstricion:
  - Pulmonary hypertension
  - Right-to-left shunting
  - Worsening hypoxia
  - Pulmonary hypoperfusion

Etiology

TTN commonly is seen in near-term or full-term infants of normal size and gestational age. TTN occurs in about 11 out of every 1000 births and is more common in boys. The infant's history often includes maternal analgesia or anesthesia during labor and delivery or episodes of intrauterine hypoxia. TTN also is commonly associated with maternal bleeding, maternal diabetes, cesarean section, and prolapsed cord.

Although the precise mechanism is not known, it is believed that TTN is due to a delayed absorption of fetal lung fluid. The delayed absorption of lung fluid is thought to be caused by any condition that increases the central venous pressure, which in turn slows the clearance of lung fluid by the lymphatic system. Infants with TTN are often lethargic at birth, resulting in a depressed cough effort and accumulation of airway secretions and mucus. The typical baby with TTN usually has good Apgar scores at birth. During the next several hours, however, signs and symptoms of respiratory distress develop. Within 24 to 48 hours, the clinical manifestations of respiratory distress usually disappear. As the process resolves, the absorption of excessive lung fluid occurs through lymphatic clearance.

OVERVIEW
of the Cardiopulmonary Clinical Manifestations Associated with
TRANSIENT TACHYPNEA OF THE NEWBORN

The following clinical manifestations result from the pathologic mechanisms caused (or activated) by **Increased Alveolar-Capillary Membrane Thickness** (see Figure 9-9) and **Excessive Bronchial Secretions** (see Figure 9-11)—the major anatomic alterations of the lungs associated with transient tachypnea of the newborn (see Figure 34-1).

CLINICAL DATA OBTAINED AT THE PATIENT'S BEDSIDE

The Physical Examination
Vital Signs

Increased respiratory rate (see page 31 ◆▶)
Infants with TTN frequently breathe quickly and then swallow. In fact, this rapid and shallow breathing

OVERVIEW

of the Cardiopulmonary Clinical Manifestations Associated with
TRANSIENT TACHYPNEA OF THE NEWBORN (Continued)

pattern often is considered a hallmark clinical manifestation of TTN. Normally, a newborn infant's respiratory rate is about 40 to 60 breaths per minute. During the early stages of TTN, the respiratory rate generally is well over 60 breaths per minute. Several pathophysiologic mechanisms operating simultaneously may lead to an increased ventilatory rate:

- Stimulation of the peripheral chemoreceptors (hypoxemia)
- Decreased lung compliance/increased ventilatory rate relationship
- Stimulation of the central chemoreceptors

Increased heart rate (pulse), cardiac output, and blood pressure (see pages 11 and 99 ◆)

Clinical Manifestations Associated With Increased Negative Intrapleural Pressure During Inspiration (see page 429 ◆)

Intercostal retractions

- Substernal retraction/abdominal distention ("seesaw" movement)
- Cyanosis of the dependent portions of the thoracic and abdominal areas
- Flaring nostrils

Chest Assessment Findings (see page 22 ◆)

- Wheezes
- Rhonchi
- Crackles

Expiratory Grunting (see page 430 ◆)

Cyanosis (see page 45 ◆)

CLINICAL DATA OBTAINED FROM LABORATORY TESTS AND SPECIAL PROCEDURES

Pulmonary Function Study Findings (extrapolated data for instructional purposes)

Expiratory Maneuver Findings (see page 61 ◆)

FVC	FEV$_T$	FEF$_{25\%-75\%}$	FEF$_{200-1200}$
↓	N or ↓	N or ↓	N
PEFR	MVV	FEF$_{50\%}$	FEV$_{1\%}$
N	N or ↓	N	N or ↑

Lung Volume and Capacity Findings (see page 62 ◆)

V$_T$	RV*	FRC*	TLC
N or ↓	↓	↓	↓
VC	IC	ERV	RV/TLC%
↓	↓	↓	N

*When airways are partially obstructed.

Arterial Blood Gases

Mild to Moderate Transient Tachypnea of the Newborn

Acute Alveolar Hyperventilation with Hypoxemia (see page 70 ◆)

pH	Paco$_2$	HCO$_3^-$	Pao$_2$
↑	↓	↓ (Slightly)	↓

Advanced Stages of Transient Tachypnea of the Newborn

Acute Ventilatory Failure with Hypoxemia (see page 73 ◆)

pH*	Paco$_2$	HCO$_3^-$*	Pao$_2$
↓	↑	↑(Slightly)	↓

*When tissue hypoxia is severe enough to produce lactic acid, the pH and HCO$_3^-$ values will be lower than expected for a particular Paco$_2$ level.

Oxygenation Indices (see page 82 ◆)

$\dot{Q}_S/\dot{Q}_T$	Do$_2$†	$\dot{V}$o$_2$	C(a-$\bar{v}$)o$_2$
↑	↓	Normal	Normal
O$_2$ER	S$\bar{v}$o$_2$		
↑	↓		

†The Do$_2$ may be normal in patients who have compensated to the decreased oxygenation status with an increased cardiac output. When the Do$_2$ is normal, the O$_2$ER is usually normal.

RADIOLOGIC FINDINGS

Chest Radiograph

Initially, the chest radiograph appears normal. Over the next 12 hours, however, signs of pulmonary vascular congestion develop. This is revealed on the chest radiograph as prominent perihilar streakings and fluid in the interlobular fissures. Air trapping and hyperinflation may occur and are manifested by peripheral hyperlucency, flattened diaphragms, and bulging intercostal spaces. Patches of infiltrates may be seen in some infants. Mild cardiomegaly and pleural effusions also may be seen (Figure 34-2).

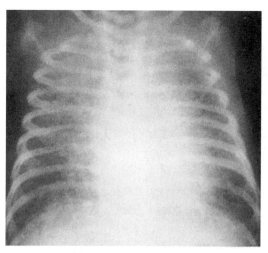

Figure 34–2 Chest X-ray of full-term infant with TTN.

General Management of TTN

RESPIRATORY CARE TREATMENT PROTOCOLS

Oxygen Therapy Protocol

Oxygen therapy is used to treat hypoxemia, decrease the work of breathing, and decrease myocardial work. Because of the hypoxemia that often develops in TTN, supplemental oxygen may be required (see Oxygen Therapy Protocol, Protocol 9-1).

Bronchopulmonary Hygiene Therapy Protocol

Because of the excessive airway secretions and accumulation associated with TTN, a number of bronchial hygiene treatment modalities may be used to enhance the mobilization of bronchial secretions (see Bronchopulmonary Hygiene Therapy Protocol, Protocol 9-2).

Hyperinflation Therapy Protocol

Hyperinflation measures commonly are administered to offset the pulmonary capillary congestion and interstitial edema associated with TTN (see Hyperinflation Therapy Protocol, Protocol 9-3).

Mechanical Ventilation Protocol

Mechanical ventilation may be necessary to provide and support alveolar gas exchange and eventually return the patient to spontaneous breathing. Patients with TTN rarely require mechanical ventilation (see Mechanical Ventilation Protocol, Protocol 9-5).

Case Study: TRANSIENT TACHYPNEA OF THE NEWBORN

Admitting History and Physical Examination

This 27-year-old woman in the thirty-fifth week of her second pregnancy awakened at 2 am with sudden lower abdominal pain and some bleeding. She had no contractions at the time. She woke her husband, who in turn called the obstetrician. The doctor instructed him to bring his wife to the hospital. On arrival at the hospital, she was immediately taken to the labor and delivery room. The nurse on duty placed an oxygen mask on the patient's face and started an intravenous (IV) line. The patient's vital signs were monitored closely. An ultrasound Doppler belt also was placed around the mother's lower abdominal area to monitor the baby's heart rate. Over the next 20 minutes, the mother continued to bleed (saturating two pads with numerous blood clots), her blood pressure fell, and her heart rate increased. The baby's heart rate had increased from 155/min to 170/min.

The obstetrician called the operating room and asked the staff to prepare for an emergency cesarean section.

The doctor also called for the neonatal resuscitation team (which consisted of a neonatologist, nurse, and respiratory therapist) and asked that they be on standby. The cesarean section was uneventful. The baby was a 7-pound girl. The neonatologist assessed the baby and gave a 1-minute Apgar score of 8 (2 heart rate, 2 respiratory rate, 1 tone, 1 reflex irritability, and 2 skin color). The baby, however, was clearly having difficulty breathing. Auscultation revealed mild bilateral rhonchi and crackles. The baby was transferred to the neonatal intensive care unit (NICU).

In the NICU, the baby was placed in a warmed isolette, and an umbilical artery catheter was inserted. An IV line and nasogastric tube also were inserted. Warm, humidified oxygen was started via a hood at an F_{IO_2} of 0.5. Ten minutes later, the infant's vital signs were as follows: heart rate 155/min, blood pressure 75/40, and respiratory rate 75/min. The infant's ventilatory pattern was described by the neonatologist as a "quiet-tachypnea" respiratory rate (fast and shallow ventilatory rate). In other words, even though the infant was breathing fast and not very deeply, she did not appear to be working hard to breathe. She had no intercostal retractions or nasal flaring at this time. Arterial blood gas values were as follows: pH 7.33, $Paco_2$ 31, HCO_3^- 21, and Pao_2 42. The baby's Spo_2 was 75%.

About 2 hours later, however, the baby started to show signs of distress. Her vital signs were as follows: heart rate 170/min, blood pressure 75/45, and respiratory rate 110/min. She demonstrated intercostal retractions, seesaw chest and abdomen movements, and nasal flaring. Her skin appeared pale and blue. Auscultation revealed moderate to severe bilateral rhonchi and crackles. Her Spo_2 was 58%. Arterial blood gas values were as follows: pH 7.52, $Paco_2$ 28, HCO_3^- 22 , and Pao_2 35. A chest X-ray showed areas of infiltrates and microatelectasis throughout both lung fields, as well as prominent white lined lung fissures (indicating fluid in the fissures). A starburst pattern was seen at the hilum of the lungs (indicating increased lymphatic fluid). The chest X-ray also showed air trapping and hyperinflation in the lower lobes (indicating fluid in the airways). The infant's diaphragms were flattened. The neonatologist charted a diagnosis of TTN in the baby's progress notes. The doctor also stated that he did not want to mechanically ventilate the baby at this time. The respiratory therapist entered the following assessment in the baby's chart:

Respiratory Assessment and Treatment Plan

S N/A

O Vital signs: HR 170/min, BP 75/45, and RR 110/min. Chest retractions, nasal flaring.

Skin pale and blue. Moderate to severe bilateral rhonchi and crackles. CXR: Infiltrates & micro-atelectasis over both lungs, generalized hyperinflation. ABGs on F_{IO_2} 0.5: pH 7.52, $Paco_2$ 28, HCO_3^- 22, Pao_2 35, Spo_2 58%.

A • TTN (neonatologist, x-ray, history)
  • Infiltrates and atelectasis (X-ray)
  • Air trapping (X-ray)
  • Excessive bronchial secretions (rhonchi and crackles)
  • Acute alveolar hyperventilation with severe hypoxemia (ABG)

P Hyperinflation Therapy Protocol (nasal CPAP at 3 to 4 cm H_2O). Increase Oxygen Therapy Protocol (F_{IO_2} 0.6 via CPAP set-up). Bronchopulmonary Hygiene Therapy Protocol (CPT Q2h). Continue to monitor closely.

Over the next 48 hours, the baby improved progressively. She no longer required oxygen therapy, and her breath sounds were normal. Her last room air arterial blood gas values showed a pH of 7.38, $Paco_2$ 39, HCO_3^- 24, and Pao_2 73. Her chest X-ray was normal. The baby was discharged the next day.

Discussion

This case reinforces the importance of observation and inspection in the assessment process. The respiratory care practitioner must continuously inspect and analyze infants with TTN. This baby, for example, born at 35 weeks, may have had infant respiratory distress syndrome (IRDS; see Chapter 35), but the clinical symptoms ruled out the diagnosis. For example, babies with IRDS have alveolar collapse and consolidation, whereas babies with TTN have airway trapping and alveolar hyperinflation. In addition, babies with IRDS generally *breathe hard, quickly,* and *deeply,* whereas infants with TTN usually *breathe quickly* and then *swallow.* In fact, this rapid and shallow breathing pattern often is considered a hallmark of TTN. Certainly, the rapid shallow breathing seen in this baby was caused, in part, by the **Increased Capillary Membrane Thickness**—and decreased lung compliance—associated with TTN (see Figure 9-9).

Although apnea may occur in these babies, it is not common. Therapeutically, most do quite well with just an oxygen hood. Occasionally, nasal continuous positive airway pressure (CPAP) may be used. Caution, however, must be taken not to give the baby too much CPAP. The lungs of these babies are usually already hyperinflated. Too much CPAP expands the baby's lungs even more and may cause a tension pneumothorax. CPAP at 3 to 4 cm H_2O is usually safe. Mechanical ventilation rarely is needed for babies with TTN.

SELF-ASSESSMENT QUESTIONS

True or False

True ☐ False ☐ **1.** TTN is most commonly seen in premature infants.

True ☐ False ☐ **2.** PPHN is commonly associated with TTN.

True ☐ False ☐ **3.** The clinical manifestations associated with TTN usually disappear 24 to 48 hours after birth.

True ☐ False ☐ **4.** TTN produces clinical symptoms similar to those seen in infant respiratory distress syndrome.

True ☐ False ☐ **5.** Therapeutically, most babies with TTN do well with just an oxygen hood.

True ☐ False ☐ **6.** The Do_2 is increased in infants with TTN.

True ☐ False ☐ **7.** TTN also is called type II respiratory distress syndrome.

True ☐ False ☐ **8.** The $S\bar{v}o_2$ is decreased in TTN.

True ☐ False ☐ **9.** Mechanical ventilation is rarely needed for babies with TTN.

True ☐ False ☐ **10.** A rapid and shallow breathing pattern is considered the hallmark clinical manifestation of TTN.

Answers appear in Appendix XI.

CHAPTER 35

Idiopathic (Infant) Respiratory Distress Syndrome

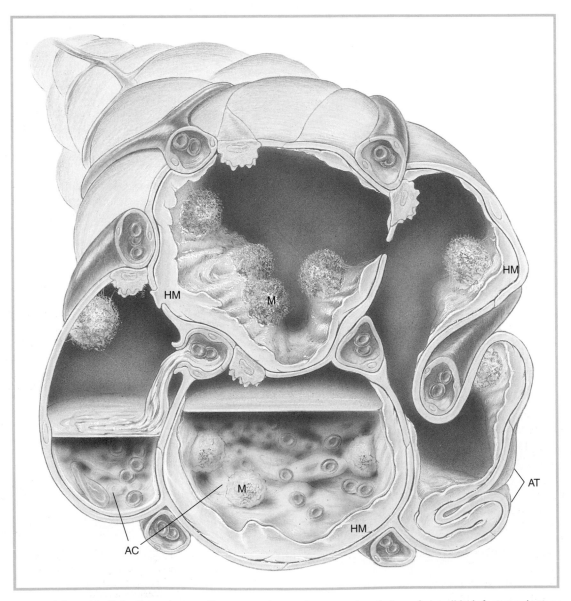

Figure 35–1 Idiopathic (infant) respiratory distress syndrome. Cross-sectional view of alveoli in infant respiratory distress syndrome. *HM,* Hyaline membrane; *AT,* atelectasis; *AC,* alveolar consolidation; *M,* macrophage. See also Plate 26.

Anatomic Alterations of the Lungs

On gross examination the lungs of an infant with *idiopathic respiratory distress syndrome (IRDS)* are dark red and liverlike. Under the microscope the lungs appear solid because of countless areas of alveolar collapse. The pulmonary capillaries are congested, and the lymphatic vessels are distended. Extensive interstitial and intra-alveolar edema and hemorrhage are evident.

In what appears to be an effort to offset alveolar collapse, the respiratory bronchioles, alveolar ducts, and some alveoli dilate. As the disease intensifies, the intra-alveolar walls become lined with a dense, rippled hyaline membrane identical to the hyaline membrane that develops in *acute respiratory distress syndrome (ARDS)* (see Chapter 27). The membrane contains fibrin and cellular debris.

During the later stages of the disease, leukocytes are present, and the hyaline membrane is often fragmented and partially ingested by macrophages. Type II cells begin to proliferate, and secretions begin to accumulate in the tracheobronchial tree. The anatomic alterations in IRDS produce a restrictive type of lung disorder (Figure 35-1).

As a consequence of the anatomic alterations associated with IRDS, babies with this disorder often develop hypoxia-induced pulmonary arterial vasoconstriction and vasospasm, causing a state of pulmonary hypertension. This results in blood shunting from right to left through the ductus arteriosus and foramen ovale; occasionally, intrapulmonary shunts may also occur. As a consequence, the blood flow is diverted away from the lungs (pulmonary hypoperfusion), which worsens the hypoxemia. Clinically, this condition is referred to as *persistent pulmonary hypertension of the neonate ([PPHN]; previously called persistent fetal circulation [PFC])*.

The major pathologic or structural changes associated with IRDS are as follows:

- Interstitial and intra-alveolar edema and hemorrhage
- Alveolar consolidation
- Intra-alveolar hyaline membrane
- Pulmonary surfactant deficiency or qualitative abnormality
- Atelectasis
- Hypoxia-induced vasospasm and vasoconstriction:
  Pulmonary hypertension
  Right-to-left shunting
  Worsening hypoxia
  Pulmonary hypoperfusion

Etiology

Although the exact cause of IRDS is controversial, the most popular theory suggests that the disorder develops as a result of (1) a pulmonary surfactant abnormality or deficiency and (2) pulmonary hypoperfusion evoked by hypoxia. The pulmonary hypoperfusion evoked by hypoxia is probably a secondary response to the surfactant abnormality. The probable steps in the development of IRDS are as follows:

1. Because of the pulmonary surfactant abnormality, alveolar compliance decreases, resulting in alveolar collapse.
2. The pulmonary atelectasis causes the infant's work of breathing to increase.
3. Alveolar ventilation decreases in response to the decreased lung compliance and infant fatigue, causing the alveolar oxygen tension (PA_{O_2}) to decrease.
4. The decreased PA_{O_2} (alveolar hypoxia) stimulates a reflex pulmonary vasoconstriction.
5. Because of the pulmonary vasoconstriction, blood bypasses the infant's lungs through fetal pathways—the patent ductus and the foramen ovale.
6. The lung hypoperfusion in turn causes lung ischemia and decreased lung metabolism.
7. Because of the decreased lung metabolism, the production of pulmonary surfactant is reduced even further, and a vicious cycle develops (Figure 35-2).

Approximately 250,000 premature infants are born each year in the United States. Of this group, about 50,000 will develop IRDS and about 10% will die. IRDS occurs more often in boys and more often in Caucasians than babies of other races. It usually is seen in infants younger than 37 weeks' gestation, babies of diabetic mothers, multiple births, cesarean births, prenatal asphyxia, prolonged labor, maternal bleeding, and second-born twins.

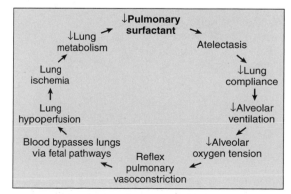

Figure 35–2 Probable etiologic steps in the development of IRDS.

OVERVIEW

of the Cardiopulmonary Clinical Manifestations Associated with
INFANT RESPIRATORY DISTRESS SYNDROME

The following clinical manifestations result from the pathologic mechanisms caused (or activated) by **Atelectasis** (see Figure 9-7), **Alveolar Consolidation** (see Figure 9-8), and **Increased Alveolar-Capillary Membrane Thickness** (see Figure 9-9)—the major anatomic alterations of the lungs associated with IRDS (see Figure 35-1).

CLINICAL DATA OBTAINED AT THE PATIENT'S BEDSIDE

The Physical Examination
Vital Signs
Increased respiratory rate (see page 31 ◆▶)
Normally, a newborn infant's respiratory rate is about 40 to 60 breaths per minute. During the early stages of IRDS, the respiratory rate is generally well over 60 breaths per minute. The respiratory pattern of the IRDS baby commonly is described as "hard, fast, and deep breathing." Several pathophysiologic mechanisms operating simultaneously may lead to an increased ventilatory rate:

- Stimulation of peripheral chemoreceptors (hypoxemia)
- Decreased lung compliance/increased ventilatory rate relationship
- Stimulation of central chemoreceptors

Increased heart rate (pulse), cardiac output, and blood pressure (see pages 11 and 99 ◆▶)

Apnea (see page 430 ◆▶)

Clinical Manifestations Associated With Increased Negative Intrapleural Pressures During Inspiration
(see page 429 ◆▶)

- Intercostal retractions
- Substernal retraction/abdominal distention ("seesaw" movement)
- Cyanosis of the dependent portions of the thoracic and abdominal areas
- Flaring nostrils

Chest Assessment Findings
(see page 22 ◆▶)

- Bronchial (or harsh) breath sounds
- Fine crackles

Expiratory grunting (see page 430 ◆▶)
Cyanosis (see page 45 ◆▶)

CLINICAL DATA OBTAINED FROM LABORATORY TESTS AND SPECIAL PROCEDURES

Pulmonary Function Study Findings
(extrapolated data for instructional purposes)

Expiratory Maneuver Findings (see page 61 ◆▶)

FVC	FEV_T	$FEF_{25\%-75\%}$	$FEF_{200-1200}$
↓	N or ↓	N or ↓	N
PEFR	MVV	$FEF_{50\%}$	$FEV_{1\%}$
N	N or ↓	N	N or ↑

Lung Volume and Capacity Findings (see page 62 ◆▶)

V_T	RV	FRC	TLC
N or ↓	↓	↓	↓
VC	IC	ERV	RV/TLC%
↓	↓	↓	N

Arterial Blood Gases
Mild to Moderate IRDS
Acute Alveolar Hyperventilation with Hypoxemia
(see page 70 ◆▶)

pH	$Paco_2$	HCO_3^-	Pao_2
↑	↓	↓ (Slightly)	↓

Advanced Stages of IRDS
Acute Ventilatory Failure with Hypoxemia
(see page 73 ◆▶)

pH*	$Paco_2$	HCO_3^-*	Pao_2
↓	↑	↑(Slightly)	↓

*When tissue hypoxia is severe enough to produce lactic acid, the pH and HCO_3^- values will be lower than expected for a particular $Paco_2$ level.

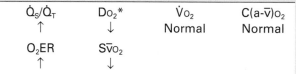

OVERVIEW
of the Cardiopulmonary Clinical Manifestations Associated with
INFANT RESPIRATORY DISTRESS SYNDROME (Continued)

Oxygenation Indices (see page 82 ◆▷)

$\dot{Q}_S/\dot{Q}_T$	Do_2*	$\dot{V}o_2$	$C(a-\bar{v})o_2$
↑	↓	Normal	Normal
O_2ER	$S\bar{v}o_2$		
↑	↓		

*The Do_2 may be normal in patients who have compensated to the decreased oxygenation status with an increased cardiac output. When the Do_2 is normal, the O_2ER is usually normal.

RADIOLOGIC FINDINGS

Chest Radiograph

• Increased opacity (ground-glass appearance)
On chest X-ray of infants with IRDS, the air-filled tracheobronchial tree typically stands out against a dense opaque (or white) lung. This white density is often described as having a fine ground-glass appearance throughout the lung fields. Because of the pathologic processes, the density of the lungs is increased. Increased lung density resists X-ray penetration and is revealed on X-ray as increased opacity. Therefore the more severe the IRDS, the whiter the X-ray image (Figure 35-3).

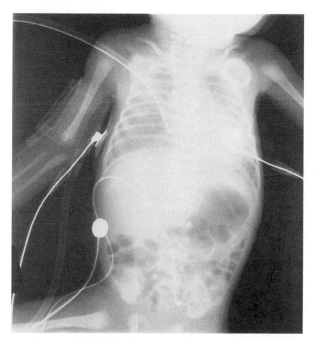

Figure 35–3 Whole body X-ray of an infant with IRDS. Note the "white out," particularly of the left lower and right upper lobes.

General Management of IRDS

During the early stages of IRDS, continuous positive airway pressure (CPAP) is the treatment of choice. Mechanical ventilation usually is avoided as long as possible. CPAP generally works well with these patients because it (1) increases the functional residual capacity, (2) decreases the work of breathing, and (3) works to increase the Pao_2 while the infant is receiving a lower inspired concentration of oxygen. A Pao_2 between 40 and 70 mm Hg is normal for newborn infants. No effort should be made to get an infant's Pao_2 within the normal adult range (80 to 100 mm Hg). Special attention should be given to the thermal environment of the infant with IRDS because the infant's oxygenation could be further compromised if the body temperature is above or below normal.

Finally, because of the decreased pulmonary surfactant associated with IRDS, the administration of exogenous surfactant preparations such as *beractant (Survanta)* or *colfosceril (Exosurf)* is helpful. The calculated dose of beractant is administered to the infant in quarters, one fourth at a time. Each quarter dose is instilled directly into the trachea through a 5-F catheter placed into the endotracheal tube. The catheter is removed after each administration, and the infant is manually ventilated or returned to the ventilator for 30 seconds or until stable.

Exosurf (composed of colfosceril palmitate, cetyl alcohol, and tyloxapol) is instilled directly into the endotracheal tube through a side-port adapter. Exosurf is administered in two stages. The first half of the dose is given in short bursts, timed to correlate with inspiration. This first half of the dose is administered with the infant in the supine position. After the first half of the dose has been given, the infant is rotated to the right and ventilated for about 30 seconds. The second half of the dose is then administered with the patient in the supine position, again in short bursts that coincide with inspiration. After the second half of the dose has been given, the infant is rotated to the left and ventilated for about 30 seconds. A new exogenous surfactant preparation called *cafactant (Infasurf)* has been approved for clinical use. Figure 35-4 provides comparison chest radiographs of an infant without exogenous surfactant and the same infant 45 minutes after treatment.

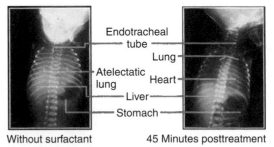

Surfactant function
Exogenous surfactant

Without surfactant   45 Minutes posttreatment

Figure 35–4   Chest X-rays of an infant with IRDS before and after exogenous surfactant treatments.

Case Study: IDIOPATHIC (INFANT) RESPIRATORY DISTRESS SYNDROME

Admitting History and Physical Examination

This premature male infant was delivered after 30 weeks' gestation. The mother was a 19-year-old, unmarried primigravida patient who claimed to be in good health during the entire pregnancy until 6 hours before admission. At that time, she noticed the onset of painless vaginal bleeding. She called her obstetrician, who told her he would meet her in the emergency department of the medical center.

On examination she was found to be a healthy young woman, approximately 30 weeks pregnant, in early labor, and bleeding slightly from the vagina. Her vital signs were stable and within normal limits. A diagnosis of premature separation of the placenta was made. Because bleeding was minimal and both mother and fetus seemed to be doing well, it was decided to deliver the baby vaginally. She was monitored very closely, and labor progressed satisfactorily for about 8 hours, at which time she delivered the infant under epidural anesthesia without any obstetric complications. The baby weighed 2100 grams. The Apgar scores were 7 after 1 minute and 9 after 5 minutes. Physical examination was entirely normal for an infant of this size.

On admission to the newborn nursery 30 minutes after delivery, the infant was noted to have some moderate respiratory distress. His respiratory rate was 40/min. There was flaring of the nostrils. A chest X-ray obtained at this time suggested the presence of left upper lobe atelectasis, but no other pulmonary abnormality was noted.

During the next 5 hours, the infant deteriorated rapidly and the respiratory distress became markedly accentuated. The baby was cyanotic, retracting, and using the accessory muscles of respiration. The respiratory rate was 64/min, and respirations were described as "grunting." His heart rate was 165/min. Crackles were heard bilaterally. A chest X-ray taken at this time revealed generalized haziness that one radiologist described as "ground glass." Arterial blood gases on an F_{IO_2} of 0.30 were pH 7.25, Pa_{CO_2} 52, HCO_3^- 21, and Pa_{O_2} 35. The Sa_{O_2} was 60%. At this time, the respiratory therapist working with the baby recorded the following assessment and plan:

Respiratory Assessment and Plan

S N/A (newborn)

O Dyspneic and cyanotic. Retracting and using accessory muscles. Flaring of nostrils. RR 64 with "grunting." HR 165. Bilateral crackles. CXR: Bilateral "ground glass" haziness. ABGs on 30% O_2: pH 7.25, $Paco_2$ 52, HCO_3^- 21, Pao_2 35, and Sao_2 60%.

A • Infant respiratory distress syndrome (history)
   • Alveolar hyaline membrane/atelectasis (CXR)
   • Acute ventilatory failure with severe hypoxemia (ABG)
     • Lactic acid likely (pH and HCO_3^- lower than expected)

P Mechanical Ventilation Protocol: Intubate/ventilate/positive end-expiratory pressure (PEEP) per neonatal intensive care unit (NICU) protocol. Oxygen Therapy Protocol: Continuous transcutaneous oximetry. Exosurf per protocol.

The baby was intubated by the therapist and put on a ventilator with PEEP ranging from +4 to +10 cm H_2O. Artificial surfactant (Exosurf) therapy was begun. The inspired oxygen concentration varied from 30% to 50%. Adjustments were made on the basis of numerous arterial blood gas and electrolyte determinations. Fluid and electrolyte balance was maintained within normal levels. Extracorporeal membrane oxygenation (ECMO) was considered, but because the baby was doing well on a more conservative regimen, it was decided not to use it at the time. On this management the baby was weaned from PEEP in 72 hours and from artificial ventilation in 96 hours. Chest X-ray examination on the seventh day was unremarkable. The baby was discharged on the fifteenth day and has been healthy ever since.

Discussion

IRDS is a fascinating disorder in which meticulous respiratory care of the infant is crucial. Most respiratory therapy students greatly look forward to and enjoy their NICU rotation. In these units the expertise of the respiratory care practitioner is crucial to the functioning of the unit because the majority of patients there have respiratory disorders. Indeed, many of the first reports of therapist-driven protocols came from this setting.

Many of the clinical manifestations seen in this case are associated with **Atelectasis** (see Figure 9-7) and **Increased Alveolar-Capillary Membrane Thickness** (see Figure 9-9). For example, the use of accessory muscles of inspiration was likely a compensatory mechanism activated to offset the increased stiffness of the lungs (decreased lung compliance) caused by the atelectasis and alveolar hyaline membrane. The atelectasis and alveolar hyaline membrane were objectively verified by the chest X-ray. In addition, the *severity level* of the anatomic alterations and clinical manifestations seen in this case was very high. This was objectively confirmed by the arterial blood gas analysis that identified the acute ventilatory failure with severe hypoxemia.

Thus the aggressive implementation of mechanical ventilation and use of artificial surfactant were certainly justified. Neonatal intensive care units usually are staffed by an in-house neonatologist, who can guide the respiratory therapist through the intricacies of therapy. Artificial surfactant has markedly improved the outlook for these infants As in adults with acute respiratory distress syndrome (ARDS), in which the pathology is very similar, constant attention must be given to the possibility of nosocomial infection, fluid overload, and cardiovascular instability. In addition, lung protection strategies such as PEEP, permissive hypercapnia, and use of small ventilator tidal volumes are commonly used in IRDS cases.

SELF-ASSESSMENT QUESTIONS

Multiple Choice

1. When persistent fetal circulation exists in IRDS, blood bypasses the infant's lungs through which of the following structures?

    I. Ductus venosus
    II. Umbilical vein
    III. Ductus arteriosus
    IV. Foramen ovale

    a. I only
    b. I and II only
    c. I and III only
    d. II and III only
    e. III and IV only

2. It is suggested that IRDS is a result of which of the following?

    I. Vernix membrane
    II. Decreased perfusion of the lungs
    III. Pulmonary surfactant abnormality
    IV. Congenital alveolar dysplasia

    a. I and III only
    b. II and III only
    c. I and IV only
    d. II, III, and IV only
    e. I, II, III, and IV

3. When an infant with IRDS creates a greater-than-normal negative intrapleural pressure during inspiration, which of the following occurs?

    I. The soft tissue between the ribs bulges outward.
    II. The substernal area protrudes.
    III. The abdominal area retracts.
    IV. The dependent blood vessels dilate and pool blood.

    a. II only
    b. IV only
    c. II and III only
    d. I, III, and IV only
    e. II, III, and IV only

4. Infants with severe IRDS often have which of the following?

    I. Diminished breath sounds
    II. Bronchial breath sounds
    III. Hyperresonant percussion notes
    IV. Fine crackles

    a. I only
    b. I and IV only
    c. III and IV only
    d. II and III only
    e. II and IV only

5. Continuous positive airway pressure (CPAP) often is administered to infants with IRDS in an effort to do which of the following?

    I. Increase the infant's FRC
    II. Decrease the infant's work of breathing
    III. Increase the infant's Pa_{O_2}
    IV. Decrease the $F_{I_{O_2}}$ necessary to oxygenate the infant

    a. I and III only
    b. II and III only
    c. III and IV only
    d. II, III, and IV only
    e. I, II, III, and IV

True or False

True ☐ False ☐ **1.** The intra-alveolar hyaline membrane seen in IRDS is identical to the hyaline membrane seen in adult respiratory distress syndrome (ARDS).

True ☐ False ☐ **2.** Alveolar consolidation develops in IRDS.

True ☐ False ☐ **3.** When activated, the dilator naris muscle widens the glottis.

True ☐ False ☐ **4.** Chest X-ray films of infants with severe IRDS appear more translucent.

True ☐ False ☐ **5.** The Pa_{O_2} of infants with IRDS should be maintained between 80 and 100 mm Hg.

Fill in the Blank

1. A premature birth is said to occur when the infant's weight is less than _____.

Answers appear in Appendix XI.

CHAPTER 36

Pulmonary Air Leak Syndromes

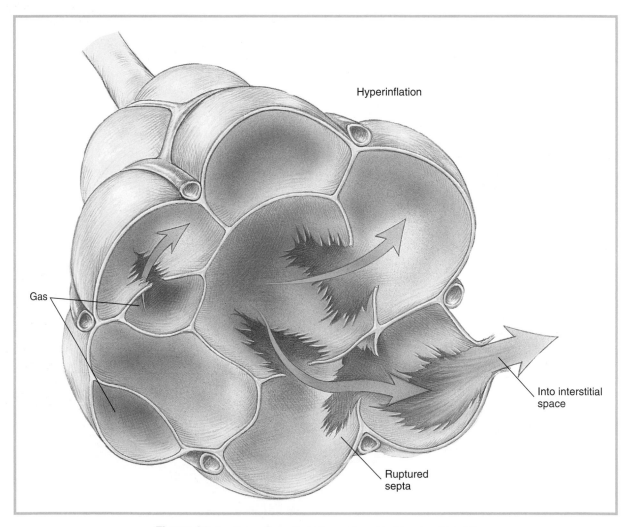

Figure 36–1 Pulmonary air leak syndromes. See also Plate 27.

Anatomic Alterations of the Lungs

Pulmonary air leak syndromes in the infant comprise a large spectrum of clinical entities, including pulmonary interstitial emphysema (PIE), pneumothorax, pneumomediastinum, and, in rare cases, intravascular systemic air embolism. Pulmonary air leak syndromes are common complications of mechanical ventilation in premature infants, especially when very high pressures are used. They are often seen in infants being treated for *infant respiratory distress syndrome* (IRDS; see Chapter 35).

All pulmonary air leak syndromes follow a common pathophysiologic pathway. When high transpulmonary pressures are applied to an infant's lungs, the distal airways and alveoli often become overdistended and rupture. The ruptured alveoli in turn allow air to leak into the interstitium, producing PIE, a condition characterized by diffuse gas-filled blebs within the interstitium of the lung ("emphysema-like" lung areas).

As shown in Figure 36-1, if a high transpulmonary pressure persists, the gas may do one of the following: (1) remain local and restrict the airway lumens; (2) continue to spread peripherally by dissecting along the peribronchial and perivascular spaces toward the visceral pleura and pulmonary hila; (3) rupture the visceral pleura and cause a pneumothorax; or (4) continue to accumulate, moving medially and dissecting out from the hila, causing a pneumomediastinum or pneumopericardium. If air under pressure accumulates in the mediastinum, it may dissect into the pleural space, the fascial planes of the neck and skin (subcutaneous emphysema), or the retroperitoneum (pneumoperitoneum) and end up in the scrotum in male babies or the labia in females. During the late stages, inflammatory changes of the airways lead to increased capillary leakage and excessive bronchial secretions.

As a consequence of the hypoxemia associated with pulmonary air leak syndromes, babies with these conditions often develop hypoxia-induced pulmonary arterial vasoconstriction and vasospasm, causing a state of pulmonary hypertension. This results in blood shunting from right to left through the ductus arteriosus and the foramen ovale; occasionally, intrapulmonary shunts may also form. Blood flow is diverted from the lungs (pulmonary hypoperfusion), worsening the hypoxemia. Clinically, this condition is referred to as *persistent pulmonary hypertension of the neonate (PPHN)*—previously called *persistent fetal circulation (PFC)*.

The major pathologic changes associated with pulmonary air leak syndromes are as follows:

- Atelectasis, caused by the following:
    Blebs ("emphysema-like")
    Pneumothorax
    Pneumomediastinum
- Airway obstruction
- Excessive bronchial secretions (late stages)
- Hypoxia-induced pulmonary vasospasm and vasoconstriction:
    Pulmonary hypertension
    Right-to-left shunting
    Worsening hypoxia
    Pulmonary hypoperfusion

Etiology

Preterm infants who weigh less than 1000 g at birth have an increased risk for the early occurrence of pulmonary air leak syndromes (often within the first 24 to 48 hours of life), especially because of the weak noncartilaginous structures of their distal airways. The most frequent etiologic factor causing air leak syndromes in preterm infants is the use of mechanical ventilation. It commonly results from the use of high levels of positive end-expiratory pressure (PEEP), high peak inspiratory pressures (PIPs), and prolonged inspiratory times (ITs).

OVERVIEW

of the Cardiopulmonary Clinical Manifestations Associated with PULMONARY AIR LEAK SYNDROMES

The following clinical manifestations result from the pathologic mechanisms caused (or activated) by **Atelectasis** (see Figure 9-7)—the major anatomic alteration of the lungs associated with pulmonary air leak syndromes (see Figure 36-1).

CLINICAL DATA OBTAINED AT THE PATIENT'S BEDSIDE

The Physical Examination

Vital Signs

Increased respiratory rate (see page 31 ◆➤)
Normally, a newborn's respiratory rate is about 40 to 60 breaths per minute. During the early stages of pulmonary air leak syndromes, the respiratory rate generally is well over 60 breaths per minute. Several pathophysiologic mechanisms operating simultaneously may lead to an increased ventilatory rate:
- Stimulation of peripheral chemoreceptors (hypoxemia)
- Decreased lung compliance/increased ventilatory rate relationship
- Stimulation of central chemoreceptors

Increased heart rate (pulse), cardiac output, and blood pressure (see pages 11 and 99 ◆➤)

Apnea (see page 430 ◆➤)

Clinical Manifestations Associated with Increased Negative Intrapleural Pressures During Inspiration (see page 429 ◆➤)
- Intercostal retractions
- Substernal retraction/abdominal distention ("seesaw" movement)
- Cyanosis of the dependent portions of the thoracic and abdominal areas
- Flaring nostrils

Chest Assessment Findings (see page 22 ◆➤)
- Wheezes
- Rhonchi
- Crackles
- Change in point of maximum impulse (PMI)

The PMI is defined as the point at which the sounds of the heart can be heard the loudest. When gas accumulates in the chest, the heart is pushed to the unaffected side, and the PMI changes. Often, the presence of a pneumothorax can be identified by PMI changes long before a chest X-ray can be obtained.

Expiratory Grunting (see page 430 ◆➤)

Cyanosis (see page 45 ◆➤)

CLINICAL DATA OBTAINED FROM LABORATORY TESTS AND SPECIAL PROCEDURES

Pulmonary Function Study Findings (extrapolated data for instructional purposes)

Expiratory Maneuver Findings (see page 61 ◆➤)

FVC	FEV_T	$FEF_{25\%-75\%}$	$FEF_{200-1200}$
↓	N or ↓	N or ↓	N
PEFR	MVV	$FEF_{50\%}$	$FEV_{1\%}$
N	N or ↓	N	N or ↑

Lung Volume and Capacity Findings (see page 62 ◆➤)

V_T	RV	FRC	TLC
N or ↓	↓	↓	↓
VC	IC	ERV	RV/TLC%
↓	↓	↓	N

Arterial Blood Gases

Mild to Moderate Pulmonary Air Leak Syndromes
Acute Alveolar Hyperventilation with Hypoxemia (see page 70 ◆➤)

pH	$Paco_2$	HCO_3^-	Pao_2
↑	↓	↓ (Slightly)	↓

Advanced Pulmonary Air Leak Syndromes
Acute Ventilatory Failure with Hypoxemia (see page 73 ◆➤)

pH*	$Paco_2$	HCO_3^-*	Pao_2
↓	↑	↑(Slightly)	↓

*When tissue hypoxia is severe enough to produce lactic acid, the pH and HCO_3^- values will be lower than expected for a particular $Paco_2$ level.

Oxygenation Indices (see page 82 ◆➤)

$\dot{Q}_S/\dot{Q}_T$	Do_2†	$\dot{V}o_2$	$C(a-\bar{v})o_2$
↑	↓	Normal	Normal
O_2ER	$S\bar{v}o_2$		
↑	↓		

†The Do_2 may be normal in patients who have compensated to the decreased oxygenation status with an increased cardiac output. When the Do_2 is normal, the O_2ER is usually normal.

OVERVIEW
of the Cardiopulmonary Clinical Manifestations Associated with
PULMONARY AIR LEAK SYNDROMES (Continued)

Increased Transillumination

Transillumination is performed by placing a high-intensity fiberoptic light source against the infant's chest in a dark room. When air is present in the chest cavity, an increased illumination is seen on the affected side.

RADIOLOGIC FINDINGS
Chest Radiograph

The chest X-ray may show focal or generalized problem areas. When significant partial airway obstruction, air trapping, and alveolar hyperinflation are present, the chest X-ray appears hyperlucent and the diaphragms may be depressed (Figure 36-2). The practitioner should always be alert for the sudden development of a pneumothorax or pneumomediastinum in infants with pulmonary air leak syndromes. When alveolar atelectasis is present, the chest X-ray shows irregular densities throughout the lungs. Although the chest X-ray picture is clearly different from that of IRDS, it is difficult to differentiate the atelectasis of the pulmonary air leak syndromes from the consolidation of pneumonia.

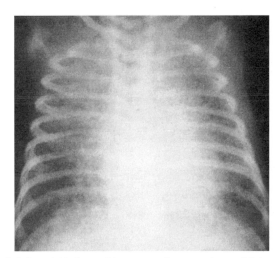

Figure 36–2 A 2-day-old infant with acute pulmonary interstitial emphysema (PIE).

General Management of Pulmonary Air Leak Syndromes

Prevention is the best treatment for pulmonary air leak syndromes. These syndromes may be prevented by the use of low mechanical ventilator pressures and the maintenance of good ventilation and oxygenation. Selective intubation of the unaffected or less affected lung may allow the injured lung time to heal. High-frequency ventilation has been successful in treating infants with pulmonary air leak syndromes. Survivors of pulmonary air leak syndromes often develop bronchopulmonary dysplasia (see Chapter 39) as a result of overly vigorous mechanical ventilation.

RESPIRATORY CARE TREATMENT PROTOCOLS

Oxygen Therapy Protocol

Oxygen therapy is used to treat hypoxemia, decrease the work of breathing, and decrease myocardial work. Because of the hypoxemia that often develops in pulmonary air leak syndromes, supplemental oxygen may be required (see Oxygen Therapy Protocol, Protocol 9-1).

Bronchopulmonary Hygiene Therapy Protocol

Because of the excessive airway secretions and mucus accumulation associated with pulmonary air leak syndromes, a number of bronchial hygiene treatment modalities may be used to enhance the mobilization of bronchial secretions (see Bronchopulmonary Hygiene Therapy Protocol, Protocol 9-2).

Hyperinflation Therapy Protocol

Hyperinflation measures commonly are administered to offset the pulmonary capillary congestion and interstitial edema and atelectasis associated with pulmonary air leak syndromes (see Hyperinflation Therapy Protocol, Protocol 9-3).

Mechanical Ventilation Protocol

Mechanical ventilation may be necessary to provide and support alveolar gas exchange and eventually return the patient to spontaneous breathing. As previously mentioned, prevention is the best treatment for pulmonary air leak syndromes. Selective intubation of the unaffected or less affected lung may allow the injured lung time to heal. High-frequency ventilation has been successful in treating infants with pulmonary air leak syndromes (see Mechanical Ventilation Protocol, Protocol 9-5).

Case Study: PULMONARY AIR LEAK SYNDROMES

Admitting History and Physical Examination

This 32-week-gestation, preterm female infant was delivered by emergency cesarean section to a healthy 25-year-old mother. The infant weighed 2750 g. The mother's admitting history showed her to be a primigravida with normal prenatal care and no history of illness during her pregnancy. The cesarean section was performed because of repeated and prolonged fetal heart rate decelerations that did not improve with maternal positioning or oxygen administration. At delivery, the infant was found to have the umbilical cord twice wrapped tightly around her neck. She was limp, appeared pale and cyanotic, and was apneic. She showed no response to tactile stimuli, and her heart rate was 65/min. Her 1-minute Apgar score was 1 (color 0, pulse 1, grimace 0, reflex irritability 0, muscle tone 0, respiratory 0).

Immediately, the neonatologist, nurse, and respiratory therapist started cardiopulmonary resuscitation (CPR) procedures, including ventilation with a bag-valve-mask at an FIO_2 of 1.0 and vigorous chest compressions. The 5-minute Apgar was 5 (color 1, pulse 2, grimace 0, reflex irritability 0, muscle tone 1, respiratory 1). Despite the fact that the baby had started to improve, she suddenly took a turn for the worse. Her heart rate started to drop; she again appeared cyanotic, and her muscle tone decreased.

At this time, the respiratory therapist noted that the baby's breath sounds were absent over the right lung and severely decreased over the left upper and middle lobes. Her heart sounds were muffled and faint, and the PMI was displaced to the left. Transillumination showed a large right pneumothorax. This was later confirmed by chest X-ray as a right tension pneumothorax. The neonatologist inserted a chest tube, and the baby was placed on a mechanical ventilator with the following settings: IMV rate 30, FIO_2 1.0, PIP 25 cm H_2O, PEEP 5 cm H_2O, IT 0.35, and flow 6 L/min.

Moments later, an umbilical artery catheter (UAC) was inserted; it showed the following values: pH 7.19, $Paco_2$ 77, HCO_3^- 19, and Pao_2 31. The ventilator rate was increased immediately to 40 breaths per minute. ABG values 20 minutes later were as follows: pH 7.33, $Paco_2$ 43, HCO_3^- 21, and Pao_2 47.

A second chest X-ray an hour later showed that the right lung had re-expanded, with segmental atelectasis throughout. At this time, the infant appeared pink and her vital signs were stable, with a heart rate of 155/min and blood pressure of 68/35.

Breath sounds revealed bilateral crackles and rhonchi. ABG values were as follows: pH 7.34, $Paco_2$ 42, HCO_3^- 22, and Pao_2 53. The respiratory therapist recorded the following in the baby's chart:

Respiratory Assessment and Plan

S   N/A

O   Skin: Pink. HR 155/min, BP 68/35.
Crackles and rhonchi throughout. ABGs: pH 7.34, $Paco_2$ 42, HCO_3^- 22, and Pao_2 53.
CXR: Re-expanded right lung with segmental atelectasis.

A   • Preterm infant in severe respiratory distress
• Atelectasis—right lung (X-ray)
• Adequate ventilation and oxygenation on present ventilator settings (ABG)
• Excessive airway secretions (crackles and rhonchi)

P   • Continue Mechanical Ventilation Protocol. Attempt to reduce FIO_2 per Oxygen Therapy Protocol. Continue Hyperinflation Therapy Protocol (PEEP + 5 cm H_2O). Start Bronchopulmonary Hygiene Therapy Protocol (chest physical therapy [CPT] qid). Monitor closely (vital signs, color, ABGs, transillumination).

Discussion

An iatrogenic tension pneumothorax caused by a resuscitation effort is not uncommon during resuscitation of the newborn. This is especially true when the staff is inexperienced or performs resuscitation too aggressively because of the anxiety and urgency of the situation. Respiratory care practitioners must be prepared to attend deliveries, manage the airways, and provide ventilatory support as requested by the other members of the health-care team. Such members of the respiratory care department are often called *designated neonatal resuscitators.*

Because of the risk of cerebral interventricular hemorrhage, many centers would not perform CPT on the infant. Proper positioning of the infant for CPT (head down) would increase the risk for IVH. Since the advent of surfactant therapy, pneumothoraces in mechanically ventilated infants in neonatal intensive care units (NICUs) have decreased. Tension pneumothorax is a potentially life-threatening emergency, and the respiratory therapist should always be alert for any signs or symptoms associated with this condition. In this case, the clinical manifestations associated with **Atelectasis** (see Figure 9-7) were quickly identified when the respiratory therapist noted the possibility of a pneumothorax by pointing out that the baby's breath sounds were absent over the right lung and severely decreased over the left upper and middle lobes. Transillumination further supported the presence of a pneumothorax. The chest radiograph confirmed a right lung pneumothorax. To help in the monitoring and the identification of a possible pneumothorax, the respiratory care practitioners often make a simple ballpoint pen mark at the PMI on the chests of infants at risk for pneumothorax. The PMI is the point at which the heart tones are most audible. If the PMI moves away from the mark, the practitioner has a good and timely clinical indication that the baby has developed a pneumothorax—even before a chest X-ray can be obtained.

Finally, it is not uncommon for infants with pulmonary air leak syndromes to develop fluid in their lungs shortly after a pneumothorax has resolved (i.e., the chest tube is no longer sucking any air out of the baby's chest). When this occurs, these infants gain weight, demonstrate rhonchi and crackles, and require a higher F_{IO_2} to maintain their desired Pa_{O_2} levels. The reason for this is that babies who have iatrogenic tension pneumothoraces often develop what is called a transient *syndrome of inappropriate antidiuretic hormone (SIADH)*. In other words, the pneumothorax causes the release of antidiuretic hormone, which inhibits urination. Some of the retained fluid accumulates in the baby's lungs. Often, a diuretic (such as furosemide), a little more airway pressure, an increased F_{IO_2}, or an increased ventilator rate may be administered to offset this transient problem. The condition usually lasts only about 24 hours. The respiratory practitioner should expect this condition and should not be overly concerned.

SELF-ASSESSMENT QUESTIONS

True or False

True ☐ False ☐ **1.** Pulmonary air leak syndromes in the newborn are associated with a number of clinical entities, including intravascular systemic air embolism.

True ☐ False ☐ **2.** The most frequent etiologic factor causing air leak syndromes in preterm infants is the use of mechanical ventilation.

True ☐ False ☐ **3.** When a pulmonary air leak syndrome affects the chest cavity of the newborn, a decreased transillumination is seen on the affected side.

True ☐ False ☐ **4.** Prevention is the best treatment for pulmonary air leak syndromes.

True ☐ False ☐ **5.** During the advanced stages of pulmonary air leak syndromes, the infant's Pa_{CO_2} is lower than normal.

True ☐ False ☐ **6.** Hypoxia-induced pulmonary arterial vasoconstriction and vasospasm are associated with pulmonary air leak syndromes.

True ☐ False ☐ **7.** When a pulmonary air leak syndrome is present, the PMI remains the same.

True ☐ False ☐ **8.** A pulmonary air leak syndrome causes an infant's $S\bar{v}_{O_2}$ to increase.

True ☐ False ☐ **9.** Urine output often decreases in infants with pulmonary air leak syndromes because of the release of antidiuretic hormone.

True ☐ False ☐ **10.** A pulmonary air leak syndrome causes the infant's $\dot{Q}s/\dot{Q}\tau$ to decrease.

Answers appear in Appendix XI.

CHAPTER 37

Respiratory Syncytial Virus (Bronchiolitis or Pneumonitis)

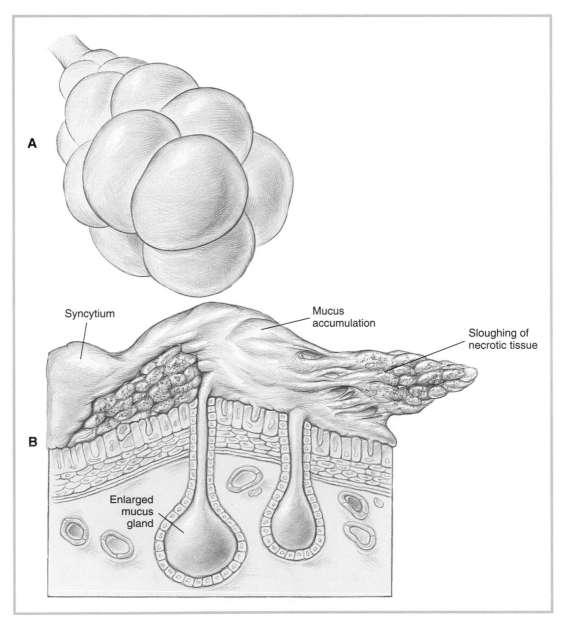

Figure 37–1 Bronchiolitis caused by respiratory syncytial virus (RSV). **A,** Partial airway obstruction and alveolar hyperinflation. **B,** Cross-section of inflamed airway. See also Plate 28.

Anatomic Alterations of the Lungs

Respiratory syncytial virus (RSV) moves down the respiratory tract by means of cell-to-cell transfer, causing bronchiolitis and, later, atelectasis and pneumonia in the child. The *syncytium* is defined as a "multinucleate mass of protoplasm produced by the merging of cells." At the level of the bronchioles the virus causes neighboring cells to fuse to form a syncytium, hence the name *respiratory syncytial virus*. The lower airways may also become infected when secretions from RSV-infected upper airways are aspirated.

RSV infection causes peribronchiolar mononuclear infiltration and necrosis of the epithelium of the small airways. This condition leads to edema of the small airways and increased mucus production. As the condition worsens, the epithelium of the small airways becomes necrotic and proliferates into the airway lumen. The combination of sloughing necrotic tissue, airway edema, and mucus accumulation leads to (1) a decreased airway lumen, (2) a partially obstructed airway, or (3) a completely obstructed airway. Partial airway obstruction leads to alveolar hyperinflation as a result of a "ball-valve" mechanism (Figure 37-1). Complete airway obstruction leads to alveolar collapse or atelectasis. Pneumonic consolidation is common. RSV is also referred to as bronchiolitis or pneumonitis.

The following major pathologic or structural changes are associated with RSV infection:

- Inflammation and swelling of the peripheral airways
- Excessive airway secretions
- Sloughing of necrotic airway epithelium
- Partial airway obstruction and alveolar hyperinflation
- Complete airway obstruction and atelectasis
- Consolidation

Etiology

RSV is the most common viral respiratory pathogen seen in infancy and early childhood. More than 50% of infants experience RSV infections within the first year of life. Virtually all children experience an RSV infection by 3 years of age. RSV outbreaks are seasonal and usually occur during the fall and winter months. In the northern hemisphere, the RSV season usually is between October and March. Between 0.5% and 2% of infants with severe lower respiratory tract RSV require hospitalization and medical intervention. Most of these infants are younger than 6 months of age.

A child commonly is exposed to the virus by an older sibling or another child who is demonstrating coldlike symptoms. Common modes of transmission are large aerosol particles generated by coughs from infected individuals and direct physical contact with contaminated secretions. For example, RSV remains infectious on clothes or paper for about 30 minutes. RSV may remain infectious in nasal secretions for as long as 6 hours. Although RSV infection can occur at any age, children younger than 1 year of age tend to be more severely affected, possibly because infants have reduced immune systems and smaller airways.

RSV infection should be suspected when the clinical manifestations correlate to the time of year (midwinter and spring months), the presence of a local outbreak, the age of the patient, and history of the illness. The physician confirms the diagnosis by isolating the virus or its antigens in the patient's sputum sample or from oropharyngeal or nasopharyngeal secretions. At the patient's bedside the respiratory practitioner can obtain a specimen by means of nasopharyngeal aspiration, nasal swabs, or nasal lavage. The virus also may be found via immunofluorescence staining (a method using an antibody labeled with a fluorescent dye). Results usually can be obtained within 2 to 4 hours.

OVERVIEW
of the Cardiopulmonary Clinical Manifestations Associated with
RESPIRATORY SYNCYTIAL VIRUS

The following clinical manifestations result from the pathologic mechanisms caused (or activated) by **Atelectasis** (see Figure 9-7), **Alveolar Consolidation** (see Figure 9-8), and **Excessive Bronchial Secretions** (see Figure 9-11)—the major anatomic alterations of the lungs associated with respiratory syncytial virus infection (see Figure 37-1).

CLINICAL DATA OBTAINED AT THE PATIENT'S BEDSIDE

The Physical Examination

Vital Signs

Increased respiratory rate (see page 31 ◆▷)
Normally, a newborn's respiratory rate is about 40 to 60 breaths per minute. During the early stages of RSV the respiratory rate generally is well over 60 breaths per minute. Several pathophysiologic mechanisms operating simultaneously may lead to an increased ventilatory rate:
- Stimulation of peripheral chemoreceptors (hypoxemia)
- Decreased lung compliance/increased ventilatory rate relationship
- Stimulation of central chemoreceptors

Increased heart rate (pulse), cardiac output, and blood pressure (see pages 11 and 99 ◆▷)

Apnea (see page 430 ◆▷)

Clinical Manifestations Associated With Increased Negative Intrapleural Pressures During Inspiration (see page 429 ◆▷)
- Intercostal retractions
- Substernal retraction/abdominal distention ("seesaw" movement or paradoxical chest motion)
- Cyanosis of the dependent portions of the thoracic and abdominal areas
- Flaring nostrils

Chest Assessment Findings (see page 22 ◆▷)
- Wheezes
- Rhonchi
- Crackles

Respiratory Secretions (copious)

Expiratory Grunting (see page 430 ◆▷)

Cyanosis (see page 45 ◆▷)

CLINICAL DATA OBTAINED FROM LABORATORY TESTS AND SPECIAL PROCEDURES

Pulmonary Function Study Findings (extrapolated data for instructional purposes)

Expiratory Maneuver Findings (see page 61 ◆▷)

FVC	FEV$_T$	FEF$_{25\%-75\%}$	FEF$_{200-1200}$
↓	N or ↓	N or ↓	N
PEFR	MVV	FEF$_{50\%}$	FEV$_{1\%}$
N	N or ↓	N	N or ↑

Lung Volume and Capacity Findings (see page 62 ◆▷)

V$_T$	RV*	FRC*	TLC
N or ↓	↓	↓	↓
VC	IC	ERV	RV/TLC%
↓	↓	↓	N

*↑ When airways are partially obstructed.

Arterial Blood Gases

Mild to Moderate RSV Infection
Acute Alveolar Hyperventilation with Hypoxemia (see page 70 ◆▷)

pH	Paco$_2$	HCO$_3^-$	Pao$_2$
↑	↓	↓ (Slightly)	↓

Advanced Stages of RSV Infection
Acute Ventilatory Failure with Hypoxemia (see page 73 ◆▷)

pH[†]	Paco$_2$	HCO$_3^-$[†]	Pao$_2$
↓	↑	↑ (Slightly)	↓

†When tissue hypoxia is severe enough to produce lactic acid, the pH and HCO$_3^-$ values will be lower than expected for a particular Paco$_2$ level.

Oxygenation Indices (see page 82 ◆▷)

Q̇$_S$/Q̇$_T$	Do$_2$[‡]	V̇o$_2$	C(a-v̄)o$_2$
↑	↓	Normal	Normal
O$_2$ER	Sv̄o$_2$		
↑	↓		

‡The Do$_2$ may be normal in patients who have compensated to the decreased oxygenation status with an increased cardiac output. When the Do$_2$ is normal, the O$_2$ER is usually normal.

RADIOLOGIC FINDINGS

Chest Radiograph

RSV appears as both bronchiolitis and bronchopneumonia in infants and young children. The chest radiograph commonly shows streaky peribronchial opacities associated with air trapping and hyperinflation. Lobar atelectasis frequently is seen, and alveolar and lobar pneumonic consolidation occasionally may be seen as well (Figure 37-2).

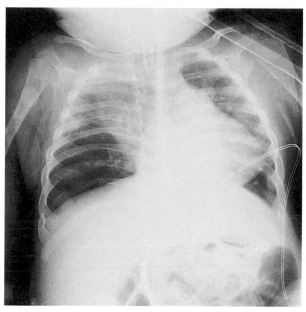

Figure 37–2   Chest X-ray of a 6-month-old child with RSV.

General Management of RSV (Broncholitis, Pneumonitis)

RESPIRATORY CARE TREATMENT PROTOCOLS

Oxygen Therapy Protocol

Oxygen therapy is used to treat hypoxemia, decrease the work of breathing, and decrease myocardial work. The hypoxemia that develops in RSV most commonly is caused by the excessive airway fluid, atelectasis, and consolidation associated with the disorder. Hypoxemia caused by capillary shunting is often partially refractory to oxygen therapy (see Oxygen Therapy Protocol, Protocol 9-1).

Bronchopulmonary Hygiene Therapy Protocol

Because of the excessive airway secretions associated with RSV infection, bronchial hygiene treatment modalities often are used to enhance the mobilization of bronchial secretions (see Bronchopulmonary Hygiene Therapy Protocol, Protocol 9-2).

Aerosolized Medication Protocol

Both sympathomimetic and parasympatholytic agents may be used to induce bronchial smooth muscle relaxation (see Aerosolized Medication Protocol, Protocol 9-4).

Antiviral Aerosol

Ribavirin. Ribavirin (Virazole) is effective in treating children with RSV infection. Ribavirin is supplied as 6 g of lyophilized powder in a 100-ml vial, which is reconstituted in 300 ml of sterile water, making a 2% (20 mg/ml) solution. The solution is aerosolized and delivered to the patient by means of a device called a *small particle aerosol generator* (SPAG). The aerosol is administered continuously for 12 to 18 hours per day for 3 to 7 days through an oxyhood, face tent, or oxygen tent. Because of the potential side effects and hazards (e.g., ribavirin is cytotoxic and is an environmental pollutant), however, ribavirin usually is administered only as a last resort in more severe cases.

Palivizumab. As a preventive measure against RSV, health-care guidelines recommend that some high-risk babies (e.g., premature babies, infants on long-term ventilator care) be injected with an agent called *palivizumab (Synagis)*—an immune globulin prophylaxis—once a month.

Case Study: RESPIRATORY SYNCYTIAL VIRUS INFECTION

Admitting History and Physical Examination

This premature baby boy was born in mid-November at 31 weeks' gestation. He weighed 1300 g at birth and immediately demonstrated respiratory distress that rapidly progressed into infant respiratory distress syndrome (IRDS; see Chapter 35). During the first hour after delivery, the baby was intubated, placed on a mechanical ventilator, and given a dose of pulmonary surfactant. An umbilical artery line was inserted, and antibiotics were given for several days. Over the next 10 days, the baby was slowly weaned off the ventilator and started on feedings. Both the umbilical artery and intravenous (IV) lines were discontinued. Over the next week, the baby gained weight and appeared to be doing well.

Two days later, however, the baby started to demonstrate more periods of apnea and signs of respiratory distress. His vital signs were as follows: heart rate 165/min, blood pressure 85/55, respiratory rate 65, and temperature 37° C. He demonstrated nasal flaring and intercostal retractions. Wheezing and rhonchi could be auscultated over both lung fields. His skin appeared cyanotic, and his oxygen saturation by pulse oximetry decreased from 90% to 83%. A chest X-ray revealed bilateral streaky infiltrates and scattered areas of atelectasis.

Because of the baby's history, the time of year, and the increased number of colds and flu reported throughout the medical community, the neonatologist suspected RSV infection. The baby was placed in an oxygen hood at an F_{IO_2} of 0.5, and a nasopharyngeal swab was obtained and sent to the laboratory. The smear was positive for RSV. Because apnea is commonly associated with RSV infection, the baby was re-intubated and placed back on the ventilator for support. The ventilator settings were as follows: IMV mode 15, inspiratory pressure 20 cm H_2O, PEEP 4 cm H_2O, flow 6 L/min, and F_{IO_2} 0.4. His saturation increased to 88%. At this time, the respiratory therapist charted the following SOAP note:

Respiratory Assessment and Plan

S   N/A

O   Apnea. Positive RSV smear. Vital signs: HR 165/min, BP 85/55, RR 65, T 37° C. Nasal flaring, intercostal retractions, and cyanosis. Wheezing and rhonchi. CXR: Atelectasis. Spo_2 on F_{IO_2} 0.4: 88%. Ventilator settings: IMV rate 15, PIP 20, PEEP 4, flow 6 Lpm.

A   • Atelectasis (X-ray)
  • Bronchospasm (wheezing)
  • Excessive airway secretions (rhonchi)
  • Hypoxemia (Spo_2 and cyanosis)

P   Continue Mechanical Ventilation Protocol. Begin Bronchopulmonary Hygiene Therapy Protocol (CPT and suction prn). Begin Aerosolized Medication Therapy Protocol (0.25 mg albuterol per kg with 2 ml normal saline q 3 h, in-line with the ventilator). Oxygen therapy per Mechanical Ventilation Protocol. Continue to monitor closely. Obtain ABG via capillary heel stick and reevaluate.

Because the neonatologist preferred to use ribavirin only as a last resort (because of the potential environmental pollutant hazards associated with the agent), he fully agreed with the respiratory therapist's assessment. Over the next 7 days, the baby was slowly weaned off the bronchopulmonary hygiene therapy, bronchodilator therapy, oxygen therapy, and mechanical ventilator. The baby was monitored closely over the next week and discharged in good health.

Discussion

The value of routine bronchodilator therapy has been questioned in the treatment of RSV. Many centers implement a short trial period of bronchodilator therapy and then re-assess. Respiratory care practitioners must recognize their potential role in transmitting RSV. Any infected health-care practitioners or family members can easily transmit the virus through aerosolized sprays generated by a cough, a sneeze, or even the secretions from the mucous membranes of the eyes that have been rubbed and transmitted by hand to the infant. Therefore the mainstay of treatment for RSV infection clearly is *prevention*.

Medical personnel who can recognize infants at risk for RSV (e.g., premature babies, babies on ventilators for long periods, babies on oxygen, babies who have bronchopulmonary dysplasia) also can easily take extra preventive measures, including the use of hand washing, gloves, gowns, and masks. As previously mentioned in the treatment section, babies at high risk for RSV are injected with a dose of palivizumab—an immune globulin prophylaxis—once a month. In most cases, however, the anatomic alterations of the lung and the clinical manifestations that ensue can be effectively treated by good respiratory therapy (i.e., appropriate oxygen therapy, bronchopulmonary hygiene therapy, and bronchodilator therapy). For example, the implementation of the *Bronchopulmonary Hygiene Therapy Protocol* to offset the **Excessive Airway Secretions** (see Figure 9-11) and the administration of the *Aerosolized Medication Therapy Protocol* (albuterol) to offset the **Bronchospasm** (see Figure 9-10) demonstrated in this case were clearly justified. Because of the potential side effects and hazards, ribavirin is generally used only for the most severe cases.

SELF-ASSESSMENT QUESTIONS

Multiple Choice

1. Which of the following are associated with RSV infection?

      I. Alveolar hyperinflation
      II. Atelectasis
      III. Excessive bronchial secretions
      IV. Pneumonic consolidation

   a. I and IV only
   b. II and IV only
   c. III and IV only
   d. II, III, and IV only
   e. I, II, III, and IV

2. In the northern hemisphere, the RSV season is usually between:

   a. January and April
   b. October and March
   c. May and June
   d. July and September
   e. November and December

3. How long may RSV remain infectious in nasal secretions?

   a. 3 hours
   b. 6 hours
   c. 12 hours
   d. 18 hours
   e. 24 hours

4. Although the RSV infection can occur at any age, children younger than what age tend to be more severely affected?

   a. Less than 1 year
   b. Less than 2 years
   c. Less than 3 years
   d. Less than 4 years
   e. Less than 5 years

5. Which of the following agents is/are used to prevent RSV infection in high-risk babies?

      I. Virazole
      II. Synagis
      III. Streptomycin
      IV. Ribavirin

   a. I only
   b. II only
   c. III only
   d. I and IV only
   e. I, II, and IV only

True or False

True ☐ False ☐ 1. RSV is the most common viral respiratory pathogen seen in infancy and early childhood.

True ☐ False ☐ 2. RSV infection often leads to airway obstruction by a "ball-valve" mechanism.

True ☐ False ☐ 3. RSV remains infectious on clothes or paper for as long as 6 hours.

True ☐ False ☐ 4. RSV can be revealed via immunofluorescence.

True ☐ False ☐ 5. RSV outbreaks generally last between 6 and 12 months.

Answers appear in Appendix XI.

CHAPTER 38

Bronchopulmonary Dysplasia

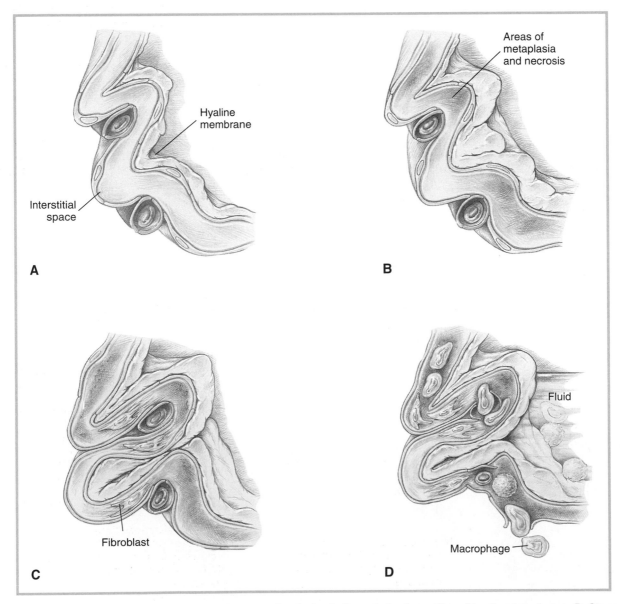

Figure 38–1 The four stages of bronchopulmonary dysplasia. **A**, Stage I, the formation of hyaline membrane. **B**, Stage II, the development areas of metaplasia and necrosis. **C**, Stage III, extensive metaplasia, hyperplasia, and interstitial fibrosis. **D**, Stage IV, progressive destruction of alveoli and airways. See also Plate 29.

Anatomic Alterations of the Lungs

Bronchopulmonary dysplasia (BPD) is a chronic lung disorder characterized by bronchiolar metaplasia and interstitial fibrosis. Histologically, BPD commonly is described in terms of the following four stages:

Stage I (also called the *exudative phase*) occurs during the first 2 to 3 days of life. This stage is often indistinguishable from infant respiratory distress syndrome (IRDS). During this period, alveolar hyaline membranes, patches of atelectasis, and lymphatic dilation are seen. In addition, early signs of bronchial mucosal necrosis appear during this time (Figure 38-1, *A*).

Stage II is seen between 4 and 10 days after birth. This stage entails widespread necrosis of the alveolar epithelium. Persistent alveolar hyaline membranes and atelectasis remain a problem. Early signs of bronchial smooth muscle metaplasia are seen during Stage II. *Metaplasia* is the reversible conversion of normal tissue cells into other, less differentiated cell types in response to chronic stress or injury. This process leads to bronchial necrosis, cellular debris, partial airway obstruction, air trapping, and alveolar hyperinflation. As this condition intensifies, emphysematous coalescence of the alveoli ensues (Figure 38-1, *B*).

Stage III occurs between 10 and 20 days after birth. Pathologic findings include continued injury to the alveolar epithelium, interstitial edema, septal thickening, bronchial mucosal metaplasia and hyperplasia (an increased number of cells), interstitial fibrosis, and excessive bronchial airway secretions. In addition, the alveolar hyperinflation continues to form circular groups of emphysematous bullae that are surrounded by patches of atelectasis (Figure 38-1, *C*).

Stage IV occurs beyond 30 days of life. This stage is characterized by the development of bronchial and interstitial fibrosis and the progressive destruction of alveoli, airways, and pulmonary blood vessels. Areas of emphysematous, or cystlike, areas continue to increase in size and number. Thin strands of atelectasis and normal alveoli are interspersed around emphysematous areas. In addition, pulmonary hypertension often develops, lymphatic and bronchial mucous gland deformation occurs, and excessive bronchial secretions continue to be a problem (Figure 38-1, *D*). Table 38-1 provides a summary of the BPD stages, with pathologic and radiologic correlates.

TABLE 38–1   Bronchopulmonary Dysplasia Staging

Stage	Days After Birth	Radiologic Findings of Lung	Pathologic Findings of Lung
I	2-3	Granular pattern Air bronchograms Small lung volume	Atelectasis Hyaline membranes Lymphatic dilation
II	4-10	Opacification	Widespread necrosis of alveolar epithelium Persistent alveolar hyaline membranes and atelectasis Metaplasia of bronchiolar smooth muscles Bronchial necrosis Emphysematous coalescence of alveoli
III	10-20	Circular, or cystlike, areas of lucency, surrounded by patches of irregular density	Persisting injury to alveoli Interstitial edema and septal thickening Bronchial mucosal metaplasia and hyperplasia Emphysematous areas surrounded by atelectasis Excessive airway secretions
IV	>30	Increased size and numbers of cystlike areas of hyperlucency, surrounded by thinner stands of radiodensity	Increased size and numbers of emphysematous areas, next to collapsed alveoli and normal alveoli Septal fibrosis Pulmonary hypertension, lymphatic and bronchial mucous gland deformation Excessive airway secretions

The major pathologic or structural changes of the lungs associated with BPD are as follows:

- Hyaline membrane formation
- Atelectasis
- Bronchial mucosal necrosis
- Excessive bronchial secretions
- Chronic alveolar fibrosis and bronchial smooth muscle hypertrophy
- Bronchial mucosal metaplasia and hyperplasia
- Alveolar hyperinflation
- Emphysematous areas surrounded by areas of atelectasis and normal alveoli

Before the mid-1960s, a pulmonary disease similar to BPD, called *Wilson-Mikity syndrome* (also called *pulmonary dysmaturity*), was often seen in preterm infants. This was before high positive-pressure ventilation was routinely used on preterm babies. Today, high positive-pressure ventilation used in combination with high oxygen concentrations is considered a major etiologic factor for BPD. The onset of Wilson-Mikity syndrome generally occurred during the first week of life, with streaks of bilateral infiltrates developing throughout the upper lobes. This was followed by the development of alternating areas of alveolar

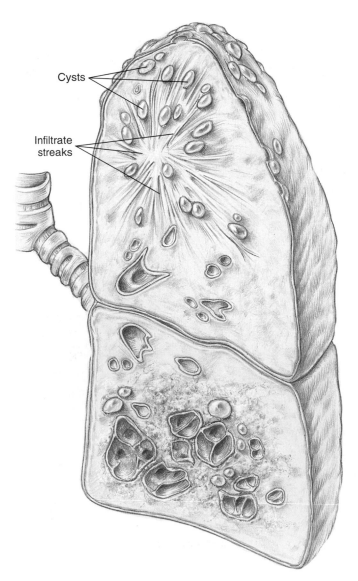

Cysts

Infiltrate
streaks

Figure 38–2 Wilson-Mikity syndrome. See also Plate 30.

hyperinflation and atelectasis and small cystic foci throughout all lung lobes. During the late stages, the cystic areas in the lower lobes enlarged and caused distention at the lung bases. The streaks of infiltrates persisted in the upper lung lobes. In the age of modern respiratory care, Wilson-Mikity syndrome is extremely rare (Figure 38-2).

Etiology

The precise cause of BPD is not known. However, low gestational age, mechanical ventilation, high mean airway pressures, and high oxygen concentrations are all believed to be fundamental etiologic factors.

For example, BPD commonly is seen in infants with a history of IRDS who weigh less than 1500 g and are treated with high concentrations of oxygen and high positive-pressure mechanical ventilation. A precise clinical assessment of the time at which a baby developed BPD is often difficult because the baby often is in the midst of being treated for IRDS and receiving mechanical ventilation and high oxygen concentrations. In general, however, the normal recovery time for IRDS is between 4 and 5 days. If the infant continues to require high concentrations of oxygen and mechanical ventilation after this period, the onset of BPD is likely. In most survivors, clinical and radiologic clinical manifestations of BPD resolve within 2 to 3 years.

OVERVIEW
of the Cardiopulmonary Clinical Manifestations Associated with BRONCHOPULMONARY DYSPLASIA

The following clinical manifestations result from the pathologic mechanisms caused (or activated) by **Atelectasis** (see Figure 9-7), **Increased Alveolar-Capillary Membrane Thickness** (see Figure 9-9), and **Excessive Bronchial Secretions** (see Figure 9-11)— the major anatomic alterations of the lungs associated with bronchopulmonary dysplasia (see Figure 38-1).

CLINICAL DATA OBTAINED AT THE PATIENT'S BEDSIDE

The Physical Examination
Vital Signs

Increased respiratory rate (see page 31 ◆▶)
Normally, a newborn's respiratory rate is about 40 to 60 breaths per minute. During the early stages of BPD, the respiratory rate is generally well over 60 breaths per minute. Several pathophysiologic mechanisms operating simultaneously may lead to an increased ventilatory rate:
- Increased stimulation of peripheral chemoreceptors (hypoxemia)
- Decreased lung compliance/increased ventilatory rate relationship
- Stimulation of central chemoreceptors

Increased heart rate (pulse), cardiac output, and blood pressure (see pages 11 and 99 ◆▶)

Clinical Manifestations Associated with Increased Negative Intrapleural Pressures During Inspiration (see page 429 ◆▶)
- Intercostal retractions
- Substernal retraction/abdominal distention ("seesaw" movement)

- Cyanosis of the dependent portions of the thoracic and abdominal areas
- Flaring nostrils

Chest Assessment Findings (see page 22 ◆▶)
- Wheezes
- Rhonchi
- Crackles

Expiratory Grunting (see page 430 ◆▶)

Cyanosis (see page 45 ◆▶)

CLINICAL DATA OBTAINED FROM LABORATORY TESTS AND SPECIAL PROCEDURES

Pulmonary Function Study Findings (extrapolated data for instructional purposes)

Expiratory Maneuver Findings (see page 61 ◆▶)

FVC	FEV$_T$	FEF$_{25\%-75\%}$	FEF$_{200-1200}$
↓	N or ↓	N or ↓	N
PEFR	MVV	FEF$_{50\%}$	FEV$_{1\%}$
N	N or ↓	N	N or ↑

Lung Volume and Capacity Findings (see page 62 ◆▶)

V$_T$	RV*	FRC*	TLC
N or ↓	↓	↓	↓
VC	IC	ERV	RV/TLC%
↓	↓	↓	N

*↑When airways are partially obstructed.

OVERVIEW

of the Cardiopulmonary Clinical Manifestations Associated with *TRANSIENT TACHYPNEA OF THE NEWBORN* (Continued)

Arterial Blood Gases

Mild to Moderate BPD
Acute Alveolar Hyperventilation with Hypoxemia
   (see page 73 ◆)

pH	Pa_{CO_2}	HCO_3^-	Pa_{O_2}
↑	↓	↓(Slightly)	↓

Advanced BPD
Chronic Ventilatory Failure with Hypoxemia
   (see page 73 ◆)

pH*	Pa_{CO_2}	HCO_3^-*	Pa_{O_2}
Normal	↑	↑(Significantly)	↓

*When tissue hypoxia is severe enough to produce lactic acid, the pH and HCO_3^- values will be lower than expected for a particular Pa_{CO_2} level.

Oxygenation Indices (see page 82 ◆)

$\dot{Q}_S/\dot{Q}_T$	D_{O_2}†	$\dot{V}_{O_2}$	$C(a-\bar{v})_{O_2}$
↑	↓	Normal	Normal
O_2ER	$S\bar{v}_{O_2}$		
↑	↓		

†The D_{O_2} may be normal in patients who have compensated to the decreased oxygenation status with an increased cardiac output. When the D_{O_2} is normal, the O_2ER is usually normal.

RADIOLOGIC FINDINGS

During Stage I, the radiologic findings are analogous to those of severe IRDS, showing a ground-glass pattern, air bronchograms, and small lung volume (Figure 38-3). During Stage II, a bilateral diffuse haziness and opacification develop. Identifying the precise cause of the haziness, whether pulmonary edema, alveolar consolidation, or atelectasis, is usually difficult (Figure 38-4).

The radiologic findings during Stage III are more specific to BPD. Circular areas of hyperlucency begin to appear that are surrounded by patches of irregular density areas caused by atelectasis. This condition generates a spongelike appearance of the lungs on the chest X-ray (Figure 38-5).

Stage IV reveals an increase in the size and number of cystlike areas of hyperlucency (emphysematous bullae), surrounded by thin strands of radiodensity (atelectasis and interstitial fibrosis). The emphysematous bullae and interstitial fibrosis around the bullae create a honeycomb appearance on the chest X-ray (see Table 38-1 for a radiologic summary). Cor pulmonale may be seen during the advanced stages of BPD.

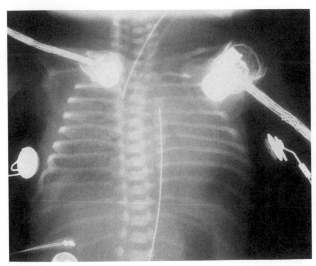

Figure 38–3   Infant with Stage I BPD.

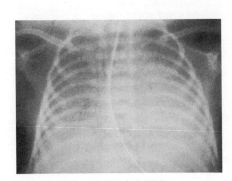

Figure 38–4   Infant with Stage II BPD.

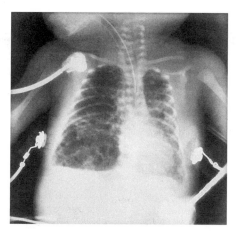

Figure 38–5   Infant with Stage III BPD.

General Management of BPD

All the major respiratory care protocols usually are needed when treating infants with BPD. Supportive care is the primary treatment. During mechanical ventilation, adequate ventilation and oxygenation should be maintained with the lowest possible oxygen concentrations and ventilator pressures. Because of the high incidence of mucus plugging of the airways and endotracheal tubes, adequate humidification of the inspired gas is important. Postural drainage, percussion, and vigorous suctioning also are extremely beneficial. Bronchodilator therapy also may be helpful, but it is of questionable value in infants with interstitial fibrosis.

The infant's fluid balance should be monitored closely. Digitalis preparations and diuretics may be required for infants with excessive interstitial fluid, pulmonary congestion, and cor pulmonale. Surgical ligation of a patent ductus arteriosus may be helpful with infants who are difficult to wean from the ventilator. In general, weaning infants with BPD from mechanical ventilation is a very slow and gradual process. Often, the infant requires high concentrations of oxygen for prolonged periods after extubation. In fact, many infants are sent home on oxygen therapy.

Case Study: BRONCHOPULMONARY DYSPLASIA

Admitting History and Physical Examination

This 1100-gram baby boy was born at 28 weeks' gestation to a mother who received no prenatal care. The mother had used cocaine and marijuana and may have had a vaginal infection during her pregnancy. Because of the baby's history and condition, mechanical ventilation was started moments after birth. Pulmonary surfactant was given. Within 24 hours the baby developed IRDS; needed numerous lines for vascular access (e.g., feeding tube, intravenous [IV] line, and umbilical artery catheter); and required high concentrations of oxygen, positive end-expiratory pressure (PEEP), and continuous positive airway pressure (CPAP). Over the next 4½ weeks, he developed pneumonia and was aggressively treated for atelectasis and excessive bronchial secretions. At this time, the baby was considered to have a chronic case of BPD.

At 5 weeks the baby was still on the mechanical ventilator with the following settings: peak inspiratory pressure (PIP) 25 cm H_2O, respiratory rate 35/min, inspiratory time 0.5 sec, FIO_2 0.6, and PEEP 7 cm H_2O. His pulmonary mechanics showed increased airway resistance and decreased lung compliance. He demonstrated coarse bilateral rhonchi and some wheezes. His chest radiograph had the classic Stage III BPD appearance, with bilateral patches of bullae and areas of atelectasis. The X-ray also showed interstitial emphysema and areas of pulmonary fibrosis. His arterial blood gases on an FIO_2 of 0.4 were pH 7.36, $PaCO_2$ 55, HCO_3^- 30, and PaO_2 51. The doctor wrote the following order in the baby's chart: "Respiratory therapy to assess patient and begin to wean from ventilator." The respiratory care practitioner charted the following assessment at this time:

Respiratory Assessment and Plan

S N/A

O Marginal pulmonary mechanics—decreased compliance and increased airway resistance. Coarse rhonchi and wheezes. CXR: BPD—interstitial emphysema and fibrosis. ABG on ventilator and 40% oxygen: pH 7.36, $Paco_2$ 55, HCO_3^- 30, and Pao_2 51.

A • Stiff lung with airway obstruction (pulmonary mechanics)
   • Chronic ventilatory failure with moderate hypoxemia (ABGs)
   • Excessive bronchial secretions (rhonchi and suctioning results)
   • Possible bronchospasm (wheezes—may be caused by bronchial secretions)
   • Appears ready for slow weaning trial

P Wean slowly per Mechanical Ventilation Protocol (decrease respiratory rate slowly—decrease need for pressure and rate). Continue Oxygen Therapy Protocol (do not attempt to wean from oxygen therapy until rate is down to about 5 breaths per minute). Continue aggressive Bronchopulmonary Hygiene Therapy per protocol (CPT q 2 h and suction prn). Continue Bronchodilator Therapy Protocol (in-line neb with 0.15 cc albuterol in 2 cc normal saline q 4 h). Continue to monitor closely and assess frequently.

Over the next 10 weeks, the baby slowly improved. Five days before discharge, the mother was trained on several respiratory and nursing procedures for home care. Over the following 4 years, the child's lungs continued to improve even though he often had pneumonia and was unstable during the first 6 months. On one occasion, the baby was re-admitted to the hospital for a week. However, he recovered and currently is doing well. He now is of normal weight and height for his age, runs and plays well with other children, and is about to enter preschool.

Discussion

Several comments should be made regarding this challenging pulmonary disorder of the newborn. *First*, infants with BPD have limited pulmonary reserves. Their lungs are seriously damaged, scarred, and fibrotic. They have increased airway resistance and decreased lung compliance. Because their lung tissues are constantly being bombarded by inflammatory stimuli, their hearts and lungs have a limited ability to recover from stress. These infants may require hours to recover from such procedures as tracheal or nasal suctioning, chest physical therapy, or pulmonary surfactant administration. Therefore health-care personnel should perform all therapeutic procedures as quickly and efficiently as possible.

Second, every attempt should be made to wean the baby off the ventilator because the ventilator pressures, rates, and high oxygen concentrations are the main factors causing the pulmonary damage. The longer the baby is on the ventilator, the more the lungs are being damaged. Also, because chronic ventilatory failure with hypoxemia commonly occurs in infants with chronic BPD, the respiratory therapist should not hurry to decrease the infant's $Paco_2$ to the "normal" 35 to 45 mm Hg range. Infants in the acute and chronic stages of BPD often have a high $Paco_2$ and normal pH (compensated). A $Paco_2$ of 60 or 70 mm Hg often is tolerated well. Therefore the therapist must be prepared to accept chronically high $Paco_2$ levels. As the lungs worsen, moreover, the ability of blood to flow easily through the lungs progressively declines. As the condition worsens, the work of the right side of the heart increases. If the BPD does not resolve, cor pulmonale may develop.

BPD is a disorder that requires a great deal of parental education and support at the time of the baby's discharge from the hospital. The respiratory therapist can be instrumental in working with the family both in the hospital and in the home to ensure that the parents are prepared to support the child's respiratory care needs. For example, the parents must understand the procedures of tracheal and nasal suctioning, chest physical therapy, and aerosolized medication administration at home. Infants with BPD who have been discharged from the hospital commonly return to the hospital once or twice a year in acute respiratory distress. Therefore the importance of aggressive, long-term respiratory care in the home must be stressed to the family. For example, the value of good *Bronchopulmonary Hygiene Therapy* at home to offset the clinical manifestations associated with the accumulation of **Excessive Bronchial Secretions** (see Figure 9-11) cannot be overly emphasized.

SELF-ASSESSMENT QUESTIONS

True or False

True ☐ False ☐ **1.** BPD commonly is seen in infants with a history of IRDS.

True ☐ False ☐ **2.** Histologically, BPD is commonly described in terms of five stages.

True ☐ False ☐ **3.** In BPD the formation of alveolar hyaline membranes occurs in Stage III.

True ☐ False ☐ **4.** BPD commonly is seen in infants treated with high concentrations of oxygen and high positive-pressure mechanical ventilation.

True ☐ False ☐ **5.** The recovery period for babies with BPD is between 2 and 3 years.

Complete the Following

During the advanced stage of BPD, the:
1. pH _____ increases _____ decreases _____ is normal
2. $Paco_2$ _____ increases _____ decreases _____ is normal
3. HCO_3^- _____ increases _____ decreases _____ is normal
4. $S\bar{v}o_2$ _____ increases _____ decreases _____ is normal
5. $C(a-\bar{v})o_2$ _____ increases _____ decreases _____ is normal

Answers appear in Appendix XI.

CHAPTER 39

Diaphragmatic Hernia

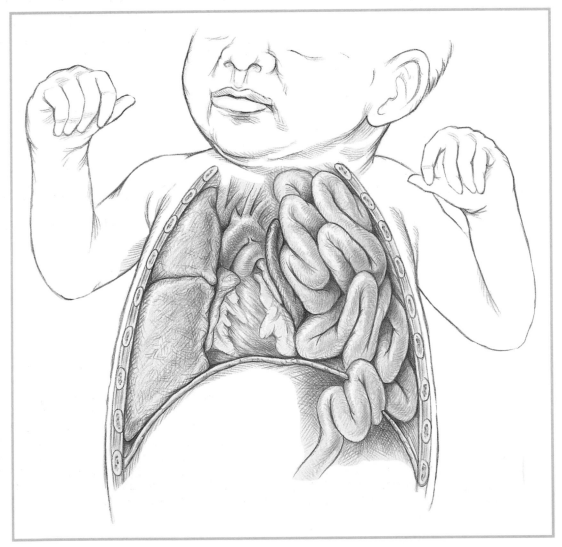

Figure 39–1 Diaphragmatic hernia. See also Plate 31.

Anatomic Alterations of the Lungs

During fetal development, the diaphragm initially appears anteriorly as a septum between the heart and liver but then continues to develop posteriorly. It closes last at the left *Bochdalek foramen*, between the eighth and tenth week of gestation. At about the tenth week of gestation, the intestines and stomach migrate from the yolk sac. If, however, the bowels reach this area before the foramen closes, a hernia results—a congenital diaphragmatic hernia. In this condition, the abdominal contents communicate directly with the thoracic cavity. As the fetus develops, the intestines—and in some cases the stomach—protrude through the defect and compress the lung. A congenital diaphragmatic hernia most commonly occurs on the left side.

As shown in Figure 39-1, the effects of a diaphragmatic hernia are similar to the effects of a pneumothorax or hemothorax—the lungs are compressed. As the condition becomes more severe, atelectasis and complete lung collapse may occur. When this happens, the heart and mediastinum are pushed to the right side of the chest (dextrocardia). In addition, long-term lung compression *in utero* causes pulmonary hypoplasia, which is most severe on the affected (ipsilateral) side but also occurs on the unaffected (contralateral) side. This pathologic process causes a marked reduction in the number of bronchial generations and alveoli per acinus. The concomitant increased muscularity of the small pulmonary arteries may contribute to the increased pulmonary vascular resistance and hypertension commonly seen in these patients. Respiratory distress usually develops soon after birth. As the infant struggles to inhale, the increased negative intrathoracic pressure generated during each inspiration causes more bowel to be sucked into the thorax. Further compression of the heart occurs as the infant cries and swallows air, causing the intestine and stomach to distend further.

Finally, as a consequence of the hypoxemia associated with diaphragmatic hernia, these babies often develop hypoxia-induced pulmonary arterial vasoconstriction and vasospasm, which produces a state of pulmonary hypertension. This results in blood shunting from right to left through the ductus arteriosus and foramen ovale; occasionally, intrapulmonary shunting may occur. Blood flow is diverted away from the lungs (pulmonary hypoperfusion), worsening the hypoxemia. Clinically, this condition is referred to as *persistent pulmonary hypertension of the neonate (PPHN)*—previously called *persistent fetal circulation (PFC)*.

The major pathologic or structural changes associated with diaphragmatic hernia may include the following:

- Failure of the Bochdalek foramen of the diaphragm to close:
  - Migration of intestines and stomach into thorax
- Atelectasis
- Complete lung collapse
- Mediastinum shift to the unaffected side of the thorax
- Reduction in bronchial generations and alveoli per acinus
- Hypoxia-induced pulmonary vasospasm and vasoconstriction:
  - Pulmonary hypertension
  - Right-to-left-shunting
  - Worsening hypoxia
  - Pulmonary hypoperfusion

Etiology

A congenital diaphragmatic hernia occurs in 1 out of 2500 live births. The baby is usually mature, and two thirds of affected infants are male. Approximately 90% of diaphragmatic cases occur on the left side through the Bochdalek foramen. The mortality rate is about 50% within 6 hours after delivery. The prognosis depends on (1) the size of the defect, (2) the degree of hypoplasia, (3) the condition of the lung on the unaffected side, and (4) the success of the surgical diaphragmatic closure.

OVERVIEW

of the Cardiopulmonary Clinical Manifestations Associated with DIAPHRAGMATIC HERNIA

The following clinical manifestations result from the pathologic mechanisms caused (or activated) by **Atelectasis** (see Figure 9-7)—the major anatomic alteration of the lungs associated with diaphragmatic hernia (see Figure 39-1).

CLINICAL DATA OBTAINED AT THE PATIENT'S BEDSIDE

THE PHYSICAL EXAMINATION

Vital Signs

Increased respiratory rate (see page 31 ◆▶)
Normally, a newborn's respiratory rate is about 40 to 60 breaths per minute. When a diaphragmatic hernia is present, the respiratory rate is generally well over 60 breaths per minute. Several pathophysiologic mechanisms operating simultaneously may lead to an increased ventilatory rate:

- Stimulation of peripheral chemoreceptors (hypoxemia)
- Decreased lung compliance/increased ventilatory rate relationship
- Stimulation of central chemoreceptors

Increased heart rate (pulse), cardiac output, and blood pressure (see pages 11 and 99 ◆▶)

Clinical Manifestations Associated with Increased Negative Intrapleural Pressures During Inspiration (see page 429 ◆▶)

- Intercostal retraction
- Substernal retraction
- Cyanosis of the dependent portions of the thoracic and abdominal areas
- Flaring nostrils

Chest Assessment Findings (see page 22 ◆▶)

- Diminished or absent breath sounds over the affected side
- Bowel sounds over the affected side
- Apical heartbeat heard over the unaffected side (usually right)

Expiratory Grunting (see page 430 ◆▶)

Cyanosis (see page 45 ◆▶)

Barrel Chest (see page 45 ◆▶)

When the intestines are in the chest and distended with gas, the baby often demonstrates a barrel chest.

Scaphoid Abdomen

Depending on the degree of intestinal displacement into the thorax, the infant's abdomen often appears flat or concave.

CLINICAL DATA OBTAINED FROM LABORATORY TESTS AND SPECIAL PROCEDURES

Pulmonary Function Study Findings (extrapolated data for instructional purposes)

Expiratory Maneuver Findings (see page 61 ◆▶)

FVC	FEV_T	$FEF_{25\%-75\%}$	$FEF_{200-1200}$
↓	N or ↓	N or ↓	N
PEFR	MVV	$FEF_{50\%}$	$FEV_{1\%}$
N	N or ↓	N	N or ↑

Lung Volume and Capacity Findings (see page 62 ◆▶)

V_T	RV	FRC	TLC
N or ↓	↓	↓	↓
VC	IC	ERV	RV/TLC%
↓	↓	↓	N

Arterial Blood Gases

Mild to Moderate Diaphragmatic Hernia
Acute Alveolar Hyperventilation with Hypoxemia
(see page 70 ◆▶)

pH	$Paco_2$	HCO_3^-	Pao_2
↑	↓	↓ (Slightly)	↓

Severe Diaphragmatic Hernia
Acute Ventilatory Failure with Hypoxemia
(see page 73 ◆▶)

pH*	$Paco_2$	HCO_3^-*	Pao_2
↓	↑	↑(Slightly)	↓

*When tissue hypoxia is severe enough to produce lactic acid, the pH and HCO_3^- values will be lower than expected for a particular $Paco_2$ level.

Oxygenation Indices (see page 82 ◆▶)

$\dot{Q}_S/\dot{Q}_T$	Do_2†	$\dot{V}o_2$	$C(a-\bar{v})o_2$
↑	↓	Normal	Normal
O_2ER	$S\bar{v}o_2$		
↑	↓		

†The Do_2 may be normal in patients who have compensated to the decreased oxygenation status with an increased cardiac output. When the Do_2 is normal, the O_2ER is usually normal.

OVERVIEW

of the Cardiopulmonary Clinical Manifestations Associated with DIAPHRAGMATIC HERNIA (Continued)

RADIOLOGIC FINDINGS

Chest Radiograph

A typical radiograph shows fluid- and air-filled loops of intestine in the chest and a shift of the heart and mediastinum to the unaffected side. Atelectasis and complete lung collapse may be present. The lungs may appear hypoplastic and may not expand to meet the chest wall. A nasogastric tube (hopefully, in the infant's stomach) may be seen on the chest radiograph. It is used to decompress the abdominal viscera. The presence of a diaphragmatic hernia on a chest X-ray usually confirms the need for surgery (Figure 39-2).

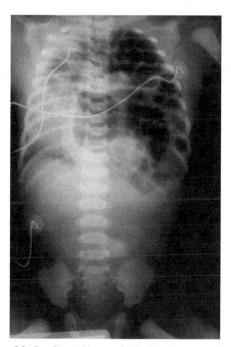

Figure 39–2   Chest X-ray of left diaphragmatic hernia.

General Management of a Diaphragmatic Hernia

Severe diaphragmatic hernia is one of the most urgent neonatal surgical emergencies. Although prompt surgical repair is imperative, a number of therapeutic measures may be instituted until the baby is stabilized for surgery. The baby may not be stable enough for surgery for several days— especially if PPHN is present.

As soon as the diagnosis of a diaphragmatic hernia is made, a double-lumen oral gastric tube should be inserted with intermittent or low continuous suction. This reduces the amount of gas in the bowels and thereby reduces lung compression. Oxygen therapy should be started immediately. The infant also may be placed in the semi-Fowler's position, which reduces the intrathoracic pressure and facilitates the downward positioning of the abdominal viscera. Placing the infant on the affected side aids expansion of the good lung. *The infant must not be manually ventilated with a bag and mask.*

The infant may, however, need to be intubated and ventilated. Mechanical ventilation should be applied with low peak airway pressures (<30 cm H_2O) and rapid respiratory rates. A typical set of ventilator parameters would be as follows: peak inspiratory pressure (PIP) 18 to 20 cm H_2O, respiratory rate (RR) 40, F_{IO_2} 100%, positive end-expiratory pressure (PEEP) 2 to 3 cm H_2O, and inspiratory time (IT) 0.4. High-frequency oscillatory ventilation and jet ventilation are sometimes successful. Because the infant's lungs are fragile and rupture easily, the incidence of pneumothorax is high. Therefore the physician may need to insert one or more chest tubes during mechanical ventilation. Paralysis with pancuronium and sedation with morphine are helpful at times. Paralysis eliminates the swallowing of air, which helps to keep the bowels compressed. These infants are commonly treated with extracorporeal membrane oxygenation (ECMO) while on the ventilator. While on ECMO, the infant is usually ventilated only three or four times per minute to keep the lung inflated.

The surgical procedure entails repositioning the abdominal contents into the abdomen and closing the diaphragmatic defect. In some infants, the peritoneal cavity may be too small to contain the abdominal contents. In these cases, the surgeon leaves the fascia open and closes only the skin. This results in a ventral hernia that is repaired several months after the initial surgery. After surgery, the baby is placed back on the ventilator and weaned per ventilator protocol. Mechanical ventilation with PEEP and continuous positive airway pressure (CPAP) commonly are required to offset the atelectasis and hypoplasia associated with the disorder. Often, the lung on the affected side is hypoplastic and may require days or weeks of therapy for full expansion to occur.

Occasionally, certain pharmacologic agents may be administered to offset the infant's pulmonary hypertension. Such drugs include tolazoline, digitalis agents, diuretics, nitroglycerin, and inhaled nitric oxide (INO). The physiologic action of INO is believed to be similar to the vasoactive substance endothelium-derived relaxing factor (ERF) (see persistent pulmonary hypertension of the newborn [PPHN], page 430). ECMO may be indicated to treat circulatory and respiratory complications after surgery for infants who do not respond favorably to conventional medical therapy. Pulmonary surfactant usually is administered because the lungs are immature and hypoplastic. The administration of pulmonary surfactant may not only offset the infant's surfactant deficiency and improve compliance but may also lower pulmonary vascular resistance and improve pulmonary blood flow.

Case Study: DIAPHRAGMATIC HERNIA

Admitting History and Physical Examination

This full-term baby boy was delivered at 2:25 AM with no remarkable problems to a mother who had received no prenatal care. After delivery, however, the baby made one cry and quickly became blue and limp, started to have bradycardia, and became apneic. The baby's 1-minute Apgar score was 3 (heart rate 1, respiration 0, tone 1, reflex irritability 1, color 0). The nurse handed the baby to a student intern, who immediately began to ventilate the baby manually. Both the respiratory therapist and nurse noted that the baby's abdomen was scaphoid; the therapist stated that the baby might have a diaphragmatic hernia and that bagging should be stopped immediately. Moments later, the neonatologist entered the room, confirmed the scaphoid abdomen, noted that the lungs were very stiff in response to the bagging, and ordered a stat intubation with a 3.5-mm tube and a chest X-ray.

The infant was then transferred to the neonatal intensive care unit (NICU). The chest X-ray confirmed a left diaphragmatic hernia and hypoplastic left lung. At this time, a nasogastric tube was inserted, and suction was begun. The baby was sedated and placed on a mechanical ventilator. An intravenous (IV) line and umbilical artery catheter were then secured. The initial ventilatory settings were RR 30/min, IT 1:2, PEEP 4, PIP 25, and F_{IO_2} 1.0. Initial arterial blood gases were pH 7.19, Pa_{CO_2} 63, HCO_3^- 21, and Pa_{O_2} 24. No breath sounds could be heard over the infant's left lung. The neonatologist diagnosed persistent pulmonary hypertension of the neonate (PPHN). The respiratory therapist then adjusted the ventilatory settings as follows: RR 35/min, IT 0.6 second, PEEP 5, PIP 28 cm H_2O, and F_{IO_2} 1.0. A second set of arterial blood gases taken 15 minutes later showed pH 7.29, Pa_{CO_2} 49, HCO_3^- 23, and Pa_{O_2} 44.

To decrease the PPHN, the baby was placed on ECMO, with the ventilator set to minimal settings. Even though the ECMO was doing all the oxygenation, the baby's lungs were expanded by the ventilator about four times a minute. Four days later, the baby's pulmonary artery pressure was determined to be low enough for surgery. The diaphragmatic hernia was repaired, and the baby was returned to the NICU with a chest tube in the left side of the chest. The baby was again placed on a ventilator.

The ventilator settings 3 days later were RR 8/min, IT 1:2, PIP 20, PEEP and CPAP 4, and F_{IO_2} 0.45. His vital signs were heart rate 145/min, blood pressure 70/45, RR 65 (between ventilator breaths), and temperature 37° C (96.8° F). His skin was pink and normal. Good breath sounds were auscultated over the right lung, and diminished breath sounds could be heard over the left lung. Arterial blood gases at this time were as follows: pH 7.36, Pa_{CO_2} 44, HCO_3^- 23, and Pa_{O_2} 73. The baby's chest X-ray showed good lung expansion on the right side. Although the upper half of the left lung was well expanded, atelectasis and hypoplasia were still seen over the lower half of the left lung. Rhonchi and crackles were auscultated over the left lower lung field, but bubbles were no longer coming from the left-sided chest tube. A small amount of thin, clear secretions was suctioned from the baby's endotracheal tube three or four times an hour. At this time, the respiratory therapist wrote the following assessment in the infant's chart:

Respiratory Assessment and Plan

S N/A

O Vital signs: On ECMO HR 145, BP 70/45, RR 65 (8 mechanical breaths), T 37° C (96.8° F). Skin: Pink and normal. Breath sounds: Right and upper left lung—normal; left lower lung—rhonchi and crackles. No chest tube bubbles. ABGs: pH 7.36, Pa_{CO_2} 44, HCO_3^- 23, and Pa_{O_2} 73. CXR: Right lung normal; atelectasis and hypoplasia in left lower lung.

A • On ECMO, ventilator-dependent, but improving (ventilator)
• Mild amount of large and small airway secretions (crackles, rhonchi)
• Atelectasis and hypoplasia of the left lower lobe (X-ray)
• May be ready to wean from ECMO—check with physician

P Mechanical ventilation Protocol (continue to wean per protocol—wean pressures first, then F_{IO_2}). Hyperinflation Therapy Protocol (continue PEEP and CPAP per Ventilator Protocol). Bronchopulmonary Hygiene Therapy Protocol (continue suction and CPT prn). Oxygen Therapy Protocol (keep Sp_{O_2} at 97% or more as the F_{IO_2} is decreased. Do not decrease F_{IO_2} more than 10% per hour).

ECMO was discontinued. The baby continued to improve over the next 5 days. On day 6, the baby was off the ventilator. The baby was discharged from the hospital 1 week later. The baby continued to develop normally over the next 4 years; at the time of this writing, he was about to enter kindergarten.

Discussion

This case nicely illustrates the importance of good assessment skills. Most diaphragmatic hernias are identified before the baby is born by abdominal ultrasound of the abdomen during routine prenatal care. Unfortunately, this mother had no prenatal care, and as a result, the baby's diaphragmatic hernia was a surprise. Fortunately, the respiratory care practitioner and nurse in this case quickly and correctly identified the possibility of the diaphragmatic hernia by noting the scaphoid abdomen. Had the student intern continued to bag the baby manually, more gas would have entered the stomach and intestines, compressing and compromising the infant's lungs even more. The **Atelectasis** (see Figure 9-7) caused by the enlarged intestines was objectively confirmed on the chest radiograph. The *Hyperinflation Therapy Protocol* was clearly justified to offset the atelectasis after the diaphragmatic hernia was repaired.

This case further illustrates that the first objective in the management of the infant born with a diaphragmatic hernia is the correction of the PPHN. Often, as in this case, treatment requires that the infant be treated with ECMO for 3 or 4 days before surgery. After the PPHN is controlled, the second objective is surgical repair of the hernia. Mechanical ventilation with PEEP and CPAP are usually required after surgery to correct the atelectasis and hypoplasia associated with the disorder. Typically, weaning involves decreasing the F_{IO_2} while monitoring the baby's pulse oximetry. Ideally, the ventilator pressures are decreased first, and then the ventilatory rates are decreased. A target Pa_{CO_2} of 40 mm Hg or less is commonly used. An infant on a ventilatory rate of 12/min, a peak inspiratory pressure of 15 cm H_2O or less, and a PEEP of 3 cm H_2O or less is usually ready for a weaning trial.

SELF-ASSESSMENT QUESTIONS

True or False

True ☐ False ☐ **1.** The Bochdalek foramen closes between the fifteenth and twentieth week of gestation.

True ☐ False ☐ **2.** The pathophysiologic effects of a diaphragmatic hernia are similar to the effects of a pneumothorax or hemothorax.

True ☐ False ☐ **3.** The incidence of diaphragmatic hernia is higher in female subjects.

True ☐ False ☐ **4.** Ninety percent of all diaphragmatic hernias occur on the right side.

True ☐ False ☐ **5.** Depending on the degree of intestinal displacement into the thorax, the infant's abdomen often appears convex.

True ☐ False ☐ **6.** When PPHN is present, the baby may not be stable enough for surgery for several days.

True ☐ False ☐ **7.** Before surgery, the infant may benefit from being placed on the affected side.

True ☐ False ☐ **8.** Before surgery, mechanical ventilation may be necessary. When this is the case, the mechanical ventilator should be applied with high peak pressures and slow rates.

True ☐ False ☐ **9.** Babies with diaphragmatic hernias are commonly treated with ECMO while on the ventilator.

True ☐ False ☐ **10.** The physiologic action of inhaled nitric oxide (INO) is believed to be similar to the vasoactive substance endothelium-derived relaxing factor (ERF).

Answers appear in Appendix XI.

CHAPTER 40

Croup Syndrome: Laryngotracheobronchitis and Acute Epiglottitis

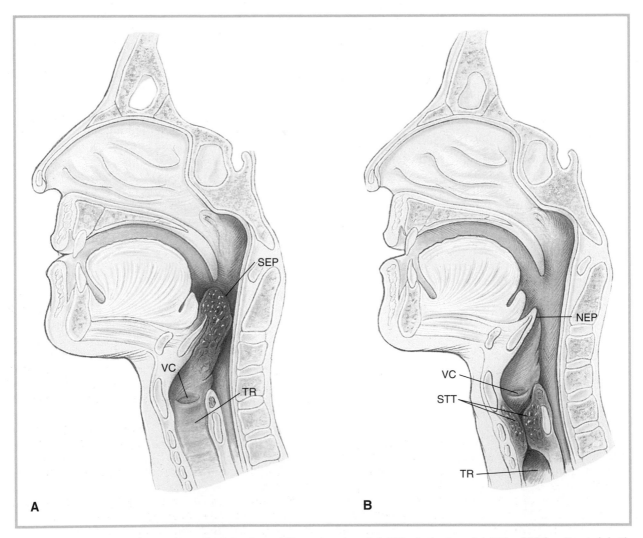

Figure 40–1 Croup syndrome: laryngotracheobronchitis and acute epiglottitis. **A,** Acute epiglottitis. *SEP,* Swollen epiglottis; *VC,* vocal cords; *TR,* trachea. **B,** Laryngotracheobronchitis. *NEP,* Normal epiglottis; *VC,* vocal cords; *STT,* swollen trachea tissue; *TR,* trachea. See also Plate 32.

Croup is a general term used to describe the inspiratory, barking sound associated with the partial upper airway obstruction that develops in laryngotracheobronchitis (subglottic croup) and acute epiglottitis (supraglottic croup) (Figure 40-1). Clinically, the inspiratory sound heard in croup also is called *inspiratory stridor*.

Anatomic Alterations of the Upper Airway

LARYNGOTRACHEOBRONCHITIS

Because this disease entity can affect the lower laryngeal area, trachea, and occasionally the bronchi, the term *laryngotracheobronchitis (LTB)* is used as a synonym for "classic" subglottic croup. Pathologically, LTB is an inflammatory process that causes edema and swelling of the mucous membranes. Although the laryngeal mucosa and submucosa are vascular, the distribution of the lymphatic capillaries is uneven or absent in this region. Consequently, when edema develops in the upper airway, fluid spreads and accumulates quickly throughout the connective tissues, which causes the mucosa to swell and the airway lumen to narrow. The inflammation also causes the mucous glands to increase their production of mucus and the cilia to lose their effectiveness as a mucociliary transport mechanism.

Because the subglottic area is the narrowest region of the larynx in an infant or small child, even a slight degree of edema can cause a significant reduction in cross-sectional area. The edema in this area is further aggravated by the rigid cricoid cartilage, which surrounds the mucous membrane and prevents external swelling as fluid engorges the laryngeal tissues. The edema and swelling in the subglottic region decrease the ability of the vocal cords to abduct (move apart) during inspiration. This further reduces the cross-sectional area of airway in this region.

ACUTE EPIGLOTTITIS

Acute epiglottitis is a life-threatening emergency. In contrast to LTB, epiglottitis is an inflammation of the supraglottic region, which includes the epiglottis, aryepiglottic folds, and false vocal cords (see Figure 40-1). Epiglottitis does not involve the pharynx, trachea, or other subglottic structures. As the edema in the epiglottis increases, the lateral borders curl and the tip of the epiglottis protrudes posteriorly and inferiorly. During inspiration the swollen epiglottis is pulled (or sucked) over the laryngeal inlet. In severe cases, this may completely block the laryngeal opening. Clinically, the classic finding is a swollen, cherry-red epiglottis.

The major pathologic or structural changes associated with croup are as follows:

- LTB—Airway obstruction caused by tissue swelling just below the vocal cords
- Epiglottitis—Airway obstruction caused by tissue swelling just above the vocal cords

Etiology

LARYNGOTRACHEOBRONCHITIS

More than 40,000 children are admitted to the hospital with LTB annually. The parainfluenza viruses 1, 2, and 3, transmitted via aerosol droplets, are the most frequently identified etiologic agents, with type 1 being the most prevalent. LTB also may be caused by influenza A and B, respiratory syncytial virus (RSV), herpes simplex virus, *Mycoplasma pneumoniae*, rhinovirus, and adenoviruses.

LTB is primarily seen in children between 6 months and 6 years of age. Boys are affected slightly more often than girls. The onset of LTB is slow (i.e., symptoms progressively increase over 24 to 48 hours), and it is most common during the fall and winter. A brassy or barking cough is commonly present. The child's voice is hoarse, and the inspiratory stridor is typically loud and high in pitch. The patient usually does not have a fever, drooling, swallowing difficulties, or a toxic appearance.

ACUTE EPIGLOTTITIS

Acute epiglottitis is a bacterial infection that is almost always caused by *Haemophilus influenzae* B. It is transmitted via aerosol droplets. Since 1985, when vaccinations with *H. influenzae* type B vaccine became widespread, the number of reported cases of epiglottitis has decreased by over 95%. *H. influenzae* type B, however, is still responsible for 75% of the epiglottitis cases. Since the vaccination program was initiated, the cause of epiglottis is often the non–*H. influenzae* type B, with primarily group A β-hemolytic streptococcal being the infectious organism. Other causes of epiglottitis include aspiration of hot liquid and trauma from repeated intubation attempts.

Epiglottitis has no clear-cut geographic or seasonal incidence. Although acute epiglottitis may develop in all age groups (neonatal to adulthood), it most often occurs in children between 2 and 6 years of age. Boys are affected more often than girls. The onset of epiglottitis is usually abrupt. Although the initial clinical manifestations are usually mild, they progress rapidly over a 2- to 4-hour period. A common scenario includes a sore throat or mild upper respiratory problem that quickly progresses to a high fever, lethargy, and difficulty in swallowing and handling secretions. The child usually appears pale. As the supraglottic area becomes swollen, breathing becomes noisy, the tongue is often thrust forward during inspiration, and the child may drool. Compared with LTB, the inspiratory stridor is usually softer and lower in pitch. The voice and cry are usually muffled rather than hoarse. Older children commonly complain of a sore throat during swallowing. A cough is usually absent in patients with epiglottitis.

The general history and physical findings of LTB and epiglottitis are compared and contrasted in Table 40-1.

TABLE 40–1   General History and Physical Findings of Laryngotracheobronchitis and Epiglottitis

Clinical Finding	LTB	Epiglottitis
Age	6 months-6 years	2-6 years
Onset	Slow (24-48 hours)	Abrupt (2-4 hours)
Fever	Absent	Present
Drooling	Absent	Present
Lateral neck X-ray	Haziness in subglottic area	Haziness in supraglottic area
Inspiratory stridor	High-pitched and loud	Low-pitched and muffled
Hoarseness	Present	Absent
Swallowing difficulty	Absent	Present
White blood count	Normal (viral)	Elevated (bacterial)

OVERVIEW
of the Cardiopulmonary Clinical Manifestations Associated with LARYNGOTRACHEOBRONCHITIS AND EPIGLOTTITIS

The following clinical manifestations result from the pathologic mechanisms caused (or activated) by an **Upper Airway Obstruction**—the major anatomic alteration of the lungs associated with laryngotracheobronchitis (LTB) and epiglottitis (see Figure 40-1). (Upper Airway Obstruction is not one of the major clinical scenarios discussed in Chapter 9.)

CLINICAL DATA OBTAINED AT THE PATIENT'S BEDSIDE

The Physical Examination

Vital Signs

Increased respiratory rate (see page 31 ◀▶)
Several pathophysiologic mechanisms operating simultaneously may lead to an increased ventilatory rate:
- Increased stimulation of peripheral chemoreceptors
- Anxiety

Increased heart rate (pulse), cardiac output, and blood pressure (see pages 11 and 99 ◀▶)

Chest Assessment Findings (see page 22 ◀▶)
- Diminished breath sounds

Inspiratory Stridor
Under normal circumstances, the slight narrowing of the upper (extrathoracic) airway that naturally occurs during inspiration is insignificant. Because the upper airway is relatively small in infants and children, however, even a slight degree of edema may become significant. Thus when the cross-section of the upper airway is reduced because of the edema, the child will generate stridor during inspiration, when the upper airway naturally becomes smaller. It also should be noted that if the edema becomes severe, the patient may generate both inspiratory and expiratory stridor.

Cyanosis (see page 45 ◀▶)

Use of Accessory Muscles During Inspiration (see page 40 ◀▶)

Substernal and Intercostal Retraction (see page 43 ◀▶)

CLINICAL DATA OBTAINED FROM LABORATORY TESTS AND SPECIAL PROCEDURES

Arterial Blood Gases

Mild to Moderate LTB or Epiglottitis
Acute Alveolar Hyperventilation with Hypoxemia (see page 70 ◀▶)

pH	Paco$_2$	HCO$_3^-$	Pao$_2$
↑	↓	↓ (Slightly)	↓

OVERVIEW

of the Cardiopulmonary Clinical Manifestations Associated with LARYNGOTRACHEOBRONCHITIS AND EPIGLOTTITIS *(Continued)*

Severe LTB or Epiglottitis
Acute Ventilatory Failure with Hypoxemia (see page 73 ◄►)

pH	$Paco_2$	HCO_3^-*	Pao_2
↓	↑	↑(Slightly)	↓

*When tissue hypoxia is severe enough to produce lactic acid, the pH and HCO_3^- values will be lower than expected for a particular $Paco_2$ level.

Oxygenation Indices (see page 82 ◄►)

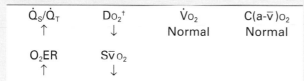

$\dot{Q}_s/\dot{Q}_T$	Do_2†	$\dot{V}o_2$	$C(a-\bar{v})o_2$
↑	↓	Normal	Normal
O_2ER	$S\bar{v}o_2$		
↑	↓		

†The DO_2 may be normal in patients who have compensated to the decreased oxygenation status with an increased cardiac output. When the Do_2 is normal, the O_2ER is usually normal.

LATERAL NECK X-RAY

- Haziness in the subglottic area (LTB)
- "Steeple point" or "pencil point" narrowing of the upper airway (LTB)
- Haziness in the supraglottic area (epiglottitis)
- Classic "thumb sign" (epiglottitis)

Although the diagnosis of epiglottitis or LTB can generally be made on the basis of the patient's clinical history, a lateral neck X-ray sometimes is used to confirm the diagnosis. When the patient has LTB, a white haziness is demonstrated in the subglottic area. When the patient has acute epiglottitis, a white haziness is evident in the supraglottic area. In addition, epiglottitis often appears on a lateral neck X-ray as the classic "thumb sign." The epiglottis is swollen and rounded, giving it an appearance of the distal portion of a thumb (Figure 40-2).

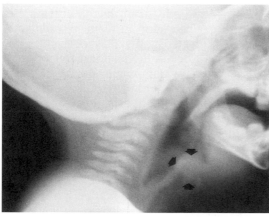

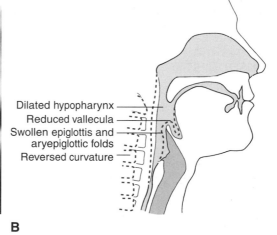

Dilated hypopharynx
Reduced vallecula
Swollen epiglottis and aryepiglottic folds
Reversed curvature

A   **B**

Figure 40–2   The classic "thumb sign" of an edematous epiglottis is evident in this lateral neck film (see *arrows* in **A**). The schematic illustrates the findings to look for in a lateral film of a patient with suspected epiglottitis **(B)**. Such films are unnecessary in a child with the classic history, signs, and symptoms of epiglottitis; they can be of tremendous help, however, in diagnosing mild or questionable cases and explaining to parents the need for aggressive treatment. (From Ashcraft CK, Steele RW: *J Respir Dis* 9:48, 1988.)

General Management of Laryngotracheobronchitis and Epiglottitis

The treatment of mild cases of LTB primarily is supportive. Care includes temperature control, adequate hydration, and humidification of inspired air. The patient's vital signs, degree of retractions, mental status, and ventilatory and oxygenation status are closely monitored. Early recognition of epiglottitis may save a patient's life. A history of upper airway obstruction requires a general examination as soon as possible. Under no circumstances should the mouth or throat be examined unless personnel and equipment are available to rapidly intubate or tracheostomize the patient. In cases of suspected epiglottitis, examination or inspection of the pharynx and larynx is absolutely contraindicated, except in the operating room with a fully trained team. This is because direct examination of the throat (even though depression of the tongue may reveal a bright red epiglottis and confirm the diagnosis) often results in a sudden and complete closure of the upper airway. A lateral neck radiograph may be necessary to differentiate LTB, epiglottitis, or some other upper airway obstruction. After the diagnosis is established, the general management of LTB and acute epiglottitis is as follows.

SUPPLEMENTAL OXYGEN

Because hypoxemia is associated with both LTB and epiglottitis, supplemental oxygen is required (see Oxygen Therapy Protocol, Protocol 9-1).

COOL AEROSOL MIST

Cool aerosol mist therapy (with oxygen) either by face mask or tent is the primary mode of treatment for LTB. It liquifies thick secretions and cools and reduces subglottic edema. Generations of mothers have learned this homespun therapy, and it usually (although not always) works. Warm aerosols also are often effective.

RACEMIC EPINEPHRINE (MICRO-NEFRIN, VAPONEFRIN)

Aerosolized racemic epinephrine usually is administered to children with LTB. This adrenergic agent is used for its mucosal vasoconstriction and is recognized as an effective and safe aerosol decongestant (see Aerosolized Medication Protocol, Protocol 9-4).

CORTICOSTEROIDS

Corticosteroids have been shown to reduce the severity and duration of LTB. They generally are prescribed when the patient does not respond to cool mist and racemic epinephrine therapy (see Appendix II).

ANTIBIOTIC THERAPY

Because acute epiglottitis almost always is caused by *H. influenzae,* appropriate antibiotic therapy should be part of the treatment plan. Ampicillin and chloramphenicol often are prescribed to cover the most common organisms that cause acute epiglottitis.

ENDOTRACHEAL INTUBATION OR TRACHEOSTOMY

In cases of suspected epiglottitis, examination or inspection of the pharynx and larynx is absolutely contraindicated, except in the operating room with a fully trained surgical team in attendance. This is because the epiglottis may obstruct completely in response to even the slightest touch during inspection. The physician, nurse, and respiratory care practitioner should not leave the patient's bedside until the endotracheal tube is secured. If the patient is anxious, restless, or uncooperative, restraints may be needed to prevent accidental extubation. After intubation, the patient should be transferred to the intensive care unit (ICU), sedated, and placed on continuous positive airway pressure (CPAP).

Case Study 1: LARYNGOTRACHEOBRONCHITIS

Admitting History and Physical Examination

A 3-year-old boy had a mild viral upper respiratory infection and some hoarseness; at 10 PM on the third day of his illness, he rapidly developed a brassy cough and high-pitched inspiratory stridor. He became moderately dyspneic. The child was restless and appeared frightened. Rectal temperature was 37° C. The mother claimed that the child was "blue" on two occasions during this episode. She was going to take the child to the emergency room, but the grandmother suggested that she try steam inhalation first. Accordingly, the child was taken to the bathroom, where the shower was turned on full force. The child was comforted by the grandmother and urged to breathe slowly and deeply. As the bathroom became filled with steam, the respiratory distress abated and within a few minutes the child was free of stridor, breathing essentially normally. The next day the same symptoms recurred, and the patient was taken to the emergency department. The respiratory therapist documented the following assessment and plan:

Respiratory Assessment and Plan

S Mother reports patient had cough and inspiratory stridor.

O Confirms above. Lungs clear except for stridor and tracheal breath sounds throughout. RR 50/min. Circumoral pallor noted. O₂ sat 92% on room air. CXR and soft tissue X-ray of neck suggests laryngotracheobronchitis.

A Croup, moderate (history and inspiratory stridor)

P Cool mist aerosol treatment. Med. neb. treatment with racemic epinephrine per protocol. Will obtain throat culture if okay with the physician

The patient did well, and at discharge, the patient's mother was instructed in home treatment of croup, using aerosolized racemic epinephrine prn.

Discussion

Home remedies sometimes do work. Any parent who has had a child with croup will find this scenario familiar. What may not be as widely recognized is that sometimes warm and sometimes cool aerosols improve this syndrome. When this approach failed, the parents were wise to bring their son to the emergency department for prompt vasoconstrictive therapy accompanied by a cool mist aerosol. This resulted in prompt improvement. In most pediatric units, decongestant aerosol therapy and mist inhalation are part of the *Aerosolized Medication Protocol* (see Protocol 9-4).

Note the emphasis on family education, including the use of racemic epinephrine aerosolization for outpatients. These instructions may have kept the patient from ever returning again to the emergency department to be treated for such an episode.

Case Study 2: ACUTE EPIGLOTTITIS

Admitting History and Physical Examination

This 2-year-old girl appeared quite well in the evening and was put to bed at the usual time. She woke up 2 hours later, and her parents were immediately aware that she was in serious respiratory distress. She was sitting up in bed, drooling, unable to speak or cry, and breathing noisily.

The parents wrapped the child in warm blankets and drove her to the emergency department of the nearest hospital. On inspection, the child demonstrated a puffy face, drooling, inspiratory stridor, and cyanotic nail beds. The emergency physician looked at the girl and listened to her chest but did not examine her mouth. Respiratory rate was 42/min, blood pressure was 80/50, and pulse was 140/min. The physician ordered a lateral soft tissue X-ray of the neck, but while waiting for the X-ray, the child became increasingly dyspneic and more cyanotic. Her Spo₂ on room air was 70%. At this time, the following respiratory SOAP note was charted:

Respiratory Assessment and Plan

S Mother states that patient is in severe respiratory distress.

O RR 42/min, BP 80/50, P 140 regular. Child's face puffy, drooling. Inspiratory stridor (worsening). Nail beds cyanotic. Room air Spo₂ 70%. Soft tissue X-ray of neck pending.

A • Probable acute epiglottitis. No history of foreign body aspiration (general history)
  • Impending acute ventilatory failure (history, drooling, inspiratory stridor, and cyanosis)
P Anesthesiologist and ENT surgeon paged. Mask with 100% oxygen and cool mist pending their arrival.

The emergency physician placed an emergency page for the anesthesiologist on call and for an ENT surgeon. Immediately, a nonrebreathing oxygen mask was lightly held to the patient's face by the respiratory therapist. As soon as the physicians arrived (after about 10 minutes), the child was taken to the operating room. The surgeon stood by to perform an emergency cricothyrotomy while the anesthesiologist attempted to intubate the child.

Fortunately, the anesthesiologist was successful in spite of an enlarged, cherry-red epiglottis partially obstructing the larynx. As soon as the endotracheal tube was in place, the child relaxed and soon went to sleep. She was admitted to the ICU, sedated, and placed on 5 cm H_2O CPAP. She was extubated the next day and discharged on the third hospital day. A throat culture taken in the ICU was positive for *H. influenzae*. She was treated orally with amoxicillin.

Discussion

Acute epiglottitis is a life-threatening condition. The key point to remember is to refrain from examining the throat until a staff member qualified in pediatric intubation is nearby. Such manipulation often is unsuccessful, and unless qualified assistance is at hand, the child may asphyxiate.

The treatment suitably selected here was placement of a nonrebreathing oxygen mask while the appropriate team was assembled. Typical of this disease is its abrupt onset and, under appropriate therapy, the rapid manner in which it subsides.

SELF-ASSESSMENT QUESTIONS

True or False

True ☐ False ☐ **1.** LTB is supraglottic croup.

True ☐ False ☐ **2.** Acute epiglottitis is a life-threatening emergency.

True ☐ False ☐ **3.** Acute epiglottitis predominantly is seen in children between 2 and 6 years of age.

True ☐ False ☐ **4.** Acute epiglottitis is usually caused by *H. influenzae* B.

True ☐ False ☐ **5.** The onset of LTB is relatively slow (24 to 48 hours).

True ☐ False ☐ **6.** Drooling is usually present in LTB.

True ☐ False ☐ **7.** A fever is associated with acute epiglottitis.

True ☐ False ☐ **8.** The inspiratory stridor is usually low pitched and muffled in LTB.

True ☐ False ☐ **9.** The white blood count is usually elevated in LTB.

True ☐ False ☐ **10.** Swallowing is usually difficult in patients with LTB.

Answers appear in Appendix XI.

CHAPTER 41

Cystic Fibrosis

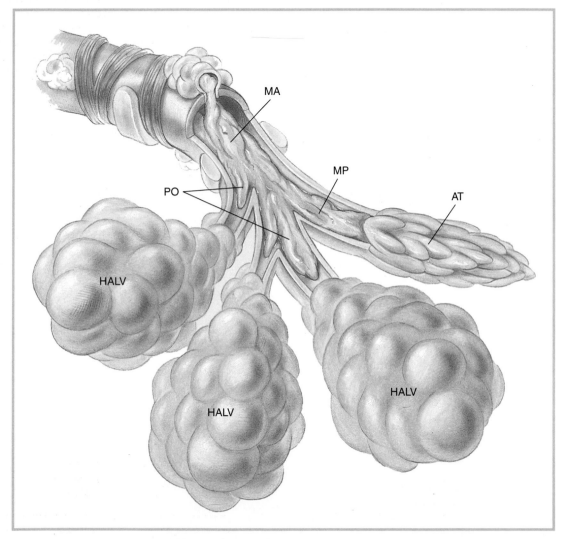

Figure 41–1   Cystic fibrosis. *MA,* Mucus accumulation; *MP,* mucus plug; *AT,* atelectasis; *PO,* partial obstruction of the airways; *HALV,* hyperinflation of alveoli. See also Plate 33.

Anatomic Alterations of the Lungs*

Although the lungs of patients with cystic fibrosis appear normal at birth, abnormal structural changes develop quickly. Initially, there is bronchial gland hypertrophy and metaplasia of goblet cells, which secrete large amounts of thick, tenacious mucus. Because the mucus is particularly tenacious, impairment of the normal mucociliary clearing mechanism ensues, and many small bronchi and bronchioles become partially or totally obstructed (mucus plugging). Partial obstruction leads to overdistention of the alveoli, and complete obstruction leads to patchy areas of atelectasis. Bronchial obstruction and hyperinflation of the lungs are the predominant features of cystic fibrosis in the advanced stages.

The abundance of stagnant mucus in the tracheobronchial tree also serves as an excellent culture medium for bacteria, particularly *Staphylococcus aureus*, *Haemophilus influenzae*, and *Pseudomonas aeruginosa*. The infection stimulates additional mucus production and further compromises the mucociliary transport system. This condition may lead to secondary bronchial smooth muscle constriction. Finally, as the disease progresses, the patient may develop signs and symptoms of recurrent pneumonia, chronic bronchitis, bronchiectasis, and lung abscesses (Figure 41-1).

The major pathologic or structural changes associated with cystic fibrosis are as follows:

- Excessive production and accumulation of thick, tenacious mucus in the tracheobronchial tree
- Partial or total bronchial obstruction (mucus plugging)
- Atelectasis
- Hyperinflation of the alveoli

Etiology

Cystic fibrosis is a genetic disease caused by mutations in a pair of genes located on chromosome 7. Under normal conditions, every cell in the body (except the sex cells) has 46 chromosomes—23 pairs (one half inherited from father and the other half from mother). In the patient with cystic fibrosis, however, an abnormal gene is located on each number 7 chromosome. Over 700 different cystic fibrosis mutations have been identified on chromosome 7. The most common mutation is ΔF508. The mutated genes

associated with cystic fibrosis are responsible for the production of a protein called *cystic fibrosis transmembrane regulator (CFTR)*.

The absence—or abnormal production or function—of the CFTR leads to abnormal electrolyte and water movement in and out of the epithelial cells, including those lining the bronchial airways, intestines, pancreas, liver ducts, sweat glands, and vas deferens. As a result, thick, viscous mucus accumulates in the lungs, and mucus blocks the passageways of the pancreas, preventing enzymes from the pancreas from reaching the intestines. This condition inhibits the digestion of protein and fat, which in turn leads to deficiencies of vitamins A, D, E, and K. In addition, diarrhea, malnutrition, and weight loss are also common. Some infants with cystic fibrosis develop a blockage of the intestine shortly after birth—a condition called meconium ileus. Most men with cystic fibrosis are infertile as a result of a missing or an underdeveloped vas deferens. Infertility is not common in women with cystic fibrosis.

Other than the fact that the carrier of the cystic fibrosis gene may be identified through genetic testing, the carrier (heterozygotes) does not demonstrate evidence of the disease. If both parents carry the cystic fibrosis gene, the possibility of their children having cystic fibrosis (regardless of gender) follows the standard Mendelian pattern: There is a 25% chance that each child will have cystic fibrosis, a 25% chance that each child will be completely normal (and not carry the gene), and a 50% chance that each child will be a carrier (Figure 41-2). About 1 in 29 Caucasians in the United States carry the cystic fibrosis gene.

---

*Cystic fibrosis does not affect the lungs exclusively. It also affects the function of exocrine glands in other parts of the body. In addition to being characterized by abnormally viscid secretions in the lungs, the disease is clinically manifested by pancreatic insufficiency and high sodium concentrations in the sweat.

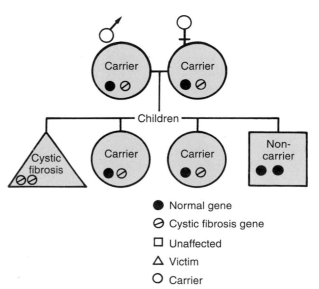

Figure 41-2 Standard Mendelian pattern of inheritance of cystic fibrosis.

In the United States, about 1000 new cases of cystic fibrosis are reported annually. Caucasians are most often affected (1 in 3500). Cystic fibrosis is less common in Hispanics (1 in 9500), African-Americans (1 in 15,000), and Asians (1 in 31,000). Approximately 70% of the cystic fibrosis cases are confirmed before the subject reaches 1 year of age; most are diagnosed within the first several months. About 7% of the newly diagnosed patients with cystic fibrosis are adults. The median life expectancy is 31 years. Some live beyond 50 years of age. Death usually is caused by pulmonary complications.

BOX 41–1

Clinical Indicators Justifying the Evaluation for Cystic Fibrosis

Pulmonary
Wheezing
Chronic cough
Sputum production
Frequent respiratory infections *(Staphylococcus aureus, Pseudomonas aeruginosa, Haemophilus influenzae)*
Abnormal chest radiograph
Nasal polyps
Parasinusitis
Digital clubbing

Gastrointestinal
Failure to thrive
Foul-smelling, greasy stools
Voracious appetite
Milk and formula intolerance
Rectal prolapse
Meconium ileus
Meconium peritonitis
Distal intestinal obstruction syndrome
Pancreatic insufficiency
Pancreatitis

Hepatobiliary
Hepatomegaly
Focal biliary cirrhosis
Prolonged neonatal jaundice
Cholelithiasis

Nutritional Deficits
Fat-soluble vitamin deficiency (vitamins A, D, E, K)
Hypoproteinemia
Hypochloremia (metabolic alkalosis)

Infertility (male)
Obstructive azoospermia

BOX 41–2

Diagnosis of Cystic Fibrosis

The diagnosis of cystic fibrosis is confirmed when at least one item from each of the following areas is established:

Laboratory
Sweat chloride level (> 60 mEq/L in children)
or
Two CFTR mutations
or
Elevated levels of serum trypsinogen
or
Abnormal difference in voltage potential across the nasal epithelium

History or Clinical Manifestations
Clinical manifestations associated with cystic fibrosis
or
Family history of cystic fibrosis

Screening and Diagnosis

Box 41-1 provides common clinical indicators that justify evaluation for cystic fibrosis. The diagnosis of cystic fibrosis is based on the existence of one or more distinctive phenotypic features or a family history of the disease. As shown in Box 41-2, the diagnosis of cystic fibrosis requires both positive laboratory testing results and a history or a clinical presentation that is consistent with cystic fibrosis.

SWEAT TEST

The *sweat test* is the standard diagnostic test for cystic fibrosis. This test measures the amount of sodium and chloride in the patient's sweat. During the procedure, a small amount of sweat-producing chemical, called *pilocarpine,* is applied to the patient's arm or leg—usually the forearm. An electrode is attached to the chemically prepared area, and a mild electric current is applied to stimulate sweat production. To collect the sweat, the area is covered with a gauze pad or filter paper and wrapped in plastic. After about 30 minutes, the plastic is removed, and the sweat collected in the pad or paper is sent to the laboratory for analysis.

Although the sweat glands of patients with cystic fibrosis are microscopically normal, the glands secrete up to four times the normal amount of sodium and chloride. The actual volume of sweat, however, is no greater than that produced by a normal individual. In children, a sweat chloride concentration greater than 60 mEq/L is considered to be a diagnostic sign of the disease. In adults, a sweat chloride concentration greater than 80 mEq/L usually is required to confirm the diagnosis. The sweat chloride level in the patient with cystic fibrosis may be up to five times greater than normal.

CFTR GENE ANALYSIS

The diagnosis of cystic fibrosis can made when two mutated CFTR alleles are identified. Even though more than 700 mutations have been identified, current genotyping methods are able to identify fewer than 100 mutated alleles. The most common mutation in cystic fibrosis is ΔF508. Although gene analysis for cystic fibrosis is considered a valuable diagnostic tool, it does have its limitations. For example, some individuals have CFTR mutations but demonstrate no typical clinical manifestations of cystic fibrosis. In addition, some patients may have two CFTR mutations, but the mutations cannot be identified with the gene analysis methods presently available. In view of these limitations, genetic testing is used to make the diagnosis of cystic fibrosis but not to rule it out completely on the basis of a negative test result.

IMMUNOREACTIVE TRYPSINOGEN TEST

Because babies may not produce enough sweat for a reliable test during the first few months of life, the physician usually does not order the test until the baby is at least several months old. In these cases, the doctor may order the *immunoreactive trypsinogen test (IRT)*. During this procedure, a heel-stick blood sample is analyzed twice for a specific protein called *trypsinogen*. Elevated levels of serum trypsinogen are associated with pancreatic insufficiency and cystic fibrosis. Two positive test results indicate cystic fibrosis. The diagnosis is confirmed with a sweat chloride test or the presence of two CFTR mutated genes.

NASAL ELECTRICAL POTENTIAL DIFFERENCE

The measurement of certain alterations in the difference in voltage potential across the nasal epithelium can be used to identify cystic fibrosis is some patients. However, this diagnostic tool is relatively new, and its availability is limited.

OVERVIEW

of the Cardiopulmonary Clinical Manifestations Associated with CYSTIC FIBROSIS

The following clinical manifestations result from the pathophysiologic mechanisms caused (or activated) by **Atelectasis** (see Figure 9-7), **Bronchospasm** (see Figure 9-10), and **Excessive Bronchial Secretions** (see Figure 9-11)—the major anatomic alterations of the lungs associated with cystic fibrosis (see Figure 41-1).

CLINICAL DATA OBTAINED AT THE PATIENT'S BEDSIDE

The Physical Examination

Vital Signs

Increased respiratory rate (see page 31 ◆►)
Several pathophysiologic mechanisms operating simultaneously may lead to an increased ventilatory rate:
- Stimulation of peripheral chemoreceptors (hypoxemia)
- Decreased lung compliance/increased ventilatory rate relationship
- Anxiety

Increased heart rate (pulse), cardiac output, and blood pressure (see pages 11 and 99 ◆►)

Use of Accessory Muscles During Inspiration (see page 40 ◆►)

Use of Accessory Muscles During Expiration (see page 42 ◆►)

Pursed-Lip Breathing (see page 42 ◆►)

Increased Anteroposterior Chest Diameter (Barrel Chest) (see page 45 ◆►)

Cyanosis (see page 45 ◆►)

Digital Clubbing (see page 46 ◆►)

Peripheral Edema and Venous Distention (see page 47 ◆►)

Because polycythemia and cor pulmonale are associated with cystic fibrosis, the following may be seen:
- Distended neck veins
- Pitting edema
- Enlarged and tender liver

Cough, Sputum Production, and Hemoptysis (see page 47 ◆►)

Chest Assessment Findings (see page 22 ◆►)
- Decreased or increased tactile and vocal fremitus
- Hyperresonant percussion note
- Diminished breath sounds
- Diminished heart sounds
- Crackles, rhonchi, and wheezing

Spontaneous Pneumothorax (see Chapter 22)
Spontaneous pneumothorax commonly is seen in patients with cystic fibrosis. The incidence is greater than 20% in adults with CF. When a patient with cystic fibrosis has a pneumothorax, there is about a 50% chance that it will recur. The respiratory care practitioner must be alert for the signs and symptoms of this complication (e.g., pleuritic pain, shoulder

OVERVIEW

of the Cardiopulmonary Clinical Manifestations Associated with CYSTIC FIBROSIS (Continued)

pain, sudden shortness of breath). Precipitating factors include excessive exertion, high altitude, and positive-pressure breathing.

CLINICAL DATA OBTAINED FROM LABORATORY TESTS AND SPECIAL PROCEDURES

Pulmonary Function Study Findings

Expiratory Maneuver Findings
(see page 62 ◆▶)

FVC	FEV$_T$	FEF$_{25\%-75\%}$	FEF$_{200-1200}$
↓	↓	↓	↓
PEFR	MVV	FEF$_{50\%}$	FEV$_{1\%}$
↓	↓	↓	↓

Lung Volume and Capacity Findings
(see page 66 ◆▶)

V$_T$	RV	FRC	TLC
N or ↑	↑	↑	N or ↑
VC	IC	ERV	RV/TLC ratio
↓	N or ↓	N or ↓	↑

Arterial Blood Gases

Mild to Moderate Cystic Fibrosis
Acute Alveolar Hyperventilation with Hypoxemia
(see page 70 ◆▶)

pH	Paco$_2$	HCO$_3^-$	Pao$_2$
↑	↓	↓ (Slightly)	↓

Severe Cystic Fibrosis
Chronic Ventilatory Failure with Hypoxemia
(see page 73 ◆▶)

pH	Paco$_2$	HCO$_3^-$	Pao$_2$
Normal	↑	↑ (Significantly)	↓

Acute Ventilatory Changes Superimposed on Chronic Ventilatory Failure
(see page 75 ◆▶)

Because acute ventilatory changes frequently are seen in patients with chronic ventilatory failure, the respiratory care practitioner must be familiar with and alert for (1) acute alveolar hyperventilation superimposed on chronic ventilatory failure and (2) acute ventilatory failure superimposed on chronic ventilatory failure.

Oxygenation Indices (see page 82 ◆▶)

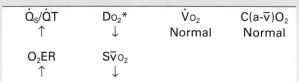

$\dot{Q}_S/\dot{Q}T$	Do$_2$*	$\dot{V}o_2$	C(a-$\bar{v}$)O$_2$
↑	↓	Normal	Normal
O$_2$ER	S$\bar{v}$o$_2$		
↑	↓		

*The Do$_2$ may be normal in patients who have compensated to the decreased oxygenation status with (1) an increased cardiac output, (2) an increased hemoglobin level, or (3) a combination of both. When the Do$_2$ is normal, the O$_2$ER is usually normal.

Hemodynamic Indices (Severe) (see page 99 ◆▶)

CVP	RAP	$\overline{PA}$	PCWP
↑	↑	↑	Normal
CO	SV	SVI	CI
Normal	Normal	Normal	Normal
RVSWI	LVSWI	PVR	SVR
↑	Normal	↑	Normal

LABORATORY FINDINGS

- Complete blood count (CBC)—Elevated hemoglobin concentration and hematocrit
- Increased white cells with superimposed infections

RADIOLOGIC FINDINGS

Chest Radiograph
- Translucent (dark) lung fields
- Depressed or flattened diaphragms
- Right ventricular enlargement
- Areas of atelectasis and fibrosis
- Pneumothorax (spontaneous)
- Abscess formation (occasionally)

During the late stages of cystic fibrosis, the alveoli become hyperinflated, which causes the residual volume and functional residual capacity to increase. This condition decreases the density of the lungs. Consequently, the resistance to X-ray penetration is not as great, and the X-ray film becomes darker.

Because of the increased residual volume and functional residual capacity, the diaphragm is depressed and appears so on the radiograph (Figure 41-3). Because right ventricular enlargement and failure often develop as secondary problems during the advanced stages of cystic fibrosis, an enlarged heart may be identified on the radiograph. In some patients, areas of atelectasis, abscess formation, or a pneumothorax may be seen.

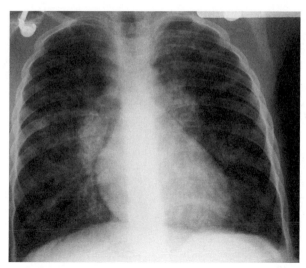

Figure 41–3 Chest X-ray of a patient with cystic fibrosis. Note the pulmonary hyperexpansion and the large main pulmonary artery segments.

Common Nonrespiratory Clinical Manifestations

MECONIUM ILEUS

Meconium ileus is an obstruction of the small intestine of the newborn that is caused by the impaction of thick, dry, tenacious meconium, usually at or near the ileocecal valve. This results from a deficiency in pancreatic enzymes and is the earliest manifestation of cystic fibrosis. The disease is suspected in newborns who demonstrate abdominal distention and fail to pass meconium within 12 hours after birth. Meconium ileus may occur in as many as 25% of infants with cystic fibrosis.

MECONIUM ILEUS EQUIVALENT

Meconium ileus equivalent is an intestinal obstruction (similar to meconium ileus in neonates) that occurs in older children and young adults with cystic fibrosis.

MALNUTRITION AND POOR BODY DEVELOPMENT

In cystic fibrosis, the pancreatic ducts become plugged with mucus, which leads to fibrosis of the pancreas. The pancreatic insufficiency that ensues inhibits the digestion of protein and fat, and this results in deficiencies of vitamins A, D, E, and K. Vitamin K deficiency may be the cause of easy bruising and bleeding. Approximately 80% of all patients with cystic fibrosis have vitamin deficiencies and therefore show signs of malnutrition and poor body development throughout life.

NASAL POLYPS AND SINUSITIS

About 20% of patients with cystic fibrosis have nasal polyps and sinusitis. The polyps are usually multiple and may cause nasal obstruction; in some cases, they cause distortion of the normal facial features.

INFERTILITY

Approximately 99% of men with cystic fibrosis are sterile. Women with cystic fibrosis who become pregnant are not likely to carry the infant to term. An infant who is carried to term will either have cystic fibrosis or be a carrier.

General Management of Cystic Fibrosis

The patient and the patient's family should be instructed regarding the disease and the way it affects bodily functions. They should be taught home care therapies, the goals of these therapies, and the way to administer medications. Patients with severe cystic fibrosis commonly are managed by a pulmonary rehabilitation team. Such teams include a respiratory therapist, a physical therapist, a respiratory nurse specialist, an occupational therapist, a dietitian, a social worker, and a psychologist. A pediatrician or an internist trained in respiratory rehabilitation outlines and orchestrates the patient's therapeutic program.

Patients with cystic fibrosis should have regular medical checkups for comparative purposes to determine their general health, weight, height, pulmonary function abilities, and sputum culture. In addition, time-released pancreatic enzymes, such as pancreatic lipase, are prescribed for patients with cystic fibrosis to aid food digestion. Patients also are encouraged to replace body salts either by heavily salting their food or by taking sodium supplements. Supplemental multivitamins and minerals also are important.

RESPIRATORY CARE TREATMENT PROTOCOLS

Oxygen Therapy Protocol

Oxygen therapy is used to treat hypoxemia, decrease the work of breathing, and decrease myocardial work. The hypoxemia that develops in cystic fibrosis is caused by the pulmonary shunting associated with the disorder and is often refractory to oxygen therapy. When the patient demonstrates chronic ventilatory failure during the advanced stages of cystic fibrosis, caution must be taken not to overoxygenate the patient (see Oxygen Therapy Protocol, Protocol 9-1).

Bronchopulmonary Hygiene Therapy Protocol

Because of the excessive mucus production and accumulation associated with cystic fibrosis, a number of respiratory therapy modalities are used to enhance the mobilization of bronchial secretions. Aggressive and vigorous bronchial hygiene—especially chest physical therapy and postural drainage—should be performed regularly on patients both in the hospital and at home (see Bronchopulmonary Hygiene Therapy Protocol, Protocol 9-2).

Hyperinflation Therapy Protocol

Hyperinflation techniques often are administered to offset the alveolar atelectasis associated with cystic fibrosis (see Hyperinflation Therapy Protocol, Protocol 9-3).

Aerosolized Medication Protocol

Various sympathomimetic, parasympatholytic, and mucolytic agents are commonly used to induce bronchial smooth muscle relaxation and mucus thinning. Dornase alpha (Pulmozyme—also known as rhDNase or DNase) has been shown to be especially helpful in the management of cystic fibrosis. This aerosolized agent is an enzyme that breaks down the deoxyribonucleic acid (DNA) of the thick bronchial mucus associated with cystic fibrosis. Dornase alpha has shown good results in improving the lung function of patients with cystic fibrosis while reducing the frequency and severity of respiratory infections (see Aerosolized Medication Protocol, Protocol 9-4).

Mechanical Ventilation Protocol

Because acute ventilatory failure superimposed on chronic ventilatory failure often is seen in patients with severe cystic fibrosis, mechanical ventilation may at these times be required to maintain an adequate ventilatory status. Continuous mechanical ventilation is justified when the acute ventilatory failure is thought to be reversible (see Mechanical Ventilation Protocol, Protocol 9-5), for example, when pneumonia complicates the condition.

MEDICATION AND SPECIAL PROCEDURES PRESCRIBED BY THE PHYSICIAN

Xanthines

Xanthines are occasionally used to enhance bronchial smooth muscle relaxation (see Appendix II).

Expectorants

Expectorants often are used when water alone or aerosolized mucolytics are not sufficient to facilitate expectoration (see Appendix II).

Antibiotics

Antibiotics commonly are administered to prevent or combat secondary respiratory tract infections (see Appendix II).

Lung or Heart/Lung Transplantation

Several large organ transplant centers currently are performing lung or heart/lung transplantations in selected patients with cystic fibrosis whose general body condition is good.

Case Study: CYSTIC FIBROSIS

Admitting History

A 27-year-old man has a long history of respiratory problems caused by cystic fibrosis. Even though his medical records are incomplete, he reported on admission that his parents told him that he had suffered several episodes of pneumonia during his early years. He is an adopted child and therefore does not know his biologic family history. His parents are actively involved in his general care, which entails the home care suggestions or therapeutic procedures presented by the pulmonary rehabilitation team. He takes supplemental multivitamins and timed-release oral pancreatic enzymes regularly, as prescribed by his doctor.

During his teens he had fewer respiratory symptoms than he has today and was able to lead a relatively normal life. During that time, he took up water-skiing and became proficient in the slalom event. He is known to most of his associates as a "wonder." Although he qualifies for disability income because of his continual shortness of breath, he is able to do various small jobs, which always relate to water-skiing. He is well known throughout the water-skiing circuit as an excellent chief judge at national and regional tournaments. In addition, he is a certified driver for jump-trick and slalom events and recently has become involved in selling water-ski tournament ropes and handles, which provides him with a small additional income.

Over the past 3 years, his cough has become more persistent and increasingly productive, with about a cupful of sputum noted daily. Over the same period, he has noted intermittent hemoptysis and has become short of breath when climbing stairs. Even though the man has a normal appetite, he has lost a great deal of weight over the past 2 years. On admission, he denied experiencing any recent changes in bowel habits, despite his weight loss, but said that he has noticed a tendency to pass rather pale stools. Much to the chagrin of his doctor, 3 years ago he began smoking about 10 cigarettes a day, his reason being that the cigarettes help him cough up the sputum.

Physical Examination

On examination, the patient appeared pale, cyanotic, and thin. He had a barrel chest and was using his accessory muscles of respiration. Clubbing of the fingers was present. He demonstrated a frequent, productive cough. His sputum was sweet smelling, thick, and yellow-green. His neck veins were distended, and he showed mild-to-moderate peripheral edema. He stated that he had not been this short of breath in a long time.

He had a blood pressure of 142/90, a heart rate of 108 bpm, and a respiratory rate of 28/min. He was afebrile. Palpation of the chest was unremarkable. Expiration was prolonged. Hyperresonant notes were elicited bilaterally during percussion. Auscultation revealed diminished breath sounds and heart sounds. Crackles and rhonchi were heard throughout both lung fields.

His chart showed that during his last medical checkup (about 10 months before this admission) a pulmonary function test (PFT) was conducted. Results revealed moderate-to-severe airway obstruction. No blood gases were analyzed.

His chest X-ray on this admission revealed hyperlucent lung fields, depressed hemidiaphragms, and right ventricular enlargement (Figure 41-4). His arterial blood gas values (ABGs) on 1.5 L/min oxygen by nasal cannula were as follows: pH 7.51, $Paco_2$ 58 mm Hg, HCO_3^- 43 mMol/L, and Pao_2 66 mm Hg. His hemoglobin oxygen saturation measured by pulse oximetry (Spo_2) was 94%. On the basis of these clinical data, the following SOAP was documented:

Respiratory Assessment and Plan

S   "I've not been this short of breath in a long time."

O   Skin: pale, cyanotic; barrel chest and use of accessory muscles of respiration; digital clubbing; cough frequent and productive; sputum: sweet-smelling, thick, yellow-green; distended neck veins and peripheral edema; vital signs: BP 142/90, HR 108, RR 28, T normal; bilateral

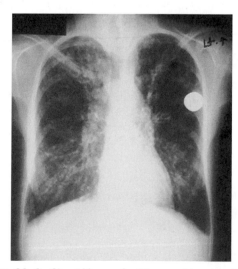

Figure 41–4   Chest X-ray of a 27-year-old man with cystic fibrosis.

hyperresonant percussion notes; diminished breath sounds; crackles and rhonchi; CXR: hyperlucency, flattened diaphragms, and right ventricular enlargement; ABGs (1.5 L/min O_2 by nasal cannula): pH 7.51, $Paco_2$ 58, HCO_3^- 43, Pao_2 66; Spo_2 94%

A
- Respiratory distress (general appearance, vital signs)
- Excessive tracheobronchial tree secretions (productive cough)
- Infection likely (yellow-green sputum)
- Hyperinflated alveoli (barrel chest, use of accessory muscles, CXR)
- Acute alveolar hyperventilation superimposed on chronic ventilatory failure with mild hypoxemia (history, ABGs)
  - Possible impending acute ventilatory failure
- Cor pulmonale (distended neck veins, peripheral edema, CXR)

P Bronchopulmonary Hygiene Therapy Protocol (cough and deep breathe Tx q 4 h), sputum culture). Oxygen Therapy Protocol (2 L by nasal cannula). Monitor possible impending ventilatory failure closely (pulse oximetry, vital signs, ABGs).

• • • • •

48 Hours After Admission

The respiratory therapist from the consult service noted that the patient was again in respiratory distress. The man stated that he could not get enough air to sleep even 10 minutes. He appeared cyanotic and was using his accessory muscles of respiration. His vital signs were as follows: blood pressure 147/95, heart rate 117 bpm, respiratory rate 32/min, and temperature 37° C (98.6° F).

He coughed frequently, and although his cough was weak, he produced large amounts of thick, green sputum. Hyperresonant notes were produced during percussion over both lung fields. On auscultation, breath sounds and heart sounds were diminished. Crackles, rhonchi, and wheezing were heard throughout both lung fields. No recent chest X-ray was available. A sputum culture confirmed the presence of *Pseudomonas aeruginosa*. His Spo_2 was 92% and his ABGs were as follows: pH 7.55, $Paco_2$ 54 mm Hg, HCO_3^- 45 mMol/L, and Pao_2 57 mm Hg. On the basis of these clinical data, the following SOAP was documented:

Respiratory Assessment and Plan

S "I can't get enough air to sleep 10 minutes!"

O Cyanosis and use of accessory muscles of respiration; vital signs: BP 147/95, HR 117, RR 32, T 37° C (98.6° F); cough: frequent, weak, and productive of large amounts of thick,

green sputum; *Pseudomonas aeruginosa* cultured; bilateral hyperresonant notes and diminished breath sounds; crackles, rhonchi, and wheezes; Spo_2 92%; ABGs: pH 7.55, $Paco_2$ 54, HCO_3^- 45, Pao_2 57

A
- Continued respiratory distress (general appearance, vital signs, use of accessory muscles)
- Excessive bronchial secretions (cough, sputum, breath sounds)
- Poor ability to mobilize secretions (weak cough)
- Acute alveolar hyperventilation superimposed on chronic ventilatory failure with mild-to-moderate hypoxemia (ABGs)
- Possible impending ventilatory failure

P Start Aerosolized Medication Protocol (0.5 cc albuterol in 2 cc rhDNase q 4 h). Up-regulate Bronchopulmonary Hygiene Therapy per protocol (CPT and PEP therapy q 2 h). Up-regulate oxygen therapy per protocol (HAFOE mask at Fio_2 0.35). Continue to monitor possible impending ventilatory failure closely.

• • • • •

64 Hours After Admission

The respiratory care practitioner noted that the patient was in obvious respiratory distress. The patient said he could not find a position that allowed him to breathe comfortably. He appeared cyanotic and was using pursed-lip breathing, using his accessory muscles of respiration. His vital signs were as follows: blood pressure 145/90, heart rate 120 bpm, respiratory rate 22/min, and oral temperature 38° C (100.5° F). Palpation was normal, but bilateral hyperresonant percussion notes were elicited. Auscultation revealed crackles, rhonchi, and wheezing bilaterally. No recent chest X-ray was available. His Spo_2 was 65%, and his ABGs were as follows: pH 7.33, $Paco_2$ 79 mm Hg, HCO_3^- 41 mMol/L, and Pao_2 37 mm Hg%. On the basis of these clinical data, the following SOAP was entered in the patient's chart:

Respiratory Assessment and Plan

S "I can't get into a comfortable position to breathe."

O Cyanosis; pursed-lip breathing and use of accessory muscles of respiration; vital signs: BP 145/90, HR 120, RR 22, T 38° C (100.5° F); bilateral hyperresonant percussion notes, crackles, rhonchi, and wheezing; Spo_2 65%; ABGs: pH 7.33, $Paco_2$ 79, HCO_3^- 41, Pao_2 37

A
- Continued respiratory distress (general appearance, vital signs, use of accessory muscles, pursed-lip breathing)

- Excessive bronchial secretions
  (cough, sputum, breath sounds)
- Acute ventilatory failure superimposed
  on chronic ventilatory failure with severe
  hypoxemia (ABGs, vital signs)

P Contact physician stat. Consider intubation
and mechanical ventilation. Continue bronchial
hygiene therapy per protocol (after patient has
been placed on ventilator). Up-regulate oxygen
therapy per protocol (initially, F_{IO_2} 0.50 on
ventilator). Monitor closely.

Discussion

The science of respiratory care has advanced over
the years, and the prognosis for patients with this
multisystem genetic disorder has improved. In this
patient's lifetime, at least four therapeutic landmarks
can be noted:

1. Vigorous use of chest physical therapy
   (percussion and postural drainage)
2. Intermittent treatment of secretions with
   antibiotics and mucolytic enzymes, such as
   rhDNase
3. Positive expiratory pressure (PEP) therapy
4. Lung transplantation (when all else fails)

This patient had received at least three of these
treatments and was in the hands of caring parents.
His own stubborn nature and interest in athletics
were clearly helpful in his prolonged survival.
Important to note are the circumstances surrounding
his admission, especially the fact that he had
experienced hemoptysis, dyspnea, and weight loss
during the several years preceding his admission.
Note also that he had started smoking cigarettes.

In this case study, the patient's chief complaints
purposely have been buried in the admitting history
by the authors. The reader should have discerned
that the patient was coughing productively and had
hemoptysis, dyspnea, and weight loss. The recommended therapeutic strategy arises from recognition
of these four presenting complaints. Note also that

on admission the patient presented with neck vein
distention and peripheral edema, suggesting cor
pulmonale. If the experience with chronic obstructive pulmonary disease can be translated to patients
with cystic fibrosis, this is a bad prognostic sign
and one that clearly calls for intensification of the
therapeutic regimen.

Note that on the **initial physical examination**,
the patient demonstrated **Excessive Bronchial
Secretions** and a productive cough; no baseline arterial blood gases existed with which to compare his
current values (see Figure 9-11). Thus the observation of an elevated Pa_{CO_2} should be taken very, very
seriously since (at least initially) whether this value
is a "chronic" arterial blood gas value is unclear.

At the time of the **second evaluation** the
patient clearly is not improving. The up-regulation
of bronchial hygiene therapy at this point was
appropriate—the increased chest physical therapy
(along with PEP therapy) q 2 h, and rhDNase
therapy. A repeat chest X-ray would not be out of
order at this time.

The **third assessment** suggests that the patent
clearly is deteriorating despite vigorous noninvasive
therapy. At this point, the patient was placed on an
F_{IO_2} of 0.5, but the stat call to the physician regarding
the acute ventilatory failure was clearly justified.
The addition of intubation and mechanical ventilation at this time prevents fatigue, allows deep nasal
tracheal suctioning, and facilitates repeat bronchoscopy if it becomes necessary.

Despite this initial downhill course, the patient
was placed on a ventilator and slowly improved.
Over the next 7 days, the patient was extubated. The
therapist should note that despite all the "good"
things the patient and family did to treat his illness,
the patient's initiation of smoking clearly could be
a "last-straw" phenomenon. The patient should be
placed on a smoking-cessation program. This step is
as important for the long-term prognosis as is the
skill of the practitioner caring for him during this
bout of acute ventilatory failure.

SELF-ASSESSMENT QUESTIONS

Multiple Choice

1. Which of the following organisms is/are commonly found in the tracheobronchial tree secretions of patients with cystic fibrosis?

   I. *Staphylococcus*
   II. *Haemophilus influenzae*
   III. *Streptococcus*
   IV. *Pseudomonas aeruginosa*

   a. I only
   b. II only
   c. IV only
   d. I and IV only
   e. I, II, and IV only

2. When two carriers of cystic fibrosis produce children, there is a:

   I. 75% chance that the baby will be a carrier
   II. 25% chance that the baby will be completely normal
   III. 50% chance that the baby will have cystic fibrosis
   IV. 25% chance that the baby will have cystic fibrosis

   a. I only
   b. III only
   c. II and IV only
   d. I and II only
   e. I, III, and IV only

3. The cystic fibrosis gene is located on which chromosome?

   a. 5
   b. 6
   c. 7
   d. 8
   e. 9

4. In cystic fibrosis the patient commonly demonstrates which of the following?

   I. Increased FEV_T
   II. Decreased MVV
   III. Increased RV
   IV. Decreased FEV_1/FVC ratio

   a. I only
   b. II only
   c. III only
   d. III and IV only
   e. II, III, and IV only

5. During the advanced stages of cystic fibrosis, the patient generally demonstrates which of the following?

   I. Bronchial breath sounds
   II. Dull percussion notes
   III. Diminished breath sounds
   IV. Hyperresonant percussion notes

   a. I and III only
   b. II and IV only
   c. I and IV only
   d. III and IV only
   e. II and III only

6. Approximately 80% of all patients with cystic fibrosis demonstrate a deficiency in which of the following vitamins?

   I. A
   II. B
   III. D
   IV. E
   V. K

   a. III and IV only
   b. I, IV, and V only
   c. II, III, and IV only
   d. I, III, IV, and V only
   e. I, II, III, IV, and V

7. In children, which of the following sweat chloride concentration values is diagnostic of cystic fibrosis?

   a. 50 mEq/L
   b. 60 mEq/L
   c. 70 mEq/L
   d. 80 mEq/L
   e. 90 mEq/L

8. Which of the following is/are a mucolytic agent(s)?

   I. N-acetylcysteine
   II. Aristocort
   III. rhDNase
   IV. Aldactone

   a. I only
   b. II only
   c. III only
   d. II and IV only
   e. I and III only

9. In regard to the secretion of sodium and chloride, the sweat glands of patients with cystic fibrosis secrete up to:

   a. 3 times the normal amount
   b. 5 times the normal amount
   c. 7 times the normal amount
   d. 10 times the normal amount
   e. 15 times the normal amount

10. Which of the following clinical manifestations are associated with severe cystic fibrosis?

   I. Decreased hemoglobin concentration
   II. Increased central venous pressure
   III. Decreased breath sounds
   IV. Increased pulmonary vascular resistance

   a. I and III only
   b. II and III only
   c. III and IV only
   d. II, III, and IV only
   e. I, II, III, and IV

Answers appear in Appendix XI.

PART XIII

Other Important Topics

CHAPTER 42

Near Drowning

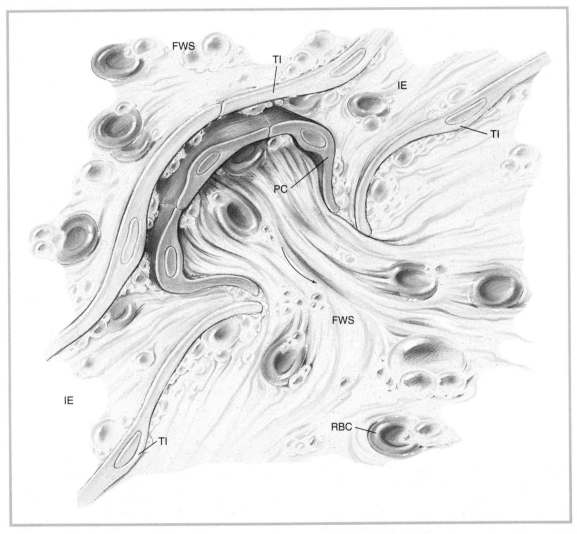

Figure 42–1 Near wet drowning. Cross-sectional, microscopic view of the alveolar-capillary unit. Illustration shows fluid moving from a pulmonary capillary to an alveolus. *PC*, Pulmonary capillary; *FWS*, frothy white secretions; *RBC*, red blood cell; *TI*, type I alveolar cell; *IE*, interstitial edema. See also Plate 34.

Anatomic Alterations of the Lungs

Drowning is defined as suffocation and death as a result of submersion in liquid. Drowning may be classified further as *near drowning, dry drowning,* and *wet drowning. Near drowning* refers to the situation in which a victim survives a liquid submersion, at least temporarily. In *dry drowning,* the glottis spasms and prevents water from passing into the lungs. The lungs of dry drowning victims are usually normal.

In *wet drowning* the glottis relaxes and allows water to flood the tracheobronchial tree and alveoli. When fluid initially is inhaled, the bronchi constrict in response to a parasympathetic-mediated reflex. As fluid enters the alveoli, the pathophysiologic processes responsible for noncardiogenic pulmonary edema begin—that is, fluid from the pulmonary capillaries moves into the perivascular spaces, peribronchial spaces, alveoli, bronchioles, and bronchi. As a consequence of this fluid movement, the alveolar walls and interstitital spaces swell, pulmonary surfactant concentration decreases, and the alveolar surface tension increases.

As this condition intensifies, the alveoli shrink and atelectasis develops. Excess fluid in the interstitital spaces causes the lymphatic vessels to dilate and the lymph flow to increase. In severe cases, the fluid that accumulates in the tracheobronchial tree is churned into a frothy, white (sometimes blood-tinged) sputum as a result of air moving in and out of the lungs (generally by means of mechanical ventilation).

Finally, if the victim was submerged in unclean water (e.g., swamp, pond, sewage, or mud), a number of pathogens (e.g., *Pseudomonas*) and solid material may be aspirated. When this happens, pneumonia may occur, and in severe cases, adult respiratory distress syndrome (ARDS) may develop. Although the theory has been controversial in the past, it is now believed that the major pathologic changes of the lungs are essentially the same in fresh water and sea water wet drownings; both result in a reduction in pulmonary surfactant, alveolar injury, atelectasis, and pulmonary edema (Figure 42-1).

The major pulmonary pathologic and structural changes associated with wet drowning are as follows:

- Laryngospasm and bronchial constriction
- Interstitial edema, including engorgement of the perivascular and peribronchial spaces, alveolar walls, and interstitial spaces
- Decreased pulmonary surfactant
- Increased surface tension of alveolar fluid
- Alveolar shrinkage and atelectasis
- Frothy, white secretions throughout the tracheobronchial tree

Etiology

Between 6000 and 8000 people drown each year in the United States. Children under the age of 5 account for about 40% of these deaths. An additional 20% of the drowning deaths occur in persons between 5 and 20 years of age. About 8000 victims of near drownings are hospitalized annually. The peak incidence of drownings occurs at 4 years of age for both boys and girls; usually, these accidents are related to poor adult supervision. In fact, it is estimated that the drowning of younger children is witnessed in fewer than 20% of the cases, yet up to 85% of the victims are supposedly receiving responsible supervision.

Male victims have a second peak incidence between 15 and 19 years of age; usually, the accidents are related to alcohol intoxication and risk-taking behavior (e.g., diving into shallow water, engaging in horseplay, and operating powerboats). African-American children drown at a rate of 4.5 per 100,000, usually in freshwater lakes and ponds. Caucasian children drown at a rate of 2.5 per 100,000, usually in home pools. Box 42-1 summarizes the general sequence of events that occurs in drowning or near drowning. Victims submerged in cold water generally demonstrate a much higher survival rate than victims submerged in warm water. Table 42-1 lists favorable prognostic factors in cold-water near drowning.

BOX 42–1

Drowning or Near Drowning Sequence

1. Panic and violent struggle to return to the surface
2. Period of calmness and apnea
3. Swallowing of large amounts of fluid, followed by vomiting
4. Gasping inspirations and aspiration
5. Convulsions
6. Coma
7. Death

TABLE 42–1 **Favorable Prognostic Factors in Cold-Water Near Drowning**

Age	The younger, the better
Submersion time	The shorter, the better (60 minutes appears to be the upper limit in cold-water submersions)
Water temperature	The colder, the better (range, 27° F to 70° F)
Water quality	The cleaner, the better
Other injuries	None serious
Amount of struggle	The less struggle, the better
Cardiopulmonary resuscitation (CPR) quality	Good CPR technique increases the survival rate
Suicidal intent	Lower survival rate among victims who attempted suicide than among victims of accidental submersion

OVERVIEW
of the Cardiopulmonary Clinical Manifestations Associated with NEAR WET DROWNING

The following clinical manifestations result from the pathologic mechanisms caused (or activated) by **Atelectasis** (see Figure 9-7), **Alveolar Consolidation** (see Figure 9-8), **Increased Alveolar-Capillary Membrane Thickness** (see Figure 9-9), and **Bronchospasm** (see Figure 9-10)—the major anatomic alterations of the lungs associated with near wet drowning (see Figure 42-1).

CLINICAL DATA OBTAINED AT THE PATIENT'S BEDSIDE

The Physical Examination

Apnea is directly related to the length of time the victim is submerged. The longer the submersion, the more likely it is that the victim will not have spontaneous respiration. When spontaneous breathing is present, the respiratory rate is usually increased.

Vital Signs

Increased respiratory rate (see page 31 ◆)

Several pathophysiologic mechanisms operating simultaneously may lead to an increased ventilatory rate:
- Stimulation of peripheral chemoreceptors (hypoxemia)
- Decreased lung compliance/increased ventilatory rate relationship
- Stimulation of J receptors
- Anxiety (conscious patient)

Increased heart rate (pulse), cardiac output, and blood pressure (see pages 11 and 99 ◆)

Cyanosis (see page 45 ◆)

Cough and Sputum Production (Frothy, Pink, Stable Bubbles) (see page 47 ◆)

Chest Assessment Findings (see page 22 ◆)
- Crackles and rhonchi

CLINICAL DATA OBTAINED FROM LABORATORY TESTS AND SPECIAL PROCEDURES

Pulmonary Function Study Findings (extrapolated data for instructional purposes)

Expiratory Maneuver Findings (see page 61 ◆)

FVC	FEV$_T$	FEF$_{25\%-75\%}$	FEF$_{200-1200}$
↓	N or ↓	N or ↓	N
PEFR	**MVV**	**FEF$_{50\%}$**	**FEV$_{1\%}$**
N	N or ↓	N	N or ↑

Lung Volume and Capacity Findings (see page 62 ◆)

V$_T$	RV	FRC	TLC
N or ↓	↓	↓	↓
VC	**IC**	**ERV**	**RV/TLC%**
↓	↓	↓	N

Arterial Blood Gases

Early and Advanced Stages of Near Drowning
Acute Ventilatory Failure with Hypoxemia (see page 73 ◆)

pH*	Paco$_2$	HCO$_3^-$*	Pao$_2$
↓	↑	↓ (lactic acidosis is common)	↓

*When tissue hypoxia is severe enough to produce lactic acid, the pH and HCO$_3^-$ values will be lower than expected for a particular Paco$_2$ level.

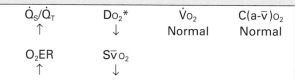

OVERVIEW
of the Cardiopulmonary Clinical Manifestations Associated with
NEAR WET DROWNING (Continued)

Oxygenation Indices (see page 82 ◆▶)

$\dot{Q}_S/\dot{Q}_T$	D_{O_2}*	$\dot{V}_{O_2}$	$C(a-\bar{v})_{O_2}$
↑	↓	Normal	Normal

O_2ER	$S\bar{v}_{O_2}$
↑	↓

*The D_{O_2} may be normal in patients who have compensated to the decreased oxygenation status with an increased cardiac output. When the D_{O_2} is normal, the O_2ER is usually normal.

RADIOLOGIC FINDINGS

Chest Radiograph

- Fluffy infiltrates
- Pneumothorax and pneumomediastinum

The initial appearance of the radiograph may vary from being completely normal to showing varying degrees of pulmonary edema (Figure 42-2). It should be emphasized, however, that an initially normal chest radiograph still may be associated with significant hypoxemia, hypercapnia, and acidosis. In any case, radiographic deterioration may occur in the first 48 to 72 hours. Because a pneumothorax or pneumomediastinum often occurs in near drowning patients who are on ventilator support, the respiratory care practitioner must be alert for this condition.

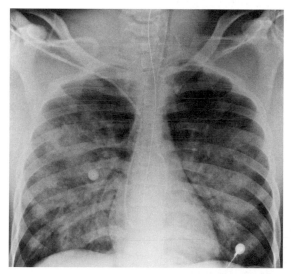

Figure 42–2 This radiograph of a young man, taken just after an episode of near drowning, shows a pulmonary edema pattern. (From Armstrong P et al: *Imaging of diseases of the chest*, ed 2, St Louis, 1995, Mosby.)

General Management

THE FIRST RESPONDER

The first objectives in treating a drowning victim are to remove the person from the water and, if the patient has no spontaneous ventilation and pulse, to call for help and immediately initiate cardiopulmonary resuscitation (CPR). When the patient has been submerged for less than 60 minutes in cold water, fixed and dilated pupils do not necessarily indicate a poor prognosis. Because water is an excellent conductor of body heat (cold water can cool the body 25 times faster than air at the same temperature) and because evaporation further reduces an individual's body heat, the victim's wet clothing should immediately be removed and replaced with warm, dry coverings.

MANAGEMENT DURING TRANSPORT

The primary goal in treating near drowning victims during transport is high-quality CPR, with 100% oxygen. The victim's body heat should be conserved by removing any wet garments and covering high heat-loss areas with warm, dry coverings. High heat-loss areas of the body include the head and neck, axillae, and inguinal areas. The victim's vital signs, including rectal temperature, should be monitored closely while traveling to the hospital. The victim's body temperature frequently falls during transport, and measures to conserve the patient's body heat are extremely important. Victims with spontaneous ventilation should be monitored with pulse oximetry during transport, if at all possible.

MANAGEMENT AT THE HOSPITAL

Treatment at the hospital is an extension of prehospital management. Virtually every near drowning victim suffers from hypoxemia, hypercapnia, and acidosis (acute ventilatory failure). Hypoxemia generally persists after aspiration of fluids in the airway (wet drowning) because of alveolar capillary damage and continued intrapulmonary shunting. The degree of hypoxemia is directly related to the amount of alveolar-capillary damage. A chest radiograph should be obtained to help evaluate the magnitude of the alveolar-capillary injury. However, a normal chest radiograph does not rule out the possibility of alveolar-capillary deterioration during the first 24 hours.

Intubation and mechanical ventilation should be performed immediately for any victim with no spontaneous ventilations and for victims who are breathing spontaneously but are unable to maintain a Pao_2 of 60 mm Hg with an Fio_2 of 0.5 or lower. Because of the nature of the alveolar-capillary injury seen in most wet drowning victims, mechanical ventilation with positive end-expiratory pressure (PEEP) or continuous positive airway pressure (CPAP) should be administered. It should be noted, however, that barotrauma is a common complication of ventilatory therapy in these patients. The patient also may benefit from inotropic agents and diuretics.

Finally, warming the victim should progress concomitantly with all the other treatment modalities. Nearly all near drowning victims are hypothermic to some degree. Depending on the severity of the hypothermia and on the available resources, a number of warming techniques may be employed. For example, the body temperature can be increased by the intravenous administration of heated solutions; by heated lavage of the gastric, intrathoracic, pericardial, and peritoneal spaces; or by the administration of heated lavage to the bladder and rectum. Additional external heat techniques include heating blankets, warm baths, and immersion in a heated Hubbard tank. In rare cases, extracorporeal circulation, with complete cardiopulmonary bypass, has been successful.

Case Study: NEAR DROWNING

Admitting History and Physical Examination

This 12-year-old boy had a history of a seizure disorder but had not taken his medication for almost a year. On the morning of admission, he participated in a regular swimming class in the junior high school pool. According to the coach on duty, there had been a "pool check" 30 seconds before the patient's partner reported that the patient seemed to stay under water "too long."

When taken from the water, he was unconscious and "blue." He was given mouth-to-mouth resuscitation, and by the time the EMT squad arrived about 20 minutes later, he was breathing at a rate of 10/min, although his lips and fingers were still cyanotic. He remained comatose and was taken to the nearest hospital.

An X-ray showed bilateral, diffuse increase in density, which suggested pulmonary edema or possible hemorrhage. His oxygen saturation on 5 Lpm O_2 was 72%. Plans were made to transfer him to a nearby tertiary care medical center.

The respiratory therapist in the emergency department entered the following assessment:

Respiratory Assessment and Plan

S   N/A (patient comatose). History of near drowning.

O   Comatose. Spontaneous breathing at 10/min, BP 100/60, P 140. Crackles bilaterally. Nasotracheal suctioning yields clear fluid. Cyanotic. Spo_2 on 5 Lpm O_2: 72%.

A   • Near drowning. R/O seizure disorder (history)
    • Increased airway secretions (suctioning of clear fluid)
    • Poor oxygenation (cyanosis, Spo_2)

P   Stat ABG on 100% oxygen, then titrate per Oxygen Therapy Protocol. Have equipment to intubate on standby. Bag, ventilate, and suction. Provide continuous pulse oximetry. Continue nasotracheal suctioning. Take seizure precautions. Will accompany on transfer.

• • • • •

On admission to the medical center, the patient was described as a well-developed, slightly obese adolescent in obvious respiratory distress. He was now alert, oriented, but extremely apprehensive. His vital signs were: temperature (rectal) 100.8° F, blood pressure 112/70, pulse 140/min, and respirations 60/min. The lips and fingertips were cyanotic. The respirations were paradoxical. There was marked substernal retraction. Breath sounds were diminished bilaterally, and loud crackles were heard over both lungs anteriorly.

Laboratory examination revealed a leukocytosis of 21,000/mm³ and 2+ albumin in the urine but was otherwise within normal limits. There was no evidence of hemolysis. On an F_{IO_2} of 0.8, the arterial blood gases were pH 7.29, $Paco_2$ 52, HCO_3^- 25, and Pao_2 38. The patient's condition was rapidly deteriorating, and he developed even more severe crackles. He now had a spontaneous cough with frothy sputum production. The chest X-ray revealed pulmonary edema and nearly complete opacification of both lungs. The following was entered in the patient's chart:

Respiratory Assessment and Plan

S Anxious, dyspneic, crying. "I can't get my breath. Where am I? Am I going to die?"

O Afebrile. BP 112/70, P 140/min, RR 60/min. Cyanotic. Paradoxical chest/abdomen movements, sternal retraction. Crackles in both lungs anteriorly. Spontaneous cough with frothy sputum production, WBC 21,000/mm³. On 80% oxygen: pH 7.29, $Paco_2$ 52, HCO_3^- 25, Pao_2 38. CXR: "White-out."

A • Pulmonary edema secondary to near drowning (frothy sputum)
• Acute ventilatory failure with metabolic acidosis (likely lactic acid) with severe hypoxemia (ABG)

P Place on 100% O_2. Page physician stat. Obtain intubation equipment and prepare to place patient on ventilator. Follow oximetry. Prepare to assist in placement of Swan-Ganz catheter.

• • • • •

The patient was intubated with thiopental sodium and paralyzed with succinylcholine. As soon as he was intubated, copious pink foam was aspirated from the endotracheal tube. He was alternately suctioned and ventilated with an Ambu bag. He was given 7 mg of morphine for sedation and was mechanically ventilated at a rate of 10 breaths per minute. On an F_{IO_2} of 0.6 and PEEP of +10 cm H_2O, his blood gases were pH 7.44, $Paco_2$ 43, HCO_3^- 24, and Pao_2 109. Because he was still fighting the respirator, he was paralyzed with pancuronium.

After several hours, the lungs were clear, the secretions were no longer present, and his blood gases returned to normal on an F_{IO_2} of 0.5 and PEEP of 10 cm H_2O (pH 7.42, $Paco_2$ 42, HCO_3^- 24, Pao_2 98). His hemodynamic status was normal. The chest X-ray revealed considerable clearing of the earlier noted bilateral pulmonary infiltrates.

Respiratory Assessment and Plan

S N/A (patient sedated, paralyzed)

O Lungs clear. No secretions. On 50% O_2 and +10 PEEP: pH 7.42, $Paco_2$ 42, HCO_3^- 24, and Pao_2 98. CXR: Considerable improvement in bilateral infiltrates. No cardiomegaly. PCWP 10 mm Hg.

A • Considerable improvement on CMV and PEEP (general improvement of clinical indicators)
• Acceptable ventilatory and oxygenation status on present ventilatory settings (ABG)
• Frothy airway secretions no longer present (clear lungs and no secretions)

P Contact physician to wean from muscle relaxant. Wean from mechanically ventilated breaths, F_{IO_2}, and PEEP per Mechanical Ventilation Protocol. Change ventilator to Synchronized Intermittent Mandatory Ventilation (SIMV).

The patient was weaned from the ventilator over a period of 6 hours, after which he was extubated. The following morning, arterial blood gases on a 28% HAFOE oxygen mask were as follows: pH 7.37, $Paco_2$ 35, HCO_3^- 23, and Pao_2 158. X-ray examination of the lungs was normal. An oxygen titration protocol was performed. He was discharged 2 days later.

Discussion

This case demonstrates initial worsening of the near drowning victim despite intensive respiratory care. The initial ABGs showed severe hypoxemia as a result of **Alveolar-Capillary Thickening** and alveolar flooding (see Figures 9-9 and 42-1), as well as acute ventilatory failure and metabolic (probably lactic) acidosis. Bronchospasm never developed, and aggressive respiratory care prohibited the development of atelectasis and aspiration pneumonia. When suctioning, supplemental oxygen, and bag ventilation were no longer successful, the patient was intubated and mechanical ventilation with PEEP was begun.

Even on these modalities, the patient remained anxious and was ultimately paralyzed to allow better respiratory synchrony and diminish the chance for barotrauma. Morphine was used for its sedative qualities and as an afterload reducer.

This case demonstrates again the necessity for frequent reassessment of the patient and therapeutic adjustments to follow the findings so observed.

SELF-ASSESSMENT QUESTIONS

Fill in the Blanks

1. The situation in which a victim survives a liquid submersion, at least temporarily, is called _____ drowning.

2. In _____ drowning, the glottis spasms and prevents water from passing into the lungs.

3. In _____ drowning, the glottis relaxes and allows water to flood the tracheobronchial tree and alveoli.

4. In wet drowning, as fluid enters the alveoli, the pathophysiologic processes responsible for _____ begin.

5. Cold water can cool the body _____ times faster than air at the same temperature.

Complete the Following

In near drowning, the:

1. pH _____ increases _____ decreases _____ is normal

2. Pa_{CO_2} _____ increases _____ decreases _____ is normal

3. D_{O_2} _____ increases _____ decreases _____ is normal

4. Q_S/Q_T _____ increases _____ decreases _____ is normal

5. FRC _____ increases _____ decreases _____ is normal

Answers appear in Appendix XI.

CHAPTER 43

Smoke Inhalation and Thermal Injuries

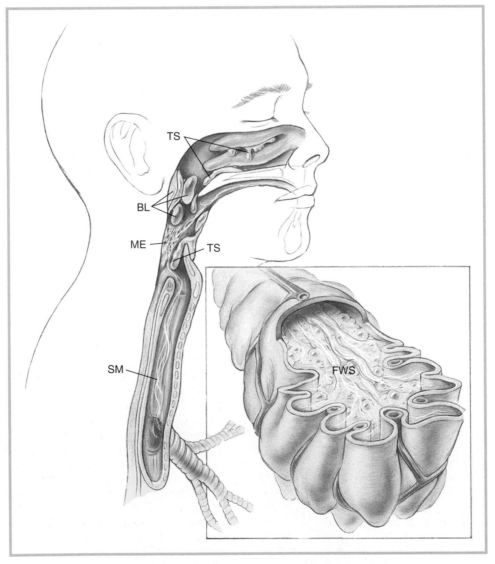

Figure 43–1 Smoke inhalation and thermal injuries. *TS,* Thick secretions; *BL,* airway blister; *ME,* mucosal edema; *SM,* smoke (toxic gas); *FWS,* frothy white secretions (pulmonary edema). See also Plate 35.

Anatomic Alterations of the Lungs

The inhalation of smoke and hot gases and body surface burns—in any combination—continue to be a major cause of morbidity and mortality among fire victims and firefighters. In general, fire-related pulmonary injuries can be divided into thermal and smoke (toxic gases) injuries.

THERMAL INJURY

Thermal injury refers to injury caused by the inhalation of hot gases. Thermal injuries are usually confined to the upper airway—the nasal cavity, oral cavity, nasopharynx, oropharynx, and larynx. The airways distal to the larynx and the alveoli are usually spared serious injury because of (1) the remarkable ability of the upper airways to cool hot gases, (2) reflex laryngospasm, and (3) glottic closure. The upper airway is an extremely efficient "heat sink." In fact, in 1945, Moritz and associates demonstrated that the inhalation of hot gases alone did not produce significant damage to the lung. Anesthetized dogs were forced to breathe air heated to 500° C through an insulated endotracheal tube. The researchers' results showed that the air temperature dropped to 50° C by the time it reached the level of the carina. No histologic damage was noticed in the lower trachea or lungs.

Even though thermal injury may occur with or without surface burns, the presence of facial burns is a classic predictor of thermal injury. Thermal injury to the upper airway results in blistering, mucosal edema, vascular congestion, epithelial sloughing, and accumulation of thick secretions. An acute upper airway obstruction (UAO) occurs in about 20% to 30% of hospitalized patients with thermal injury and is usually most marked in the supraglottic structures. When body surface burns require the rapid administration of resuscitative fluids, a UAO may develop rapidly (Figure 43-1).

It should be noted that the inhalation of steam at 100° C or greater usually results in severe damage at all levels of the respiratory tract. This damage occurs because steam has about 500 times the heat energy content of dry gas at the same temperature. Thermal injury to the distal airways results in mucosal edema, vascular congestion, epithelial sloughing, obliterative bronchiolitis, atelectasis, and pulmonary edema.

Therefore direct thermal injuries usually do not occur below the level of the larynx, except in the rare instance of steam inhalation. Damage to the distal airways mostly is caused by a variety of harmful products found in smoke.

SMOKE INHALATION INJURY

The pathologic changes in the distal airways and alveoli are mainly caused by the irritating and toxic gases, suspended soot particles, and vapors associated with incomplete combustion and smoke. Many of the substances found in smoke are extremely caustic to the tracheobronchial tree and poisonous to the body. The progression of injuries that develop from smoke inhalation and burns is described as the early stage, intermediate stage, and late stage.

Early Stage (0 to 24 Hours Postinhalation)

The injuries associated with smoke inhalation do not always appear right away, even when extensive body surface burns are evident. During the first 24 hours, however, the patient's pulmonary status often changes markedly. Initially, the tracheobronchial tree becomes more inflamed. This process causes an overabundance of bronchial secretions to move into the airways, resulting in bronchospasm. In addition, the toxic effects of smoke often slow the activity of the mucosal ciliary transport mechanism, causing further mucus retention.

Smoke inhalation also may cause noncardiogenic high-permeability pulmonary edema—commonly referred to in smoke inhalation cases as "leaky alveoli." Pulmonary edema also may be caused by overhydration resulting from overzealous fluid resuscitation (see insert panel in Figure 43-1). In severe cases, adult respiratory distress syndrome (ARDS) also may occur early in the course of the pathology.

Intermediate Stage (2 to 5 Days Postinhalation)

Whereas upper airway thermal injuries usually begin to improve during this period, the pathologic changes deep in the lungs associated with smoke inhalation usually peak. Mucus production continues to increase, while mucosal ciliary transport activity continues to decrease. The mucosa of the tracheobronchial tree frequently becomes necrotic and sloughs (usually between 3 and 4 days). The necrotic debris, excessive mucus production, and mucus retention lead to mucus plugging and atelectasis. In addition, the mucus accumulation often leads to bacterial colonization, bronchitis, and pneumonia. Organisms commonly cultured include gram-positive *Staphylococcus aureus* and gram-negative *Klebsiella, Enterobacter, Escherichia coli,* and *Pseudomonas.* If not already present, both *noncardiogenic pulmonary edema* and *acute respiratory distress syndrome* may develop at any time during this period.

When chest wall (thorax) burns are present, the situation may be further aggravated by the patient's inability to breathe deeply and cough as a result of

(1) pain, (2) the use of narcotics, (3) immobility, (4) increased airway resistance, and (5) decreased lung and chest compliance.

Late Stage (5 or More Days Postinhalation)

Infections resulting from burn wounds on the body surface are the major concern during this period. These infections often lead to sepsis and multiorgan failure. Sepsis-induced multiorgan failure is the primary cause of death in seriously burned patients during this stage.

Pneumonia continues to be a major problem during this period. Pulmonary embolism also may develop within 2 weeks after serious body surface burns. Pulmonary embolism may develop from deep venous thrombosis secondary to a hypercoagulable state and prolonged immobility.

Finally, the long-term effects of smoke inhalation can result in restrictive and obstructive lung disorders. In general, a restrictive lung disorder develops from alveolar fibrosis and chronic atelectasis. An obstructive lung disorder generally is caused by increased and chronic bronchial secretions, bronchial stenosis, bronchial polyps, bronchiectasis, and bronchiolitis.

The major pathologic and structural changes of the respiratory system caused by thermal or smoke inhalation injuries are as follows:

Thermal injury (upper airway—nasal cavity, oral cavity, and pharynx):

- Blistering
- Mucosal edema
- Vascular congestion
- Epithelial sloughing
- Thick secretions
- Acute UAO

Smoke inhalation injury (tracheobronchial tree and alveoli):

- Inflammation of the tracheobronchial tree
- Bronchospasm
- Excessive bronchial secretions and mucus plugging
- Decreased mucosal ciliary transport
- Atelectasis
- Alveolar edema and frothy secretions (pulmonary edema)
- ARDS (severe cases)
- Bronchiolitis obliterans with organizing pneumonia (BOOP)
- Alveolar fibrosis, bronchial stenosis, bronchial polyps, bronchiolitis, and bronchiectasis (severe cases)

Pneumonia (Chapter 15) and pulmonary embolism (Chapter 20) often complicate smoke inhalation injury.

Etiology

Fire-related death is the third most common cause of accidental death in the United States. According to some estimates, thermal injury results in about 60,000 hospitalizations and 6000 deaths annually. Children account for about 50% of these deaths. Mortality rates are highest among very young children and older individuals. Flame burns account for up to 15% of thermal injuries and, when associated with smoke inhalation, are the cause of most deaths. Scalding burns account for up to 80% of the thermal injuries among children. The prognosis of fire victims usually is determined by the (1) extent and duration of smoke exposure, (2) chemical composition of the smoke, (3) size and depth of body surface burns, (4) temperature of gases inhaled, (5) age (the prognosis worsens in the very young or old), and (6) pre-existing health status. When smoke inhalation injury is accompanied by a full-thickness or third-degree skin burn, the mortality rate almost doubles.

Smoke can result from either pyrolysis (smoldering in a low-oxygen environment) or combustion (burning, with visible flame, in an adequate-oxygen environment). Smoke is composed of a complex mixture of particulates, toxic gases, and vapors. The composition of smoke varies according to the chemical makeup of the material that is burning and the amount of oxygen being consumed by the fire. Table 43-1 lists some of the more common toxic substances produced by burning products that frequently are found in office, industrial, and residential buildings.

Although in some instances the toxic components of the smoke may be obvious, in most cases the precise identification of the inhaled toxins is not feasible. In general, the inhalation of smoke with toxic agents that have high water solubility (e.g., ammonia, sulfur dioxide, and hydrogen fluoride) affects the structures of the upper airway. In contrast, the inhalation of toxic agents that have a low water solubility (e.g., hydrogen chloride, chlorine, phosgene, and oxides of nitrogen) affects the distal airways and alveoli. Many of the substances in smoke are caustic and can cause significant injury to the tracheobronchial tree (e.g., aldehydes [especially acrolein], hydrochloride, oxides of sulfur).

Body Surface Burns

Because the amount and severity of body surface burns play a major role in the patient's risk of mortality and morbidity, an approximate estimate of the percentage of the body surface area burned is important. Table 43-2 lists the approximate percentage of surface area for various body regions of adults

TABLE 43–1 **Toxic Substances and Sources Commonly Associated with Fire and Smoke**

Substance	Source
Aldehydes (acrolein, acetaldehyde, formaldehyde)	Wood, cotton, paper
Organic acids (acetic and formic acids)	
Carbon monoxide, hydrogen chloride, phosgene	Polyvinylchloride (PVC)
Hydrogen cyanide, isocyanate	Polyurethanes
Hydrogen fluoride, hydrogen bromide	Fluorinated resins
Ammonia	Melamine resins
Oxides of nitrogen	Nitrocellulose film, fabrics
Benzene	Petroleum products
Carbon monoxide, carbon dioxide	Organic material
Sulfur dioxide	Sulfur-containing compounds
Hydrogen chloride	Fertilizer, textiles, rubber manufacturing
Chlorine	Swimming pool water
Ozone	Welding fumes
Hydrogen sulfide	Metal works, chemical manufacturing

TABLE 43–2 **The Approximate Percentage of Body Surface Area (BSA) for Various Body Regions of Adults and Infants**

Anatomic Region	Adult % of BSA	Infant % of BSA
Entire head and neck	9	18
Each arm	9	9
Anterior trunk	18	18
Posterior trunk	18	18
Genitalia	1	1
Each leg	18	13.5

Note: The "rule of nines" is used to estimate percentage of injury; each of the areas listed here represents about 9% or 18% of the body surface area. This rule does not apply to the legs of infants.

and infants. The severity and depth of burns usually are defined as follows:

First degree (minimal depth in skin): Superficial burn, damage limited to the outer layer of epidermis. This burn is characterized by reddened skin, tenderness, and pain. Blisters are not present. Healing time is about 6 to 10 days. The result of healing is normal skin.

Second degree (superficial to deep thickness of skin): Burns in which damage extends through the epidermis and into the dermis but is not of sufficient extent to interfere with regeneration of epidermis. If secondary infection results, the damage from a second-degree burn may be equivalent to that of a third-degree burn. Blisters usually are present. Healing time is between 7 and 21 days. The result of healing ranges from normal to a hairless and depigmented skin with a texture that is normal, pitted, flat, or shiny.

Third degree (full thickness of skin including tissue beneath skin): Burns in which both epidermis and dermis are destroyed, with damage extending into underlying tissues. Tissue may be charred or coagulated. Healing may occur after 21 days or may never occur without skin grafting if the burned area is large. The resultant damage heals with hypertrophic scars (keloids) and chronic granulation.

The following clinical manifestations result from the pathologic mechanisms caused (or activated) by **Atelectasis** (see Figure 9-7), **Alveolar Consolidation** (see Figure 9-8), **Increased Alveolar-Capillary Membrane Thickness** (see Figure 9-9), **Bronchospasm** (see Figure 9-10), and **Excessive Airway Secretions** (see Figure 9-11)—the major anatomic alterations of the lungs associated with smoke inhalation and thermal injuries (see Figure 43-1).

CLINICAL DATA OBTAINED AT THE PATIENT'S BEDSIDE

The Physical Examination

Vital Signs

Increased respiratory rate (see page 31 ◆►)
Several pathophysiologic mechanisms operating simultaneously may lead to an increased ventilatory rate:
- Stimulation of peripheral chemoreceptors (hypoxemia)
- Decreased lung compliance/increased ventilatory rate relationship
- Stimulation of J receptors
- Pain/anxiety

Increased heart rate (pulse), cardiac output, and blood pressure (see pages 11 and 99 ◆►)

Assessment of Acute Upper Airway Obstruction (Thermal Injury)

- Obvious pharyngeal edema and swelling
- Inspiratory stridor
- Hoarseness
- Altered voice
- Painful swallowing

Because the inhalation of hot gases often results in severe upper airway edema, the respiratory care practitioner always should be alert for any clinical manifestations of acute upper airway obstruction, even when the patient shows no remarkable upper airway problems or upper body burns at admission.

Cyanosis (see page 45 ◆►)

Cough and Sputum Production
(see page 47 ◆►)

When the patient suffers upper airway thermal injuries, an excessive amount of thick secretions usually is present. During the early stage of recovery from smoke inhalation, the patient generally expectorates a small amount of black, sooty sputum (carbonaceous sputum). During the intermediate stage, the patient may produce moderate to large amounts of frothy secretions. During the late stage, purulent mucus is common.

Chest Assessment Findings (see page 22 ◆►)
- Usually normal breath sounds (early stage)
- Wheezing
- Crackles
- Rhonchi

CLINICAL DATA OBTAINED FROM LABORATORY TESTS AND SPECIAL PROCEDURES

Pulmonary Function Study Findings

Expiratory Maneuver Findings (see page 61 ◆►)

FVC	FEV_T	$FEF_{25\%-75\%}$	$FEF_{200-1200}$
↓	N or ↓	N or ↓	N
PEFR	**MVV**	**$FEF_{50\%}$**	**$FEV_{1\%}$**
N	N or ↓	N	N or ↑

Lung Volume and Capacity Findings
(see page 62 ◆►)

V_T	RV*	FRC*	TLC
N or ↓	↓	↓	↓
VC	**IC**	**ERV**	**RV/TLC%**
↓	↓	↓	N

*↑When airways are partially obstructed.

Decreased Diffusion Capacity (DL_{CO})
(see page 67 ◆►)

Arterial Blood Gases

Early Stages of Smoke Inhalation
Acute Alveolar Hyperventilation with Hypoxemia
(see page 70 ◆►)

pH	$Paco_2$	HCO_3^-	Pao_2
↑	↓	↓ (Slightly)	↓/Normal

Severe Smoke Inhalation and Burns with Metabolic Acidosis (see page 77 ◆►)

COHb	pH	$Paco_2$	HCO_3^-	Pao_2
↑	↓ (lactic acidemia)	↓	↓ (but patient has tissue hypoxia)	Normal (but tissue hypoxia)

When carbon monoxide or cyanide poisoning is present, the pH may be decreased during the early stages of smoke inhalation. This decrease in pH occurs because patients with severe carbon monoxide or cyanide poisoning commonly have lactic acidemia as a result of tissue hypoxia—even in the presence of a normal Pao_2. Therefore when carbon monoxide or cyanide poisoning is present, the patient may demonstrate the following arterial blood gas values:

Late Stages of Smoke Inhalation
Acute Ventilatory Failure with Hypoxemia
(see page 73 ◆►)

pH	$Paco_2$	HCO_3^-*	Pao_2
↓	↑	↑(Slightly)	↓

*When tissue hypoxia is severe enough to produce lactic acid, the pH and HCO_3^- values will be lower than expected for a particular $Paco_2$ level.

Oxygenation Indices (Smoke Inhalation and Burns) (see page 82 ◆▶)

	Early and Intermediate Stages	Late Stage
Do_2	↓	↓
$\dot{V}o_2$	↑	↓
$C(a-\bar{v})o_2$	↑	↓
O_2ER	↑	↓
$S\bar{v}o_2$	↓	↓

When carbon monoxide or cyanide poisoning is present, the oxygenation indices are unreliable because the Pao_2 often is normal in the presence of carbon monoxide poisoning, and when cyanide poisoning is present, the tissue cells are prevented from consuming oxygen. Both of these conditions cause false oximeter readings. For example, when carbon monoxide is present, a normal Do_2 value may be calculated when, in reality, the patient's oxygen transport status is extremely low. When cyanide poisoning is present, the patient's $\dot{V}o_2$ may appear normal or increased when in actuality the tissue cells are extremely hypoxic. Typically, these problems are not present during the intermediate and late stages in the presence of appropriate treatment.

Hemodynamic Indices (Cardiogenic Pulmonary Edema) (see page 99 ◆▶)

	Early Stage	Intermediate Stage	Late Stage
CVP	↓	Normal	↓
RAP	↓	Normal	↓
$\bar{PA}$	↓	Normal	↓
PCWP	↓	Normal	↓
CO	↓	Normal	↓
SV	↓	Normal	↓
SVI	↓	Normal	↓
CI	↓	Normal	↓
RVSWI	↓	Normal	↓
LVSWI	↓	Normal	↓
PVR	Normal	Normal	↑
SVR	↑	Normal	↑

In general, the hemodynamic profile seen in patients with body surface burns relates to the amount of intravascular volume loss (hypovolemia) that occurs as a result of third-space fluid shifts. For example, during the early stage, the decreased values shown for the CVP, RAP, PA, CWP, CO, SV, SVI, CI, RVSWI, and LVSWI reflect the reduction in pulmonary intravascular and cardiac filling volumes. Hypovolemia causes a generalized peripheral vasoconstriction, which is reflected in an elevated SVR. When appropriate fluid resuscitation is administered, the patient's hemodynamic indices usually are normal during the intermediate stage.

CARBON MONOXIDE POISONING

When a patient has been exposed to smoke, *carbon monoxide (CO) poisoning must be assumed!* Although CO has no direct injurious effect on the lungs, it can greatly reduce the patient's oxygen transport because CO has an affinity for hemoglobin that is about 210 times greater than that of oxygen. CO attached to hemoglobin is called *carboxyhemoglobin (COHb)*. Breathing CO at a partial pressure of less than 2 mm Hg can result in a COHb of 40% or more. In other words, 40% or more of the oxygen transport system is inactivated.

In addition, high concentrations of COHb cause the oxyhemoglobin dissociation curve to move markedly to the left, which makes it more difficult for oxygen to leave the hemoglobin at the tissue sites. In essence, the tissue cells are better oxygenated when 40% of the hemoglobin is absent (anemia) than when a COHb of 40% is present. Table 43-3 lists the clinical manifestations associated with carbon monoxide poisoning.

A COHb level in excess of 20% is usually considered CO poisoning, and a COHb level of 40% or greater is considered severe. A COHb level in excess of 50% may cause irreversible damage to the central nervous system (CNS). Pulse oximetry and Pao_2 measurements are unreliable in the presence of COHb. Arterial blood gas measurements, however, do provide important information regarding the presence of hypoxemia, widened alveolar-arterial oxygen gradient, and acid-base status. If available, hyperbaric oxygen (HBO) therapy is usually used at a COHb $\geq$ 10%.

CYANIDE POISONING

When smoke contains cyanide, oxygen transport may be further impaired. Cyanide poisoning should be suspected in comatose patients who have inhaled fumes from burning plastic (polyurethane) or other synthetic materials. Inhaled cyanide is easily transported in the blood to the tissue cells, where it bonds to the cytochrome oxidase enzymes of the mitochondria. This inhibits the metabolism of oxygen and causes the tissue cells to shift to an inefficient anaerobic form of metabolism. The end product

OVERVIEW

of the Cardiopulmonary Clinical Manifestations Associated with SMOKE INHALATION AND THERMAL INJURIES (Continued)

of anerobic metabolism is lactic acid. Cyanide poisoning may result in lactic acidemia, which is normally caused by an inadequate tissue oxygen level, even though the Pao_2 is normal or above normal. Clinically, cyanide concentrations are easily measured with commercially available kits. A cyanide blood level in excess of 1 mg/L usually is fatal.

RADIOLOGIC FINDINGS

Chest Radiograph
• Usually normal (early stage)

• Pulmonary edema/ARDS (intermediate stage)
• Patchy or segmental infiltrates (late stage)

During the early stage, the radiograph is generally normal. Signs of pulmonary edema and ARDS may be seen during the intermediate and late stages. The chest X-ray reveals dense, fluffy opacities and patchy or segmental infiltrates (Figure 43-2).

TABLE 43–3 Blood COHb Levels and Clinical Manifestations

COHb (%)	Clinical Manifestations
0 to 10	Usually no symptoms
10 to 20	Mild headache, dilation of cutaneous blood vessels
	Cherry red skin—but not always
20 to 30	Throbbing headache, nausea, vomiting, impaired judgment
30 to 50	Throbbing headache, possible syncope, increased respiratory and pulse rates
50 to 60	Syncope, increased respiratory and pulse rates, coma, convulsions, Cheyne-Stokes respiration
60 to 70	Coma, convulsions, cardiovascular and respiratory depression, and possible death
70 to 80	Cardiopulmonary failure and death

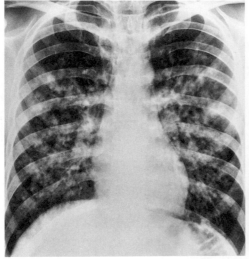 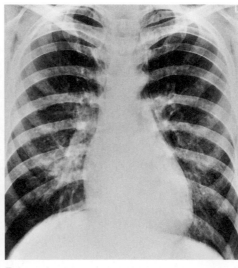

A   B

Figure 43–2   **A,** Radiograph of a young man admitted after accidentally setting his kitchen on fire while intoxicated. **B,** Prompt recovery after 72 hours. (Courtesy Dr. K. Simpkins, Leeds, England. From Armstrong P et al: *Imaging of diseases of the chest*, ed 2, St. Louis, 1995, Mosby.)

General Management of Hot Gas and Smoke Inhalation

GENERAL EMERGENCY CARE

The principal goals in the initial care of patients suffering from smoke inhalation and burns include the immediate assessment of the patient's airway and respiratory status, cardiovascular status, the percentage of body burned, and the depth of burns. An intravenous (IV) line should be started immediately to administer medications and fluids. Easily separated clothing should be removed. Any remaining clothing should be soaked thoroughly. When present, burn wounds should be covered to prevent shock, fluid loss, heat loss, and pain. Infection control includes isolation, room pressurization, air filtration, and wound coverings.

Fluid resuscitation with Ringer's lactate solution is usually initiated according to the Parkland formula—4 ml/kg of body weight for each percent of body surface area burned over a 24-hour period. The patient's hemodynamic status will usually remain stable at this fluid replacement rate, with an average urine output target of 30 to 50 ml/hr and a central venous pressure (CVP) target of 2 to 6 mm Hg. Because this process often leads to overhydration and acute upper airway obstruction and pulmonary edema, the patient's fluid and electrolyte status (weight, input and output, and laboratory values) must be monitored carefully.

Finally, knowledge of the exposure characteristics of the fire-related accident may be helpful in assessing the potential clinical complications. For example, did the accident involve a closed-space setting or entrapment? The amount and concentration of smoke usually are much greater in these conditions. What type of material was burning in the fire? Are the inhaled toxins known? Was CO or cyanide produced by the burning substances? Was the patient unconscious before entering the hospital?

AIRWAY MANAGEMENT

Early elective endotracheal intubation should be performed on the patient who has inhaled hot gases and demonstrates any signs of impending UAO (e.g., upper airway edema, blisters, inspiratory stridor, thick secretions). *This is a medical emergency!* Even though acute UAO is considered one of the most treatable complications of smoke inhalation, death still occurs from UAO (hence the well-supported clinical guideline that states "When in doubt, intubate").

Securing an endotracheal tube often is difficult in the presence of facial burns (typically wet wounds). Adhesive tape may cause further trauma to the burn wounds. The ingenuity and creativity of the respiratory care practitioner may be required. The securing of the endotracheal tube without traumatizing the patient has been successful with the use of umbilical tape and a variety of helmets, halo traction devices, and Velcro straps.

Because of the infections associated with body surface burns and smoke inhalation, a tracheostomy should be reserved for conditions in which an airway cannot be established otherwise or for the patient who will require prolonged mechanical ventilation.

BRONCHOSCOPY

Bronchoscopy often is used to clear the airways of mucus plugs and eschar. In addition, early bronchoscopy often is performed for inspection and evaluation of the upper airways. Mucosal changes distal to the larynx serve as good predictors of subsequent respiratory problems.

HYPERBARIC OXYGEN

Hyperbaric oxygenation (HBO) therapy may be useful in the rapid elimination of CO and the enhancement of skin graft viability. Although a Pao_2 greater than 1500 mm Hg can be achieved with a hyperbaric chamber, it often is not possible or practical to institute this therapy. The chamber may not be immediately available. Can the patient be transported safely? Will the interruption of immediate therapy be detrimental?

TREATMENT FOR CYANIDE POISONING

The treatment for cyanide poisoning includes amyl nitrite inhalation and intravenous sodium thiosulfate.

Antibiotic Agents

Antibiotics may be used to treat burn wounds and pulmonary infections (see Appendix II).

Expectorants

Expectorants may be administered to facilitate expectoration (see Appendix II).

Analgesic Agents

Analgesics generally are ordered when surface burns are present.

Prophylactic Anticoagulants

Heparin and other anticoagulants often are administered to patients with severe, long-term fire-related injuries to reduce the risk of pulmonary embolism. Immobile patients also are treated with this therapy.

RESPIRATORY CARE TREATMENT PROTOCOLS

Oxygen Therapy Protocol

Oxygen therapy is used to treat hypoxemia, decrease the work of breathing, and decrease myocardial work. Because of the hypoxemia and CO poisoning associated with smoke inhalation, a high concentration of oxygen always should be administered immediately. The COHb half-life when a patient is breathing room air at 1 atmosphere is approximately 5 hours. In other words, a 40% COHb decreases to about 20% in 5 hours and about 10% in another 5 hours. Breathing 100% oxygen at 1 atmosphere reduces the HbCO half-life to less than 1 hour (see Oxygen Therapy Protocol, Protocol 9-1).

Bronchopulmonary Hygiene Therapy Protocol

Because of the excessive mucus production and accumulation in the intermediate and late stages of smoke inhalation injuries, a number of respiratory therapy modalities may be used to enhance the mobilization of bronchial secretions. However, even though chest physical therapy is an excellent treatment modality to mobilize secretions, patients with severe chest burns or recent skin grafts do not tolerate chest percussion and vibration (see Bronchopulmonary Hygiene Therapy Protocol, Protocol 9-2).

Hyperinflation Therapy Protocol

Hyperinflation techniques commonly are used to offset the alveolar atelectasis and consolidation associated with smoke inhalation injuries. The administration of continuous positive airway pressure (CPAP) via an endotracheal tube or mask (when the patient has no facial or neck burns) may help minimize the development of pulmonary edema. CPAP also supports the edematous airway and maintains or increases the patient's functional residual capacity (see Hyperinflation Therapy Protocol, Protocol 9-3).

Aerosolized Medication Protocol

Both sympathomimetic and parasympatholytic agents commonly are used to produce vasoconstriction of the mucosa and to offset bronchial smooth muscle constriction. Mucolytics and antiinflammatory agents also may be administered as part of the Aerosolized Medication Protocol (see Protocol 9-4).

Mechanical Ventilation Protocol

Mechanical ventilation with positive end-expiratory pressure (PEEP) usually is required for patients who develop pulmonary edema, ARDS, and pneumonia. Mechanical ventilation should be implemented in the presence of acute or impending ventilatory failure (see Mechanical Ventilation Protocol, Protocol 9-5).

Case Study: SMOKE INHALATION AND THERMAL INJURY

Admitting History and Physical Examination

A 21-year-old male was in excellent health until a few hours before admission when, after smoking marijuana and falling asleep, he suffered second- and third-degree burns on his face, chest, and abdomen as a result of his bed catching fire. The extent of second- and third-degree burns was only 6% to 8% of his total body surface.

Shortly after admission, he developed respiratory distress and pulmonary edema. His blood pressure was 110/60, pulse 100/min, and respiratory rate 30/min. His oral temperature was 98.8° F. Bilateral crackles, rhonchi, and occasional wheezing were present. Spontaneous cough produced large amounts of thick whitish-grey sputum. The chest radiograph revealed bilateral patchy infiltrates and consolidation. On 4 L/min oxygen, his arterial blood gas values were pH 7.51, $Paco_2$ 28, HCO_3^- 21, and Pao_2 45.

He was treated conservatively, and the pulmonary edema cleared in 48 hours. However, the respiratory distress and hypoxemia persisted, even on 50%

oxygen by HAFOE mask. Fiberoptic bronchoscopy revealed extensive thermal damage to the trachea and large bronchi.

Three days after treatment was administered, the patient's condition was worsening. At this time, the following respiratory assessment was documented:

Respiratory Assessment and Plan

S   Complains of productive cough, substernal chest pain when coughing, and moderate dyspnea.

O   Afebrile. BP 120/65, P 119 and regular, RR 35. Bilateral crackles, rhonchi, and expiratory wheezing. On 50% O_2: pH 7.54, $Paco_2$ 25, HCO_3^- 20, and Pao_2 38. CXR: Bilateral patchy infiltrates and consolidation. No cardiomegaly. Bronchoscopy—blackish eschar in oropharynx; reddened and inflamed larynx, trachea, and large airways. Thick, whitish-grey secretions noted.

A   • Smoke inhalation with thermal burns of the oropharynx, larynx, and large airways (history and bronchoscopy)

- Alveolar infiltrates and consolidation (CXR)
- Acute alveolar hyperventilation with severe hypoxemia (ABG)
- Impending ventilatory failure (general history and clinical trends)
- Excessive and thick airway secretions (sputum)

P Confer with attending physician to intubate and initiate ventilator care per protocol. Oxygen Therapy Protocol: FIO_2 at 1.0 via nonrebreather mask. Aerosolized Medication and Bronchopulmonary Hygiene Protocols: albuterol premix 2.0 cc via med neb q 2 h (alternate with epinephrine 6 drops in 2.0 cc normal saline). Gentle nasotracheal and oral suctioning after med neb treatments and prn. Check I&O status and daily weights. If doctor commits patient to ventilator, consider in-line ultrasonic nebulizer treatments, for 30 min q 4 h.

The patient was intubated and started on intravenously administered steroids. He was ventilated with an FIO_2 of 0.50, rate of 12, and PEEP of +10 cm H_2O. Because of the upper body burns, chest physical therapy and postural drainage were prohibited. The bronchial secretions, however, were loosened and mobilized adequately with an in-line ultrasonic nebulizer and frequent endotracheal suctioning. In-line aerosolized steroids also were administered at this time.

• • • • •

The patient's vital signs and blood gases improved on this regimen. After 12 days of respiratory care, he was weaned to room air and extubated. He continued to complain of exertional dyspnea with transfer activities but denied dyspnea at rest. Crackles were improved but still easily auscultated throughout all lung fields when the patient took deep breaths. Occasional expiratory wheezes also were heard.

Three days after extubation, on room air his pH was 7.46, $Paco_2$ 38, HCO_3^- 24, and Pao_2 59. On exercise, the Spo_2 fell to 85%. His PEFR was 40% of predicted. At this time, the respiratory therapist recorded the following assessment in the patient's chart:

Respiratory Assessment and Plan

S Complains of shortness of breath with any activity.

O Vital signs stable. Crackles heard over both lung bases. Some expiratory prolongation. Room air: pH 7.46, $Paco_2$ 38, HCO_3^- 24, and Pao_2 59. Room air Spo_2 falls to 85% with exercise. PEFR 40% of predicted. CXR: Improvement in patchy lung infiltrates.

A • Moderate hypoxemia secondary to thermal injury to lung (ABG and history)

- Moderate obstructive pulmonary disease (PEFR)

P Complete pulmonary function tests ordered. Oxygen per Oxygen Therapy Protocol. If obstructive pulmonary disease is confirmed, start Bronchial Hygiene and Aerosolized Medication Protocols.

Pulmonary function studies showed severely reduced expiratory flows and a sharply decreased diffusion capacity. Chest X-rays taken at regular intervals thereafter began to show emphysematous changes. The diaphragms were flattened, and bilateral coarse reticular infiltrates were evident. In spite of vigorous therapy over the next 6 weeks, the patient's cardiopulmonary status continued to worsen. The patient died on day 56, 2 months after his original thermal and inhalational injury. The antemortem diagnosis, confirmed by autopsy, was bronchiolitis fibrosa obliterans.

Discussion

At the time of the **first assessment**, the patient demonstrated most of the pathophysiologic correlates of smoke inhalation and thermal injuries to the lung. His dyspnea reflected the increased work of breathing associated with **Bronchospasm** (see Figure 9-10), **Increased Alveolar-Capillary Thickening** (see Figure 9-9), and **Excessive Bronchial Secretions** (see Figure 9-11). The first of these problems was treated with the vigorous use of both bronchodilator (albuterol) and decongestant (epinephrine) aerosols; the excessive bronchial secretions were treated with ultrasonic bland aerosols and airway suctioning. No specific treatment was available for the changes that occurred in the alveolar-capillary membrane

This interesting case is instructive for several additional reasons. The first is that all patients with burns of the upper chest, neck, or face should have a careful oropharyngeal examination to determine whether burns have indeed occurred in the upper airway. The presence of soot or eschar in the oropharynx is diagnostic of this problem; respiratory distress almost certainly will ensue if such findings are present, although this does not happen immediately. A 24- to 72-hour lag may occur between the burn and clinical obstruction of the airway.

Second, a dreaded complication of smoke and heat inhalation is bronchiolitis fibrosa obliterans, which developed in this patient and ultimately was responsible for his demise.

These days, the patient might be considered a candidate for lung transplantation. This case study should remind the respiratory care practitioner that immediate intubation over the diagnostic bronchoscope may be necessary and that he or she should prepare accordingly.

SELF-ASSESSMENT QUESTIONS

Multiple Choice

1. About what percentage of hospitalized patients with thermal injury have an acute upper airway obstruction (UAO)?

   a. 0% to 10%
   b. 10% to 20%
   c. 20% to 30%
   d. 30% to 40%
   e. 40% to 50%

2. Except for the rare instance of steam inhalation, direct thermal injuries usually do not occur below the level of which of the following structures?

   a. Oral pharynx
   b. Larynx
   c. Carina
   d. Bronchi
   e. Bronchioles

3. When chest burns are present, the patient's pulmonary condition may be further aggravated by which of the following?

   I. Decreased lung and chest compliance
   II. Increased airway resistance
   III. The use of narcotics
   IV. Immobility

   a. I and III only
   b. II and III only
   c. I, II, and III only
   d. II, III, and IV only
   e. I, II, III, and IV

4. Which of the following is/are the pulmonary-related pathologic change(s) associated with smoke inhalation?

   I. Alveolar hyperinflation
   II. Bronchospasm
   III. Pulmonary edema
   IV. Pulmonary embolism

   a. I only
   b. II only
   c. III and IV only
   d. II, III, and IV only
   e. I, II, III, and IV

5. Which of the following produce carbon monoxide when burned?

   I. Polyurethanes
   II. Wood, cotton, paper
   III. Organic material
   IV. Polyvinylchloride (PVC)

   a. I only
   b. II only
   c. III and IV only
   d. I, II, and III only
   e. I, II, III, and IV

6. Which of the following oxygenation indices is/are associated with smoke inhalation and burns during the early and intermediate stages?

   I. Increased $\dot{V}_{O_2}$
   II. Decreased $C(a\text{-}\bar{v})_{O_2}$
   III. Increased D_{O_2}
   IV. Decreased $S\bar{v}_{O_2}$

   a. II only
   b. IV only
   c. II and III only
   d. I and IV only
   e. II, III, and IV only

7. Which of the following hemodynamic indices is/are associated with body surface burns during the early stage?

   I. Decreased CO
   II. Increased SVR
   III. Decreased $\overline{PA}$
   IV. Increased PCWP

   a. I only
   b. III only
   c. II and IV only
   d. I, II, and III only
   e. I, II, III, and IV

8. If an adult's entire right arm, right leg, and anterior trunk have been burned, approximately what percentage of the patient's body surface area is burned?

   a. 15%
   b. 25%
   c. 35%
   d. 45%
   e. 55%

9. Healing time for a second-degree burn is between:

   a. 1 and 7 days
   b. 7 and 21 days
   c. 21 and 31 days
   d. 1 and 2 months
   e. 2 and 3 months

10. Breathing 100% oxygen at 1 atmosphere reduces the carboxyhemoglobin (COHb) half-life to less than:

   a.   1 hour
   b.   2 hours
   c.   3 hours
   d.   4 hours
   e.   5 hours

Answers appear in Appendix XI.

CHAPTER 44

Postoperative Atelectasis

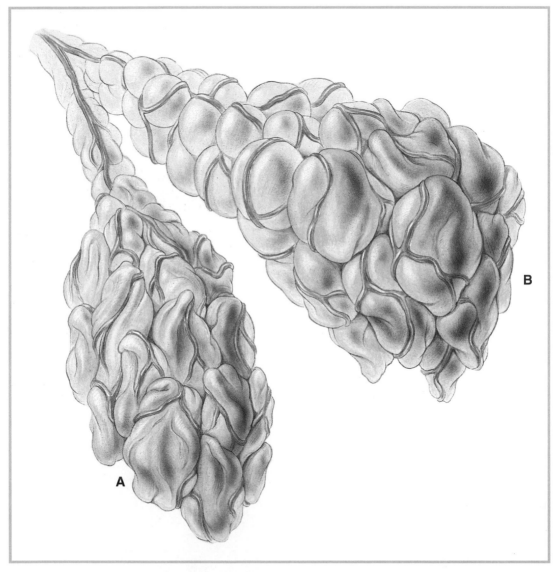

Figure 44–1   Alveoli in postoperative atelectasis. **A,** Total alveolar collapse. **B,** Partial alveolar collapse. See also Plate 36.

Anatomic Alterations of the Lungs

Postoperative atelectasis commonly is seen after upper abdominal and thoracic surgical procedures. *Atelectasis,* in the strict sense of the term, is defined as the condition in which the lungs of the newborn remain unexpanded (airless) at birth. In the clinical setting, however, the meaning of *atelectasis* in all age groups generally is broadened to include partial or total collapse of previously expanded lung regions. Atelectasis may be limited to the smallest lung unit (i.e., alveolus or primary lobule*; Figure 44-1) or may involve an entire lung or a segment or lobe of the lung.

The major pathologic and anatomic alterations associated with postoperative atelectasis include partial or total collapse of the following:

- Alveoli of primary lobules (micro-atelectasis or subsegmental atelectasis)—very common
- Lung segment—fairly common
- Lung lobe—less common
- Entire lung—rare

Etiology

Postoperative atelectasis develops when lung expansion is decreased or when excess airway secretions cause mucus plugs, which in turn produce distal "degassing" of lung units.

DECREASED LUNG EXPANSION

Good lung expansion depends on the patient's intact chest cage and his or her ability to generate an appropriate negative intrapleural pressure. Thoracic and upper abdominal procedures often result in a reduction in the patient's ability to generate good lung expansion and therefore are considered as high-risk factors for subsequent development of postoperative atelectasis.

Other precipitating factors that decrease the patient's ability to generate a negative intrapleural pressure include (1) anesthesia, (2) postoperative pain, (3) supine position, (4) obesity, (5) advanced age, (6) inadequate tidal volumes during mechanical ventilation, (7) malnutrition, (8) ascites, (9) diaphragmatic apraxia (e.g., topical cooling of the left phrenic nerve often occurs during cardiac surgery and may lead to an inadequate diaphragmatic movement and left lower lobe atelectasis), and (10) the presence of restrictive lung disorders (e.g., pleural effusion, pneumothorax, acute respiratory distress syndrome [ARDS], pulmonary edema, chronic interstitial lung disease, and pleural masses).

ALVEOLAR DEGASSING DISTAL TO AIRWAY SECRETIONS AND MUCUS PLUGS (AIRWAY OBSTRUCTION)

Postoperative atelectasis often is associated with retained airway secretions and mucus plugs. Precipitating factors for retained secretions include (1) decreased mucociliary transport, (2) excessive secretions, (3) inadequate hydration, (4) weak or absent cough, (5) general anesthesia, (6) smoking history, (7) gastric aspiration, and (8) certain pre-existing conditions (e.g., bronchiectasis, chronic bronchitis, cystic fibrosis, asthma). When total airway obstruction develops, alveolar oxygen is absorbed into the pulmonary circulation and alveolar degassing ensues. The breathing of high oxygen concentrations favors this pathologic process.

---

*A primary lobule is a cluster of alveoli that originates from a single terminal bronchiole. Each primary lobule is about 3.5 mm in diameter and contains about 2000 alveoli. Each lung contains about 150,000 primary lobules. A primary lobule also is called an *acinus, terminal respiratory unit, lung parenchyma,* or *functional lung unit.* The lung parenchyma consist of the terminal respiratory units.

OVERVIEW
of the Cardiopulmonary Clinical Manifestations Associated with POSTOPERATIVE ATELECTASIS

The following clinical manifestations result from the pathological mechanisms caused (or activated) by **Atelectasis** (see Figure 9-7)—the major anatomic alterations of the lungs associated with postoperative atelectasis (see Figure 44-1).

CLINICAL DATA OBTAINED AT THE PATIENT'S BEDSIDE

The Physical Examination
Vital Signs

Increased respiratory rate (see page 31 ◆►)
Several pathophysiologic mechanisms operating simultaneously may lead to an increased ventilatory rate:

- Stimulation of peripheral chemoreceptors (hypoxemia)
- Decreased lung compliance/increased ventilatory rate relationship
- Stimulation of J receptors
- Pain/anxiety/fever

Increased heart rate (pulse), cardiac output, and blood pressure (see pages 11 and 99 ◆►)

Cyanosis (see page 45 ◆►)

Chest Assessment Findings (see page 22 ◆►)

- Increased tactile and vocal fremitus
- Dull percussion note
- Bronchial breath sounds
- Diminished breath sounds (common when atelectasis in caused by mucus plugs)
- Crackles (usually heard initially in the dependent lung regions and during late inspiration)
- Whispered pectoriloquy

CLINICAL DATA OBTAINED FROM LABORATORY TESTS AND SPECIAL PROCEDURES

Pulmonary Function Study Findings
Expiratory Maneuver Findings (see page 61 ◆►)

FVC	FEV$_T$	FEF$_{25\%-75\%}$	FEF$_{200-1200}$
↓	N or ↓	N or ↓	N
PEFR	MVV	FEF$_{50\%}$	FEV$_{1\%}$
N	N or ↓	N	N or ↑

Lung Volume and Capacity Findings (see page 62 ◆►)

V$_T$	RV	FRC	TLC
N or ↓	↓	↓	↓
VC	IC	ERV	RV/TLC%
↓	↓	↓	N

Arterial Blood Gases

Small or Localized Postoperative Atelectasis
Acute Alveolar Hyperventilation with Hypoxemia (see page 70 ◆►)

pH	Paco$_2$	HCO$_3^-$	Pao$_2$
↑	↓	↓ (Slightly)	↓

Widespread Postoperative Atelectasis
Acute Ventilatory Failure with Hypoxemia (see page 73 ◆►)

pH	Paco$_2$	HCO$_3^-$*	Pao$_2$
↓	↑	↑(Slightly)	↓

*When tissue hypoxia is severe enough to produce lactic acid, the pH and HCO$_3^-$ values will be lower than expected for a particular Paco$_2$ level.

Oxygenation Indices (see page 82 ◆►)

$\dot{Q}_S/\dot{Q}_T$	Do$_2$†	$\dot{V}_{O_2}$	C(a-$\bar{v}$)o$_2$
↑	↓	Normal	Normal
O$_2$ER	S$\bar{v}$o$_2$		
↑	↓		

†The Do$_2$ may be normal in patients who have compensated to the decreased oxygenation status with an increased cardiac output. When the Do$_2$ is normal, the O$_2$ER is usually normal.

RADIOLOGIC FINDINGS

Chest Radiograph
- Increased density in areas of atelectasis
- Air bronchograms
- Elevation of the hemidiaphragm on the affected side
- Mediastinal shift toward the affected side

Areas of increased density generally appear initially in dependent lung regions, such as the lower lobes, or posteriorly in patients who must recline in the supine position. Air bronchograms can be seen when large areas of atelectasis are present. An elevation of the hemidiaphragm or mediastinal shift toward the affected side often is seen when large areas of atelectasis exist. Figure 44-2, *A* shows left lung atelectasis caused by a misplaced endotracheal tube in the right main stem bronchus. Figure 44-2, *B* shows the same patient 20 minutes after the endotracheal tube was pulled back above the carina.

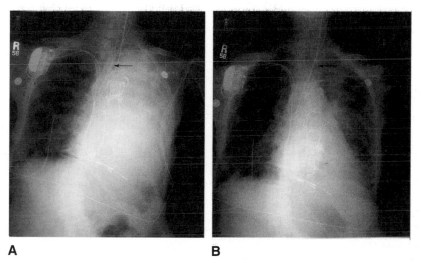

A   **B**

Figure 44–2 **A,** Endotracheal tube tip misplaced in the right main stem bronchus (see *arrow*). Note that the left lung has collapsed completely (i.e., white fluffy appearance in the left lung). **B,** The same patient 20 minutes after the endotracheal tube was pulled back above the carina (see *arrow*). Note that the left lung is better ventilated (i.e., appears darker). (From Des Jardins T: *Cardiopulmonary anatomy and physiology: essentials for respiratory care,* ed 4, Albany, 2002, Delmar.)

General Management of Postoperative Atelectasis

Precipitating factors for postoperative atelectasis should be identified during the preoperative and postoperative assessments (see the previous section on etiology). High-risk patients should be monitored closely. For example, bedside spirometry (vital capacity and inspiratory capacity) is useful in the early detection of atelectasis. Preventive measures often are prescribed for high-risk patients. For example, incentive spirometry frequently is prescribed to encourage good lung expansion. Chest physical therapy also may be given to the patient with mild to moderate preoperative or postoperative bronchial secretions to offset the development of mucus plugs and atelectasis. Patients who demonstrate combined obstructive and restrictive pulmonary disease preoperatively generally are thought to be at extremely high risk for atelectasis. When the diagnosis of postoperative atelectasis has been made, the following respiratory care procedures may be prescribed.

GENERAL CONSIDERATIONS

Whenever possible, treatment of the underlying cause of the postoperative atelectasis should be prescribed immediately (e.g., medication for pain, correction of inadequate tidal volumes during mechanical ventilation, repositioning of an endotracheal tube in the right mainstem bronchus, or withdrawal of air or fluid from the pleural cavity).

RESPIRATORY CARE TREATMENT PROTOCOLS

Oxygen Therapy Protocol

Oxygen therapy is used to treat hypoxemia, decrease the work of breathing, and decrease myocardial work. Because of the hypoxemia that may develop in atelectasis, supplemental oxygen may be required. However, the hypoxemia that develops in postoperative atelectasis is caused by capillary shunting and therefore is refractory to oxygen therapy (see Oxygen Therapy Protocol, Protocol 9-1).

Bronchopulmonary Hygiene Therapy Protocol

When atelectasis is caused by mucus accumulation and mucus plugs, a number of bronchial hygiene treatment modalities may be used to enhance the mobilization of airway secretions (see Bronchopulmonary Hygiene Therapy Protocol, Protocol 9-2).

Hyperinflation Therapy Protocol

Hyperinflation measures commonly are administered to offset atelectasis and reinflate collapsed lung areas (see Hyperinflation Therapy Protocol, Protocol 9-3).

Mechanical Ventilation Protocol

Short-term mechanical ventilation often is prescribed after major surgery, especially if the patient demonstrates one or more high-risk factors for postoperative atelectasis. For example, in patients undergoing cardiac surgery, mechanical ventilation generally is maintained until the cardiopulmonary parameters are stable (see Mechanical Ventilation Protocol, Protocol 9-5).

Case Study: POSTOPERATIVE ATELECTASIS

Admitting History and Physical Examination

This 62-year-old man with a 35-pack/year smoking history had his left lower lobe resected for small-cell carcinoma. Anesthesia had been performed using a right-sided double-lumen endotracheal tube. At the end of the procedure, the patient was breathing well and the tube was removed.

In the recovery room, 30 minutes after arrival, his respiratory rate increased from 22/min to 34/min. His pulse increased from 70 to 130 beats/min with regular rhythm, and his blood pressure decreased from 115/85 to 100/60 mm Hg. His peripheral oxygen saturation dropped from 97% to 92% while on an FIO_2 of 0.30. Breath sounds were decreased in the left lower anterior chest. A chest X-ray showed atelectasis of the left lower lobe. Arterial blood gas values on 1 L/min O_2 per cannula were pH 7.29, $Paco_2$ 63, HCO_3^- 25, and Pao_2 55. At this time, the respiratory therapist recorded the following SOAP note:

Respiratory Assessment and Plan

S N/A. Patient still sedated from anesthesia.

O RR 34/min, P 130 and regular, BP 100/60. Breath sounds decreased in left lower chest anteriorly. CXR: Left lower lobe atelectasis. On 1 L/min O_2: pH 7.29, $Paco_2$ 63, HCO_3^- 25, and Pao_2 55.

A • Left lower lobe atelectasis; rule out mucus plugs (CXR and decreased breath sounds)

• Acute ventilatory failure with moderate hypoxemia (ABG)

P Contact physician regarding intubation and mechanical ventilation (SIMV mode). Oxygen Therapy per Protocol (FIO_2 0.5). Bronchopulmonary Hygiene Therapy Protocol (encourage cough and deep breathing, suction frequently, discuss with physician the possibility of respiratory therapist assistance with therapeutic bronchoscopy). Hyperinflation Therapy Protocol postintubation (PEEP based on titration study). Aerosolized Medication Therapy Protocol (in-line albuterol 0.5 cc in 2.0 cc 20% acetylcysteine q 2 h, then decrease or increase according to reassessment). Repeat ABG in 30 minutes, and reevaluate.

The patient was reintubated, ventilated, and oxygenated according to protocol. A mucolytic (acetylcysteine) was aerosolized and also directly instilled into the patient's endotracheal tube. Aggressive tracheobronchial suctioning was performed. This produced small amounts of secretions with little or no benefit to the patient.

In view of this, a fiberoptic bronchoscope was inserted through the endotracheal tube, and a large mucus plug was identified in the orifice of the left lower lobe bronchus. The plug was removed under direct vision. After the bronchoscopy, the patient improved rapidly and could be extubated after about 60 minutes. A chest X-ray taken before this time showed full expansion of the left lower lobe. The patient was discharged on the sixth postoperative day.

Discussion

Care of postoperative **Atelectasis** (see Figure 9-7) is one of the day-to-day responsibilities of the respiratory care practitioner. Accordingly, the respiratory care practitioner must be extremely adept in the assessment and management of such patients. The development of immediate postoperative atelectasis almost always is related to **Excessive Bronchial Secretions** (see Figure 9-11)—in this case caused by a large mucus plug obstructing the left lower lobe. Because such patients (in the immediate postoperative period) often cannot cough vigorously, particularly after thoracotomy, the decision to initiate

bronchoscopy immediately rather than to rely on physical therapy and mucolytics was certainly in order.

In patients who have undergone abdominal surgery or those who develop atelectasis later, the simpler approaches should certainly be tried first. Atelectasis has a tendency to recur, and these patients need to be followed at least 72 hours postoperatively to ensure that this has not happened. Therefore the therapist's suggestion to follow pulse oximetry is entirely appropriate.

As important as treatment is, prevention is better, and in this regard the bronchopulmonary hygiene and volume expansion protocols ordered are very important. Indeed, institution of these simple protocols often prevents the late development of atelectasis in postoperative patients.

SELF-ASSESSMENT QUESTIONS

Complete the Following

1. List the two types of surgery that are considered high risks for postoperative atelectasis.

    A.

    B.

2. List five precipitating factors that decrease the patient's ability to generate negative intrapleural pressure.

    A.

    B.

    C.

    D.

    E.

3. List five precipitating factors associated with airway secretions and mucus plugs.

    A.

    B.

    C.

    D.

    E.

Answers appear in Appendix XI.

CHAPTER 45

Respiratory Failure*

The amount of knowledge regarding pathophysiology, technical jargon, and the frequently changing status of the patient required for the provision of cost-effective *mechanical ventilation* is generally so daunting that optimal care requires more than the service of one practicing respiratory care practitioner (RCP). Despite this, many centers have started their therapist-driven protocol (TDP) programs with Mechanical Ventilation Protocols rather than with the more simple protocols described elsewhere in this text (see Chapter 9). The decision to proceed in this manner tends to be based on humanistic, pathophysiologic, and economic grounds. Indeed, who could defend practices that are unnecessary (if not actually harmful), uncomfortable, and costly to patients requiring ventilator support? The need for a standardized approach to ventilator management therefore has necessitated the development of a "Fifth Protocol" that systematically details the care of patients requiring ventilator support (see Figure 9-5).

Mechanical ventilation may be delivered by endotracheal tube (most common) or by tracheostomy, face mask, or a cuirass-type device. Ventilator modes consist of assist-control (A/C) and synchronized intermittent mandatory ventilation (SIMV) with or without pressure support (PS). Much less commonly used modes include SIMV alone, inverse-rate ventilation (IRV), and airway pressure release ventilation (APRV). This chapter does not review or discuss these various ventilator and weaning modes, although most Mechanical Ventilation Protocols require the RCP to choose ventilator modes on the basis of patient need.

The goal of mechanical ventilation is to totally or partially replace the gas exchange function of the lungs—with as few complications as possible. The objectives of mechanical ventilation are to improve and maintain alveolar ventilation; to ensure adequate CO_2 and pH homeostasis, oxygenation, and lung inflation; and to reduce the work of breathing. Achievement of these objectives reverses acute respiratory acidosis (also called acute ventilatory failure) and hypoxemia, relieves patient discomfort, reverses or prevents atelectasis, reverses respiratory muscle fatigue, stabilizes the chest wall, allows sedation and/or neuromuscular blockade, and decreases systemic or myocardial oxygen consumption in cases of acute respiratory distress syndrome (ARDS) or cardiogenic shock—a daunting list, indeed!

Achievement of these goals and objectives results from an intelligent assessment of patient needs, understanding of the pertinent pathophysiology, and application of ventilator management techniques most likely to meet the needs of the moment. This is the cornerstone of the "assess and treat" paradigm of protocol ventilator therapy.

Etiology and Pathogenesis

Literally any of the numerous illnesses described in this text can worsen to the point at which alveolar gas exchange is so impaired that near-terminal and ultimately fatal respiratory failure may occur. Oxygen desaturation that is resistant to therapeutic oxygen delivery may occur alone or in conjunction with respiratory acidosis. In severe cases, metabolic acidosis resulting from lactic acidosis may be present.

A recent multicenter prevalence study from intensive care units (ICUs) in the United States and Canada documented four conditions that commonly required mechanical ventilation in respiratory failure:

Acute respiratory failure (ARF)	74%
Exacerbation of chronic obstructive pulmonary disease (COPD)	16% (see Chapters 11 through 13)
Coma	7%
Neuromuscular disease	3% (see Chapters 29 and 30)

*The authors wish to thank John E. Scaggs, BS, RRT, Clinical Supervisor of Cardiopulmonary Medicine at Memorial Medical Center, Springfield, Illinois, for his assistance in preparing this chapter. His department has been extremely successful in using Therapist-Driven Protocols in ventilator management and weaning.

539

The causes of ARF include the following:

Postoperative complications	17% (see Chapter 44)
Sepsis	17%
Trauma	13% (see Chapters 21 and 22)
Pneumonia	13% (see Chapter 15)
Heart failure	13% (see Chapter 20)
ARDS	9% (see Chapter 27)
Aspiration	3% (see Chapters 15 and 33)
Other (miscellaneous)	16%

All of the clinical scenarios described in Chapter 9 may (and do, if left untreated) lead to respiratory failure. As discussed in Chapter 9, it is crucial that the RCP be able to recognize the clinical scenarios caused by (1) the six most common anatomic alterations of the lungs and (2) the respiratory disorders that produce them (Table 45-1).

Deterioration Despite Intensive Respiratory Care

The respiratory care student must also understand the fragile nature of patients who require mechanical ventilation. The causes of ARF listed above are very similar to a list of conditions that complicate in-hospital management of ventilated patients; RCPs should keep these diseases in mind at all times when caring for patients requiring ventilatory support. Ventilator management and weaning are much easier when problems do not arise, and success in the work is directly proportional to the RCP's identification of complicating conditions. For example, when RCPs use the Bronchopulmonary Hygiene Protocol to control secretions in ventilated patients, they also must employ the Mechanical Ventilation Protocol to achieve the optimal result.

A mnemonic to aid the RCP in recognizing complicating conditions in patients receiving ventilator support (CAP PNEUMONIA) may be helpful, especially in cases in which a ventilated patient either is not improving or is worsening (Box 45-1).

BOX 45–1

Conditions That May Develop in the Hospital and Complicate the Management of Patients Receiving Mechanical Ventilation

C   Cardiovascular events (e.g., hypotension, arrhythmia, myocardial infarction, congestive heart failure)
A   Acute respiratory distress syndrome and barotrauma
P   Pulmonary—embolism/infarction

P   Pneumothorax
N   Neuropsychiatric complication (e.g., stroke, psychosis)
E   Electrolyte and fluid imbalance (e.g., hypokalemia, hypophosphatemia)
U   Upper airway obstruction (e.g., tracheal stenosis)
M   Malnutrition
O   Oxygen toxicity (rare)
N   Nonsense data (e.g., erroneous data input, loose leads, poor-quality chest radiographs)
I   Infection (e.g., nosocomial infection, pneumonia, staphylococcal sepsis)
A   Atelectasis

The Fifth Protocol—General Management

After assessing the patient and identifying the nature and severity of the respiratory failure as described previously, the RCP must ask a second question: Do any contraindications to invasive mechanical ventilation exist? Such contraindications include the

---

TABLE 45–1   Common Anatomic Alterations of the Lungs Resulting in Respiratory Failure

Anatomic Alteration of the Lung	Examples of Respiratory Disorders
Atelectasis (see Figure 9-7)	Mucus plugging (e.g., chronic bronchitis)
Alveolar consolidation (see Figure 9-8)	Pneumonia
Increased alveolar-capillary membrane thickness (see Figure 9-9)	Acute respiratory distress syndrome, pulmonary edema
Bronchospasm (see Figure 9-10)	Asthma
Excessive bronchial secretions (see Figure 9-11)	Chronic bronchitis, asthma, pulmonary edema
Distal airway and alveolar weakening (see Figure 9-12)	Emphysema

OVERVIEW
of the Cardiopulmonary Clinical Manifestations Associated with ACUTE RESPIRATORY FAILURE

At the right side of each of the clinical scenarios (see Figures 9-7 through 9-12) is an overview of the signs and symptoms of the various diseases that, when allowed to proceed to their "worst case scenario," end in acute respiratory failure. The reader will note a certain sameness to each of these descriptions. When taken together, they describe the clinical findings in the whole gamut of conditions that can end in the death of the patient unless they are treated quickly and correctly.

The following are clinical manifestations of acute respiratory failure that are indications for mechanical ventilation:

- Somnolence proceeding to coma (an indication of alveolar hypoventilation)

- Severe and worsening hypoxemia
- Excessive work of breathing
- Inadequate lung expansion

Clinical indicators: respiratory acidosis (acute ventilatory failure) ($\uparrow$ $Paco_2$, $\downarrow$ pH, $\downarrow$ Spo_2, $\downarrow$ Pao_2)

Clinical indicators: agitation, tachycardia, pulse >120, $\uparrow$ A-ao_2, $\downarrow$ Pao_2/Fio_2, $\uparrow$ shunt fraction, venous admixture

Clinical indicators: dyspnea, $\uparrow$ ventilatory effort (VE), $\uparrow$ physiologic dead space (PDS), $\uparrow$ respiratory rate (RR), diaphoresis, extreme use of accessory muscles, abdominal paradox

Clinical indicators: atelectasis, $\downarrow$ ventilatory capacity (VC), $\downarrow$ maximum inspiratory pressure (MIP), $\downarrow$ maximum voluntary ventilation (MVV)

---

availability of noninvasive modes of ventilation (e.g., noninvasive positive-pressure ventilation [NIPPV], continuous positive-pressure ventilation [CPPV], cuirass-aided ventilation), patient wishes to the contrary, and the fact that intubation and mechanical ventilation would be futile and would needlessly prolong the patient's life.

The selection of the mode of ventilation depends on the goals of mechanical ventilation. For example, the *National Heart, Lung, and Blood Institute (NHLBI) ARDS Clinical Trials Network* recently chose the following goals when ventilating patients suffering from ARDS:

Oxygenation goal—Pao_2 55-80 mm Hg, or Spo_2 88%-95%

pH goal—7.30-7.45

Ventilator plateau pressure (PP) goal $\leq$30 cm H_2O

Inspiratory/expiratory (I:E) ratio goal—1:1.0-1:1.3

Because clinical objectives vary among the various conditions, a variety of modes of ventilation, suggested tidal volumes, positive end-expiratory pressure (PEEP) settings, and weaning strategies are appropriate.

Ventilator Management and Ventilator Weaning Modes (see Table 9-3)

More than 90% of patients requiring ventilatory support in the United States are ventilated with (A/C) alone or in combination with (PS) ventilation. Initial tidal volume (V_T) settings of 6 to 10 ml/kg

ideal body weight traditionally are used, with recent "lung protective strategies" favoring smaller V_T settings in the range of 5 to 6 ml/kg.

In routine cases (e.g., postoperative ventilator support, drug overdoses), focal or unilateral lung disease (e.g., lobar pneumonia, atelectasis), acute brain injury, and flail chest without acute lung injury, tidal volumes of 10 to 12 ml/kg are used routinely. In cases of obstructive lung disease and ARDS, 5 to 8 ml/kg settings usually are ordered. Tidal volumes as great as 16 ml/kg have been used to minimize dyspnea and prevent atelectasis in acute neuromuscular diseases such as Guillain-Barré syndrome or cervical spinal cord injury. An initial PEEP setting of 5.0 cm H_2O is used in most cases. However, PEEP should not be used in patients with acute brain injury and should be used only with great caution in patients with obstructive lung disease (in which dynamic hyperinflation may exist) or acute lung injury (in which barotrauma may result).

Except in patients with anoxic brain or myocardial injuries, permissive hypercapnia is allowed. The initial RR is set to approximate the initial baseline ventilatory rate but should not be greater than 35 breaths/minute. V_T and RR are adjusted to achieve the predetermined pH and plateau pressure goals, and the inspiratory flow is set above spontaneous breathing patient demand.

Each weaning mode has its advocates. In the United States, SIMV with PS ventilation and PS ventilation alone are used more often than spontaneous breathing ("T-piece") trials (SBT). The selection of weaning mode does not appear to be as crucial as the clinical skills of the person doing the weaning. Aggressive weaning techniques have resulted in tremendous shortening of ventilator hours in most centers, particularly in the postoperative setting (e.g., in patients recovering from open-heart surgery).

Use of Other Protocols

In addition to understanding any Mechanical Ventilation Protocols or Weaning Protocols that are in use,

the RCP must be cognizant of situations requiring the use of other protocols or protocol contents. Especially important are the Bronchopulmonary Hygiene Therapy Protocol (see Protocol 9-2), Hyperinflation Therapy Protocol (see Protocol 9-3), and Aerosolized Medication Protocol (see Protocol 9-4). Intubation and ventilator management of patients in no way bypasses the need for such therapies. Indeed, they may be needed in greater-than-usual intensity in some patients.

Case Study: ACUTE RESPIRATORY FAILURE*

Admitting History and Physical Examination

A 49-year-old homosexual African-American man arrived at the hospital complaining of exertional dyspnea of gradual onset. The condition had been troubling him for the past 3 months. The dyspnea had worsened over the 3 weeks before admission and was associated with a nonproductive cough and streaky hemoptysis. He had recently lost weight and currently weighed 68 kg. On admission, the patient appeared well nourished and was in no acute distress. His blood pressure was 152/75 mm Hg; heart rate, 119/min; RR, 18/min; and temperature, 97.6° F. Lung examination revealed diffuse coarse crackles. Cardiac, extremity, and abdominal examinations were unremarkable. A chest radiograph (Figure 45-1) demonstrated bilateral interstitial infiltrates. His arterial blood gas values were as follows: pH 7.46, Pa_{CO_2} 39, HCO_3^- 27, Pa_{O_2} 34, and Sa_{O_2} 69% on room air. The patient's white blood cell count (WBC) was 13,400 cells/cm^3 (79% neutrophils, 2% bands); hemoglobin, 13 g/dl; hematocrit, 42%; and platelet count, 348,000/cm^3. Electrolytes, blood urea nitrogen (BUN), and creatinine were normal. Lactate dehydrogenase (LDH) was 1007 U/L (with normal being 313 to 618 U/L), and all other liver chemistry tests were normal.

---

*The authors wish to express their appreciation to Timothy G. Janz, MD, and the other authors of an article presenting this case in the literature (Schnader J, editor: Clinical conference on management dilemmas: progressive infiltrates and respiratory failure, *Chest* 117:562, 2000). The authors of this text have altered the original case presentation slightly for teaching purposes.

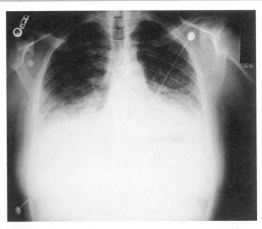

Figure 45–1 Admission anteroposterior chest X-ray showing bilateral infiltrates, which are more pronounced in the perihilar and lower lung fields. The infiltrate has a reticular pattern suggesting interstitial lung disease.

The patient was treated with intravenous (IV) piperacillin/tazobactam, erythromycin, furosemide, and cotrimoxazole, as well as oral prednisone 60 mg twice a day (BID). Blood and sputum cultures were negative. A two-dimensional echocardiogram showed mild biventricular hypertrophy, right atrial enlargement, and normal systolic ventricular function. Initially, administration of 2 L/min of oxygen via nasal cannula resulted in an Sa_{O_2} of 91%; however, over the next 2 days the RR increased to 34 breaths/min, and the Sa_{O_2} fell to 84%. The fraction of inspired oxygen (Fi_{O_2}) was increased to 0.40 via mask, causing the Sa_{O_2} to improve to 93%.

The patient was transferred to the medical intensive care unit (ICU), and on the fourth hospital day, bronchoscopy demonstrated normal bronchial mucosa, minimal secretions, and no endobronchial lesions. Stains and cultures of bronchial washings were negative for *Pneumocystis carinii*, acid-fast bacilli, fungi, other pathogenic bacteria, and viruses. Because of complications during the procedure, including unstable cardiorespiratory parameters, bronchoalveolar lavage (BAL) and transbronchial biopsy were judged too dangerous and were not performed. A human immunodeficiency virus-1 (HIV-1) titer was negative, and cotrimoxazole and prednisone were discontinued. The erythrocyte sedimentation rate (ESR) was 78 mm/h (with normal being 0 to 15 mm/h). The antinuclear antibody (ANA) titer was 1:80 with a cytoplasmic pattern; the antineutrophilic cytoplasmic antibody (ANCA) test was negative. Serum IgG and IgA levels were 2598 mg/dl (with normal being 564 to 1765 mg/dl) and 616 mg/dl (with normal being 85 to 385 mg/dl), respectively; serum IgM, C3, and C4 levels were normal. Antiglomerular basement membrane antibodies were not present.

The patient complained of severe dyspnea. His RR increased to 32 to 40 breaths/min, requiring an F_{IO_2} of 0.60 to maintain an Sao_2 greater than 90%. The chest radiograph showed worsening infiltrates. On the sixth hospital day, a right-sided heart catheter was placed to confirm that the infiltrates were noncardiogenic in nature. Table 45-2 summarizes the patient's hemodynamic data. The patient was afebrile. The pulmonary artery catheter was removed on the eighth hospital day.

The patient's dyspnea became even more severe. On the ninth hospital day, his RR rose to 60 breaths/min and his heart rate to 130 beats/min. Auscultation of the chest revealed persistent, widespread crackles.

His Spo_2 was 90%. Arterial blood gases on an F_{IO_2} of 0.55 were as follows: pH 7.41, $Paco_2$ 39, Pao_2 54, HCO_3^- 26, and Sao_2 88%. He developed a fever, which rose to 102° F; the chest radiograph revealed worsening infiltrates. The WBC count increased from 17,000 to 27,000 cells/cm³. At this time, the respiratory therapist recorded the following SOAP note in the patient's record:

Respiratory Assessment and Plan

S Patient complains of severe shortness of breath.
O T 102° F, RR 60, HR 130, Spo_2 90%. Diffuse crackles in all lung fields. ABGs on 55% O_2: pH 7.41, $Paco_2$ 39, Pao_2 54, HCO_3^- 26, Sao_2 via co-oximetry 88%. WBC 27,000; CXR: bilateral diffuse infiltrates, worse at the bases.
A • Impending respiratory failure (ABGs)
 • Widespread pulmonary infiltrate—rule out pneumonitis (fever, WBC, CXR) versus ARDS (infiltrates, hemodynamic data)
P Elective semi-urgent intubation. Titrate F_{IO_2} with pulse oximetry. Initial ventilator settings: F_{IO_2} 1.0, SIMV mode, back-up rate (BUR) 12/min, V_T 700 cc; CXR and ABG 30 minutes after intubation.

• • • • •

Assessment 20 Minutes Later

The patient was intubated and mechanically ventilated in the A/C mode with a V_T of 800 cc, an RR of 12/min, and an F_{IO_2} of 1.00. A chest X-ray was taken 30 minutes later (Figure 45-2). Arterial blood gases were as follows: pH 7.21, $Paco_2$ 51, HCO_3^- 21, Pao_2 34, and Sao_2 52%. PEEP was administered incrementally to 17 cm H_2O, and midazolam and vecuronium were infused for sedation and paralysis. Arterial blood gases measured at this point were as follows: pH 7.26, $Paco_2$ 53, HCO_3^- 23, Pao_2 76,

TABLE 45–2 **Hemodynamics on Hospital Day 6**		
	Time	
Parameter	**8 AM (Initial Reading)**	**10 PM**
Heart rate (beats/min)	96	118
Central venous pressure (mm Hg)	6	9
Mean pulmonary artery pressure (mm Hg)	31	41
Pulmonary artery occlusion wedge pressure (mm Hg)	13	12
Mean systemic arterial pressure (mm Hg)	96	84
Cardiac output (L/min)	9.7	17.6
Cardiac index (L/min/m²)	4.7	8.5
Stroke volume (ml)	101.0	149.2
Systemic vascular resistance (dyne/s/cm⁻⁵)	742	341
Pulmonary vascular resistance (dyne/s/cm⁻⁵)	148	132

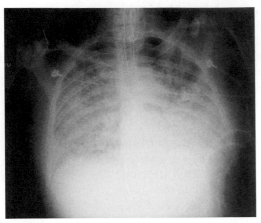

Figure 45–2   Chest X-ray on the fourth hospital day, with worsening, homogenous, near-confluent infiltrates.

and Sao_2 93%. Levofloxacin was added to the other antibiotics being given. Blood, urine, and deep tracheal suction–obtained sputum cultures were repeated, but these again tested negative.

Several hours after the initiation of mechanical ventilation (by 6 PM on day 9) the patient's blood pressure fell to 89/48 mm Hg, prompting the administration of fluids, 5 mg/kg/min of dopamine, and 5 mg/kg/min of dobutamine. The patient remained febrile, with a temperature of 101° F. A Swan-Ganz pulmonary artery catheter was inserted for better management of her hypotension. Table 45-3 summarizes the patient's hemodynamic data. With a set rate of 16 breaths/min on a V_T of 800 cc and a PEEP of 14 cm H_2O, the peak airway pressure was 84 cm H_2O;

plateau pressure was 82 cm H_2O; and respiratory dynamic and static compliances were 11.4 and 11.8 ml/cm H_2O, respectively. The Spo_2 was 91%. Breath sounds were diminished, with underspread crackles. Arterial blood gases on 100% O_2 were as follows: pH 7.25, $Paco_2$ 55, HCO_3^- 22, Pao_2 70 mm Hg, and Sao_2 90%. At this point, the ICU respiratory therapist recorded the following SOAP note in the patient's record:

Respiratory Assessment and Plan

S   N/A (intubated)

O   T 101° F, BP 89/48, RR 16/min on A/C mode, HR 134, Spo_2 91%. Breath sounds decreased. Persistent underspread crackles. Ventilator settings: Fio_2 1.0, A/C 16/min, PEEP 14 cm H_2O, peak airway pressure 84 cm H_2O, plateau pressure 82 cm H_2O, dynamic compliance 11.4 ml/cm H_2O, static compliance 11.8 cm H_2O. CXR: worsening bilateral infiltrates; ABGs on 100% O_2: pH 7.25, $Paco_2$ 55, HCO_3^- 22, Pao_2 70; Sao_2 via co-oximetry 90%, HCO_3^- 15.5.

A   • Acute ventilatory failure with mild hypoxemia, worsening, with CO_2 retention and metabolic acidosis (ABGs)
- Diffuse pulmonary infiltrates, worsening (CXR), with poorly compliant lung mechanics (ventilator graphics) requiring high airway pressures
- Hypermetabolic state (hemodynamics)
- Possible sepsis
- Risk of barotrauma (ventilator and airway pressures)
- Low cardiac output state (hemodynamic monitoring)

TABLE 45–3 **Hemodynamics on Hospital Day 9**		
	Time	
Parameter	**6 PM (Initial Reading, Patient on Dopamine and Dobutamine)**	**10 PM (After Increased Dopamine, IV Fluids, and No Dobutamine)**
Heart rate (beats/min)	134	113
Central venous pressure (mm Hg)	13	17
Mean pulmonary artery pressure (mm Hg)	42	51
Pulmonary artery occlusion wedge pressure (mm Hg)	16	18
Mean systemic arterial pressure (mm Hg)	63	94
Cardiac output (L/min)	10.0	6.3
Cardiac index (L/min/m²)	4.8	3.0
Stroke volume (ml)	74.6	55.8
Systemic vascular resistance (dyne/s/cm⁻⁵)	400	977
Pulmonary vascular resistance (dyne/s/cm⁻⁵)	208	419

P Discuss case with pulmonologist attending. Consider increasing PEEP, with pneumothorax precautions. Consider permissive hypercapnia and reducing V_T to 6 ml/kg (400 to 500 cc).

Subsequent Hospital Course

The patient became unresponsive, and his neurologic status worsened. Because of the high airway pressures, the V_T was reduced to 700 cc, the PEEP was increased to 17 cm H_2O, and the inspiratory/expiratory ratio was changed from 1:1.7 to 1:1. However, the patient's Pao_2 subsequently fell to 51 mm Hg and the oxygen saturation to 79%. In response, the V_T was changed back to 800 cc, and the Pao_2 and oxygen saturation returned to 70 mm Hg and 90%, respectively. Open-lung biopsy was considered, but the patient was believed to be too unstable to undergo the procedure.

On the tenth hospital day, subcutaneous emphysema was noted on physical examination, and the chest radiograph and computed tomography (CT) scan again showed diffuse alveolar infiltrates, extensive pneumomediastinum, pneumoperitoneum, and a small right pneumothorax (Figure 45-3). A right-sided chest tube was placed. The patient's temperature dipped to 94.0° F, his Pao_2 fell to 43 mm Hg, and his creatinine rose to 2.6 mg/dl. Methylprednisolone was begun empirically, and midazolam and vecuronium infusions were discontinued. In spite of this, the patient remained comatose—he was unresponsive to stimuli and diffusely flaccid, lacking light, corneal, and oculocephalic reflexes. On hospital day 12, his arterial blood gases were as follows: pH 7.22; $Paco_2$ 44; HCO_3^- 18; Pao_2 59; and Sao_2 88% on a V_T of 800 cc, an RR of 22/min, an Fio_2 of 1.00, and a PEEP of 20 cm H_2O. On day 15, a right-sided

chest tube was inserted to treat a tension pneumothorax (Figure 45-4). On the following day, a nuclear brain scan was performed; it revealed no cerebral blood flow. The regional organ procurement organization was consulted; however, the patient was refused as an organ donor. After the family was consulted, the patient was removed from life support, whereupon he died.

Note: *The decision not to perform bronchoscopic lavage, transbronchial biopsy, and open-lung biopsy in this case was not made by the authors of this case report.*

Discussion

The patient's hypoxemic respiratory failure despite therapy suggested that an exact cause for his illness had not yet been determined. While attempts were being made to do this, his respiratory failure worsened and his toxic state became more severe. Tachycardia, tachypnea, and anxiety resulted from his hypoxemia. The pulmonary crackles heard on auscultation and the infiltrates observed on his chest X-ray suggest the possibility of an infectious process (i.e., **Alveolar Consolidation** [see Figure 9-8], or **Increased Alveolar-Capillary Membrane Thickness** [see Figure 9-9]), as does the leukocytosis. No sputum had been obtained for analysis, and his hemodynamic parameters confirmed a hypermetabolic state.

The normal pulmonary capillary wedge pressures argued against left ventricular failure. The 3-month prodrome suggested that more than just acute and usual pneumonia may have been present, but his acutely ill state precluded open-lung or transbronchial lung biopsy.

The negative HIV-1 titer and negative bronchial washings argued against a diagnosis of acquired

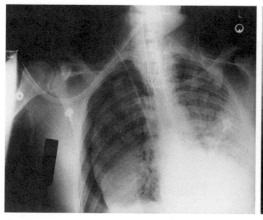
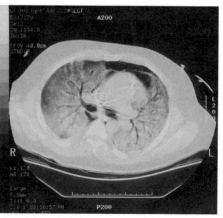

A **B**

Figure 45–3 Chest X-ray and CT scan on the tenth hospital day. Note the development of a right pneumothorax, and the presence of widespread pulmonary consolidation and air bronchograms in the CT scan.

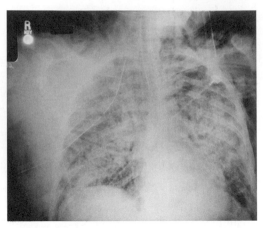

Figure 45–4   Chest X-ray on the fifteenth hospital day. Note the bilateral, dense, diffuse infiltrates. Bilateral chest tubes are evident, and subcutaneous emphysema is visible.

immunodeficiency syndrome (AIDS). A CD4 count and helper/suppressor lymphocyte ratio would have been helpful.

The patient was intubated after the first assessment because of his distress, increased work of breathing, and progressive hypoxemia. The need to control the airway before any diagnostic lung biopsy procedure could be performed probably influenced the team toward that intervention rather than toward providing F_{IO_2} therapy by mask.

At autopsy the lungs were heavy and edematous, the bronchi contained large amounts of bloody mucus, and thromboemboli were found. Microscopic examination revealed diffuse proliferation of fibroblasts with thickening of the alveolar septa. (The student should review Figure 9-9, which illustrates in detail the pathophysiologic changes seen in **Alveolar-Capillary Membrane Thickening**.) Bronchial and mycobacterial cultures were negative. The final diagnosis was acute interstitial pneumonitis.

SELF-ASSESSMENT QUESTIONS

Complete the Following

In the space to the right of each mnemonic letter, list the conditions that may develop in the hospital setting and complicate the management of patients receiving mechanical ventilation.

C _____

_____

A _____

_____

P _____

_____

P _____

_____

N _____

_____

E _____

_____

U _____

_____

M _____

_____

O _____

_____

N _____

_____

I _____

_____

A _____

_____

PART XIV

Selected Practice Case Studies

Using the SOAP format, the reader is challenged to write on a separate piece of paper the assessments and treatments for each of the practice case studies provided in this section. The assessment and treatment selection scenario areas throughout each case are designated as follows:

■ ■ SOAP 1, 2, OR 3 ■ ■

To facilitate the assessment process, a predesigned SOAP form is provided at the end of this section. The reader may wish to copy this form for use in writing his or her assessments and treatment selections for each case study. Answers are provided in Appendix XII.

Case 1: CHRONIC BRONCHITIS

ADMITTING HISTORY

A 68-year-old retired geologist arrived in the emergency room with his daughter. Well-known to the respiratory care consult team, he has a 40-year history of smoking a pack of cigarettes a day, is widowed, lives alone, and has difficulty managing his daily activities. For the past week, the man has experienced increased dyspnea and cough and has been unable to care for himself. His personal hygiene appeared to have deteriorated. He stated that he has been unable to get his breath or inhale deeply enough to cough up secretions. He complained of mild nausea without abdominal pain or vomiting. His physician had given him an unknown oral antibiotic 3 days before this admission.

The patient was diagnosed with severe chronic bronchitis approximately 6 years ago and had an acute myocardial infarction 2 years ago. His pulmonary function studies (completed 1 year before this admission) showed severe airway obstruction and air trapping. He has a history of high blood pressure, congestive heart failure, chronic dyspnea on exertion, and chronic cough, and he experienced two episodes of pneumonia within the last year. According to a neighbor, he has become increasingly depressed in recent months.

According to his daughter, his physical activity is minimal. He generally spends most of his days watching television, smoking, and napping. All his children, none of whom live in the immediate area, have tried to coax him to move to a boardinghouse environment, but he has adamantly refused. The advantages of pulmonary rehabilitation were discussed with him during his last admission. The patient said that he had no need for pulmonary education or the services of other agencies or organizations that would monitor his condition through home visits.

PHYSICAL EXAMINATION (TIME: 1730)

Inspection revealed a barrel chest, clubbing of fingers and toes, cyanotic skin, and pitting edema (2+) around the ankles. The patient's breathing was labored; he pursed his lips to breathe, using his accessory muscles of respiration, and he appeared weak. He had a frequent, weak cough productive of large amounts of thick, yellow sputum.

Vital signs were as follows: blood pressure 190/115, heart rate 125 bpm, respiratory rate 30/min, and oral temperature 37° C (98.6° F). Tactile fremitus was present over both lung fields, and hyperresonant percussion notes were produced both anteriorly and posteriorly. Bilateral rhonchi were auscultated. His abdomen was soft and not tender. Bowel sounds were active.

On room air his arterial blood gas values (ABGs) were as follows: pH 7.53, $Paco_2$ 56 mm Hg, HCO_3^- 33 mMol/L, and Pao_2 43 mm Hg. On his last hospital discharge his baseline ABGs on 2 L/min oxygen were as follows: pH 7.39, $Paco_2$ 85 mm Hg, HCO_3^- 38 mMol/L, and Pao_2 64 mm Hg. His carboxyhemoglobin level was 6%. His chest X-ray on this admission showed severe hyperinflation with depressed hemidiaphragms. No acute infiltrates were apparent. His heart size was normal. His complete blood count values were all normal except for a hematocrit of 58%. The attending physician ordered a respiratory care consult. The following order was written in the patient's chart: "All efforts should be made to keep the patient off the ventilator."

■ ■ **SOAP 1** ■ ■

EARLY MORNING, NEXT DAY (TIME: 0230)

The floor nurse called the on-duty respiratory care practitioner to evaluate the patient. The nurse reported that the patient had said that he was having a bad period. The nurse added that the patient appeared restless and short of breath and was coughing excessively.

On inspection the patient could be seen using his accessory muscles of respiration. He demonstrated pursed-lip breathing. In addition, he demonstrated a weak, productive cough and expectorated large amounts of thick, yellow secretions. The patient's vital signs were as follows: blood pressure 185/135, heart rate 130 bpm, respiratory rate 28/min, and oral temperature 37° C (98.6° F). Bilateral rhonchi were auscultated over the lung bases. His ABGs were as follows: pH 7.55, $Paco_2$ 53 mm Hg, HCO_3^- 32 mMol/L, Pao_2 41 mm Hg. His hemoglobin oxygen saturation measured by pulse oximetry (Spo_2) was 83%.

■ ■ **SOAP 2** ■ ■

LATE AFTERNOON, SAME DAY (TIME: 1415)

Although the patient had been resting comfortably for several hours, he suddenly became short of breath and difficult to arouse, directly before a scheduled bronchial hygiene treatment. The respiratory therapist on duty noted that the patient said that he was "doing worse again." He was sitting up in bed, using his accessory muscles of respiration, and demonstrating pursed-lip breathing. His breathing was rapid and shallow. His cough continued to be weak. No sputum production was noted at this time. Expiration was prolonged.

His vital signs were as follows: blood pressure 150/95, heart rate 140 bpm, respiratory rate 25/min, and temperature 37° C (98.6° F). He had bilateral wheezes and rhonchi. A recent chest X-ray was unavailable. His ABGs were as follows: pH 7.28, $Paco_2$ 105 mm Hg, HCO_3^- 41 mMol/L, and Pao_2 44 mm Hg. His carboxyhemoglobin level was 2.5%. A toxic drug blood screen was negative.

■ ■ **SOAP 3** ■ ■

Case 2: EMPHYSEMA

ADMITTING HISTORY

A 62-year-old man has a history of cough and shortness of breath, coupled with multiple hospitalizations. He was admitted because of severe, worsening dyspnea. He lived and worked in Pittsburgh, Pennsylvania, for 35 years as a foundry worker in a steel manufacturing plant. His wife died 10 years ago. After his wife's death, he lived alone for 9 years and managed his daily activities with progressive difficulty.

Approximately 2 years before this admission, he was forced to retire early because of declining health. His doctor told him that he had chronic emphysema. For the past year, he has been living with his brother's family in Chicago. The patient's brother indicated during the interview that the patient might "have the flu again." The patient has a 35-pack/year history of smoking unfiltered cigarettes, but he stopped smoking at the time of his forced retirement.

His last hospitalization was 9 weeks before this admission. At that time, he was hospitalized for 2 days for cough, muscle aches and pains, fever, and respiratory distress. He underwent a complete pulmonary function study and received bronchial hygiene therapy, oxygen therapy, and instruction in at-home breathing exercises.

Also at this time, hospital personnel noted that the patient's expiratory flow rate measurements had declined significantly since his pulmonary function tests (PFTs) a year earlier. In fact, in the past year his forced expiratory volume in 1 second (FEV_1) had declined from 70% of that predicted to 45% of that predicted. At discharge 9 weeks before this admission and on 1.5 L/min oxygen by nasal cannula, the patient's ABGs were as follows: pH 7.37, $Paco_2$ 67 mm Hg, HCO_3^- 36 mM/L, and Pao_2 63 mm Hg. He had received influenza vaccine 6 months earlier and pneumococcal vaccine 2 years earlier.

At the time of discharge 9 weeks earlier, he was demonstrating pursed-lip breathing and using his accessory muscles of inspiration at rest. He demonstrated no spontaneous cough or sputum production. His bronchodilator therapy was discontinued 1 year ago because it had been "found to be ineffective" during his PFT. He was strongly encouraged to perform his pulmonary rehabilitation exercises daily. A weekly exercise diary was given to him by the respiratory care department at discharge.

PHYSICAL EXAMINATION

In the emergency room, the patient was febrile, cyanotic, and in obvious respiratory distress. He appeared malnourished. He was 180 cm (6 feet tall) and weighed 66 kg (146 lb). His skin was cool and clammy. The patient said, "I'm so short of breath!"

His vital signs were as follows: blood pressure 155/110, heart rate 95 bpm, respiratory rate 25/min, and oral temperature 38.3° C (101° F). He was using his accessory muscles of inspiration and breathing through pursed lips. An increased anteroposterior diameter of the chest was easily visible. Percussion revealed that he had low-lying, poorly mobile hemidiaphragms. Expiration was prolonged, and his breath sounds were diminished. No wheezes were noted, but crackles could be heard over the right lower lobe.

A chest X-ray showed pulmonary hyperexpansion, severe apical pleural scarring, a large bulla in the right middle lobe, and a right lower lobe infiltrate consistent with pneumonia. On instruction the patient's forced cough was weak and productive of a small amount of yellow sputum. On 1.5 L/min oxygen by nasal cannula, his ABGs were as follows: pH 7.59, $Paco_2$ 40 mm Hg, HCO_3^- 37 mMol/L, and Pao_2 38 mm Hg. The physician ordered a pulmonary consult and stated that she did not want to commit the patient to a ventilator if possible. The patient also was started on intravenous doses of aminophylline and methylprednisolone.

■ ■ SOAP 1 ■ ■

2 DAYS LATER

At this time, the patient stated that his chest was feeling tighter and that he was even more short of breath. His vital signs were as follows: blood pressure 160/115, heart rate 97 bpm, respiratory rate 15/min and shallow, and oral temperature 37.8° C (100° F). Expectorated sputum was thick, yellow, and tenacious. He no longer was using his accessory muscles of inspiration or demonstrating pursed-lip breathing. His breath sounds were diminished bilaterally, and crackles no longer could be heard over the right lower lobe. Dull percussion notes were elicited over the right lower lobe. His ABGs were as follows: pH 7.28, $Paco_2$ 82 mm Hg, HCO_3^- 36 mMol/L, and Pao_2 41 mm Hg. His hemoglobin oxygen saturation measured by pulse oximetry (Spo_2) was 68%. A repeat chest X-ray showed more extensive pulmonary infiltrates, particularly in the right lower chest. The physician ordered subcutaneous terbutaline every 8 hours.

■ ■ SOAP 2 ■ ■

Case 3: ASTHMA

ADMITTING HISTORY

A 10-year-old girl was well known to the respiratory care protocol team. Over the past 8 years, she was hospitalized for severe asthma three or four times per year. On average, each hospital stay lasted 2 to 3 days. She required mechanical ventilation three separate times over the past 4 years. Because of her excessive absenteeism from school, the girl was held back in the second grade. At the time of this admission, the patient was in the fourth grade.

About 2 years ago, the girl's mother lost her job as a bank teller because of the many days she needed to take off from work to accompany her daughter to the doctor. For the past 15 months, the mother has been able to work only part time as a checkout clerk at a local grocery store. This turn of events led to additional financial problems, compounded by increasing medical bills.

The last time the patient was on a ventilator was about 2 years ago. After that hospitalization, her mother—a single parent—quit smoking, a habit she practiced for about 20 years, and gave away the family cat. In addition, the family's mobile home and its heating system were cleaned thoroughly, and several portable air-conditioning units were installed. For the past 6 months, the girl has been on an albuterol inhaler four times a day and as needed; a beclomethasone inhaler four times a day; and oral theophylline twice daily. Her mother was instructed in the proper way to monitor her daughter's peak expiratory flow rate (PEFR) regularly. The patient's personal best PEFR was about 290 L/min.

During a recent doctor's appointment, allergy skin tests turned up positive for ragweed and grasses. The patient was begun on a program of hyposensitization. Despite these efforts, the girl still experienced a number of serious asthmatic episodes, two of which required hospitalization. Mechanical ventilation was not required in either case.

The patient was last hospitalized 6 weeks earlier. Her PEFR on admission was 175 L/min, and she had severe hypoxemia. At that time, she received aerosolized albuterol almost continuously for 3 hours and oxygen therapy per protocol. The physician on duty treated her aggressively with intravenous aminophylline and steroids. The patient progressively improved. Her ABGs returned to normal within 6 hours of her admission. She was discharged the next afternoon. Fortunately, because the asthma episode occurred over a weekend, she did not miss any school days.

About 6 hours before the current admission, the patient had gone to bed (at 9 PM) with no respiratory complaints, although she had been achy and tired for about 1 week. At approximately 1:30 AM, she awoke short of breath. After alerting her mother, she took two puffs of her albuterol inhaler. The mother then measured her daughter's PEFR and noted that it was 235 L/min. Hoping that this asthma episode would subside soon, she instructed her daughter to take another puff of her inhaler. She then encouraged her daughter to try to go back to sleep.

Within 45 minutes, however, the girl's condition had not improved; in fact, it was becoming progressively worse. Her PEFR at this time was 210 L/min.

Again, the mother had her daughter take two puffs of her albuterol inhaler. Then, minutes later, the mother again asked her daughter to exhale forcefully into her peak flow meter. Her PEFR was 170 L/min. At this point, she put her daughter, still wearing her pajamas, into the car and drove to the hospital emergency room.

PHYSICAL EXAMINATION (TIME: 0315)

On admission to the emergency department, the patient demonstrated extreme shortness of breath. She was sitting up with her legs crossed on the hospital gurney, her hands and arms in front of her and anchored to her knees in a tripod position. She was using her accessory muscles of inspiration, demonstrating pursed-lip breathing, and crying; she appeared anxious and cyanotic. She stated, "I feel horrible, and my chest is tight." She frequently demonstrated a strong, productive cough. Her sputum was moderate in quantity and thick and white.

Her PEFR was 150 L/min. Her heart rate was 190 bpm; her blood pressure was 110/85, and she had a respiratory rate of 28/min. Her temperature was normal. Auscultation revealed diminished breath sounds, wheezing, and rhonchi bilaterally. Her chest X-ray showed severe air trapping, with depressed hemidiaphragms and hyperlucency of the lungs. Her hemoglobin oxygen saturation measured by pulse oximetry (Sp_{O_2}) on 2 L/min oxygen by nasal cannula was 77%, and her ABGs were as follows: pH 7.45, Pa_{CO_2} 28 mm Hg, HCO_3^- 19 mMol/L, and Pa_{O_2} 40 mm Hg. The physician had the patient transferred to the pediatric intensive care unit. A respiratory care consult was requested. The physician had written the following on the patient's chart: "Respiratory care— please assess and treat as aggressively as our protocol boundaries permit. I want to keep this patient off the ventilator if possible."

■ ■ **SOAP 1** ■ ■

TIME: 0530 (SAME DAY)

Since her admission, neither the patient nor her mother had been able to sleep. The patient was in a high Fowler's position, with her arms fixed to the side bedrails. She was using her accessory muscles of inspiration and breathing through pursed lips, and she was cyanotic. She had a frequent, strong cough that produced a moderate amount of thick, white secretions during each coughing episode. Her chest still appeared hyperinflated. She stated, "I'm sorry. I'm wheezing too much, and I can't go to sleep."

Her PEFR at this time was 175 L/min. Her heart rate was 180 bpm, blood pressure 105/82, and respiratory rate 24/min. Hyperresonant percussion notes were produced bilaterally. On auscultation, she demonstrated prolonged expiration, diminished breath sounds, rhonchi, and wheezing bilaterally. No follow-up chest X-ray had been taken. Her Sp_{O_2} was 95%, and her ABGs were as follows: pH 7.48, Pa_{CO_2} 34 mm Hg, HCO_3^- 24 mMol/L, and Pa_{O_2} 73 mm Hg.

■ ■ **SOAP 2** ■ ■

TIME: 0745 (SAME DAY)

The patient's assigned day-shift therapist gathered clinical data during her morning rounds. The patient stated that she felt as though a weight were on her chest. She was using her accessory muscles of inspiration and demonstrating pursed-lip breathing. Her skin was damp and cool, and she was cyanotic. No cough or sputum production was noted. Her PEFR was 145 L/min. Her vital signs were as follows: blood pressure 160/100, heart rate 185 bpm, and respiratory rate 13/min. Her breath sounds were diminished bilaterally, and no wheezes or rhonchi were audible during auscultation. Hyperresonant percussion notes were elicited bilaterally. Her Sp_{O_2} was 79% and her ABGs were as follows: pH 7.27, Pa_{CO_2} 57 mm Hg, HCO_3^- 24 mMol/L, and Pa_{O_2} 51 mm Hg.

■ ■ **SOAP 3** ■ ■

Case 4: PNEUMONIA

ADMITTING HISTORY

A 79-year-old man was admitted to the hospital because of cough, fever, and a right lower lobe infiltrate. He was born in Detroit, where he worked as a truck driver for a dry-cleaning chemicals company for 51 years. He was always a hard worker and an active member of Teamsters Local 299. As a truck driver, he was often on the road 3 to 4 days at a time.

He never married, and after his sister died when he was 55 years old, he no longer had any living relatives. He started smoking at 14 years of age and averaged about two packs of cigarettes per day.

When he was not working, he consumed alcohol regularly. Despite his smoking and drinking habits, he retired in good health at 65 years of age.

The patient was last admitted to the hospital 2 years ago for an acute inferior myocardial infarction. He was treated with medications and recovered quite well. He stopped smoking at that time but continued to consume alcohol regularly. He reported that he generally consumed about four to six bottles of beer each night at a local bar with some fellow retirees. After his myocardial infarction, he continued to manage his daily affairs without difficulty. He exercised regularly by working in his yard each day, and he power-walked every other day at the mall.

Then, 4 days before this current admission, the man reported that he began experiencing "flulike" symptoms. He had chills; a mild fever; and a hacking, nonproductive cough. Although he was not feeling good, he continued to work in his yard and power-walk at the mall. He also socialized and consumed beer with his friends each night. The evening before this admission, his friends noted that he was getting progressively worse and encouraged him to see a doctor. The patient stated that he would seek medical care if he did not feel better in a week. The next day, however, the patient was very short of breath, his cough was more frequent, and he had a temperature of 38.3° C (101° F). At that point, he drove himself to the hospital.

PHYSICAL EXAMINATION

On inspection, the patient was a well-nourished man in obvious respiratory distress on 2 L/min oxygen by nasal cannula. He was monitored by pulse oximetry. The patient stated that he was very short of breath. He had a blood pressure of 165/90, heart rate of 120 bpm, respiratory rate of 33/min, and an oral temperature of 39.5° C (103° F). He demonstrated a frequent, strong cough. His cough was hacking and productive of a small amount of white and yellow sputum. His skin appeared pale and damp. When the man repeated the phrase *ninety-nine,* increased tactile and vocal fremitus was noted over the right lower lung posteriorly. Dull percussion notes and bronchial breath sounds were noted over the right lower lung regions posteriorly. His oxygen saturation measured by pulse oximetry (Spo_2) was 87%, and his ABGs

(on a 2 L nasal cannula) were as follows: pH 7.56, $Paco_2$ 24 mm Hg, HCO_3^- 22 mMol/L, and Pao_2 56 mm Hg. His chest X-ray demonstrated a right lower lobe infiltrate consistent with pneumonia (air bronchograms, and alveolar consolidation). His white blood cell (WBC) count was 21,000/mm³.

■ ■ SOAP 1 ■ ■

6 HOURS LATER

The therapist performing assessment rounds gathered the following clinical information:

The patient stated, "My doctor is too young. I feel worse than when I came in here." The patient had a blood pressure of 140/70, a heart rate of 125 bpm, a shallow respiratory rate of 35/min, and a temperature of 38.9° C (102° F). He demonstrated a strong, "barking" cough, and during each major coughing episode he produced a small amount of blood-streaked sputum. His lips and nailbeds appeared cyanotic. Over his right lower and middle lobes and his left lower lobe, he demonstrated increased tactile and vocal fremitus, dull percussion notes, bronchial breath sounds, and crackles. His Spo_2 was 86%. His ABGs were as follows: pH 7.55, $Paco_2$ 26 mm Hg, HCO_3^- 24 mMol/L, and Pao_2 53 mm Hg.

■ ■ SOAP 2 ■ ■

THE NEXT DAY

The respiratory therapist assigned to evaluate the patient gathered the following clinical information:

The patient stated that he slept most of the night and was breathing more easily.

The patient's blood pressure was 135/85; his heart rate was 90 bpm; his respiratory rate was 19/min; and he had an oral temperature of 37.3° C (99° F).

He had a strong, nonproductive cough. His morning chest X-ray and report indicated partial resolution of the pneumonic process but persistent consolidation or atelectasis in the right lower and middle lobes and left lower lobe. In these lung areas, the tactile and vocal fremitus had increased, and dull percussion notes and bronchial breath sounds were audible. His Spo_2 was 97%. On a 3 L/min nasal cannula, his ABGs were as follows: pH 7.44, $Paco_2$ 35 mm Hg, HCO_3^- 24 mMol/L, and Pao_2 163 mm Hg.

■ ■ SOAP 3 ■ ■

Case 5: PULMONARY EDEMA

ADMITTING HISTORY

A 68-year-old hypertensive man arrived in the emergency department via ambulance at 6:45 AM. The patient's wife stated that her husband had been doing well until the evening before admission, when he complained of being tired and short of breath. She also noted that he had demonstrated a sudden onset of dry, nonproductive cough. Thinking that he was getting a "touch of the flu," she gave her husband some hot soup, two aspirins, and a tablespoon of Robitussin and made him go to bed at about 8:30 PM. She stated that she had awoken about 4:30 AM to find her husband sitting up in bed, gasping for air. Alarmed, she had called 911.

The man's history shows that he had been in fairly good health since his retirement as a plumber 2 years ago. He has smoked about one pack of cigarettes a day for the past 40 years. For the past 2 years, he and his wife had actively devoted most of their time to gardening and travel. They are planning a cross-country trailer trip to Alaska. About 1 year ago, the man underwent a physical examination in preparation for this trip. At that time, his physician placed him on digoxin and furosemide (Lasix) to treat atrial fibrillation and mild congestive heart failure, and the man quit smoking.

On the patient's arrival at the treatment room, the emergency room nurse immediately placed him in a high Fowler's position. The respiratory therapist started oxygen at 2 L/min by nasal cannula. His wife appeared anxious. She was sobbing and walking back and forth, stating repeatedly, "Bill takes a heart pill and a water pill, and he follows a low-salt diet—just like the doctor told him to do."

PHYSICAL EXAMINATION (TIME: 0700)

On inspection, the patient was in obvious respiratory distress. However, the man stated, "I don't think I'm having a serious problem." He also added, "My wife and I are only 2 days away from our dream trip to Alaska. We've been planning this trip for 8 years! I can't believe this! It is just 2 days before we are supposed to leave, and here I am on this emergency room gurney!"

His vital signs were as follows: blood pressure 100/50, heart rate 145 bpm and irregular, and respiratory rate 22/min. The man was afebrile. His throat was reddened. On 2 L/min oxygen, his oxygen saturation measured by pulse oximetry (Sp_{O_2}) was 70%. His lips were blue, his neck veins were distended, he appeared very anxious, and he was coughing frequently, producing small amounts of frothy, pink secretions. His abdomen was distended, and pitting edema was present to the midcalf area. Palpation of his chest was unremarkable. Dull percussion notes were elicited over the lower lung regions bilaterally. Auscultation revealed inspiratory crackles and expiratory wheezing over the left and right lower lung regions.

His ABGs on 2 L/min oxygen by nasal cannula were as follows: pH 7.56, Pa_{CO_2} 28 mm Hg, HCO_3^- 20 mMol/L, and Pa_{O_2} 51 mm Hg. According to the radiologist's report, his chest X-ray showed faint opacities over the lower lung areas bilaterally. The X-ray report also noted that the patient's heart was moderately enlarged, suggesting left ventricular hypertrophy.

The emergency room physician started the patient on intravenous digitalis, dobutamine, and furosemide. The physician ordered another chest X-ray and asked the respiratory care consult service to see the patient. He specifically requested that respiratory care personnel monitor the patient closely over the next several hours.

■ ■ **SOAP 1** ■ ■

TIME: 1100

The repeat bedside chest X-ray showed no remarkable improvement. The patient stated, "I still don't feel great." His vital signs were as follows: blood pressure 160/90, heart rate 105 bpm and regular rhythm, respiratory rate 20/min, and temperature 37.1° C (98.8° F). The color of his lips had improved slightly, but no improvement was apparent in the patient's distended neck veins. The nurse noted that the man's urine output over the past 2 hours had been 650 ml. The patient still coughed frequently; however, no frothy, pink sputum was noted at this time. Auscultation continued to reveal inspiratory crackles and expiratory wheezing over the lower lung lobes bilaterally. His Sp_{O_2} was 84%. His ABG study revealed a pH 7.54, Pa_{CO_2} 25 mm Hg, HCO_3^- 18 mMol/L, and Pa_{O_2} 51 mm Hg. Neither his cardiac enzymes nor his troponin levels had risen.

■ ■ **SOAP 2** ■ ■

TIME: 1630

The man stated that he was breathing better. His vital signs were as follows: blood pressure 140/115, heart rate 95 bpm and regular, respiratory rate 16/min, and oral temperature 37.3° C (99.1° F). His lips and fingertips were no longer blue. The nursing chart showed that the patient's urine output over the past 2 hours had been 850 ml. The man appeared relaxed and no longer demonstrated any significant venous distention. On request, the patient produced a strong, nonproductive cough. Auscultation revealed bilateral crackles over the lower lung lobes. His pulse oximetry showed an SpO_2 of 97%, and repeated ABGs were as follows: pH 7.44, $PaCO_2$ 36 mm Hg, HCO_3^- 24 mMol/L, and PaO_2 190 mm Hg.

■ ■ **SOAP 3** ■ ■

Case 6: FLAIL CHEST

ADMITTING HISTORY

A 22-year-old Caucasian man has a long history of alcohol abuse. While in middle school, he and his friends stole their parents' beer and drank regularly. By the time he was a senior in high school, he was drinking beer and whiskey almost daily. When he was drinking, he often became mean and got into fights. Although he was well built and considered attractive, he generally could not maintain a long-term relationship with any of the girls whom he dated in high school. At graduation, however, he was dating the woman whom he would marry 7 months later.

The marriage was a stormy one. His wife was well known to the social workers who answered the hot line at the local crisis center. On several occasions, his wife summoned the police to the couple's mobile home with reports of spousal abuse. Once the man waved a small handgun at her and accidentally shot a hole through their kitchen wall. He always apologized extensively to his wife after a major incident and promised, to no avail, to stop drinking.

Within 1 year of their marriage, he lost his job as a carpenter because he missed too many days of work. Then, 15 months after their wedding, his wife completed a restraining order against him, filed for divorce, and moved in with her parents. He continued to drink heavily as he worked various minimum-wage jobs for the next 2 years. The local union laid him off 3 months ago from his position as an unskilled laborer. Using his unemployment checks to subsidize his habits, he spent most of his days and evenings in local bars drinking, playing cards, and shooting pool.

He lost his driver's license 5 weeks before this admission for a year for hitting—and completely destroying—a parked car while he was driving under the influence of alcohol.

On the day of this admission, the man started drinking heavily around 4 PM. By 11:30 PM, he was at a local dance club, extremely intoxicated. He was using foul language, bumping into people, yelling insults at the band, and constantly trying to start fights with other customers. The bouncer quickly ushered him off the premises.

The weather was bad on this night. It was cold, raining, sleeting, and dark as he walked and hitchhiked along a country road. He stumbled and staggered and yelled profanities at the cars as they drove past. A witness later told the police that he appeared to dare the cars to hit him. Approximately 20 minutes after he was ejected from the dance club, he was hit by a pickup truck. The ambulance crew found him 35 yards from the road, lying in a cornfield.

PHYSICAL EXAMINATION

When the man was brought into the emergency room, he was unconscious but breathing on his own through a nonrebreathing mask. He had numerous scrapes and lacerations on his face, anterior chest, and legs. Both his upper and lower front teeth were broken at the gum lines. Paradoxical movement could clearly be seen over most of his anterior chest. His skin appeared pale and cyanotic, and the smell of alcohol radiated strongly from his body. His blood alcohol level was 0.34%.

The man's vital signs were as follows: blood pressure 165/92, heart rate 120 bpm, respiratory rate 26/min and shallow, and rectal temperature 36.2° C (97.2° F). His weight was approximately 86 kg (190 lb). Breath sounds were diminished bilaterally. A chest X-ray showed extensive multiple double rib fractures of the right and left anterior and lateral ribs, between ribs 4 and 9. No pneumothorax was visible. His sternum was fractured in three separate places. Increased densities, consistent with atelectasis, were visible throughout both lung fields in the chest X-ray. The patient's ABGs on an $F_{IO_2} = 0.8$ by nonrebreathing mask were as follows: pH 7.17, Pa_{CO_2} 82 mm Hg, HCO_3^- 27 mMol/L, and Pa_{O_2} 37 mm Hg. His oxygen saturation measured by pulse oximetry (Sp_{O_2}) was 59%.

■ ■ SOAP 1 ■ ■

24 HOURS AFTER ADMISSION

The patient's condition was still classified as serious and unstable. He was on a mechanical ventilator in the control mode. A pulmonary artery catheter, a central venous pressure catheter, and an arterial line were in place. Although the patient drifted in and out of consciousness, he was on a pancuronium (Pavulon) drip and was unable to move. No paradoxical movement of the chest was detected.

His skin still appeared pale and cyanotic, and his neck veins were distended. The patient's vital signs were as follows: blood pressure 100/65, heart rate 145 bpm, and a control mode mechanical ventilation respiratory rate of 12/min. His temperature was unchanged. No breath sounds could be heard over the right lung field. Diminished breath sounds were audible over the left lung lobes. Rhonchi and crackles also could be heard over the left lung fields.

A portable chest X-ray taken earlier that morning showed the left lung to be partially aerated with patches of atelectasis; the right lung was shown to be completely atelectatic. No pneumothorax was present. His hemodynamic status revealed an increased CVP,

RAP, $\overline{PA}$, RVSWI, and PVR and a decreased PCWP, CO, SV, SVI, CI, LVSWI, and SVR. His ABGs were as follows: pH 7.25, Pa_{CO_2} 65 mm Hg, HCO_3^- 25 mMol/L, and Pa_{O_2} 54 mm Hg. The patient's oxygenation status showed an increased $\dot{Q}s/\dot{Q}\tau$, $C(a-\bar{v})_{O_2}$, and O_2ER, and a decreased D_{O_2} and Sv_{O_2}. His Sp_{O_2} was 86%.

■ ■ SOAP 2 ■ ■

72 HOURS AFTER ADMISSION

The patient's condition was classified as critical and unstable. His skin still appeared cyanotic, and his neck veins were severely distended. His vital signs were as follows: blood pressure 80/32, heart rate 190 bpm, controlled mechanical ventilation respiratory rate of 14/min, and rectal temperature 38.9° C (102° F). No breath sounds could be heard over the right lung fields. Diminished breath sounds were audible over the left lung. Rhonchi and crackles also could be heard over the left lung fields. Large amounts of yellow sputum were being suctioned from the patient's endotracheal tube.

A portable chest X-ray showed the left lung to be partially aerated, with patches of atelectasis more extensive than they had been 2 days before. The right lung was still shown to be airless. The radiologist also described early signs of adult respiratory distress syndrome (ARDS). No pneumothorax was present. The patient's electrocardiogram demonstrated periodic premature ventricular contractions.

All the patient's hemodynamic values had worsened from earlier readings. His ABGs were as follows: pH 7.22, Pa_{CO_2} 71 mm Hg, HCO_3^- 24 mMol/L, and Pa_{O_2} 34 mm Hg. The man's oxygenation status had worsened progressively from readings made 2 days earlier; his Sp_{O_2} was 61%.

■ ■ SOAP 3 ■ ■

Over the next few hours, the patient's family was called, and the hospital priest was notified. He died 24 hours later.

Case 7: PNEUMOTHORAX

ADMITTING HISTORY

A 64-year-old white man is familiar to the respiratory care consult team. He has a history of chronic bronchitis and emphysema. Although he has not been hospitalized in more than 2 years, he received extensive care 4 years ago for a left lower lobe pneumonia that compromised his already severe chronic obstructive

pulmonary disease (COPD). He was placed on the ventilator for 17 days. His medical record shows that hospital personnel experienced difficulty weaning him from the ventilator for both pathophysiologic and psychologic reasons. Despite this experience, he continues to smoke about 30 cigarettes a day, a habit he started when he joined the Navy at 19 years of age.

Since the episode 4 years ago, however, the man's medical history has been essentially unremarkable. As instructed, he schedules regular (twice-yearly) appointments with his doctor. Most of the time, he demonstrates a productive cough and wheezing. The man generally takes several medications, including daily dosages of antibiotics, xanthines, expectorants, and aerosolized sympathomimetics. Three or four times a week, for about 30 minutes, the man also performs a number of breathing exercises that members of the pulmonary rehabilitation team showed him.

He has worked as a janitor for more than 30 years in the local public school system. At the time of this admission, he was 7 months from his retirement party. Even though he has suffered from chronic bronchitis and emphysema for many years, he has always been considered a reliable, hardworking employee by the school administration and his fellow workers. Although he often has gone to work feeling less than good, he always has been able to finish the day without major problems. He seldom complains about his health because he does not like to draw attention to himself.

About 4 days before the present admission, however, he started to find it difficult to endure an entire workday. He told his wife that he thought he was getting the flu, with symptoms of fatigue, chills, and a cough that was becoming worse and more productive. He nevertheless continued to go to work each day, and he made it to the end of the week. At home on Saturday, 2 hours before admission, he suddenly became very short of breath with minimal exertion. At one point, he was unable to climb the stairs to his bedroom without stopping several times to rest. Concerned, his wife helped him into the car and drove him to the hospital.

PHYSICAL EXAMINATION

The man was in obvious respiratory distress. He was sitting in a wheelchair, with his arms braced on the arms of the chair, using his accessory muscles of respiration. He was thin but well nourished. His skin appeared cyanotic, and his fingers were clubbed. He was demonstrating pursed-lip breathing, and his chest was barrel shaped. He demonstrated a frequent, strong cough productive of large amounts of thick yellow and green sputum. He stated that he had been coughing so much and so hard that his chest hurt around his left "collar bone."

His vital signs were as follows: blood pressure 145/85, heart rate 94 bpm, respiratory rate 20/min, and oral temperature 37.9° C (100.3° F). Palpation of the chest was unremarkable. Percussion revealed hyperresonant notes bilaterally. Auscultation revealed diminished breath sounds and rhonchi throughout both lung fields. His heart sounds were diminished. Expiration took him three times as long as inspiration.

His last pulmonary function test (PFT), taken about 6 months ago at his last doctor's appointment, showed a moderate-to-severe obstructive disorder. His chest X-ray in the emergency room revealed dark, translucent lung fields; depressed and flattened hemidiaphragms; and a long, narrow heart. A small anterior pneumothorax (about 10%) also was noted between the second and third ribs on the left. His ABGs on room air were as follows: pH 7.53, $Paco_2$ 48 mm Hg, HCO_3^- 38 mMol/L, and Pao_2 57 mm Hg. His baseline ABGs at his last medical appointment were as follows: pH 7.42, $Paco_2$ 69 mm Hg, HCO_3^- 41 mM/L, and Pao_2 74 mm Hg. The physician ordered guaifenesin (Robitussin), theophylline (Theo-Dur), bed rest with limited physical activity, and a respiratory care consult.

■ ■ **SOAP 1** ■ ■

3 HOURS LATER

The patient's primary nurse called a physician and paged respiratory care stat. A portable chest X-ray also was requested. The patient's respiratory distress had obviously worsened. The nurse stated that the patient had just pressed his bedside buzzer to request help for his breathing. As the respiratory therapist walked into the patient's room, the man stated that he felt "like hell."

He appeared cyanotic and was breathing through pursed lips and perspiring. He demonstrated a frequent but weak cough, and when he did cough, he pulled his left arm to his side to brace himself. Although he expectorated only a small amount of sputum, he sounded "full." Rhonchi could be heard without the aid of a stethoscope. The sputum he did produce was still thick and yellow-green. The left anterior area of his chest appeared hyperinflated and fixed compared with the right.

His vital signs were as follows: blood pressure 95/55, heart rate 125 bpm and weak, and respiratory rate 28/min and shallow. Palpation of the chest was unremarkable. Percussion revealed hyperresonant notes bilaterally. Auscultation revealed diminished breath sounds and crackles, as well as rhonchi throughout the right lung. No breath sounds were audible over the left lung fields. Heart sounds could be heard to the right of the sternum. His ABGs on 5 L/min oxygen per nasal cannula were as follows: pH 7.24, $Paco_2$ 103 mm Hg, HCO_3^- 43 mMol/L, and Pao_2 37 mm Hg. His oxygen saturation measured by pulse oximetry (Spo_2) was 62%.

The chest X-ray showed that the patient's original small, left-sided pneumothorax had increased dramatically. The entire left lung now was collapsed, the left hemidiaphragm was significantly lower than the right, the mediastinum had shifted to the right, and patches of atelectasis were visible throughout the right lung.

The attending physician, along with a physician's assistant, inserted a chest tube in the left pleural cavity and began suction with negative pressure of −10 cm H_2O. The physician stated that in light of the problems the patient had experienced in the past, he did not want to commit the man to a ventilator. He requested respiratory care to assess the patient again, with a portable chest X-ray film to follow the first respiratory therapy treatments by 30 minutes.

■   ■   **SOAP 2**   ■   ■

30 MINUTES LATER

Although the patient was still in respiratory distress, his condition had improved. Tube suction had been increased. The chest X-ray showed that his left lung had re-expanded about 75%. The right lung fields were translucent, with no signs of atelectasis. The mediastinum had moved back to its normal position. The patient stated that he was feeling better. He was breathing through pursed lips and using his accessory muscles of respiration. Although he was still perspiring, the amount was less than it had been 30 minutes earlier.

No spontaneous cough or sputum production was observed. However, auscultation revealed diminished breath sounds and rhonchi over the right lung field. Breath sounds were diminished over the left lung area. His vital signs were as follows: blood pressure 145/85, heart rate 105 bpm, respiratory rate 22/min, and oral temperature 38° C (100.5° F). He was no longer cyanotic. Palpation of the chest was unremarkable. Percussion revealed hyperresonant notes bilaterally. Heart sounds no longer were heard over the right lung area. His ABGs were as follows: pH 7.35, $Paco_2$ 85 mm Hg, HCO_3^- 41 mMol/L, and Pao_2 64 mm Hg. His Spo_2 was 90%.

■   ■   **SOAP 3**   ■   ■

Case 8: ACUTE RESPIRATORY DISTRESS SYNDROME (ARDS)

ADMITTING HISTORY

On his way to work, a 32-year-old man was involved in an automobile accident during an ice storm. His car hit a patch of ice, spun out of control, and hit a cement bridge support. A 911 team spent 90 minutes extricating him from the car. He was stabilized at the accident site and then transported to the hospital. Although he was unconscious, he started to move and speak en route to the hospital. His speech was incoherent.

On admission, he was hypotensive, conscious, and complaining of severe pain. When he was asked to identify specific pain sites, he stated that his whole body hurt. He had numerous facial lacerations and several broken teeth. The left zygomatic arch and his right maxilla were fractured. He had a compound fracture of the left humerus, a Colles' fracture of the left radius, and several simple fractures of the first, second, and third phalanges on his left hand. A large bruise in the shape of a steering wheel could be observed easily over his anterior chest. He had splintered fractures of his right tibia and fibula. Although the chest X-ray taken in the emergency room showed no rib fractures, bilateral patchy infiltrates could be seen throughout both lungs.

He was taken to surgery, where maxillofacial, plastic, and orthopedic surgeons worked to treat his multiple injuries. The patient was in the operating room for 16 hours. His surgery was described as successful, and the long-term prognosis was believed to be good. He was in the postoperative recovery room for 2 hours with no remarkable problems and then was transferred to the surgical intensive care unit (ICU).

On arrival in the ICU, the man was breathing on his own, receiving supplemental oxygen via a 2 L/min nasal cannula. His general cardiopulmonary status was stable, and his recovery for the first 24 hours was as expected. At that time, however, the patient began to show signs of respiratory distress, and the attending physician ordered a respiratory care evaluation.

PHYSICAL EXAMINATION

The respiratory therapist assigned to assess and treat the patient gathered this clinical information: On inspection in the ICU, the patient was in moderate respiratory distress. He appeared uncomfortable and complained that he could not move very well and that he was becoming short of breath. He stated that he had never been a smoker. His blood pressure was 125/78, heart rate 93 bpm, respiratory rate 21/min, and core temperature normal. His skin appeared pale, and when he was asked to cough, he demonstrated an adequate although nonproductive cough. On palpation, tenderness was noted over his anterior chest area bilaterally, and dull percussion notes were elicited over both lower lung regions. On auscultation, bilateral bronchial breath sounds were heard. His oxygen saturation measured by pulse oximetry (Spo_2) was 95%, and his arterial blood gas values (ABGs) on a 3 L/min oxygen nasal cannula were as follows: pH 7.51, $Paco_2$ 29 mm Hg, HCO_3^- 22 mMol/L, and Pao_2 68 mm Hg. His chest X-ray showed "ground-glass" infiltrates throughout both lung fields. The process was more extensive than that noted on admission to the emergency department.

■ ■ **SOAP 1** ■ ■

3 DAYS AFTER SURGERY

The patient paged the nurse and stated that he was feeling worse. Respiratory care was called. On observation, the patient appeared cyanotic. His respiratory rate was 30/min, blood pressure was 165/95, heart rate was 110 bpm, and rectal temperature was 38.8° C (101.8° F). His cough was still nonproductive, and his anterior chest was still tender. Bronchial breath sounds and crackles were heard throughout both lung fields. His Spo_2 was 75%, and his ABGs on an $Fio_2 = 0.80$ were as follows: pH 7.56, $Paco_2$ 24 mm Hg, HCO_3^- 18 mMol/L, and Pao_2 35 mm Hg. No recent chest X-ray was available, but one had been ordered.

■ ■ **SOAP 2** ■ ■

30 MINUTES LATER

The respiratory therapist assigned to monitor and evaluate the patient noted that the patient's respiratory rate was 18/min, blood pressure was 170/97, heart rate was 150 bpm, and rectal temperature was 37.8° C (100° F). He appeared cyanotic, and he no longer responded verbally when asked questions. On auscultation, bronchial breath sounds and crackles could be heard bilaterally. His Spo_2 was 69%, and his ABGs on 100% oxygen were as follows: pH 7.31, $Paco_2$ 48 mm Hg, HCO_3^- 22 mMol/L, and Pao_2 31 mm Hg. A current chest X-ray showed increased opacities throughout both lung fields.

■ ■ **SOAP 3** ■ ■

Case 9: IDIOPATHIC (INFANT) RESPIRATORY DISTRESS SYNDROME

ADMITTING HISTORY

A 1644 g (3 lb, 10 oz) boy was born 8 weeks early (at 32 weeks' gestation). The nurses were concerned about the mother's lack of interest in her baby's care. The mother is an unmarried, 17-year-old Caucasian high-school dropout who plans to put the child up for adoption. Before this admission, the mother, whose pregnancy was considered high risk, was seen for prenatal care only once. At the prenatal visit, she was accompanied by her sister, who lived with her. Shortly after this visit, the sister moved to a large nearby town, where she planned to become a certified nurse's assistant. The mother, a checkout clerk at a small grocery store, continued to live in their mobile home with her boyfriend, who was out of work.

After the baby's birth, the mother appeared moderately nervous as she sat up in bed talking to the social worker in preparation for her discharge. She appeared thin and poorly nourished and constantly asked whether she could go to the smoking room.

Because of the mother's obvious disinterest, little progress was made regarding her follow-up care, the baby's present condition, or the adoption. Despite having given birth only 5 hours previously, she appeared quite anxious to be discharged.

PHYSICAL EXAMINATION

In the neonatal intensive care unit the baby appeared to be in mild respiratory distress. His Apgar scores at delivery were 4 and 6. On observation the baby appeared mildly cyanotic and demonstrated intercostal retractions and nasal flaring with all respirations. A mild, gruntlike cry was noted.

The baby's vital signs were as follows: blood pressure 50/20, apical heart rate 180 bpm, respiratory rate 74/min, and rectal temperature 37.1° C (98.8° F). Auscultation revealed bilateral crackles and sighing breath sounds. A stat chest X-ray showed mild haziness and air bronchograms in both lung bases consistent with the onset of infant respiratory distress syndrome (IRDS). The infant was placed on an F_{IO_2} of 0.4 via an oxygen hood. Umbilical ABGs were as follows: pH 7.52, Pa_{CO_2} 29 mm Hg, HCO_3^- 21 mMol/L, and Pa_{O_2} 49 mm Hg.

■ ■ **SOAP 1** ■ ■

16 HOURS AFTER DELIVERY

At this time, the baby was placed on a time-cycled, pressure-limited synchronized intermittent mandatory ventilation (SIMV) rate of 30/min, inspiratory time of 0.5 seconds, peak inspiratory pressure (PIP) of 20 cm H_2O, F_{IO_2} of 0.6, and positive end-expiratory pressure (PEEP) of 3 cm H_2O. The baby had no spontaneous breaths. His blood pressure was 60/40, and the apical heart rate was 184 bpm. On auscultation, harsh bronchial breath sounds and fine crackles could be heard bilaterally. A chest X-ray revealed a dense, "ground-glass" appearance throughout both lung fields. Artificial surfactant was administered to

the baby. Twenty minutes later, umbilical ABGs were as follows: pH 7.28, Pa_{CO_2} 53 mm Hg, HCO_3^- 19 mMol/L, and Pa_{O_2} 57 mm Hg.

■ ■ **SOAP 2** ■ ■

48 HOURS LATER

The baby remained intubated and on mechanical ventilation. The ventilator was in the continuous positive airway pressure (CPAP) mode at a pressure setting of 3 cm H_2O, with an F_{IO_2} of 0.45. The infant's vital signs showed a blood pressure of 74/50, an apical heart rate of 120 bpm, a spontaneous respiratory rate of 42/min, and a normal temperature. On auscultation, clear, normal vesicular breath sounds were heard. A morning chest X-ray revealed substantial improvement in the lung fields. Umbilical ABGs were as follows: pH 7.42, Pa_{CO_2} 37 mm Hg, HCO_3^- 24 mMol/L, and Pa_{O_2} 162 mm Hg.

■ ■ **SOAP 3** ■ ■

Case 10: POSTOPERATIVE ATELECTASIS

ADMITTING HISTORY

A 43-year-old woman was admitted to the hospital for an exploratory thoracotomy to diagnose and excise a 1.5-cm pulmonary nodule that had resisted diagnosis by bronchoscopy and percutaneous needle biopsy. She has been a registered nurse for the past 15 years and, up until about a year ago, was the director of nursing at the admitting hospital. For the past 4 months, she has been working the night shift as a general floor nurse in a nursing home owned by the hospital. Although she is considered an attractive woman, her general appearance over the last several years has progressively declined. For the past 3 years, she has rapidly moved from a normal, healthy weight to clear obesity.

Over the last 6 months, she almost always has worn one of the same three outfits, gone without makeup, and increased her smoking from one pack to two-and-a-half packs of cigarettes a day. Her general hygiene has been poor, and her hair often appears dirty. Her estranged husband reported that she has been depressed for the past year or so. He said that he had suggested that they both see a marriage counselor, but to no avail. Frustrated, he moved into his brother's apartment a few miles away from

his wife. Despite these events, they continued to speak to each other regularly.

The patient was seen in the preoperative education area before her surgery. Her forced vital capacity (FVC) was normal, but her forced expiratory volume in 1 second (FEV_1) was 50% of the predicted value. She frequently generated a spontaneous, strong cough, producing moderate amounts of yellow sputum. She was instructed on the use of aerosolized medication therapy via metered dose inhaler (MDI) and deep breathing and coughing (C&DB) techniques. Her attention span, however, was poor, and she continually praised every employee who passed her room. She also flooded the respiratory therapist with "aren't you wonderful" phrases as the therapist tried to ask her to demonstrate the various techniques that she would be required to perform after her surgery.

After her surgery and while she was in the postanesthesia area, she continually used foul language and threatened to have everyone fired. Her physician ordered a sedative and then transferred her to the postoperative unit. Over the next 2 hours, the patient's general respiratory status declined. Concerned, the primary nurse paged the physician. Busy in another part of the hospital, the physician requested a respiratory care consult.

PHYSICAL EXAMINATION (TIME: 1330)

The respiratory care practitioner noted that the patient was awake and in obvious respiratory distress. Her vital signs were as follows: blood pressure 185/90, heart rate 130 bpm, respiratory rate 35/min, and temperature normal. She demonstrated a frequent spontaneous, weak cough. She often expectorated a moderate amount of yellow sputum during a coughing episode. She appeared cyanotic and quickly stated, "My gut really hurts, . . . and I can't seem to get any air."

Over the left lower lung, diminished breath sounds were noted. Bronchial breath sounds and dull percussion notes were noted over the right lower lung. The nurse indicated that the patient's incentive spirometry (IS) volume was only about 40% of her preoperative value (when she could get the patient to attempt to use the device). Her oxygen saturation measured by pulse oximetry (Spo_2) on a 2 L/min oxygen nasal cannula was 77%. ABGs obtained by the respiratory care practitioner were as follows: pH 7.57, $Paco_2$ 23 mm Hg, HCO_3^- 21 mMol/L, and Pao_2 43 mm Hg. No recent chest X-ray was available. As the therapist documented the data, the patient's physician entered the room and stated, "I'll do anything to keep this patient off the ventilator. Keep me informed." The physician then prescribed some medication for the patient's pain and quickly left the room.

■ ■ **SOAP 1** ■ ■

1 DAY AFTER SURGERY

Despite the patient's need for aggressive respiratory care, she was generally uncooperative or unwilling to tolerate various treatment modalities. She had not been transferred to the ICU. Her skin was blue, cool, and damp. Her eyes were closed, and she was unresponsive to questions. She still demonstrated a weak cough every few minutes. Although sputum retention was suspected, none was actually seen; the patient was believed to be swallowing any sputum produced. Her vital signs were as follows: blood pressure 188/100, heart rate 135 bpm, respiratory rate 36/min, and rectal temperature 38.1° C (100.6° F).

On chest assessment dull percussion notes, bronchial breath sounds, and crackles were noted over the right middle and both lower lobes. A portable chest X-ray revealed that she had mild atelectasis in the right middle and both lower lobes. Air bronchograms also were noted in this area. Her Spo_2 was 72%. Her ABGs were as follows: pH 7.55, $Paco_2$ 29 mm Hg, HCO_3^- 22 mMol/L, and Pao_2 46 mm Hg.

■ ■ **SOAP 2** ■ ■

7 HOURS LATER

A therapeutic bronchoscopy was performed in the ICU. The patient was not intubated. The respiratory care practitioner on the pulmonary consult team found the patient in obvious respiratory distress. Her skin was cyanotic, cool, and damp. She stated, "I think I'm dying." No cough was observed at this time. No right-sided chest excursion could be seen, and her trachea was deviated to the right.

Her vital signs were as follows: blood pressure 192/90, heart rate 142 bpm, respiratory rate 20/min, and oral temperature 37.3° C (99.1° F). Bronchial breath sounds, crackles, and dull percussion notes were found over the right middle and lower lobes. Dull percussion notes and no breath sounds were noted over the left lower lobe. Her Spo_2 was 62%. Her ABGs were as follows: pH 7.26, $Paco_2$ 53 mm Hg, HCO_3^- 22 mMol/L, and Pao_2 37 mm Hg.

■ ■ **SOAP 3** ■ ■

SOAP Form

Respiratory Assessment Flow Chart

Subjective ↑	Objective ↑	Assessment ↑	Plan ↑

Subjective ↑

Anterior

Posterior

Pt. name

| Age | Male | Female |
| Date | Time | |

Admitting diagnosis

Therapist

Hospital

Objective ↑

Vital signs: RR _____ HR _____ BP _____

Temp. _____ On antipyretic agent? ☐ Yes ☐ No

Chest assessment:

Insp. _____

Palp. _____

Perc. _____

Ausc. _____

Radiography _____

Bedside spir.: PEFR ā _____ p̄ _____ Tx

SVC _____ FVC _____ NIF _____

Cough: ☐ Strong ☐ Weak

Sputum production: ☐ Yes ☐ No

Sputum char. _____

ABG: pH _____ $Paco_2$ _____ HCO_3^- _____

Pao_2 _____ Sao_2 _____ Spo_2 _____

Neg. O_2 transport factors _____

Other: _____

Assessment ↑

Plan ↑

Present Plan

Plan Modifications

References

General Respiratory Care

FUNDAMENTALS OF RESPIRATORY CARE

Burton GG, Hodgkin JE, Ward JJ: *Respiratory care: a guide to clinical practice,* ed 4, Philadelphia, 1997, JB Lippincott.

Hess DR, MacIntyre NR, Galvin WF, Adams AB, Saposnick AB: *Respiratory care—principles and practice,* Philadelphia, 2002, WB Saunders

Kacmarek RM, Dimas S: *Essentials of respiratory care,* ed 4, St. Louis, 2005, Mosby.

Wilkins RL, Stoller JK, Scanlan CL: *Egan's fundamentals of respiratory care,* ed 8, St. Louis, 2003, Mosby.

RESPIRATORY CARE EQUIPMENT

Branson RD, Hess DR, Chatburn RL: *Respiratory care equipment,* ed 2, Philadelphia, 1998, JB Lippincott.

Cairo JM, Pilbean SP: *McPherson's respiratory therapy equipment,* ed 7, St. Louis, 2004, Mosby.

White GC: *Equipment theory for respiratory care,* ed 4, Albany, NY, 2005, Delmar Publishers.

MECHANICAL VENTILATION

Chang DW: *Clinical application of mechanical ventilation,* Albany, NY, 2006 Delmar Publishers.

Dupuis YG: *Ventilators: Theory and clinical applications,* ed 2, St. Louis, 1992, Mosby.

Hess DR, Kacmarek RM: *Essentials of mechanical ventilation,* New York, 1996, McGraw-Hill.

MacIntyre NR, Branson RD: *Mechanical ventilation,* Philadelphia, 2001, WB Saunders.

Pierce LNB: *Guide to mechanical ventilation and intensive respiratory care,* Philadelphia, 1995, WB Saunders.

Pilbeam SP: *Mechanical ventilation: Physiological and clinical applications,* ed 3, St. Louis, 1998, Mosby.

Respiratory Care Monitoring

HEMODYNAMICS

Darovic GO: *Hemodynamic monitoring: Invasive and noninvasive clinical applications,* ed 3, Philadelphia, 2002, WB Saunders.

Darovic GO: *Handbook of hemodynamic monitoring,* ed 2, Philadelphia, 2004, WB Saunders.

Hodges RK, Garrett K, Chernecky CC, Schumacher L: *Real world nursing survival guide: Hemodynamic monitoring,* Philadelphia, 2005, WB Saunders.

PULMONARY FUNCTION TESTING

Ferguson GT et al: Office spirometry for lung health assessment in adults: a consensus statement from the National Lung Health Education Program, *Chest* 117(4):1146, 2000.

Hyatt RE, Scanlon PD: *Interpretation of pulmonary function tests: a practical guide,* ed 2, Philadelphia, 2002, JB Lippincott.

Madama VC: *Pulmonary function testing and cardiopulmonary stress testing,* ed 2, Albany, NY, 1998, Delmar Publishers.

Ruppel GL: *Manual of pulmonary function testing,* ed 8, St. Louis, 2004, Mosby.

SELECTED ARTERIAL BLOOD GASES

Malley WJ: *Clinical blood gases: Applications and intervention,* ed 2, Philadelphia, 2005, WB Saunders.

Martin L: *All you really need to know to interpret arterial blood gases,* ed 2, Baltimore, 1999, Williams and Wilkins.

Shapiro BA, Peruzzi WT, Kozlowska-Templin R: *Clinical application of blood gases,* ed 5, St. Louis, 1994, Mosby.

SELECTED OXYGENATION TOPICS

Cane RD et al: Unreliability of oxygen tension-based indices in reflecting intrapulmonary shunting in critically ill patients, *Crit Care Med* 16:1243, 1988.

Hess D, Kacmarek RM: Techniques and devices for monitoring oxygenation, *Respir Care* 38(6):646, 1993.

Kandel G, Aberman A: Mixed venous oxygen saturation: Its role in the assessment of the critically ill patient, *Arch Intern Med* 143:1400, 1993.

Nelson LD: Assessment of oxygenation: Oxygenation indices, *Respir Care* 38(6):631, 1993.

Nelson LD, Rutherford EJ: Monitoring mixed venous oxygen, *Respir Care* 37(2):154, 1992.

Rasanen J et al: Oxygen tension and oxyhemoglobin saturations in the assessment of pulmonary gas exchange, *Crit Care Med* 15:1058, 1987.

SELECTED HYPOXIC-DRIVE TOPICS

Aubier M et al: Effects of the administration of oxygen on ventilation and blood gases in patients with chronic obstructive pulmonary disease during acute respiratory failure, *Am Rev Respir Dis* 122:747, 1980.

Cullen JH, Kaemmerlen JT: Effect of oxygen administration at low rates of flow in hypercapic patients, *Am Rev Respir Dis* 95:116, 1967.

Dunn WF, Nelson SB, Hubmayr RD: Oxygen-induced hypercapnia in obstructive pulmonary disease, *Am Rev Respir Dis* 144:526, 1991.

French W: Hypoxic-drive theory revisited, *RT/The Journal for Respiratory Care Practitioners,* Feb/Mar, 2000, pp. 84-85.

Sassoon CS, Hassell KT, Mahutte CK: Hyperoxic-induced hypercapnia in stable chronic obstructive pulmonary disease, *Am Rev Respir Dis* 135:907, 1987.

Respiratory Pharmacology

Bills GW, Soderberg RC: *Principles of pharmacology for respiratory care,* ed 2, Albany, NY, 1998, Delmar Publishers.

Hill F: *Delmar's respiratory care drug reference,* Albany, NY, 1999, Delmar Publishers.

Howder CL: *Cardiopulmonary pharmacology: a handbook for respiratory practitioners and other allied health personnel,* ed 2, Baltimore, 1996, Williams and Wilkins.

Rau JL: *Respiratory care pharmacology,* ed 6, St. Louis, 2002, Mosby.

Physical Examination and Assessment

GENERAL

Craven RR, Hirnle CJ: *Fundamentals of nursing: Human health and function,* ed 4, Philadelphia, 2002, JB Lippincott.

Dains J, Ciofu Baumann L, Scheibel P: *Advanced health assessment and clinical diagnosis in primary care,* ed 2, St. Louis, 2003, Mosby.

DeWet SC: *Fundamental concepts and skills for nursing,* Philadelphia, 2001, WB Saunders.

Jarvis C: *Physical examination and health assessment,* ed 4, Philadelphia, 2004, WB Saunders.

Lehrer S: *Practical guide to health assessment,* ed 2, Philadelphia, 2002, WB Saunders.

Lewis SM, Heitkemper MM, Dirksen SR: *Medical surgical nursing,* ed 6, St. Louis, 2004, Mosby.

Potter PA, Perry AG: *Basic nursing—essentials for practice,* ed 5, St. Louis, 2003, Mosby.

Taylor C, Lillis C: *Fundamentals of nursing—the art and science of nursing,* ed 5, Philadelphia, 2004, JB Lippincott.

Timby BK: *Fundamental skills and concepts,* ed 8, Philadelphia, 2004, JB Lippincott.

ASSESSMENT IN RESPIRATORY CARE

American Thoracic Society Consensus Statement: Dyspnea: Mechanisms, assessment, and management, *Am J Respir Crit Care Med* 159:321, 1999.

Wilkins RL, Hodgkin JE, Lopez B: *Fundamentals of lung and heart sounds,* ed 3, St. Louis, 2004, Mosby.

Wilkins RL, Sheldon RL: *Clinical assessment in respiratory care,* ed 5, St. Louis, 2005, Mosby.

SELECTED REFERENCES ON PHYSICAL EXAMINATION ASSESSMENT

Pilbeam SP et al: Proficiency in applying treatment algorithms: Training at clinical sites using therapist-driven protocols is associated with better performance in assessing respiratory care practitioners' assessment skills by performance on case studies: Students vs. therapists vs. instructors, *Respir Care* 38(11, abstr):1219, 1993.

Weed LL: *Medical records, medical education, and patient care,* St. Louis, 1969, Mosby.

Weed LL: *Medical records, medical education, and patient care: The problem-oriented record as a basic tool,* Cleveland, 1971, Case Western Reserve University Press.

Radiography

Christian PE, Bernier DR, Langan JK: *Nuclear medicine and PET—technology and techniques,* ed 5, St. Louis, 2004, Mosby.

Hansell DM, Armstrong P, Lynch DA, McAdams P: *Imaging of diseases of the chest,* ed 4, St. Louis, 2005, Mosby.

Mettler FA: *Essentials of radiology,* ed 2, Philadelphia, 2004, WB Saunders.

Malott JC, Fodor J, III: *The art and science of medical radiography,* St. Louis, 2002, Mosby.

Reed JC: *Chest radiology,* ed 5, St. Louis, 2003, Mosby.

Seeram E: *Computed tomography—physical principles, clinical applications, and quality control,* ed 2, Philadelphia, 2001, WB Saunders.

General Anatomy and Physiology

Guyton AC, Hall JE: *Textook of medical physiology,* ed 10, Philadelphia, 2001, WB Saunders.

Marieb EN: *Human anatomy and physiology,* ed 6, Redwood City, Calif, 2004, Benjamin Cummings.

Martini FH: *Fundamentals of anatomy and physiology,* ed 6, Redwood City, Calif, 2004, Benjamin Cummings.

Solomon EP: *Introduction to human anatomy and physiology,* ed 2, Philadelphia, 2003, WB Saunders.

Thibodeau GA, Patton KT: *Anatomy and physiology,* ed 5, St. Louis, 2003, Mosby.

Cardiopulmonary Anatomy and Physiology

Beachey W: *Respiratory care anatomy and physiology: Foundations for clinical practice,* St. Louis, 1997, Mosby.

Comroe JH: *Physiology of respiration,* ed 2, Chicago, 1974, Year Book Medical Publishers.

Conover MH, Zalis EG: *Understanding electrocardiography,* ed 8, St. Louis, 2003, Mosby.

Des Jardins TD: *Cardiopulmonary anatomy and physiology: Essentials for respiratory care,* ed 4, Albany, NY, 2001, Delmar Publishers.

Hicks GH: *Cardiopulmonary anatomy and physiology,* Philadelphia, 2000, WB Saunders.

Levitzky MG: *Pulmonary physiology,* ed 5, New York, 1999, McGraw-Hill Health Professions.

Murray JF: *The normal lung,* ed 2, Philadelphia, 1986, WB Saunders.

Murray JG, Nadel JA: *Textbook of respiratory medicine,* ed 4, Philadelphia, 2005, WB Saunders.

Slonim NB, Hamilton LH: *Respiratory physiology,* ed 5, St. Louis, 1987, Mosby.

Theodore C et al: *ECG in emergency medicine and acute care,* St. Louis, Mosby.

West JB: *Respiratory physiology: the essentials,* ed 6, Philadelphia, 2000, Lippincott, Williams and Wilkins.

Microbiology

Bauman RB: *Microbiology,* Redwood City, Calif, 2004, Benjamin Cummings.

Bergquist L, Pogosian B: *Microbiology—principles and health science applications,* Philadelphia, 2000, WB Saunders.

Burton G, Engelkirk P: *Microbiology for the health sciences,* ed 6, Philadelphia, 2000, JB Lippincott.

Forbes BA, Sahm DF: *Bailey & Scott's diagnostic microbiology,* ed 11, St. Louis, 2002, Mosby.

Mims C, Goering R, Roitt I, Wakelin D, Zuckerman M: *Medical microbiology,* ed 3, St. Louis, 2004, Mosby.

General Pathophysiology

Cotran R, Kumar V, Collins T: *Robbins' pathologic basis of disease*, ed 6, Philadelphia, 1999, WB Saunders.

Gould BE: *Pathophysiology for the health professions*, Philadelphia, 2002, WB Saunders.

McCance KL, Huether SE: *Pathophysiology: the biologic basis for disease in adults and children*, ed 3, St. Louis, 1998, Mosby.

Porth CM: *Essentials of pathophysiology: Concepts of altered health states*, Philadelphia, 2003, JB Lippincott.

Price SA, Wilson LM: *Pathophysiology: Clinical concepts of disease processes*, ed 6, St. Louis, 2003, Mosby.

General Pulmonary Disorders

Albert RK, Spiro SG, Jett JR: Clinical respiratory medicine, ed 2, Philadelphia, 2004, Mosby.

Fishman AP, Elias JA, editors: *Fishman pulmonary diseases and disorders*, ed 3, New York, 1998, McGraw-Hill.

Fraser RS, Colman NC, Nestor ML, Pare PD: *Synopsis of diseases of the chest*, ed 3, Philadelphia, 2005, WB Saunders.

Crapo JD, Glassroth JL, Karlinsky JB, King TE: *Baum's textbook of pulmonary diseases*, ed 7, Philadelphia, 2003, JB Lippincott.

George RB, Light RW, Matthay MA, Matthay RA: *Chest medicine—essentials of pulmonary and critical care medicine*, ed 4, Philadelphia, 2000, JB Lippincott.

Gibson J, Geddes D, Costabel U, Sterk P, Corrin B: *Respiratory medicine*, ed 3, Philadelphia, 2003, WB Saunders.

McCane KL, Huether SE: *Pathophysiology: the biologic basis for disease in adults and children*, ed 4, St. Louis, 2002, Mosby.

Murray JF, Nadel JA: *Textbook of respiratory medicine*, ed 4, Philadelphia, 2005, WB Saunders.

Weinberger SE: *Principles of pulmonary medicine*, ed 4, Philadelphia, 2003, WB Saunders.

West JB: *Pulmonary pathophysiology: the essentials*, ed 5, Baltimore, 1998, Williams and Wilkins.

Wilkins RL, Dexter JR: *Respiratory disease: Principles of patient care*, Philadelphia, 1993, FA Davis.

General Neonatal and Pediatric Pulmonary Disorders

Aloan CA, Hill TV: *Respiratory care of the newborn and child*, ed 2, Philadelphia, 1997, JB Lippincott.

Avory A, Martin R, Martin R: *Neonatal-perinatal medicine*, ed 7, St. Louis, 2001, Mosby.

Barnhart SL, Czervinske MP: *Perinatal and pediatric respiratory care*, ed 2, Philadelphia, 2003, WB Saunders.

Behrman RE, Kliegman RM, Arvin AM: *Nelson textbook of pediatrics*, ed 16, Philadelphia, 2000, WB Saunders.

Feischer GR, Ludwig S: *Textbook of pediatric emergency medicine*, ed 4, Baltimore, 2000, Williams and Wilkins.

Goetzman BW, Wennberg RP: *Neonatal intensive care handbook*, ed 3, St. Louis, 1999, Mosby.

MacDonald M, Mullett M, Seshia M: *Avery's neonatology pathophysiology and management of the newborn*, ed 6, Philadelphia, 2005, JB Lippincott.

Taussig LM, Landau LI: *Pediatric respiratory medicine*, St. Louis, 1999, Mosby.

Whitaker K: *Comprehensive perinatal and pediatric respiratory care*, ed 3, Albany, NY, 2001, Delmar Publishers.

Selected Pulmonary Disorders

CHRONIC OBSTRUCTIVE PULMONARY DISEASE

American Thoracic Society Position Statement: Standards for the diagnosis and care of patients with chronic obstructive pulmonary disease, *Am J Respir Crit Care Med* 152(5):S78, 1995.

Barnes PJ: New therapies for chronic obstructive pulmonary disease, *Thorax* 53:137, 1998.

Celli BR: Standards for the optimal management of COPD, *Chest* 113(4 suppl):283s, 1998.

Cohen M, Sahn SA: Bronchietasis in systemic diseases, *Chest* 116(4):1063, 1999.

Grossman RF: The value of antibiotics and the outcomes of antibiotic therapy in exacerbations of COPD, *Chest* 113:2495, 1998.

Hoo GW, Hakimian M, Santiago SM: Hypercapnic respiratory failure in COPD patients: Response to therapy, *Chest* 117(1):169, 2000.

Jeffner JE, Frye MD: Chronic obstructive pulmonary disease. In Hess DR et al: *Respiratory Care—principles and practice*, Philadelphia, 2002, WB Saunders.

Senior RM, Anthonisen NR: Chronic obstructive pulmonary disease (COPD), *Am J Respir Crit Care Med* 157:s139, 1998.

Snow V, Lascher S, Mottur-Pilson C, for the Joint Expert Panel on Chronic Obstructive Pulmonary Disease of the American College of Chest Physicians and the American College of Physicians—American Society of Internal Medicine: Evidence base for management of acute exacerbations of chronic obstructive pulmonary disease, *Ann Intern Med* 134(7):595-599, 2001 and *Chest* 119:1185-1189, 2001.

The National Lung Health Education Program (NLHEP): Strategies in preserving lung health and preventing COPD and associated diseases, *Chest* 113(2 suppl):123S, 1998.

ASTHMA

Blumenthal MN et al: A multicenter evaluation of the clinical benefits of cromolyn sodium aerosol by metered-dose inhaler in the treatment of asthma, *J Allergy Clin Immunol* 81:681, 1988.

Cardan DL et al: Vital signs including pulsus paradoxus in the assessment of acute bronchial asthma, *Ann Emergency Med* 12:80, 1983.

Cherniack RM: Physiologic diagnosis and function in asthma, *Clin Chest Med* 16:567, 1995.

Doeschug KC et al: Asthma guidelines: an assessment of physician understanding and practice, *Am J Respir Crit Care Med* 159:1735-1741, 1999.

Drazen JM, Israel E, O'Byrne PM: Drug therapy: Treatment of asthma with drugs modifying the leukotrienes, *N Engl J Med* 340(3):197, 1999.

Henkind SJ, Benis AM, Teichholz LE: The paradox of pulsus paradoxus, *Am Heart J* 114:198, 1987.

Kemp JP: Comprehensive asthma management: Guidelines for clinicians, *J Asthma* 35(8):601, 1998.

Lipworth BJ: Leukotriene-receptor antagonists, *Lancet* 353(9146):67, 1999.

Mannino DM et al: Surveillance for asthma—United States, 1960-1995, *MMWR CDC Surveil Summ* 47(1):1, 1998.

Myers TR, Chatburn RL: Asthma. In Hess DR et al: *Respiratory care—principles and practice*, Philadelphia, 2002, WB Saunders.

Nafstad P, Magnus P, Jaakkola JJK: Early respiratory infections and childhood asthma, *Pediatrics* 106(3):E38, 2000.

National Asthma Education and Prevention Program, National Heart, Lung, and Blood Institute: Guidelines for the diagnosis and management of asthma: Expert panel report 2, NIH pub. no. 97-4051, Bethesda, Md., 1997, National Institutes of Health.

Owen CL: New direction in asthma management, *Am J Nurs* 99(3):26, 1999.

Portnow J, Aggarwal J: Continuous terbutaline nebulization for the treatment of severe exacerbations of asthma in children, *Ann Allergy* 60:368, 1988.

Reed CE: The natural history of asthma in adults: the problem of irreversibility, *J Allergy Clin Immunol* 103:539, 1999.

Sly RM: Decreases in asthma mortality in the United States, *Ann Allergy Asthma Immunol* 85(2):121, 2000.

INFECTIOUS PULMONARY DISORDERS

PNEUMONIA

Afessa B, Weaver B: Pneumonia. In Hess DR et al: *Respiratory care—principles and practice,* Philadelphia, 2002, WB Saunders.

American Thoracic Society Consensus Statement: Hospital-acquired pneumonia in adults: Diagnosis, assessment of severity, initial antimicrobial therapy and preventive strategies, *Am J Respir Crit Care Med* 153:1711, 1995.

American Thoracic Society Statement: Guidelines for the initial management of adults with community-acquired pneumonia: Diagnosis, assessment of severity, and initial antimicrobial therapy, *Am Soc Respir Dis* 148:1418, 1993.

Benstein JM: Treatment of community-acquired pneumonia—IDSA guidelines, *Chest* 315(suppl):9S, 1999.

Brown PD, Lerner SA: Community acquired pneumonia, *Lancet* 352(9136):1295, 1999.

Jadavi T et al: A practical guide for the diagnosis and treatment of pediatric pneumonia, *Can Med Assoc J* 156(5) S703-S711, 1997.

Khrana S, Litaker D: The dilemma of nosocomial pneumonia: What primary care physicians should know, *Cleveland Clin J Med* 67(1):25, 2000.

Nelson S et al: Pathophysiology of pneumonia, *Clin Chest Med* 16:1, 1995.

Toumanen EI, Austrian R, Masure HR: Pathogenesis of pneumococcal infection, *N Engl J Med* 332:1280, 1995.

LUNG ABSCESS

Bartlett JG: Anaerobic bacterial infections of the lung, *Chest* 91: 901, 1987.

Bartlett JG: Lung abscess, *Johns Hopkins Med J* 15:141, 1982.

Estrera AS et al: Primary lung abscess, *J Thorac Cardiovasc Surg* 79:275, 1980.

Pohlson EC et al: Lung abscess: a changing pattern of the disease, *Am J Surg* 150:97, 1985.

FUNGAL DISORDERS OF THE LUNGS

Sarosi GA, Davies SF: *Fungal diseases of the lung,* ed 3, Philadelphia, 1999, JB Lippincott.

TUBERCULOSIS

American Thoracic Society: Control of tuberculosis in United States (ATS statement), *Am Rev Respir Dis* 146:1623, 1992.

American Thoracic Society: Diagnostic standards and classification of tuberculosis, *Am Rev Respir Dis* 142(3):725, 1990.

Barnes PF et al: Tuberculosis in patients with human immunodeficiency virus infection, *N Engl J Med* 324:1644, 1991.

Brudney K, Dobkin J: Resurgent tuberculosis in New York City: Human immunodeficiency virus, homelessness, and the decline of tuberculosis control programs, *Am Rev Respir Dis* 144:745, 1991.

Dye C et al: Global burden of tuberculosis: Estimated incidence, prevalence, and mortality by country, *JAMA* 282(7):677, 1999.

McCray E: The epidemiology of tuberculosis in the United States, *Clin Chest Med* 18:99, 1997.

Mitchison DA: How drug resistance emerges as a result of poor compliance during short-course chemotherapy for tuberculosis, *Int J Tuberculosis Lung Dis* 2:10, 1998.

Rom WN, Stuart MG: *Tuberculosis,* ed 3, Philadelphia, 2003, JB Lippincott.

Schraufnagel DE: Tuberculosis treatment for the beginning of the next century, *Int J Tuberculosis Lung Dis* 3(8):651, 1999.

Temple ME, Nahata MC: Rifapentine: Its role in the treatment of tuberculosis, *Ann Pharmacother* 33(11):1203, 1999.

PULMONARY EDEMA

American Heart Association: *Heart disease and stroke statistics— 2004 update,* Dallas, Tex., 2003, American Heart Association.

Branson RD, Hurst JM, DeHaven DB: Mask CPAP: State of the art, *Respir Care* 30:846, 1985.

Chesebro JH, Burnett JC: Cardiac failure: Characteristics and clinical manifestations. In Brandenburg RO et al, editors: *Clinical assessment in respiratory care,* St. Louis, 1990, Mosby.

Gropper MA, Wiener-Kronish JP, Hashimoto S: Acute cardiogenic pulmonary edema, *Clin Chest Med* 15:501-515, 1994.

Hunt SA, Baker DW, Chin MH, et al: ACC/AHA guidelines for the evaluation and management of chronic heart failure in the adult: Executive summary: A report of the American College of Cardiology/American Heart Association Task Force on Practice Guidelines (Committee to revise the 1995 Guidelines for the Evaluation and Management of Heart Failure), *Circulation* 104:2996-3007, 2001.

Krider SJ: Invasively monitored hemodynamic pressures. In Wilkins RI, Sheldon RL, Krider SJ, editors: *Clinical assessment in respiratory care,* St. Louis, 1990, Mosby.

Marland AM, Glauser FL: Hemodynamic and pulmonary edema protein measurements in a case of re-expansion pulmonary edema, *Chest* 81:250, 1982.

Medoff BD, DiSalvo TG: Cardiac failure. In Hess DR et al: *Respiratory care—principles and practice,* Philadelphia, 2002, WB Saunders.

Paperel A, Williamson DC, Modell JH: Effectiveness of CPAP via face mask for pulmonary edema associated with hypercarbia, *Intensive Care Med* 9:17, 1983.

Rasanen J et al: Continuous positive pressure by face mask in acute cardiogenic pulmonary edema: a randomized study, *Crit Care Med* 12:A325, 1983.

Szidon JP: Pathophysiology of the congested lung, *Cardio Clin* 7:39-48, 1989.

PULMONARY EMBOLISM

Ageno W: Treatment of venous thromboembolism, *Thrombosis Res* 97(1):V63, 2000.

Anderson DR et al: Thrombosis in the emergency department, *Arch Intern Med* 159:477, 1999.

Antman EM, Cohen M: Newer antithrombin agents in acute coronary syndromes, *Am Heart J* 138(suppl):S563, 1999.

Dalen JE: Clinical diagnosis of acute pulmonary embolism. When should a $\dot{V}/\dot{Q}$ scan be ordered? *Chest* 100(5):1185, 1991.

Heit JA et al: Predictors of recurrence after deep vein thrombosis and pulmonary embolism, *Arch Intern Med* 160:761, 2000.

Heit JA et al: Risk factors for deep vein thrombosis and pulmonary embolism, *Arch Intern Med* 160:809, 2000.

Horne MK, Chang R: Thrombolytic therapy for deep venous thrombosis? *JAMA* 282:2164, 1999.

Hull RD et al: Low-molecular-weight heparin vs heparin in the treatment of patients with pulmonary embolism: American-Canadian Thrombosis Study Group, *Arch Intern Med* 160(2): 229, 2000

Hyers TM: Venous thromboembolism, *Am J Respir Care Med* 159: 1, 1999

Indik JH, Alpert JS: Detection of pulmonary embolism by D-dimer assay, spiral computed tomography and magnetic resonance imaging, *Prog Cardiovasc Dis* 42(4):261, 2000.

Kline JA et al: New diagnostic tests for pulmonary embolism, *Ann Emerg Med* 35(2):168, 2000.

Litin SC, Heit JA, Mees KA: Use of low-molecular-weight heparin in the treatment of venous thromboembolic disease: Answers to frequently asked questions, *Mayo Clin Proc* 73:545, 1998.

Meignan M et al: Systematic lung scans reveal a high frequency of silent pulmonary embolism in patients with proximal deep venous thrombosis, *Arch Intern Med* 160(2):159, 2000.

Moser KM: Venous thromboembolism, *Am Rev Respir Dis* 141:235, 1990.

Mullins MD et al: The role of spiral volumetric computed tomography in the diagnosis of pulmonary embolism, *Arch Intern Med* 160:293, 2000.

Palmer SM, Tapson VG: Pulmonary vascular disease. In Hess DR et al: *Respiratory care—principles and practice*, Philadelphia, 2002, WB Saunders.

Silverstein MD et al: Trends in the incidence of deep vein thrombosis and pulmonary embolism, *Arch Intern Med* 158:585, 1998.

Stratton MA et al: Prevention of venous thromboembolism, *Arch Intern Med* 160:334, 2000.

West JW: Pulmonary embolism. In Wu K, editor: *Pathophysiology and management of thromboembolic disorders*, Littleton, Mass, 1984, PGS Publishing.

FLAIL CHEST

Bollinger CT, Van Eeden SF: Treatment of multiple rib fractures: Randomized controlled trial comparing ventilatory with non-ventilatory management, *Chest* 97:943, 1990.

Branson RD, Campbell RS, Hurst JM: Chest trauma. In Hess DR et al: *Respiratory care—principles and practice*, Philadelphia, 2002, WB Saunders.

Carpintero JL et al: Methods of management of flail chest, *Intensive Care Med* 6:217, 1980.

Craven KD, Oppenheimer L, Wood LD: Effects of contusion and flail chest on pulmonary perfusion and oxygen exchange, *J Appl Physiol* 47:729, 1979.

Duff JH, Goldstein M, McLean AP, et al: Flail chest: a clinical review and physiological study, *J Trauma* 8:63-74, 1986.

Freedland MA, Wilson RF, Bender J: The management of flail chest injury, *J Trauma* 30:1460-1468, 1990.

Gaillard M, Herve C, Mandin L, et al: Mortality prognosis factors in chest injury, *J Trauma* 30:93-96, 1990.

Maloney JV, Schmutzer KJ, Raschke E: Paradoxical respiration and "pendelluft," *J Thorac Cardiovasc Surg* 41:291, 1961.

Richardson JD, Adams L, Flint LM: Selective management of flail chest and pulmonary contusion, *Ann Surg* 196:481, 1982.

PNEUMOTHORAX

Baumann MH, Strange C, Heffner JE, et al, and the ACCP Pneumothorax Consensus Group: Management of spontaneous pneumothorax: an American College of Chest Physicians Delphi consensus statement, *Chest* 119:590-602, 2001.

Gustman P, Yerser L, Wanner A: Immediate cardiovascular effects of tension pneumothorax, *Am Rev Respir Dis* 127:171, 1983.

Harvery JE, Jeyasingham K: The difficult pneumothorax, *Br J Dis Chest* 81:209, 1987.

Jerkinson SG: Pneumothorax, *Clin Chest Med* 6:153, 1985.

Miller AC: Treatment of spontaneous pneumothorax: the clinician's perspective on pneumothorax management, *Chest* 113(5):1423, 1998.

O'Rourke JP, Yee ES: Civilian spontaneous pneumothorax: Treatment options and long-term results, *Chest* 96:1302, 1989.

Yamazaki S et al: Pulmonary blood flow to rapidly reexpand lung in spontaneous pneumothorax, *Chest* 81:118, 1982.

PLEURAL DISEASES

Ali I, Unruh H: Management of empyema thoracis, *Ann Thorac Surg* 50:355, 1990.

Collins TR, Sahn SA: Thoracocentesis: Clinical value, complications, technical problems, and patient experience, *Chest* 91:817, 1987.

Light RW: *Pleural disease*, Baltimore, 1995, Williams and Wilkins.

Lim TK: Management of pleural empyema, *Chest* 116(3):845, 1999.

Mehta AC, Dweik RA: Pleural diseases, *Cleveland Clinic Intensive Review of Internal Medicine*, ed 2, 40:452-466, 2000.

Sahn SA: The pathophysiology of pleural effusion, *Ann Rev Med* 41:7, 1990.

Sahn SA: The diagnostic value of pleural fluid analysis, *Seminars in Respir and Crit Care Med* 16(4):269-278, 1995.

Tarn AC, Lapworth R: Biochemical analysis of pleural fluid: What should we measure? *Annals of Clinical Biochemistry* 38:311-322, 2001.

Smyrnios NS, Jederlinic PJ, Irwin RS: Pleural effusion in an asymptomatic patient, *Chest* 97:192, 1990.

KYPHOSCOLIOSIS

Barrack R et al: Vibratory hypersensitivity in idiopathic sclerosis, *J Pediatr Orthop* 8(4):389, 1988.

Bergofsky EH: Respiratory failure in disorders of the thoracic cage, *Am Rev Respir Dis* 119:643, 1979.

Byrd J: Current theories on the etiology of idiopathic scoliosis, *Clin Orthop* 299:114, 1988.

Conti G et al: Respiratory system mechanics in early phase of acute respiratory failure due to severe kyphoscoliosis, *Intensive Care Medicine* 23(5):539-544, 1997.

Domanic U, Talu U, Dikici F, Hamzaoglu A: Surgical correction of kyphosis: Posterior total wedge resection osteotomy in 32 patients, *Acta Orthopaedic Scandinavica* 75(4):449-555, 2004.

Dunford M et al: Managing ventilatory insufficiency and failure in a patient with kyphoscoliosis: a case study, *Australian Critical Care Nurses* 14(4):165-169, 2001.

Ferris G et al: Kyphoscolisosis ventilatory insufficiency: Noninvasive management outcomes, *American Journal of Physical Medicine & Rehabilitation/Association of Academic Physiatrists* 79(1):24-29, 2000.

Gonzalez LF et al: Noninvasive mechanical ventilation and corrective surgery for treatment of a child with severe kyphoscoliosis. *Pediatric Pulmonology* 32(5):403-405, 2001.

Keim HA, Hensinger RN: Spinal deformities: Scoliosis and kyphosis, *Clin Symp* 41(4):3, 1989.

McMaster MJ, Singh H: Natural history of congenital kyphosis and kyphoscoliosis: a study of one hundred and twelve patients, *The Journal of Bone and Joint Surgery (American Volume)* 81(10):1367-1383, 1999.

Sawicka EH, Branthwaite MA: Respiration during sleep in kyphoscoliosis, 42(10):801-808, 1987.

PNEUMOCONIOSES

Harber P, Schenker M, Balmes J: *Occupational and environmental respiratory disease*, St. Louis, 1995, Mosby.

Hendrick D, Beckett W, Burge SP, Churg A: *Occupational disorders of the lung*, Philadelphia, 2002, WB Saunders.

McCunney RT, Barbanel CS: *Medical center occupational health and safety*, Philadelphia, 1999, JB Lippincott.

McCunney RT et al: *A practical approach to occupational and environmental medicine*, ed 3, Philadelphia, 2003, JB Lippincott.

Rom WN: *Environmental and occupational medicine*, ed 3, Philadelphia, 1998, JB Lippincott.

Rosenstock L, Cullen M, Bodkin C, Redlich C: *Textbook of clinical occupational and environmental medicine*, ed 2, Philadelphia, 2005, WB Saunders.

CANCER OF THE LUNG

Brown KG: Lung cancer and environmental tobacco smoke: Occupational risk to non-smokers, *Environ Health Perspect* 107(suppl 6):885, 1999.

Faber LP: Lung cancer. In Holleb AI, Fink DJ, Murphy GP, editors: *American Cancer Society textbook of clinical oncology*, Atlanta, 1991, American Cancer Society.

Greenlee RT et al: Cancer statistics, 2000, *CA Cancer J Clin* 50(1): 7, 2000.

Hecht SS: Tobacco smoke carcinogens and lung cancer, *J Natl Cancer Inst* 91(14):1194, 1999.

Malhotra A, Schwartz DR: Lung cancer. In Hess DR et al: *Respiratory care—principles and practice*, Philadelphia, 2002, WB Saunders

Mountain CF: Revisions in the international system for staging lung cancer, *Chest* 111(6):1710, 1997.

Pass HI, Carbone DP, Johnson DH, Minna JD, Turrisi AT: *Lung cancer*, ed 3, Philadelphia, 2004, JB Lippincott.

Petty TL: Screening strategies for early detection of lung cancer: The time is now, *JAMA* 284:1977, 2000.

Van Houtte P et al: Lung cancer. In Rubin P, editor: *Clinical oncology*, ed 8, Philadelphia, 2001, WB Saunders.

ACUTE RESPIRATORY DISTRESS SYNDROME

Abraham E: Toward new definitions of acute respiratory distress syndrome, *Crit Care Med* 27:237-238, 1999.

Acute Respiratory Distress Syndrome Clinical Network (ARDSnet). http://www.ardsnet.org.2001

The Acute Respiratory Distress Syndrome Network: Ventilation with lower tidal volumes as compared with traditional tidal volumes for acute lung injury and the acute respiratory distress syndrome, *N Engl J Med* 342:1301-1308, 2000.

Amato MB, Barbas CS, Medeiros DM, et al. Effect of a protective-ventilation strategy to prevent barotraumas in patients at high risk for acute respiratory distress syndrome, *N Engl J Med* 338:355-361, 1998.

American Lung Association: Fact sheet: Adult (acute) respiratory distress syndrome (ARDS), January, 2001, http://www.lungusa.org.

Artigas A, Bernard GR, Carlet J, et al: The American-European Consensus Conference on ARDS. Part 2: Ventilatory, pharmacologic, supportive therapy, study design strategies, and issues related to recovery and remodeling, *Am J Respir Crit Care Med* 157:1332-1347, 1998.

Ashbaugh DG et al: Acute respiratory distress in adults, *Lancet* 2:319, 1967.

Brochard L, Roudot-Thoraval F, Roupie E, et al: Tidal volume reduction for prevention of venilatory-induced lung injury in acute respiratory distress syndrome: The Multicenter Trial Group on Tidal Volume Reduction in ARDS, *Am J Respir Crit Care Med* 158:1831-1838, 1998.

Johannigman JA, Davis K Jr, Campbell RS, et al. Prone positioning for acute respiratory distress syndrome (ARDS) in the surgical intensive care unit: Who, when, and how long? *Surgery* 128: 708-716, 2000.

Kollef MH, Schuster DP: The acute respiratory distress syndrome, *N Engl J Med* 332:27, 1995.

McIntyre RC, Moore FA, Moore EE, et al: Inhaled nitric oxide variably improved oxygenation and pulmonary hypertension in patients with acute respiratory distress syndrome, *J Trauma* 39:418-425, 1995.

Neff MJ, Steinberg KP: Acute respiratory distress syndrome. In Hess DR et al: *Respiratory care—principles and practice*, Philadelphia, 2002, WB Saunders.

Rocker GM et al: Noninvasive positive pressure ventilation: Successful outcome in patients with acute lung injury ARDS, *Chest* 115(1):173, 1999.

Sachdeva RC, Guntapalli KK: Acute respiratory distress syndrome, *Crit Care Clin* 13(3):503, 1997.

Stewart TE, Meade MO, Cook DJ, et al: Evaluation of a ventilation strategy to prevent barotraumas in patients at high risk for acute respiratory distress syndrome. *N Engl J Med* 338:355-361, 1998.

Tomashefski JF: Pulmonary pathology of the adult respiratory distress syndrome, *Clin Chest Med* 11(4):593, 1990.

Ware LB et al: The acute respiratory distress syndrome, *N Engl J Med* 342:1334, 2000.

Wyncoll DLA, Evans TW: Acute respiratory distress syndrome, *Lancet* 354 (9177): 497, 1999.

CHRONIC INTERSTITIAL LUNG DISEASES

American Thoracic Society International Consensus Statement: Idiopathic pulmonary fibrosis: Diagnosis and treatment, *Am J Respir Crit Care Med* 161:646, 2000.

Du Bois RM: Diffuse lung disease—an approach to management, *Br Med J,* 309:175-179, 1994.

Flint A: Pathologic features of interstitial lung disease. In Schwarz MI, King TE, editors: *Interstitial lung disease,* Toronto, 1988, BC Decker.

Ghio AJ: Interstitial lung disease. In Hess DR et al: *Respiratory care—principles and practice*, Philadelphia, 2002, WB Saunders.

Gross TJ, Hunninghake GW: Idiopathic pulmonary fibrosis, *N Engl J Med* 345:517-525, 2001.

Hunninghake GW, Kalica AR: Approaches to treatment of pulmonary fibrosis, *Am J Respir Crit Care Med* 15:915-918, 1995.

Robertson HT: Clinical application of pulmonary function and exercise tests in the management of patients with interstitial lung disease. *Semin Respir Crit Care Med* 15:1-16, 1994.

Ryu JH, Colby TV, Hartman TE: Idiopathic pulmonary fibrosis: Current concepts, *Mayo Clin Proc* 73:1085-1101, 1998.

Schwarz MI: The acute (noninfectious) interstitial lung diseases, *Compr Ther* 22:622-637, 1996.

Sime PJ, O'Reilly KM: Fibrosis of the lung and other tissues: New concepts in pathogenesis and treatment, *Clin Immunol* 99:308-19, 2001.

GUILLAIN-BARRÉ SYNDROME

Asbury A, Cornblath D: Assessment of current diagnostic criteria for Guillain- Barré syndrome, *Ann Neurol* 27(suppl):S21-S24, 1990.

Cordova FC, Criner GJ: Neuromuscular dysfunction. In Hess DR et al: *Respiratory care—principles and practice,* Philadelphia, 2002, WB Saunders.

England JD: Guillain-Barré syndrome, *Ann Rev Med* 41:1, 1990.

Guillain-Barré Syndrome Study Group: Plasmapheresis and acute Guillain-Barré syndrome, *Neurology* 35:1096, 1985.

Plasma Exchange/Sandoglobulin Guillain-Barré Study Trial Group: Randomised trial of plasma exchange, intravenous immunoglobulin and combined treatment in Guillain-Barré syndromes, *Lancet* 349:225, 1997.

Schonberger LB et al: Guillain-Barré syndrome following vaccination in the National Influenza Immunization Program, United States, 1976-1977, *Am J Epidemiol* 100:105, 1979.

Van de Meche FGA, CAN Doorn PA: Guillain-Barré and chronic inflammatory demyelinaing polyneuropathy: Immune mechanisms and update on current therapies, *Ann Neurol* 30: S14, 1995

MYASTHENIA GRAVIS

Dushay KM, Aibrak JD, Jensen WA: Myasthenia gravis presenting as isolated respiratory failure, *Chest* 97:232-234, 1990.

Howard JF Jr: Intravenous immunoglobulin for the treatment of acquired myasthenia gravis, *Neurol* 51(6 suppl 5):30, 1998.

Keesey J: A treatment algorithm for autoimmune myasthenia in adults, *Ann NY Acad Sci* 841:753, 1998.

Lisak RP, editor: *Handbook of myasthenia gravis,* New York, 1994, Marcel Dekker.

Spinelli A, Marconi G, Gorini M, et al: Control of breathing in patients with myasthenia gravis, *Am Rev Respir Dis* 145:1359-1366, 1992.

SLEEP APNEA

Auckle DH, Hudgel DW: Management of obstructive sleep apnea syndrome. In Hess DR et al: *Respiratory Care—principles and practice,* Philadelphia, 2002, WB Saunders.

Handada T, Shireru S, Tateyama T, et al: Laser-assisted uvulopalatoplasty with Nd: YAG laser for sleep disorders, *Laryngoscope* 106:1531-1533, 1996.

Hudgel DW: Treatment of obstructive sleep apnea: a review, *Chest* 109:1346-1358, 1996.

Kryger MH, Roth T, Dement WC: *Principles and practice of sleep medicine,* ed 3, Philadelphia, 2000, WB Saunders.

McNicholas WT: Obstructive sleep apnea syndrome: Who should be treated? *Sleep* 23:S187-5190, 2000.

McNicholas WT, Phillipson E: *Breathing disorders in sleep,* Philadelphia, 2002, WB Saunders.

Mickelson SA: Laser-assisted uvulopalatoplasty for obstructive sleep apnea, *Laryngoscope* 106:10-13, 1996.

Schmidt-Nowara W, Lowe A, Wiegand L: Oral appliances for the treatment of snoring and obstructive sleep apnea: a review, *Sleep* 18:501-510, 1995.

Schwab RJ, Goldberg AN, Pack AJ. Sleep apnea syndromes. In Fishman AP, editor: *Fishman's pulmonary diseases and disorders,* ed 3, New York, 1998, McGraw-Hill.

Standards of Practice Committee of the American Sleep Disorders Association: Practice parameters for the treatment of obstructive sleep apnea in adults: the efficacy of surgical modifications of the upper airway, *Sleep* 19:152-156, 1996.

Young T, Palta M, Dempsey J, et al: The occurrence of sleep-disordered breathing among middle-aged adults, *N Engl J Med* 328:1230-1235, 1993.

TRANSIENT TACHYPNEA OF THE NEWBORN

Gross TL, Sokol RJ, Kwong MS: Transient tachypnea of the newborn: the relationship to preterm delivery and significant neonatal morbidity, *Am J Obstet Gynecol* 14:236, 1983.

Tudehope DI, Smith MH: Is transient tachypnea of the newborn always a benign condition? *Aust Paediatr J* 15:160, 1979.

INFANT RESPIRATORY DISTRESS SYNDROME

Barrie H: Simple method of applying continuous positive airway pressure in respiratory distress syndrome, *Lancet* 1:776, 1972.

Belani KG et al: Respiratory failure in newborns, infants, and children, *Indian J Pediatr* 48:21, 1981.

Bryan H et al: Perinatal factors associated with the respiratory distress syndrome, *Am J Obstet Gynecol* 162:476, 1990.

Carlo WA et al: The effect of respiratory distress syndrome on chest wall movements and respiratory pauses in preterm infants, *Am Rev Respir Dis* 126:103, 1982.

Chatburn R: Similarities and differences in the management of acute lung injury in neonates (IRDS) and in adults (ARDS), *Respir Care* 33:539, 1988.

Greenough A et al: Routine daily chest radiographs in ventilated, very low birthweight infants, *Eur J Pediatr* 160:147-149, 2001.

Gregory G et al: Treatment of the idiopathic respiratory-distress syndrome with continuous positive airway pressure, *N Engl J Med* 284:1333, 1971.

Hallman M, Gluck L: Respiratory distress syndrome—update 1982, *Pediatr Clin North Am* 29:1057, 1982.

Kjos S et al: Prevalence and etiology of respiratory distress in infants of diabetic mothers: Predictive values of fetal lung maturation tests, *Am J Obstet Gynecol* 163:898, 1990.

Lapido M: Respiratory distress revisited, *Neonatal Network* 8:9, 1989.

Pramanik AK, Holtzman RB, Merritt TA: Surfactant replacement therapy for pulmonary diseases, *Pediatr Clin North Am* 40:913, 1993.

Rodriguez RJ, Martin RJ: Exogenous surfactant therapy in newborns, *Respir Care Clin North Am* 5(4):595, 1999.

Seppanen MP et al: Doppler-derived systolic pulmonary artery pressure in acute neonatal respiratory distress syndrome, *Pediatrics* 93:769, 1994.

Soubani AO, Pieroni R: Acute respiratory distress syndrome: a clinical update, *South Med J* 92(5):450, 1999.

Verma RP: Respiratory distress syndrome of the newborn infant, *Obstet Gynecol Surv* 50(7):542, 1995

MECONIUM ASPIRATION SYNDROME

Altshuler G, Hyde S: Meconium-induced vasocontraction: a potential cause of cerebral and other fetal hypoperfusion and of poor pregnancy outcome, *J Child Neurol* 4:137, 1989.

Goetzman BW: Meconium aspiration, *Am J Dis Child* 146:1282, 1992.

MacFarlane PI, Heaf DP: Pulmonary function in children after neonatal meconium aspiration syndrome, *Arch Dis Child* 63:368, 1988.

Soll RF, Dargavill P: Surfactant for meconium aspiration syndrome in full term infants, *Cochrane Database Syst Rev* (2), 2000.

Swaminathan S et al: Long-term pulmonary sequelae of meconium aspiration syndrome, *J Pediatr* 114:356, 1989.

Wiswell TE: Advances in the treatment of the meconium aspiration syndrome, *Acta Paediatr Suppl* 436:28-30, 2001.

Wiswell TE et al: Delivery room management of the apparently vigorous meconium-stained neonates: Results of the multi-center, international collaborative trial, *Pediatrics* 105:1-17, 2000.

Wiswell TE, Tuggle JM, Turner BS: Meconium aspiration syndrome: Have we made a difference? *Pediatrics* 85:715, 1990.

Wiswell TE, Bent RC: Meconium staining and the meconium aspiration syndrome, *Pediatr Clin North Am* 40:955, 1993.

PULMONARY INTERSTITIAL EMPHYSEMA

Fitzgerald D et al: Dexamethasone for pulmonary interstitial emphysema in preterm infants, *Biol Neonate* 73:34-39, 1998.

Kilbride HW, Thibeault DW: Neonatal complications of preterm premature rupture of membranes: Pathophysiology and management, *Clin Perinatol* 28(4):761-785, 2001.

Morisot C et al: Risk factors for fatal pulmonary interstitial emphysema in neonates, *Eur J Pediatr* 149:493-495, 1990.

BRONCHOPULMONARY DYSPLASIA

Anderson AH et al: Systemic hypertension in infants with BPD: Associated clinical features, *Am J Perinatol* 10:190, 1993.

Bailey P, Giltman L: Bronchopulmonary dysplasia: an update, *Respir Care* 30:771, 1985.

Carey BE, Trotter C: Bronchopulmonary dysplasia, *Neonatal Net* 15(4):73, 1996.

Chernick V: Long-term pulmonary function studies in children with bronchopulmonary dysplasia: an everchanging saga, *J Pediatr* 133:171-172, 1998.

Eber E, Zach MS: Long-term sequelae of bronchopulmonary dysplasia (chronic lung diseases of infancy), *Thorax* 56(4):317, 2001.

Greenough A: Bronchopulmonary dysplasia: Early diagnosis, prophylaxis, and treatment, *Arch Dis Child* 65:1082, 1990.

Jacob SV et al: Long-term pulmonary sequelae of severe broncho-pulmonary dysplasia, *J Pediatr* 133:193-200, 1998.

Northway W: Bronchopulmonary dysplasia: Then and now, *Arch Dis Child* 65:1076, 1990.

Philip AG: Oxygen plus pressure plus time: the etiology of bronchopulmonary dysplasia, *Pediatrics* 55:44, 1975.

Ogawa Y et al: Epidemiology and classification of chronic lung disease *Pediatr Pulmonol* 16:25-26, 1997.

Rojas AM et al: Changing trends in the epidemiology and pathogenesis of neonatal chronic lung disease, *J Pediatr* 126:605-610, 1995.

Southall D, Samuels M: Bronchopulmonary dysplasia: a new look at management, *Arch Dis Child* 65:1089, 1990.

Swyer PR et al: The pulmonary syndrome of Wilson and Mikity, *Pediatrics* 36:374-383, 1965.

RESPIRATORY SYNCYTIAL VIRUS INFECTION

Long CE et al: Sequelae of respiratory syncytial virus infections: a role for intervention studies, *Am J Resp Crit Care Med* 151(5):1678, 1995.

Makela MJ et al: Respiratory syncytial virus infection in children, *Curr Opin Pediatr* 6(1):17, 1994.

McIntosh K: Respiratory syncytial virus infection infants and children: Diagnosis and treatment, *Pediatr Rev* 9:191, 1987.

Sigurs N et al: Respiratory syncytial virus bronchiolitis in infancy is an important risk factor for asthma and allergy at age 7, *Am J Respir Crit Care Med* 161(5):1501, 2000.

Stark JM et al: Respiratory syncytial virus infection enhances neutrophil and eosinophil adhesion to cultured respiratory epithelial cells: Roles of CDE18 and intercellular adhesion molecule-1, *J Immunol* 156(12):4474, 1996.

Stein RT et al: Respiratory syncytial virus in early life and risk of wheeze and allergy by age 13 years, *Lancet* 354(9178):541, 1999.

DIAPHRAGMATIC HERNIA

Bailey PV et al: A critical analysis of extracorporeal membrane oxygenation for congenital diaphragmatic hernia, *Surgery* 106-611, 1989.

Muratore CS et al: Pulmonary morbidity in 100 survivors of congenital diaphragmatic hernia in a multidisciplinary clinic, *J Pediatr Surg* 36:133-140, 2001.

Muratore CS, Wilson JM: Congenital diaphragmatic hernia: Where are we and where do we go from here? *Semin Perinatol* 24:418-428, 2000.

Wung JT et al: Congenital diaphragmatic hernia: Survival treated with very delayed surgery, spontaneous respiration and no chest tube, *J Pediatr Surg* 30:406-409, 1995.

CYSTIC FIBROSIS

Aitken ML et al: Recombinant human DNase inhalation in normal subjects and patients with cystic fibrosis, *JAMA* 267:1947, 1992.

App EM et al: Acute and long term amiloride inhalation in cystic fibrosis lung disease: a rational approach to cystic fibrosis therapy, *Am Rev Respir Dis* 141:605, 1990.

Boat TF et al: *The diagnosis of cystic fibrosis*, Bethesda, Md, 1998, Cystic Fibrosis Foundation.

Davis PB: Cystic fibrosis, *Pediatr Rev* 22:257-264, 2001.

Donaldson SH, Yankaskas JR: Cystic fibrosis. In Hess DR et al: *Respiratory care—principles and practice*, Philadelphia, 2002, WB Saunders.

Kosorok MR, Wei WH, Farrell PM: The incidence of cystic fibrosis, *Stat Med* 15(5):449, 1996.

Orenstein DM: *Cystic fibrosis—a guide for patient and family*, ed 3, Philadelphia, 2003, JB Lippincott.

Ramsey B: Management of pulmonary disease in patients with cystic fibrosis, *N Engl J Med* 335:179-188, 1996.

Rosenstein B, Cutting GR: Diagnosis of cystic fibrosis: a consensus statement, *J Pediatr* 132:589-595, 1998.

Shak S: Aerosolized recombinant human DNase I for the treatment of cystic fibrosis, *Chest* 107(2 suppl.):65s, 1995.

Statement from the National Institutes of Health workshop in population screening for the cystic fibrosis gene, *N Engl J Med* 323:70, 1990.

Steen JH et al: Evaluation of the PEP mask in cystic fibrosis, *Acta Paediatr Scand* 80:51, 1991.

Wilcken B: Newborn screening for cystic fibrosis: Its evolution and a review of the current situation, *Screening* 2:43-62, 1993.

Wilmott RW, Fiedler MA: Recent advances in the treatment of cystic fibrosis, *Pediatr Clin North Am* 41(3):431, 1994.

Wood RE, Boat TF, Doershuk CF: Cystic fibrosis, *Am Rev Respir Dis* 833-838, 1996.

Worldwide survey of the delta F508 mutation—report from the cystic fibrosis genetic analysis consortium, *Am J Hum Genet* 47:354-359, 1990.

CROUP AND EPIGLOTTITIS

Ashcroft CK, Russell WS: Epiglottitis: a pediatric emergency, *J Respir Dis* 7:40, 1988.

Breukels MA et al: Invasive infection with *Haemophilus influenzae* type B in spite of complete vaccination, *Ned Tijdschr Geneeskd* 142:586-589, 1998.

Butt W et al: Acute epiglottitis: a different approach to management, *Crit Care Med* 16:43, 1988.

Cherry JD: The treatment of croup: Continued controversy due to failure of recognition of historic, ecologic, etiological, and clinical perspectives, *J Pediatr* 94:352, 1979.

Denny FW: Croup: an 11-year study in a pediatric practice, *Pediatrics* 71:871, 1983.

Eigen H: Croup or epiglottitis: Differential diagnosis and treatment, *Respir Care* 20:1158, 1975.

Frantz TD, Rasgon BM: Acute epiglottis changing epidemiologic patterns, *Otolaryngol Head Neck Surg* 109:457-460, 1993.

Gonzalez-Valdapena H et al: Epiglottitis and *Haemophilus influenzae* immunization: the Pittsburgh experience—a five-year review, *Pediatrics* 96(3 pt 1):424, 1995.

Grad R: Acute infections producing upper airway obstruction. In Chernick V, Boat TF, Kendig EL, editors: *Disorders of the respiratory tract in children*, Philadelphia, 1998, WB Saunders.

Hickerson SL et al: Epiglottitis: a 9-year case review, *South Med J* 89(5):487, 1996.

Kaditis AG, Wald ER: Viral croup: Current diagnosis and treatment, *Pediatr Infect Dis J* 17(9):827, 1998.

Kimmons HC, Peterson BM: Management of acute epiglottitis in pediatric patients, *Crit Care Med* 14:278, 1986.

Klassen TP: Croup, a current perspective, *Pediatr Clin North Am* 46(6):1167, 1999.

Letourneau MA: Respiratory disorders. In Berkin RM et al, editors: *Pediatric emergency medicine*, St. Louis, 1992, Mosby.

Leung AKC, Cho H: Diagnosis of stridor in children, *Ann Fam Physician* 60(8):2289, 1999.

NEAR DROWNING

Conn A, Barker G: Fresh water drowning and near-drowning: an update, *Can Anaesth Soc J* 31(3):S38, 1984.

DeNicola LK et al: Submersion injuries in children and adults, *Crit Care Clin* 13:477-502, 1997.

Gilbert J, Puckett J, Smith R: Near drowning: Current concepts of management, *Respir Care* 30(2):108, 1985.

Golden FS, Tipton MJ, Scott RC: Immersion, near-drowning, and drowning, *Br J Anaesth* 79:214-225, 1997.

Gonzalez-Rothi R: Near drowning: Consensus and controversies in pulmonary and cerebral resuscitation, *Heart Lung* 16(5):474, 1987.

Habib DM et al: Near-drowning: Morbidity and mortality, *Pediatr Emerg Med* 12:255-258, 1996.

Karch SB: Pathophysiology of the lung in near drowning, *Am J Emerg Med* 4:4, 1986.

Nemiroff MJ: Near-drowning, *Respir Care* 37(6):600, 1992.

Orlowski J: Drowning, near-drowning, and ice-water submersions, *Pediatr Clin North Am* 34(1):75, 1987.

Ornato J: The resuscitation of near-drowning victims, *JAMA* 256(1):75, 1986.

Pearn J: Pathophysiology of drowning, *Med J Aust* 142:586, 1985.

Shaw K: Management of near drowning patients, *Respir Mgmt* 21(2):32, 1991.

Siebke H et al: Survival after 40 minutes' submersion without cerebral sequelae, *Lancet* 1:1275, 1975.

Weinstein MD, Krieger BP: Near-drowning: Epidemiology, pathophysiology, and initial treatment, *J Emerg Med* 14:461-467, 1996.

SMOKE INHALATION

Barillo DJ, Goode R, Esch V: Cyanide poisoning in victims of fire: Analysis of 364 cases and review of the literature, *J Burn Care Rehabil* 15:46-57, 1994.

Baud FJ et al: Elevated blood cyanide concentrations in victims of smoke inhalation, *N Engl J Med* 325:1761, 1991.

Cahalane M, Demling RF: Early respiratory abnormalities from smoke inhalation, *JAMA* 251:771, 1984.

Chu C: Early and late pathological changes in severe chemical burns to the respiratory tract complicated with acute respiratory failure, *Burns* 8:387, 1982.

Clark CJ, Campbell D, Reid WH: Blood carboxyhaemoglobin and cyanide levels in fire survivors, *Lancet* 1:1332, 1981.

Clark WR, Nieman GF: Smoke inhalation, *Burns* 14:473, 1988.

Demling RH: Management of the burn patient. In Shoemaker WC et al, editors: *Textbook of critical care,* ed 2, Philadelphia, 1989, WB Saunders.

Haponik EF: Smoke inhalation injury: Some priorities for respiratory care professionals, *Respir Care* 37(6):609, 1992.

Haponik EF et al: Smoke inhalation, *Am Rev Respir Dis* 138:1060, 1988.

Haponik EF, Lykens MG: Acute upper obstruction in burned patients, *Crit Care Report* 2:28, 1990.

Haponik EF, Summer WR: Respiratory complications in burned patients: diagnosis and management of inhalation injury, *J Crit Care* 2:121, 1987.

Hardy KR, Thom SR: Pathophysiology and treatment of carbon monoxide poisoning, *J Clin Toxicol* 32:613-629, 1994.

Herndon DN et al: Incidence, mortality, pathogenesis, and treatment of pulmonary injury, *J Burn Care Rehabil* 7:184, 1986.

Herndon DN, Spies M: Modern burn care, *Semin Pediatr Surg* 10:28-31, 2001.

Joffe MD: Burns. In Fleisher GR, Ludwig S, editors: *Textbook of pediatric emergency medicine,* ed 4, Philadelphia, 2000, Lippincott, Williams and Wilkins.

Khoo AK, Lee ST, Poh WT: Tracheobronchial cytology in inhalation injury, *J Trauma* 42:81-85, 1997.

Knaysi GA, Crikelair GF, Cosman B: The rule of nine: Its history and accuracy, *Plast Reconstr Surg* 41:560-563, 1968.

Mlcak R, Cortiella J, Desai M, et al: Lung compliance, airway resistance, and work of breathing in children after inhalation injury, *J Burn Care Rehabil* 18:531-534, 1997.

Moritz AR, Henriques FC, MacLean R: The effects of inhaled heat on the air passages and lungs: an experimental investigation, *Am J Pathol* 21:311, 1945.

Myers RAM, Synder SK, Emhoff TA: Subacute sequela of carbon monoxide poisoning, *Ann Emerg Med* 14:1163, 1985.

Nishimura N, Hiranuman N: Respiratory changes after major burn injury, *Crit Care Med* 10:25, 1982.

O'Neill JA: Advances in the management of pediatric trauma, *Am J Surg* 180:365-369, 2000.

Sheridan RL, Ritz R: Burn and inhalation injuries. In Hess DR et al: *Respiratory care—principles and practice,* Philadelphia, 2002, WB Saunders.

Sheridan RL, Schnitzer JJ: Management of the high-risk pediatric burn patient, *J Pediatr Surg* 36:1308-1312, 2001.

Sheridan RL, Tompkins RG, Burke JF: Management of burn wounds with prompt excision and immediate closure, *J Intensive Care Med* 9:6-19, 1994.

Traber DL et al: The pathophysiology of inhalation injury—a review, *Burns* 14:357, 1988.

Weaver LK, Howe S, Hopkins R, et al: Carboxyhemoglobin half-life in carbon monoxide-poisoned patients treated with 100% oxygen at atmospheric pressures, *Chest* 117:801-808, 2000.

POSTOPERATIVE ATELECTASIS

Hodgkin JE: Preoperative assessment of respiratory function, *Respir Care* 29(5):496, 1984.

Johnson NT, Pierson DJ: The spectrum of pulmonary atelectasis: Pathophysiology, diagnosis, and therapy, *Respir Care* 31:1107, 1986.

Luce JM: Clinical risk factors for postoperative pulmonary complications, *Respir Care* 29(5):484, 1984.

Marini JJ: Postoperative atelectasis: Pathophysiology, clinical importance, and principles of management, *Respir Care* 29(5):516, 1984.

Matthay MA, Wiener Kronish JP: Respiratory management after surgery, *Chest* 95:424, 1989.

Ricksten SE et al: Effects of periodic positive pressure breathing by mask on postoperative pulmonary function, *Chest* 89:774, 1986.

RESPIRATORY FAILURE

The Acute Respiratory Distress Syndrome Network: Ventilation with lower tidal volume as compared with traditional tidal volume for acute lung injury and the acute respiratory distress syndrome, *N Engl J Med* 342:1301, 2000.

Amato MB et al: Effect of a protective-ventilation strategy on mortality in the acute respiratory distress syndrome, *N Engl J Med* 338(6):347, 1998.

Blanch PB: Mechanical ventilator malfunctions, *Resp Care* 44(10):1183, 1999.

Borelli M et al: Hemodynamic and gas exchange response to inhaled nitric oxide and prone positioning in acute respiratory distress syndrome patients, *Crit Care Med* 28:2707, 2000.

Ely EW et al: Large scale implementation of a respiratory therapist-driven protocol for ventilator weaning, *Am J Respir Crit Care Med* 159:439, 1999.

Pierson DJ: Invasive mechanical ventilation. In Pierson DJ, Kacmarek RM, editors: *Foundations of respiratory care,* New York, 1992, Churchill Livingstone.

Tobin JM: Weaning from mechanical ventilation: What have we learned? *Resp Care* 45(4):417, 2000.

Clinical Practice Guidelines

American Association for Respiratory Care: Clinical practice guidelines, www.aarc.org.

Respiratory Protocols

Albin RJ, Criner GJ, Thomas S, Abou-Jaoude S: Pattern of non-ICU inpatient supplemental oxygen utilization in a university hospital, *Chest* 102(6):1672-1675, 1992.

Alexander E, Weingarten S, Mohsenifar Z: Clinical strategies to reduce utilization of chest physiotherapy without compromising patient care, *Chest* 110(3):430-432, 1996.

Bowton DL, Scuderi PE, Harris L, Haponik EF: Pulse oximetry monitoring outside the intensive care unit: Progress or problem? *Ann Intern Med* 115(6):450-454, 1991.

Brougher LI, Blackwelder AK, Grossman GD, Straton GW Jr: Effectiveness of medical necessity guidelines in reducing cost of oxygen therapy, *Chest* 90(5):646-648, 1986.

Browning JA, Kaiser DL, Durbin CG Jr: The effect of guidelines on the appropriate use of ABG analysis in the intensive care unit, *Respir Care* 34(4):269-276, 1989.

Clemmer TP, Spuhler VJ: Developing and gaining acceptance for patient care protocols, *New Horizons* (1):12-19, 1998.

Clemmer TP, Spuhler VJ, Berwick DM, Nolan TW: Cooperation: the foundation of improvement, *Ann Intern Med* 128(12 Pt 1): 1004-1009, 1998.

Ely EW et al: Large scale implementation of a respiratory therapist-driven protocol for ventilator weaning, *Am J Respir Crit Care Med* 159(2):439-446, 1999.

Ford R, Phillips J, Burns D: Early results of implementing a patient-driven protocol system [abstract], *Respir Care* 38(11):1306, 1993.

Ford RM, Phillips-Clar JE, Burns DM: Implementing therapist-driven protocols, *Respir Care Clin N Am* 2(1):51-76, 1996.

Giles D et al: A triage rating instrument for respiratory care: Description and relation to clinical outcomes, *Respir Care* 42(10):965-973, 1997.

Haney D: Therapist-driven protocols for adult non-ICU patients: Availability and efficacy. In Stoller JK, Kester L, editors: *Therapist driven protocols*, Philadelphia, 1996, WB Saunders.

Hart SK, Dubbs W, Gil A, Myers-Judy M: The effects of therapist evaluation of orders and interaction with physicians on the appropriateness of respiratory care, *Respir Care* 34(3):185-190, 1989.

Hess D: Clinical practice guidelines: Why, whence, whither? [editorial], *Respir Care* 40:1264-1268, 1995.

Hrst HM, Mouro D, Hall-Jennssens RA, Pamulov N: Decrease in ventilation time with a standardized weaning process, *Arch Surg* 133(5):483-489, 1998.

Kester L, Orens DK: Constructing a therapist-driven protocol, *Respir Care Clin N Am* 2(1):27-49, 1996.

Kester L, Stoller JK: Monitoring quality in a respiratory care protocol service: Methods and outcomes, *Respir Care* 44(5): 512-519, 1999.

Kester L, Stoller JK: Ordering respiratory care services for hospitalized patients: Practices of overuse and underuse, *Cleve Clin J Med* 59(6):581-585, 1992.

Kester L, Stoller JK: A primer on respiratory therapist-driven protocols, *Clin Pulmon Med* 1:93-99, 1994.

King T, Simon RH: Pulse oximetry for tapering supplemental oxygen in hospitalized patients: Evaluation of a protocol, *Chest* 92(4): 713-716, 1987.

Kirby EG, Durbin CG Jr: Establishment of a respiratory assessment team is associated with decreased mortality in patients re-admitted to the ICU, *Respir Care* 41(10):903-907, 1996.

Kollef MH: Outcomes research as a tool for defining the role of respiratory care practitioners in the ICU setting, *New Horizons* 6(1):91-98, 1998.

Kollef MK, Shapiro SD, Clinkscale D, Cracchiolo L, Clayton D, Wilner R, Hossin L: The effect of respiratory therapist initiated treatment protocols on outcomes and resource utilization, *Chest* 117:467-475, 2000.

Kollef MH, Shapiro SD, Silver P, St. John RE, Prentice D, Sauer S, et al: A randomized, controlled trial of protocol-directed versus physician-directed weaning from mechanical ventilation, *Crit Care Med* 25(4):567-574, 1997.

Komarra JJ Jr, Stoller JK: The impact of a postoperative oxygen therapy protocol, *Respir Care* 40(11):1125-1129, 1995.

Konschak MR, Binder A, Binder RE: Oxygen therapy utilization in a community hospital: Use of a protocol to improve oxygen administration and preserve resources, *Respir Care* 44(5): 506-511, 1999.

Lierl MB, Pettinichi S, Sebastian KD, Kotagal U: Trial of a therapist-directed protocol for weaning bronchodilator therapy in children with status asthmaticus, *Respir Care* 44(5):497-503, 1999.

Marelich GP et al: Protocol weaning of mechanical ventilation in medical and surgical patients by respiratory therapists and nurses: Effect on weaning time and incidence of ventilator-associated pneumonia, *Chest* 118(2):459-467, 2000.

Messenger R: Physicians' perceptions of a protocol program [abstract], *Respir Care* 42:A1108, 1997.

Nielson-Tietsort J, Poole B, Creagh CE, Repsher LE: Respiratory care protocol: an approach to in-hospital respiratory therapy, *Respir Care* 26(5):430-436, 1981.

Orens DK: A manager's perspective on respiratory therapy consult services, *Respir Care* 38(8):884-885, 1993.

Orens D, Stoller JK: Implementing a respiratory care protocol service: Steps and impediments, *Respir Care* 44(5):528-531, 1999.

Pilon CS et al: Practice guideline for ABG measurement in the intensive care unit decreases numbers and increases appropriateness in tests, *Crit Care Med* 25(8):1308-1313, 1997.

Rodriguez L, Kotin N, Lowenthal D, Kattan M: A study of pediatric house staff's knowledge of pulse oximetry [abstract], *Am Rev Respir Dis* 1474(4, Part 2):450-454, 1993.

Scheinhorn DJ, Chao DC, Stearn-Hassenpflug M, Wallace WA: Outcomes in post-ICU mechanical ventilation: a therapist-implemented weaning protocol, *Chest* 119:236-242, 2001.

Schultz TR et al: Weaning children from mechanical ventilation: a prospective randomized trial of protocol-directed versus physician-directed weaning, *Respir Care* 46(8):772-782, 2001.

Shapiro BA, Cane RD, Peterson J, Weber D: Authoritative medical direction can assure cost-beneficial bronchial hygiene therapy, *Chest* 93(5):1038-1042, 1988.

Shrake KL, Scaggs JE, England KR, Henkle JQ, Eagleton LE: A respiratory care assessment-treatment program: Results of a retrospective study, *Respir Care* 41(8):703-713, 1996.

Shrake KL, Scaggs JE, England KR, Henkle JQ, Eagleton LE: Benefits associated with a respiratory care assessment-treatment program: Results of a pilot study, *Respir Care* 39(7):715-724, 1994.

Small D et al: Uses and misuses of oxygen in hospitalized patients, *Am J Med* 92(6):591-595, 1992.

Smoker JM, Hess DR, Frey-Zeiler VL, Tangen MI, Rexrode WO: A protocol to assess oxygen therapy, *Respir Care* 31(1):35-39, 1986.

Stoller JK: Misallocation of respiratory care services: Time for a change [editorial], *Respir Care* 38:263-266, 1993.

Stoller JK: The rationale for therapist-driven protocols [review], *Respir Care Clin N Am* 2(1):1-14, 1996.

Stoller JK: The rationale for therapist-driven protocols, *Respir Care Clin N Am* 2:1-14, 1996.

Stoller JK: The rationale for respiratory care protocols: an update, *Respir Care* 43:719-723, 1998.

Stoller JK et al: Physician-ordered respiratory care versus physician-ordered use of a respiratory therapy consult service: Early experience at the Cleveland Clinic Foundation, *Respir Care* 38:1143-1154, 1993.

Stoller JK, Mascha E, Haney D, and the Section of Respiratory Therapy: A randomized controlled trial of respiratory therapy consult service-directed vs. physician-directed respiratory care to adult non-ICU inpatients [abstract], *Respir Care* 42(11):1111, 1997.

Stoller JK, Mascha EJ, Kester L, Haney D: Randomized controlled trial of physician-directed versus respiratory therapy consult service-directed respiratory care to adult non-ICU inpatients, *Am J Respir Crit Care Med* 158(4):1068-1075, 1998.

Stoller JK, Michnicki I: Medical house staff impressions regarding the impact of a respiratory therapy consult service, *Respir Care* 40:549-551, 1998.

Stoller JK, Orens DK, Ahmad M: Changing patterns of respiratory care service use in the era of respiratory care protocols: an observational study, *Respir Care* 43:637, 1998

Stoller JK, Skibinski CI, Giles DK, Keater LE, Haney DJ: Physician-ordered respiratory care versus physician-ordered use of a respiratory therapy consult service: Results of a prospective observational study, *Chest* 110(2):422-429, 1996.

Stoller JK, Thaggard I, Piquette C, O'Brien R: The impact of a respiratory therapy consult service on house officer's knowledge of respiratory care ordering, *Respir Care* 43(8):954-949, 2000.

Stoneham MD: Knowledge about pulse oximetry among medical and nursing staff, *Lancet* 344(8933):1339-1342, 1994.

Thaggard I, Stoller JK: Practical aspects of a respiratory care protocol service: Staffing and training, *Respir Care* 44(5):532-534, 1999.

Torrington KG: Protocol-driven respiratory therapy: Closing in on appropriate utilization at comparable cost and patient outcomes, *Chest* 110(2):313-314, 1996.

Walton JR, Shapiro BA, Harrison CH: Review of a bronchial hygiene evaluation program, *Respir Care* 28(2):174-179, 1983.

Weber K, Milligan S: Therapist-driven protocols: the state-of-the-art, *Respir Care* 39(3):746-756, 1994.

Wood G, Macleod B, Moffatt S: Weaning from mechanical ventilation: Physician-directed versus a respiratory-therapist-directed protocol, *Respir Care* 40(3):219-224, 1995.

Zibrak JD, Rossetti P, Wood E: Effect of reductions in respiratory therapy on patient outcome, *N Engl J Med* 315(5):292-295, 1986.

Medical Dictionaries

Anderson KN, Anderson LE, Walter GD: *Mosby's medical, nursing, and allied health dictionary,* ed 6, St. Louis, 2002, Mosby.

Dorland's illustrated medical dictionary, ed 30, Philadelphia, 2003, WB Saunders.

Web Sites

www.aarc.org: American Association for Respiratory Care
www.chestnet.com: American College of Chest Physician
www.lungusa.org/diseases: American Lung Association
www.americanheart.org: American Heart Association, Dallas
www.medlineplus.gov: Health Information
www.ama-assn.org: American Medical Association
www.acc.org: American College of Cardiology Resource Center
www.cdc.gov: Centers for Disease Control and Prevention, Atlanta, Ga.
www.jama.com: Journal of American Medical Association
www.emedicine.com: Medicine
www.mayoclinic.com: Mayo Clinic
www.my.webmed.com: Web MD Health
http://www.nlm.nih.gov/hinfo.html: National Library of Medicine
www.sleepapnea.org/: American Sleep Apnea Association
www.who.int: World Health Organization

Appendices

Symbols and Abbreviations Commonly Used in Respiratory Physiology

<table>
<tr><td colspan="2" align="center">Primary Symbols</td></tr>
<tr><td>Gas Symbols</td><td>Blood Symbols</td></tr>
<tr><td>P Pressure</td><td>Q Blood volume</td></tr>
<tr><td>V Gas volume</td><td>Q̇ Blood flow</td></tr>
<tr><td>V̇ Gas volume per unit of time, or flow</td><td>C Content in blood</td></tr>
<tr><td>F Fractional concentration of gas</td><td>S Saturation</td></tr>
<tr><td colspan="2" align="center">Secondary Symbols</td></tr>
<tr><td>Gas Symbols</td><td>Blood Symbols</td></tr>
<tr><td>ɪ Inspired</td><td>a Arterial</td></tr>
<tr><td>ᴇ Expired</td><td>c Capillary</td></tr>
<tr><td>ᴀ Alveolar</td><td>v Venous</td></tr>
<tr><td>ᴛ Tidal</td><td>v̄ Mixed venous</td></tr>
<tr><td>ᴅ Deadspace</td><td></td></tr>
</table>

ABBREVIATIONS

	Lung Volumes
VC	Vital capacity
IC	Inspiratory capacity
IRV	Inspiratory reserve volume
ERV	Expiratory reserve volume
FRC	Functional residual capacity
RV	Residual volume
TLC	Total lung capacity
RV/TLC (%)	Residual volume–to–total lung capacity ratio, expressed as a percentage
V_T	Tidal volume
V_A	Alveolar volume
V_D	Dead-space volume
V_L	Actual lung volume

	Respiratory Gas Flows and Rates
$\dot{V}_A$	Alveolar ventilation
$\dot{V}_D$	Dead-space ventilation
f	Frequency (i.e., respiratory rate)

ABBREVIATIONS—cont'd	
Spirometry	
FVC	Forced vital capacity with maximally forced expiratory effort
FEV_T	Forced expiratory volume, timed
$FEF_{200-1200}$	Average rate of airflow between 200 and 1200 ml of the FVC
$FEF_{25\%-75\%}$	Forced expiratory flow during the middle half of the FVC (*formerly called the maximal midexpiratory flow [MMF]*)
PEFR	Peak expiratory flow rate
$\dot{V}_{max}$	Forced expiratory flow related to the actual volume of the lungs as denoted by the subscript *x*, which refers to the amount of lung volume remaining when measurement is made
MVV	Maximal voluntary ventilation as the volume of air expired in a specified interval
Mechanics	
C_L	Lung compliance, volume change per unit of pressure change
R_{aw}	Airway resistance, pressure per unit of flow
Diffusion	
D_{LCO}	Diffusing capacity of carbon monoxide
Blood Gases	
PA_{O_2}	Alveolar oxygen tension
P_{CO_2}	Pulmonary capillary oxygen tension
Pa_{O_2}	Arterial oxygen tension
$P\bar{v}_{O_2}$	Mixed venous oxygen tension
PA_{CO_2}	Alveolar carbon dioxide tension
Pc_{CO_2}	Pulmonary capillary carbon dioxide tension
Pa_{CO_2}	Arterial carbon dioxide tension
Sa_{O_2}	Arterial oxygen saturation
$S\bar{v}_{O_2}$	Mixed venous oxygen saturation
pH	Negative logarithm of the H^1 concentration, expressed as a positive number
HCO_3^-	Plasma bicarbonate concentration
mEq/L	The number of grams of solute contained in 1 ml of a normal solution
Ca_{O_2}	Oxygen content of arterial blood
Cc_{O_2}	Oxygen content of capillary blood
$C\bar{v}_{O_2}$	Oxygen content of mixed venous blood
$\dot{V}/\dot{Q}$	Ventilation-perfusion ratio
$\dot{Q}s/\dot{Q}_T$	Shunt fraction
$\dot{Q}_T$ or CO	Total cardiac output

Medications Commonly Used in the Treatment of Cardiopulmonary Diseases

Aerosolized Medication Selections

AEROSOLIZED BRONCHODILATORS

Objective: Sympathomimetics and parasympatholytics are used to offset bronchial smooth muscle constriction. Common treatment modalities are as follows:

Sympathomimetics

- **Short-to-Intermediate Acting**
  Metaproterenol (Alupent, Metaprel)
  Terbutaline (Brethine, Brethaire)
  Pirbuterol (Maxair)
  Albuterol (Ventoline, Proventil)
  Levalbuterol (Xopenex)
- **Long Acting**
  Salmeterol (Serevent)
  Formoterol (Foradil)

Parasympatholytics (anticholinergics)

Atropine sulfate (Dey-Dose Atropine Sulfate
Ipratropium Bromide (Atrovent)
Tiotroprium (Spiriva)
Ipratropium bromide & albuterol (Combivent)

Mucolytic Agents

Objective: Mucolytic agents are used to enhance the mobilization and thinning of bronchial secretions. Common treatment modalities are as follows:

Acetylcysteine (Mucomyst)
Recombinant human deoxyribonuclease (DNase, Pulmozyme)
Sodium bicarbonate (2% solution)

Antiinflammatory Agents

Objective: Aerosolized corticosteroids are used to suppress bronchial inflammation and edema. They also are used for their ability to enhance the responsiveness of B_2 receptor sites to sympathomimetic agents. Common modalities are as follows:

Beclomethasone dipropionate (Beclovent, Vanceril)
Triamcinolone acetonide (Azmacort)

Flunisolide (AeroBid, AeroBid-M)
Fluticasone propionate (Flovent)
Budesonide (Pulmicort Turbuhaler, Pulmicort Respules)
Fluticasone propionate and salmeterol (Advair Diskus)

Xanthine Bronchodilators

Xanthine bronchodilators are used to enhance bronchial smooth muscle relaxation.

Generic Name	Trade Name
Theophylline	Bronkodyl
	Elixophyllin
	Somophyllin-T
	Slo-Phyllin
	Theolair
	Theo-Dur
	Theo-Dur Sprinkle
	Constant-T
	Quibron-T/SR
	Respbid
Theophylline sodium glycinate	Synophylate
Oxtriphylline (choline theophyllinate)	Aminophylline
	Phyllocontin
Dyphylline	Lufyllin

EXPECTORANTS

Expectorants are agents used to increase bronchial submucous gland secretion, which in turn decreases mucus viscosity. This facilitates the mobilization and expectoration of bronchial secretions.

Generic Name	Trade Name
Guaifenesin	Robitussin, Naldecon Senior EX, Humibid L.A.
Terpin hydrate	(Various)
Iodinated glycerol	Organidin
Potassium iodide (SSKI)	(Various)

ANTIBIOTIC AGENTS

Agent	Therapeutic Uses
Penicillins	Used in treating streptococcal species, staphylococcal species, *Haemophilus influenzae*; also used in treating aspiration pneumonia
Penicillin G	
Penicillin V	
Oxacillin (Prostaphilin)	
Cloxacillin (Tegopen)	
Methicillin (Staphcillin)	
Ampicillin (Omnipen)	
Amoxicillin (Polymox)	
Amoxicillin and clavulanate	
(Augmentin, Clavulin)Carbenicillin (Geopen)	
Ticarcillin (Ticar)	

ANTIBIOTIC AGENTS—cont'd

Agent	Therapeutic Uses
Cephalosporins	
First generation	Important for their broad-spectrum activity against common gram-positive
Cephalexin (Keflex)	cocci (primarily the first generation) and some gram-negative organisms
Cefadroxil (Duricef)	(primarily the second and third generations); also active against *Klebsiella*
Cephalothin (Keflin)	species, but lack efficacy against *Pseudomonas aeruginosa* and
	Haemophilus influenzae
Second generation	
Cefaclor (Ceclor)	
Cefoxitin (Mefoxin)	
Cefonicid (Monocid)	
Loracarbef (Lorabid)	
Third generation	
Cefixime (Suprax)	
Cefoperazone (Cefobid)	
Cefotaxime (Claforan)	
Ceftizoxime (Cefizox)	
Ceftazidime (Fortaz)	
Ceftriaxone (Rocephin)	
Aminoglycosides	Used for treating gram-negative organisms; commonly used to treat
Streptomycin	*Pseudomonas* in cystic fibrosis; streptomycin also is used in treating
Gentamicin (Garamycin)	*Mycobacterium tuberculosis*
Netilmicin (Netromycin)	
Amikacin (Amikin)	
Kanamycin (Kantrex)	
Neomycin (Neosporin)	
Sulfonimides	
Trimethoprim/sulfamethoxazole	Used in treating *Pneumocystis carinii pneumonia* (PCP)
(Septra-DS, Bactrim-DS)	
Tetracyclines	Used in treating mycoplasmal and other atypical pneumonias and acute
Doxycycline (Vibramycin)	infections superimposed on chronic bronchitis
Minocycline (Minocin)	
Macrolides	
Azithromycin (Zithromax)	
Clarithromycin (Biaxin)	
Telithromycin (Ketek)	
Quinolones	
Ciprofloxacin (Cipro)	
Ofloxacin (Floxin)	
Levofloxacin (Levaquin)	
Gatifloxacin (Tequin)	
Other antibiotic agents	
Vancomycin (Vancocin)	Used in treating staphylococcal infections
Chloramphenicol (Chloromycetin)	Used in treating penicillinase-producing *Staphylococcus, Klebsiella, Haemophilus influenzae*
Erythromycin (Erythrocin, Ilotycin)	Used in treating penicillin-allergic patients with pneumococcal pneumonia
Polymyxins	Used in treating *Pseudomonas* and other gram-negative organisms
Polymyxin B	
Polymyxin E	
Clindamycin (Cleocin) and lincomycin (Lincocin)	Used in treating aspiration pneumonia
Metronidazole (Flagyl, Metizol)	Active against anaerobic infections
Quinolones (levofloxacin [Levaquin], Tequin, Avelox)	Used in treating *Haemophilus influenzae, Legionella pneumophila, Mycobacterium pneumoniae, Pseudomonas aeruginosa*
Pentamidine isethionate (Pentam)	Used in treating the protozoan *Pneumocystis carinii* in patients with AIDS

Positive Inotropic Agents

Positive inotropic agents are used to increase cardiac contractility.

	Generic Name	Trade Name
	Digitalis	(Various)
	Deslanoside	Cedilanid-D
	Digoxin	Lanoxin
	Digitoxin	Crystodigin
	Amrinone	Inocor
	Dobutamine	Dobutrex
	Dopamine	Intropin
	Epinephrine	(Various)
	Isoproterenol	Isuprel

Diuretics

Diuretics are drugs used to increase urine output.

	Generic Name	Trade Name
	Furosemide	Lasix
	Ethacrynic acid	Edecrin
	Bumetanide	Bumex
	Hydrochlorothiazide	Esidrix, HydroDiuril
	Spironolactone	Aldactone

APPENDIX III

The Ideal Alveolar Gas Equation

Clinically, the alveolar oxygen tension can be computed from the ideal alveolar gas equation. A useful clinical approximation of the ideal alveolar gas equation is as follows:

$$P_{A_{O_2}} = [P_B - P_{H_2O}]\, F_{I_{O_2}} - P_{a_{CO_2}}\,(1.25)$$

where P_B is barometric pressure, $P_{A_{O_2}}$ is the partial pressure of oxygen within the alveoli, P_{H_2O} is the partial pressure of water vapor in the alveoli (at body temperature and at sea level P_{H_2O} in the alveoli is 47 mm Hg), $F_{I_{O_2}}$ is the fractional concentration of inspired oxygen, and $P_{a_{CO_2}}$ is the partial pressure of arterial carbon dioxide. The number 1.25 is a factor that adjusts for alterations in oxygen tension resulting from variations in the respiratory exchange ratio. The respiratory exchange ratio indicates that less carbon dioxide is transferred into the alveoli (about 200 cc/min) than the amount of oxygen that moves into the pulmonary capillary blood (about 250 ml/min). This ratio is normally about 0.8.

Therefore if a patient is receiving an $F_{I_{O_2}}$ of 40% on a day when the barometric pressure is 755 mm Hg and the $P_{a_{CO_2}}$ is 55 mm Hg, the patient's alveolar oxygen tension ($P_{a_{O_2}}$) can be calculated as follows:

$$P_{A_{O_2}} = (P_B - P_{H_2O})\, F_{I_{O_2}} - P_{a_{CO_2}}\,(1.25)$$
$$= (755 - 47)\,0.40 - 55\,(1.25)$$
$$= (708)\,0.40 - 68.75$$
$$= (283.2) - 68.75$$
$$= 214.45$$

The ideal alveolar gas equation is part of the clinical information needed to calculate the degree of pulmonary shunting (see Chapter 4).

Physiologic Dead Space Calculation

The amount of physiologic dead space (V_D) in the tidal volume (V_T) can be estimated by using the dead space–to–tidal volume ratio (V_D/V_T) equation. The equation is arranged as follows:

$$V_D/V_T = \frac{Pa_{CO_2} - P\bar{E}_{CO_2}}{Pa_{CO_2}}$$

For example, in a patient whose Pa_{CO_2} is 40 mm Hg and whose $P\bar{E}_{CO_2}$ is 28 mm Hg:

$$V_D/V_T = \frac{40 - 28}{40}$$

$$= \frac{12}{40}$$

$$= 0.3$$

In this case, approximately 30% of the patient's ventilation is dead–space ventilation. This is within the normal range.

APPENDIX V

Units of Measure

METRIC WEIGHT				
Grams	**Centigrams**	**Milligrams**	**Micrograms**	**Nanograms**
1	100	1000	1,000,000	1,000,000,000
0.01	1	10	10,000	10,000,000
0.001	0.1	1	1000	1,000,000
0.000001	0.0001	0.001	1	1000
0.000000001	0.0000001	0.000001	0.001	1

WEIGHT	
Metric	**Approximate Apothecary Equivalents**
Grams	*Grains*
0.0002	$1/300$
0.0003	$1/200$
0.0004	$1/150$
0.0005	$1/120$
0.0006	$1/100$
0.001	$1/60$
0.002	$1/30$
0.005	$1/12$
0.010	$1/6$
0.015	$1/4$
0.025	$3/8$
0.030	$1/2$
0.050	$3/4$
0.060	1
0.100	$1 1/2$
0.120	2
0.200	3
0.300	5
0.500	$7 1/2$
0.600	10
1	15
2	30
4	60

LIQUID MEASURE

Metric	Approximate Apothecary Equivalents
Milliliters	
1000	1 quart
750	1½ pints
500	1 pint
250	8 fluid ounces
200	7 fluid ounces
100	3½ fluid ounces
50	1¾ fluid ounces
30	1 fluid ounce
15	4 fluid drams
10	2½ fluid drams
8	2 fluid drams
5	1¼ fluid drams
4	1 fluid dram
3	45 minims
2	30 minims
1	15 minims
0.75	12 minims
0.6	10 minims
0.5	8 minims
0.3	5 minims
0.25	4 minims
0.2	3 minims
0.1	1½ minims
0.06	1 minim
0.05	¾ minim
0.03	½ minim

METRIC LIQUID

Liter	Centiliter	Milliliter	Microliter	Nanoliter
1	100	1000	1,000,000	1,000,000,000
0.01	1	10	10,000	10,000,000
0.001	0.1	1	1000	1,000,000
0.000001	0.0001	0.001	1	1000
0.000000001	0.0000001	0.000001	0.001	1

METRIC LENGTH

Meter	Centimeter	Millimeter	Micrometer	Nanometer
1	100	1000	1,000,000	1,000,000,000
0.01	1	10	10,000	10,000,000
0.001	0.1	1	1000	1,000,000
0.000001	0.0001	0.001	1	1000
0.000000001	0.0000001	0.000001	0.001	1

WEIGHT CONVERSIONS (METRIC AND AVOIRDUPOIS)

Grams	Kilograms	Ounces	Pounds
1	0.001	0.0353	0.0022
1000	1	35.3	2.2
28.35	0.02835	1	$^1/_{16}$
454.5	0.4545	16	1

WEIGHT CONVERSIONS (METRIC AND APOTHECARY)

Grams	Milligrams	Grains	Drams	Ounces	Pounds
1	1000	15.4	0.2577	0.0322	0.00268
0.001	1	0.0154	0.00026	0.0000322	0.00000268
0.0648	64.8	1	$^1/_{60}$	$^1/_{480}$	$^1/_{5760}$
3.888	3888	60	1	$^1/_8$	$^1/_{96}$
31.1	31104	480	8	1	$^1/_{12}$
363.25	373248	5760	96	12	1

APPROXIMATE HOUSEHOLD MEASUREMENT EQUIVALENTS (VOLUME)

			1 tsp =	5 ml
		1 tbsp = 3 tsp =		15 ml
	1 fl oz =	2 tbsp = 6 tsp =		30 ml
1 cup =	8 fl oz =			240 ml
1 pt = 2 cups =	16 fl oz =			480 ml
1 qt = 2 pt = 4 cups =	32 fl oz =			960 ml
1 gal = 4 qt = 8 pt = 16 cups =	128 fl oz =			3840 ml

VOLUME CONVERSIONS (METRIC AND APOTHECARY)

Milliliters	Minims	Fluid Drams	Fluid Ounces	Pints	Liters	Gallons	Fluid Quarts	Ounces	Pints
1	16.2	0.27	0.0333	0.0021	1	0.2642	1.057	33.824	2.114
0.0616	1	$^1/_{60}$	$^1/_{480}$	$^1/_{7680}$	3.785	1	4	128	8
3.697	60	1	$^1/_8$	$^1/_{128}$	0.946	$^1/_4$	1	32	2
29.58	480	8	1	$^1/_{16}$	0.473	$^1/_8$	$^1/_2$	16	1
473.2	7680	128	16	1	0.0296	$^1/_{128}$	$^1/_{32}$	1	$^1/_{16}$

LENGTH CONVERSIONS (METRIC AND ENGLISH SYSTEM)

		Millimeters	Centimeters	Inches	Feet	Yards	Meters
1 Å	=	$\dfrac{1}{10{,}000{,}000}$	$\dfrac{1}{100{,}000{,}000}$	$\dfrac{1}{254{,}000{,}000}$	$\dfrac{1}{3{,}050{,}000{,}000}$	$\dfrac{1}{9{,}140{,}000{,}000}$	$\dfrac{1}{10{,}000{,}000{,}000}$
1 nm	=	$\dfrac{1}{1{,}000{,}000}$	$\dfrac{1}{10{,}000{,}000}$	$\dfrac{1}{25{,}400{,}000}$	$\dfrac{1}{305{,}000{,}000}$	$\dfrac{1}{914{,}000{,}000}$	$\dfrac{1}{1{,}000{,}000{,}000}$
1 μm	=	$\dfrac{1}{1000}$	$\dfrac{1}{10{,}000}$	$\dfrac{1}{25{,}400}$	$\dfrac{1}{305{,}000}$	$\dfrac{1}{914{,}000}$	$\dfrac{1}{1{,}000{,}000}$
1 mm	=	1	0.1	0.03937	0.00328	0.0011	0.001
1 cm	=	10	1	0.3937	0.03281	0.0109	0.01
1 in	=	25.4	2.54	1	0.0833	0.0278	0.0254
1 ft	=	304.8	30.48	12	1	0.333	0.3048
1 yd	=	914.40	91.44	36	3	1	0.9144
1 m	=	1000	100	39.37	3.2808	1.0936	1

Poiseuille's Law

Poiseuille's Law for Flow Rearranged to a Simple Proportionality

$$\dot{V} \simeq \Delta P r^4, \text{ or rewritten as } \frac{\dot{V}}{r^4} \simeq \Delta P$$

When ΔP remains constant, then

$$\frac{\dot{V}}{r_1^4} \simeq \frac{\dot{V}}{r_2^4}$$

Example 1 — If the radius (r_1) is decreased to half its previous radius ($r_2 = \frac{1}{2}r_1$), then

$$\frac{\dot{V}}{r_1^4} \simeq \frac{\dot{V}}{(\frac{1}{2}r_1)^4}$$

$$\frac{\dot{V}_1}{r_1^4} \simeq \frac{\dot{V}_2}{(\frac{1}{16})r_1^4}$$

$$\left(r_1^4\right)\frac{\dot{V}_1}{r_1^4} \simeq \left(r_1^4\right)\frac{\dot{V}_2}{(\frac{1}{16})r_1^4}$$

$$\dot{V}_1 \simeq \frac{\dot{V}_2}{\frac{1}{16}}$$

$$\left(\frac{1}{16}\right)\dot{V}_1 \simeq \left(\frac{1}{16}\right)\frac{\dot{V}_2}{\frac{1}{16}}$$

$$\left(\frac{1}{16}\right)\dot{V}_1 \simeq \dot{V}_2$$

The gas flow ($\dot{V}_1$) is reduced to $\frac{1}{16}$ its original flow rate [$\dot{V}_2 \simeq (\frac{1}{16})\dot{V}_1$].

Example 2 — If the radius (r_1) is decreased by 16% ($r_2 = r_1 - 0.16r_1 = 0.84r_1$), then

$$\frac{\dot{V}_1}{r_1^4} \simeq \frac{\dot{V}_2}{r_1^4}$$

$$\frac{\dot{V}_1}{r_1^4} \simeq \frac{\dot{V}_2}{\left(0.84 r_1\right)^4}$$

$$\dot{V}_2 \simeq \frac{\left(0.84 r_1\right)^4 \dot{V}_1}{r_1^4}$$

$$\dot{V}_2 \simeq \frac{0.4979 \, \cancel{r_1^4} \, \dot{V}_1}{\cancel{r_1^4}}$$

$$\dot{V}_2 \simeq \tfrac{1}{2} \dot{V}_1$$

The flow rate ($\dot{V}_1$) decreases to half the original flow rate ($\dot{V}_2 \simeq \tfrac{1}{2}\dot{V}_1$).

Poiseuille's Law for Pressure Rearranged to a Simple Proportionality

$$P \simeq \frac{\dot{V}}{r^4}, \text{ or rewritten as } P \cdot r^4 \simeq \dot{V}$$

When $\dot{V}$ remains constant, then

$$P_1 \cdot r_1^4 \simeq P_2 \cdot r_2^4$$

Example 1 — If the radius (r_1) is reduced to half its original radius [$r_2 = (\tfrac{1}{2})r_1$], then

$$P_1 \cdot r_1^4 \simeq P_2 \cdot r_2^4$$

$$P_1 \cdot r_1^4 \simeq P_2[(\tfrac{1}{2})r_1]^4$$

$$P_1 \cdot r_1^4 \simeq P_2 \cdot \left(\tfrac{1}{16}\right)r_1^4$$

$$\frac{P_1 \cdot \cancel{r_1^4}}{\cancel{r_1^4}} \simeq \frac{P_2 \cdot \left(\tfrac{1}{16}\right) \cancel{r_1^4}}{\cancel{r_1^4}}$$

$$P_1 \simeq P_2 \cdot \left(\tfrac{1}{16}\right)$$

$$16 P_1 \simeq 16 \cdot P_2 \cdot \left(\tfrac{1}{16}\right)$$

$$16 P_1 \simeq P_2$$

The pressure (P_1) increases to 16 times its original level ($P_2 \simeq 16 \cdot P_1$).

Example 2 — If the radius (r_1) is decreased by 16% ($r_2 = r_1 - 0.16 r_1 = 0.84 r_1$), then

$$P_1 \cdot r_1^4 \simeq P_2 \cdot r_2^4$$

$$P_1 \cdot r_1^4 \simeq P_2(0.4979)r_1^4$$

$$\frac{P_1 \, \cancel{r_1^4}}{(0.4979 \, \cancel{r_1^4})} = P_2$$

$$2 \cdot P_1 = P_2$$

The pressure (P_1) increases to twice its original pressure ($P_2 \simeq 2 \cdot P_1$).

Pco₂/HCO₃⁻/pH Nomogram

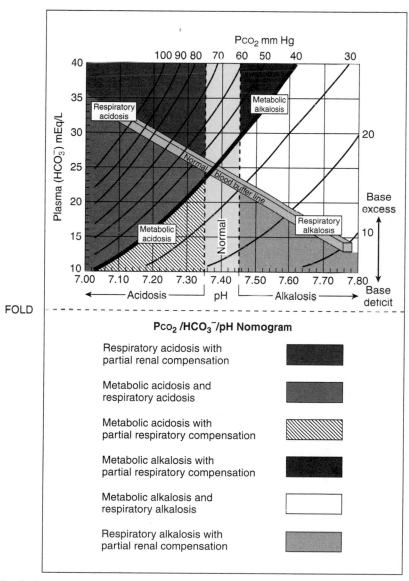

Pco₂/HCO₃⁻/pH Nomogram

Respiratory acidosis with partial renal compensation	
Metabolic acidosis and respiratory acidosis	
Metabolic acidosis with partial respiratory compensation	
Metabolic alkalosis with partial respiratory compensation	
Metabolic alkalosis and respiratory alkalosis	
Respiratory alkalosis with partial renal compensation	

(Modified from Des Jardins T: *Cardiopulmonary anatomy and physiology: essentials for respiratory care,* ed 4, Albany, NY, 2002, Delmar Publishers.)

Copy this Pco₂/HCO₃⁻/pH nomogram, color it in if you like, and have it laminated for use as a handy, pocket-size reference tool.

Calculated Hemodynamic Measurements

The following are the major hemodynamic values that can be calculated from the direct hemodynamic measurements listed in Table 6-1. The calculated hemodynamic values are easily obtained from a programmed calculator or by using the specific hemodynamic formula and a calculator. Because the calculated hemodynamic measurements vary with the size of an individual, some hemodynamic values are "indexed" by body surface area (BSA). Clinically, the BSA is obtained from a height-weight nomogram (see Appendix IX). In the normal adult, the BSA is 1.5 to 2 m^2.

Stroke Volume

The stroke volume (SV) is the volume of blood ejected by the ventricles with each contraction. The preload, afterload, and myocardial contractility are the major determinants of SV. SV is derived by dividing the cardiac output (CO) by the heart rate (HR):

$$SV = \frac{CO}{HR}$$

For example, if an individual has a cardiac output of 4 L/min (4000 ml/min) and a heart rate of 80 beats/min, the SV is calculated as follows:

$$SV = \frac{CO}{HR}$$
$$= \frac{4000 \text{ ml/min}}{80 \text{ beats/min}}$$
$$= 50 \text{ ml/beat}$$

Stroke Volume Index

The stroke volume index (SVI), also known as stroke index, is calculated by dividing the SV by the BSA:

$$SVI = \frac{SV}{BSA}$$

For example, if a patient has an SV of 50 ml and a BSA of 2 m^2, the SVI is determined as follows:

$$SVI = \frac{SV}{BSA}$$
$$= \frac{50 \text{ ml/beat}}{2 m^2}$$
$$= 25 \text{ ml/beat/}m^2$$

Assuming that the HR remains the same, as the SVI increases or decreases, the cardiac index also increases or decreases. The SVI reflects the (1) contractility of the heart, (2) overall blood volume status, and (3) amount of venous return.

Cardiac Index

The cardiac index (CI) is calculated by dividing the cardiac output (CO) by the BSA:

$$CI = \frac{CO}{BSA}$$

For example, if a patient has a CO of 6 L/min and a BSA of 2 m², the CI is computed as follows:

$$CI = \frac{CO}{BSA}$$

$$= \frac{6 \text{ L/min}}{2 \text{ m}^2}$$

$$= 3 \text{ L/min/m}^2$$

Right Ventricular Stroke Work Index

The right ventricular stroke work index (RVSWI) measures the amount of work done by the right ventricle to pump blood. The RVSWI is a reflection of the contractility of the right ventricle. In the presence of normal right ventricular contractility, increases in afterload (such as those caused by pulmonary vascular constriction) cause the RVSWI to increase until a plateau is reached. When the contractility of the right ventricle is diminished by disease states, however, the RVSWI does not appropriately increase. The RVSWI is derived from the following formula:

$$RVSWI = SVI \times (\overline{PA} - CVP) \times 0.0136 \text{ g/ml}$$

where SVI is stroke volume index, $\overline{PA}$ is mean pulmonary artery pressure, and CVP is central venous pressure. The density of mercury factor 0.0136 g/ml is needed to convert the equation to the proper units of measurement—i.e., gram meters/m² (g m/m²).

For example, if a patient has an SVI of 40 ml, a $\overline{PA}$ of 20 mm Hg, and a CVP of 5 mm Hg, the RVSWI is calculated as follows:

$$RVSWI = SVI \, (\overline{PA} - CVP) \times 0.0136 \text{ g/mL}$$

$$= 40 \text{ ml/beat/m}^2 = (15 \text{ mm Hg} - 5 \text{ mm Hg}) \times 0.0136 \text{ g/ml}$$

$$= 40 \text{ ml/beat/m}^2 \times 10 \text{ mm Hg} \times 0.0136 \text{ g/ml}$$

$$= 5.44 \text{ g m/m}^2$$

Left Ventricular Stroke Work Index

The left ventricular stroke work index (LVSWI) measures the amount of work done by the left ventricle to pump blood. The LVSWI is a reflection of the contractility of the left ventricle. In the presence of normal left ventricular contractility, increases in afterload (such as those caused by systemic vascular constriction) cause the LVSWI to increase until a plateau is reached. When the contractility of the left ventricle is diminished by disease states, however, the LVSWI does not increase appropriately. The following formula is used for determining this hemodynamic variable:

$$LVSWI = SVI \times (MAP - PCWP) \times 0.0136 \text{ g/ml}$$

where SVI is stroke volume index, MAP is mean arterial pressure, and PCWP is pulmonary capillary wedge pressure. The density of mercury factor 0.0136 g/ml is needed to convert the equation to the proper units of measurement—i.e., gram meters/m² (g m/m²).

For example, if a patient has an SVI of 40 ml, an MAP of 110 mm Hg, and a PCWP of 5 mm Hg, the patient's LVSWI is calculated as follows:

$$\text{LVSWI} = \text{SVI} \times (\text{MAP} - \text{PCWP}) \times 0.0136 \text{ g/ml}$$

$$= 40 \text{ ml/beat/m}^2 \times (110 \text{ mm Hg} - 5 \text{ mm Hg}) \times 0.0136 \text{ g/ml}$$

$$= 40 \text{ ml/beat/m}^2 \times (105 \text{ mm Hg}) \times 0.0136 \text{ g/ml}$$

$$= 59.84 \text{ g m/m}^2$$

Vascular Resistance

As blood flows through the pulmonary and systemic vascular systems, resistance to flow occurs. The pulmonary vascular system is a low-resistance system. The systemic vascular system is a high-resistance system.

PULMONARY VASCULAR RESISTANCE (PVR)

The PVR measurement reflects the afterload of the right ventricle. It is calculated by the following formula:

$$\text{PVR} = \overline{\text{PA}} - \frac{\text{PCWP}}{\text{CO}} \times 80$$

where $\overline{\text{PA}}$ is the mean pulmonary artery pressure, PCWP is the capillary wedge pressure, CO is the cardiac output, and 80 is a conversion factor for adjusting to the correct units of measurement (dyne × sec × cm⁻⁵).

For example, if a patient has a $\overline{\text{PA}}$ of 20 mm Hg, a PCWP of 5 mm Hg, and a CO of 6 L/min, the patient's PVR is calculated as follows:

$$\text{PVR} = \frac{\overline{\text{PA}} - \text{PCWP}}{\text{CO}} \times 80$$

$$= \frac{20 \text{ mm Hg} - 5 \text{ mm Hg}}{6 \text{ L/min}} \times 80$$

$$= \frac{15 \text{ mm Hg}}{6 \text{ L/min}} \times 80$$

$$= 200 \text{ dynes} \times \text{sec} \times \text{cm}^{-5}$$

SYSTEMIC OR PERIPHERAL VASCULAR RESISTANCE (SVR)

The SVR measurement reflects the afterload of the left ventricle. It is calculated by the following formula:

$$\text{SVR} = \frac{\text{MAP} - \text{CVP}}{\text{CO}} \times 80$$

where MAP is the mean arterial pressure, CVP is the central venous pressure, CO is the cardiac output, and 80 is a conversion factor for adjusting to the correct units of measurement (dyne $\times$ sec $\times$ cm^{-5}). (NOTE: The right atrial pressure [RAP] can be used in place of the CVP value.)

For example, if a patient has an MAP of 90 mm Hg, a CVP of 5 mm Hg, and a CO of 4 L/min, the patient's SVR is calculated as follows:

$$SVR = \frac{MAP - CVP}{CO} \times 80$$

$$= \frac{90 \text{ mm Hg} - 5 \text{ mm Hg}}{4 \text{ L/min}} \times 80$$

$$= \frac{85 \text{ mm Hg}}{4 \text{ L/min}} \times 80$$

$$= 1700 \text{ dynes} \times \text{sec} \times \text{cm}^{-5}$$

DuBois Body Surface Area Chart

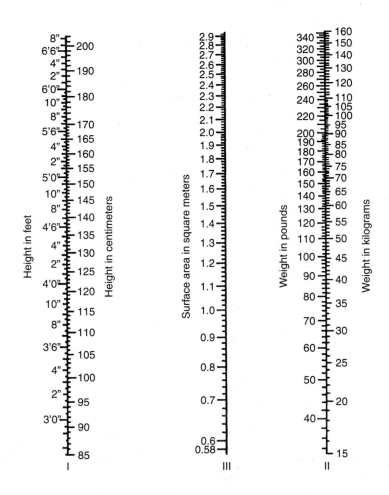

To find the body surface area of a patient, locate the height in inches (or centimeters) on Scale I and the weight in pounds (or kilograms) on Scale II, and place a straightedge (ruler) between these two points, which will intersect Scale III at the patient's surface area.

Cardiopulmonary Profile

A representative example of a cardiopulmonary profile sheet used to monitor the critically ill patient.

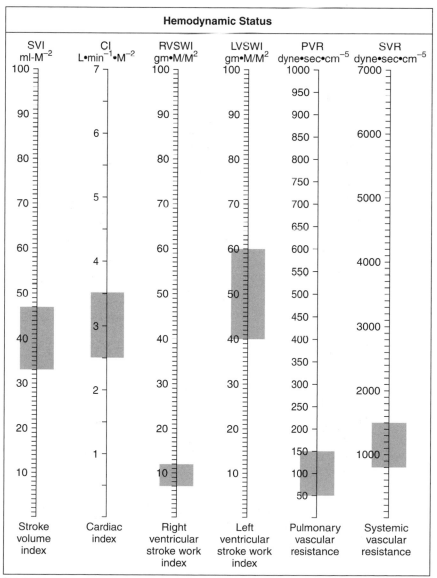

Shaded areas represent normal range.

(Modified from Des Jardins T: *Cardiopulmonary anatomy and physiology: essentials for respiratory care,* ed 4, Albany, NY, 2002, Delmar Publishers.)

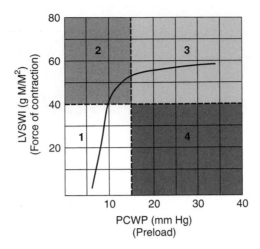

Quadrant 1: Hypovolemia
Quadrant 2: Optimal function
Quadrant 3: Hypervolemia
Quadrant 4: Cardiac failure

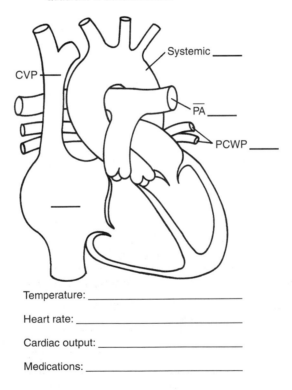

Temperature: _____

Heart rate: _____

Cardiac output: _____

Medications: _____

_____

(Modified from Des Jardins T: *Cardiopulmonary anatomy and physiology: essentials for respiratory care,* ed 4, Albany, NY, 2002, Delmar Publishers.)

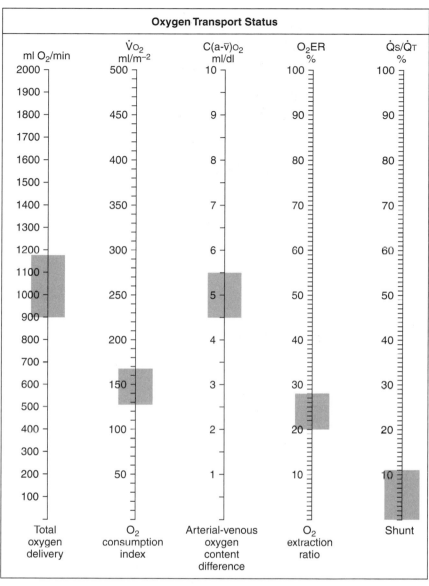

Oxygen Transport Status

ml O$_2$/min	$\dot{V}O_2$ ml/m^{-2}	C(a-$\bar{v}$)o$_2$ ml/dl	O$_2$ER %	$\dot{Q}$s/$\dot{Q}$T %
Total oxygen delivery	O$_2$ consumption index	Arterial-venous oxygen content difference	O$_2$ extraction ratio	Shunt

Blood Gas Values

pH _____

Paco$_2$ _____

HCO$_3^-$ _____

Pao$_2$ _____   P$\bar{v}$o$_2$ _____

Sao$_2$ _____ %   S$\bar{v}$o$_2$ _____ %

Fio$_2$ _____   Hb _____

Mode(s) of Ventilatory

Support: _____

_____

_____

_____

_____

Patient's Name _____

Date _____

Time _____

(Modified from Des Jardins T: *Cardiopulmonary anatomy and physiology: essentials for respiratory care,* ed 4, Albany, NY, 2002, Delmar Publishers.)

APPENDIX **XI**

Answers to the Self-Assessment Questions

Chapter 1

MATCHING

1. b
2. a
3. c
4. d
5. e

ESSAY

6. See Table 1-2

Chapter 2

1. d
2. e
3. c
4. d
5. b
6. c
7. b
8. b
9. d
10. b
11. d
12. e
13. a
14. a
15. d
16. c
17. e
18. a
19. e
20. e

Chapter 3

1. c
2. e

3. b
4. b
5. d
6. b
7. b
8. d
9. d
10. b

Chapter 4

1. d
2. e
3. c
4. b
5. b
6. e
7. a
8. b
9. d
10. e
11. d
12. a
13. c
14. d
15. e

Chapter 5

MULTIPLE CHOICE

1. e
2. a
3. b
4. d
5. a
6. c
7. e
8. b
9. c
10. e
11. b

Chapter 5—cont'd

12. c
13. c
14. d
15. b
16. e
17. c
18. e

COMPLETE THE FOLLOWING

19. $P_{AO_2} = (PB - P_{H_2O})\,F_{IO_2} - P_{aCO_2}\,(1.25)$
    $= (740 - 47)\,0.60 - 37\,(1.25)$
    $= (693)\,0.60 - 46.25$
    $= 415.8 - 46.25$
    $= 369.55$
    Answer: 369.55

20. $C_{CO_2} = (Hb \times 1.34) + (P_{aO_2} \times 0.003)$
    $= (8 \times 1.34) = (369.55 \times 0.003)$
    $= 10.72 + 11.10$
    $= 11.82$
    Answer: 11.82

21. $C_{aO_2} = (Hb \times 1.34 \times S_{aO_2}) + (P_{aO_2} \times 0.003)$
    $= (8 \times 1.34 \times 0.6) + (31 \times 0.003)$
    $= 6.43 + 0.09$
    $= 6.52$
    Answer: 6.52

22. $C\bar{v}_{O_2} = (Hb \times 1.34 \times S\bar{v}_{O_2}) + (P\bar{v}_{O_2} \times 0.003)$
    $= (8 \times 1.34 \times 51) + (21 \times 0.003)$
    $= 5.46 + 0.063$
    $= 5.52$
    Answer: 5.52

23. $\dfrac{\dot{Q}s}{\dot{Q}_T} = C_{CO_2} - \dfrac{C_{aO_2}}{C_{CO_2}} - C\bar{v}_{O_2}$

    $= \dfrac{11.82 - 6.52}{11.82 - 5.52}$

    $= \dfrac{5.3}{6.3}$

    $= 0.84$

Chapter 6

1. e
2. e
3. c
4. e
5. c
6. a
7. d
8. b
9. c
10. d

Chapter 7

1. c
2. b
3. c
4. d
5. a
6. b
7. a
8. d
9. e
10. e

Chapter 8

1. c
2. e
3. c
4. a
5. d
6. d
7. e
8. d
9. b
10. e

Chapter 9

1. a. The anatomic alterations of the lungs caused by common respiratory disorders
   b. The major pathophysiologic mechanisms activated throughout the respiratory system as a result of the anatomic alterations
   c. The common clinical manifestations that develop
   d. The treatment modalities used to correct the anatomic alterations and pathophysiologic mechanisms caused by the disorders
2. a. Quickly and systematically identify the important clinical manifestations demonstrated by the patient
   b. Formulate an accurate assessment of the clinical data—that is, identify the causes and severity of the data abnormalities
   c. Select an optimal treatment modality
   d. Document this process quickly, clearly, and precisely

Chapter 9—cont'd

3. a. Oxygen Therapy Protocol
   b. Bronchopulmonary Hygiene Therapy Protocol
   c. Hyperinflation Therapy Protocol
   d. Aerosolized Medication Protocol

Chapter 10

1. d
2. a. Summarize pertinent clinical data
   b. Analyze and assess it
   c. Record the formulation of an appropriate treatment plan
   d. Document the adjustments of the treatment plan
3. e
4. b
5. a. Subjective and objective information
   b. An assessment
   c. The treatment plan (which has measurable outcomes)
   d. An evaluation of the patient's response to the treatment plan
   e. A section to record any adjustments made to the original treatment plan
6. S Subjective information refers to information about the patient's feelings, concerns, or sensations presented by the patient.
      Examples: "I coughed hard all night!"
                 "My chest feels very tight."
   O Objective information refers to the data that the respiratory care practitioner can measure, factually describe, or obtain from other professional reports or test results.
      Examples: Heart rate
                 Respiratory rate
                 Blood pressure
   A Assessment refers to the practitioner's professional conclusion about what is the cause of the subjective and objective data presented by the patient.
      Examples: Bronchospasm
                 Atelectasis
                 Acute alveolar hyperventilation
                 Mild hypoxemia
   P Plan is the therapeutic procedure(s) selected to remedy the cause (identified in the assessment) that is responsible for the subjective and objective data demonstrated by the patient.
      Examples: Bronchodilator to offset bronchial smooth muscle constriction
                 Continuous positive airway pressure to offset atelectasis

7. e
8. a. Impending ventilatory failure
   b. Ventilatory failure
   c. Apnea
9. Impending ventilatory failure
10. S "It feels like there is a rope around my neck."
    O Heart rate, 136; blood pressure, 165/120; respiratory rate, 32; breath sounds— wheezing & rhonchi bilaterally; arterial blood gases; pH 7.56, $Paco_2$ 28, HCO_3^- 21, and Pao_2 47; strong cough effect; moderate amount of thin white secretions; peak expiratory flow rate, 185 L/min; X-ray: depressed diaphragm and hyperinflated alveoli.
    A • Acute alveolar hyperventilation with moderate hypoxemia (ABG)
       • Bronchospasm (wheezing and low peak flow)
       • Accumulation of bronchial secretions (rhonchi and sputum production)
       • Good ability to mobilize secretions (strong cough effort)
       • Hyperinflated alveoli (X-ray)
    P • Bronchodilator therapy (to offset bronchospasm, air trapping, and acute alveolar hyperventilation and hypoxemia)
       • Oxygen therapy (to offset hypoxemia and acute alveolar hyperventilation)
       • Encourage cough and deep breathing (to enhance secretion mobilization)
       • Reassess patient's response to therapy

Chapter 11

1. b
2. e
3. d
4. a
5. b
6. c
7. d
8. b
9. c
10. e

Chapter 12

1. e
2. b
3. b
4. d
5. c

Chapter 12—cont'd

6. e
7. c
8. d
9. e
10. b

Chapter 13

MULTIPLE CHOICE

1. b
2. c
3. d
4. c
5. e
6. c
7. c
8. e
9. e
10. c

TRUE OR FALSE

1. True
2. False
3. True
4. True
5. True
6. True

MATCHING

1. f
2. d
3. m
4. c
5. k
6. h
7. i
8. f
9. b
10. d
11. a
12. h
13. l

Chapter 14

1. e
2. b
3. b
4. e
5. a
6. d
7. c
8. d

9. b
10. c

Chapter 15

1. d
2. b
3. b
4. d
5. e
6. c
7. a
8. b
9. b
10. b

Chapter 16

MULTIPLE CHOICE

1. b
2. e
3. d
4. c
5. e

TRUE OR FALSE

1. True
2. False
3. True
4. True
5. False

Chapter 17

MULTIPLE CHOICE

1. e
2. d
3. e
4. d
5. c

TRUE OR FALSE

1. True
2. False
3. True
4. True
5. False

Chapter 18

MULTIPLE CHOICE

1. b
2. a

Chapter 18—cont'd

3. c
4. d
5. b

TRUE OR FALSE

1. True
2. False
3. False
4. True
5. True

Chapter 19

MULTIPLE CHOICE

1. e
2. b
3. e
4. e
5. a

TRUE OR FALSE

1. True
2. True
3. False
4. True
5. True

FILL IN THE BLANK

1. Albumin

Chapter 20

1. c
2. d
3. c
4. e
5. a
6. d
7. d
8. b

Chapter 21

MULTIPLE CHOICE

1. c
2. d
3. b
4. c
5. a

TRUE OR FALSE

1. True
2. True
3. False
4. True
5. True

Chapter 22

1. e
2. c
3. e
4. d
5. a
6. d
7. e
8. b
9. b
10. b

Chapter 23

MULTIPLE CHOICE

1. e
2. b
3. d
4. c
5. d

TRUE OR FALSE

1. True
2. False
3. True
4. True
5. True

Chapter 24

MULTIPLE CHOICE

1. a
2. c
3. c
4. a
5. e

TRUE OR FALSE

1. True
2. False
3. True
4. False
5. False

Chapter 25

MULTIPLE CHOICE

1. e
2. d
3. c
4. b
5. e

FILL IN THE BLANKS

1. the size of the dust particle
2. its chemical nature
3. its concentration
4. the time of exposure
5. the individual's susceptibility to specific inorganic dusts

Chapter 26

MULTIPLE CHOICE

1. a
2. b
3. b
4. b
5. e

TRUE OR FALSE

1. True
2. True
3. True
4. False
5. True

Chapter 27

MULTIPLE CHOICE

1. d
2. b
3. a
4. b
5. b

TRUE OR FALSE

1. True
2. False
3. True
4. False
5. False

Chapter 28

1. b
2. c

3. e
4. a
5. c
6. a
7. e
8. c
9. c
10. e

Chapter 29

MULTIPLE CHOICE

1. e
2. d
3. c
4. e
5. e

TRUE OR FALSE

1. True
2. False
3. False
4. True
5. True

Chapter 30

1. False
2. True
3. False
4. True
5. False
6. False
7. True
8. True
9. False
10. True

Chapter 31

1. d
2. e
3. e
4. b
5. e
6. d
7. c
8. b
9. a
10. d

Chapter 32

MULTIPLE CHOICE

1. e
2. c
3. b
4. d
5. b

TRUE OR FALSE

1. False
2. True
3. False
4. True
5. True

Chapter 33

MULTIPLE CHOICE

1. c
2. e
3. c
4. e
5. b

COMPLETE THE FOLLOWING

1. decreases
2. decreases
3. decreases
4. decreases
5. increases

Chapter 34

1. False
2. True
3. True
4. True
5. True
6. False
7. True
8. True
9. True
10. True

Chapter 35

MULTIPLE CHOICE

1. e
2. b

3. b
4. e
5. e

TRUE OR FALSE

1. True
2. True
3. False
4. False
5. False

FILL IN THE BLANK

1. 2.5 kg

Chapter 36

1. True
2. True
3. False
4. True
5. False
6. True
7. False
8. False
9. True
10. False

Chapter 37

MULTIPLE CHOICE

1. e
2. b
3. b
4. a
5. b

TRUE OR FALSE

1. True
2. True
3. False
4. True
5. False

Chapter 38

TRUE OR FALSE

1. True
2. False
3. False
4. True
5. True

Chapter 38—cont'd

COMPLETE THE FOLLOWING

1. is normal
2. increases
3. increases
4. decreases
5. is normal

Chapter 39

1. False
2. True
3. False
4. False
5. False
6. True
7. True
8. False
9. True
10. True

Chapter 40

1. False
2. True
3. True
4. True
5. True
6. False
7. True
8. False
9. False
10. False

Chapter 41

1. e
2. c
3. c
4. e
5. d
6. d
7. b
8. e
9. b
10. d

Chapter 42

FILL IN THE BLANKS

1. near
2. dry
3. wet
4. noncardiogenic pulmonary edema
5. 25

COMPLETE THE FOLLOWING

1. decreases
2. increases
3. decreases
4. increase
5. decrease

Chapter 43

1. c
2. b
3. e
4. d
5. c
6. d
7. d
8. d
9. b
10. a

Chapter 44

1. a. thoracic surgery
   b. upper abdominal surgery
   c. lower abdominal surgery
2. See Decreased Lung Expansion, page 533.
3. See Pulmonary Units Degassing Distal to Airway Secretions and Mucus Plugs, page 533.

Chapter 45

C
A
P

P
N   See Box 45-1, page 540.
E
U
M
O
N
I
A

Answers to Selected Practice Case Studies

Suggested SOAP Responses and Case Discussions

The SOAP responses* presented below are intended only as a guide. Depending on the specific case and severity of the clinical manifestations, other assessments and treatment selections may be appropriate. In addition, the clinical manifestations in the parentheses to the right of each assessment likely would not appear in the patient's chart. They are presented in section only to justify each assessment.

• • • • •

Case 1: Chronic Bronchitis

SOAP 1

S "I'm unable to breathe. I can't inhale deep enough to cough up secretions, and my stomach is upset."

O Vitals: BP 190/115, HR 125, RR 30, T 37° C (98.6° F). Barrel chest, labored breathing, use of accessory muscles, digital clubbing, cyanosis, and pitting ankle edema (2+); copious thick, yellow sputum; chest hyperresonant, with rhonchi heard bilaterally; CXR: lungs clear, air trapping, and depressed diaphragm; Hct 58%; COHb 6%; ABGs (room air): pH 7.53, $Paco_2$ 56, HCO_3^- 33, Pao_2 43

A • Acute exacerbation of chronic bronchitis (general presentation, sputum, vital signs, ABGs)
   • Increased work of breathing (increased heart rate, blood pressure, and respiratory rate)
   • Excessive airway secretions (sputum, rhonchi)
   • Infection likely (thick, yellow secretions)
   • Poor ability to mobilize secretions (weak cough)
   • Acute alveolar hyperventilation on top of chronic ventilatory failure (ABGs and history)
   • Possible impending ventilatory failure

P Oxygen Therapy Protocol [e.g., HAFOE (Venturi) mask, FIO_2 0.28]. Bronchopulmonary Hygiene Therapy Protocol (e.g., CPT with PD, C&DB q 6 h). Obtain sputum sample for culture. Notify physician of impending ventilatory failure. Place intubation equipment and mechanical ventilator on standby. Monitor and evaluate q 3 h (vital signs: Spo_2, ABG).

---

*ABG, Arterial blood gas; AFB, acid-fast bacilli; BAL, bronchoalveolar lavage; BP, blood pressure; BUN, blood urea nitrogen; C&DB, cough and deep breathing; CO, cardiac output; COHb, carboxyhemoglobin; CPAP, continuous positive airway pressure; CPT, chest physical therapy; CVP, central venous pressure; CXR, chest X-ray; D/C, discontinue; FEV₁, forced expiratory volume in 1 second; FVC, forced vital capacity; HBO, hyperbaric oxygen; HR, heart rate; I&O, intake and outtake; IPPB, intermittent positive pressure breathing; IS, incentive spirometry; LLL, left lower lobe; MDI, metered dose inhaler; $\overline{PA}$, pulmonary artery pressure; PCWP, pulmonary capillary wedge pressure; PD, postural drainage; PEEP, positive end-expiratory pressure; PEFR, peak expiratory flow rate; PFT, pulmonary function test; PIP, peak inspiratory pressure; prn, as required; PVR, pulmonary vascular resistance; q 2 h, every 2 hours; RAP, right arterial pressure; RLL, right lower lobe; RML, right middle lobe; RR, respiratory rate; RUL, right upper lobe; RVSWI, right ventricular stroke work index; SIMV, synchronized intermittent mechanical ventilation; SVI, stroke volume index; T, temperature; USN, ultrasonic nebulization; VT, total volume; WBC, white blood cell.

SOAP 2

S "I'm having a bad period."

O Vitals: BP 185/135, HR 130, RR 28, T 37° C (98.6° F); use of accessory muscles and pursed-lip breathing; cough weak and productive of large amounts of thick, yellow sputum; bilateral rhonchi; ABGs: pH 7.55, $Paco_2$ 53, HCO_3^- 32, Pao_2 41; Spo_2: 83%

A • Continued acute exacerbation of chronic bronchitis without improvement over the past 9 hours (general appearance and clinical data)
  • Continued increased work of breathing (general appearance, elevated heart rate, blood pressure, and respiratory rate)
  • Persistent, excessive airway secretions (sputum, rhonchi)
  • Infection likely (yellow sputum)
  • Poor ability to mobilize secretions (weak cough)
  • Acute alveolar hyperventilation on top of chronic ventilatory failure (ABGs and history)
  • Impending ventilatory failure

P Up-regulate Oxygen Therapy Protocol (e.g., Fio_2 0.40). Up-regulate Bronchopulmonary Hygiene Therapy Protocol (e.g., increasing frequency of CPT and PD to q 4 h while awake, and once on night shift). Start Aerosolized Medication Protocol (e.g., administer acetylcysteine [Mucomyst] 1.5 cc of 10% solution in 0.5 cc of albuterol in med. neb. q2h; then reevaluate). Check ABGs in 15 minutes. Notify physician of status. Continue to monitor and evaluate q 2 h. Check I&O and chart.

SOAP 3

S "I'm feeling worse again."

O Vital signs: BP 150/95, HR 140, RR 25 and shallow, T 37° C (98.6° F). Use of accessory muscles of respiration and pursed-lip breathing; cough weak and no sputum production; expiration prolonged; bilateral rhonchi; ABGs: pH 7.28, $Paco_2$ 105, HCO_3^- 41, Pao_2 44; $COHb$ 2.5%.

A • Continued exacerbation of chronic bronchitis; unimproved since last evaluation 12 hours earlier (general appearance and clinical data)
  • Excessive airway secretions (rhonchi)
  • Poor ability to mobilize secretions (weak cough)
  • Acute ventilatory failure superimposed on chronic ventilatory failure (ABGs and history)

P Page physician stat about ventilatory failure. Respiratory therapist to remain on standby for intubation and mechanical ventilation. Begin Mechanical Ventilation Protocol (e.g., initial ventilator settings: Fio_2 0.60, SIMV 12/min, V_T 12 ml/kg, PEEP 3). Continue Aerosolized Medication Therapy and Bronchopulmonary Hygiene Therapy Protocols as tolerated (e.g., CPT with PD q 4 h while awake). Monitor and evaluate per ICU standing orders.

DISCUSSION

The return to hospital of a patient with chronic bronchitis who has not complied with therapy is all too familiar to the respiratory care practitioner and physicians. This patient has persisted in smoking cigarettes, has refused pulmonary rehabilitation, and now has allowed his personal hygiene to deteriorate.

Shrugging off all this information and discharging him from the emergency room would be easy if a careful assessment were not done. This case presents several worrisome signs of impending respiratory failure, including systemic hypertension, tachycardia, increased work of breathing, decrease in cough efficiency, peripheral edema (suggesting possible cor pulmonale), and signs of pulmonary infection (with yellow sputum), all signs and symptoms (clinical manifestations) of **Excessive Bronchial Secretions** and their associated pathophysiologic mechanisms (i.e., intrapulmonary shunting, hypoxemia, and stimulation of oxygen; see Figure 9-11). If these warning signs were not enough, his admission blood gases with profound hypoxemia, despite *relative* alveolar hyperventilation, should stimulate concern. The polycythemia almost certainly reflects chronic hypoxia, and his elevated carboxyhemoglobin level reflects his cigarette smoking.

The **initial assessment** (SOAP 1) indicates the need for a specific diagnosis of the cause of his pulmonary infection (sputum culture), conservative treatment of his hypoxemia (low-flow oxygen or Venturi mask), and careful monitoring if intubation and mechanical ventilation are indicated. Before the landmark awareness of oxygen-induced hypoventilation, these patients often ended up on ventilators immediately after admission to the hospital. Today, the use of low-flow oxygen therapy and noninvasive mechanical ventilation while bronchial hygiene, aerosolized medication, and antibiotic therapy are at work often makes intubation unnecessary, thus permitting a much less expensive and more comfortable recovery. Watchful awareness of both blood pressure and ventilatory status is suggested and certainly indicated.

The **second assessment** (SOAP 2) occurs in the setting of worsening pulmonary function despite good respiratory care. Clearly, the patient has slipped from borderline to overt impending ventilatory failure in the course of his hospitalization. Several points regarding this case are instructive. First, the patient's complaints became increasingly nonspecific as his blood gas values worsened. Indeed, in the final assessment the patient's complaints of "feeling worse again" are so nonspecific as to be unhelpful. These nonspecific complaints, combined with his increasing lethargy, suggest acute respiratory failure.

The blood gas values in the **third assessment** (SOAP 3) confirm acute ventilatory failure on chronic ventilatory failure. At that time the patient's pH was 7.28, and his $Paco_2$ was 105 mm Hg. The reader should sense that the patient's cough and subjective complaint of dyspnea in the first assessment are helpful in the making of a diagnosis and should learn that the nonspecific complaints of "I'm having a bad period" and "I'm feeling worse again" really do not help hospital personnel in reaching an accurate assessment as to the nature of the patient's problem.

Another point to note in this case is the installation by the treating therapist of a series of "watchers" that allow for close monitoring of the patient. At first, these consist of the therapist's own and the nursing staff's observation, the use of a pulse oximeter, and frequent blood gas analyses. When the patient deteriorates in the last case scenario, he is transferred to the intensive care unit (ICU), where again more minute-to-minute observation is possible. At this juncture therapists would do well to ask themselves the following question: What have I done to ensure that this patient is observed carefully in the course of my care?

Two points in the admitting history are worthy of note. One is, as it turns out, a red herring; the other is not. The red herring is the patient's complaint of mild nausea without abdominal pain or vomiting. The therapist notes that the abdominal examination is negative and goes on to other things. Nausea or anorexia complicating chronic obstructive pulmonary disease (COPD) is so common as to be seen in approximately one third of admitted patients. The cause of the nausea can be peptic ulcer disease, aminophylline toxicity, medication effect, or hypoxic bowel syndrome. This patient was not receiving aminophylline-like drugs as an outpatient and was not taking oral steroids. If he were vomiting or had gastric distention, passing of a nasogastric tube would have been helpful.

That the patient had a recent history of depression, regular cigarette smoking, and disinterest in pulmonary rehabilitation is missed by the treating therapist here. The therapist fails to ascertain whether the patient has a living will or durable medical power of attorney, information that he may wish he had pursued if the patient comes to intubation and commitment to ventilator support.

Note that throughout this case, the therapist appropriately adjusts the patient's oxygen therapy, bronchial hygiene regimen, and aerosolized medication therapy and presumably uses mucolytics.

This book's purpose is not to specify precisely which treatments need to be ordered. One would imagine, however, that bronchodilator medicines, bronchopulmonary hygiene, and mucolytic therapy every 2 hours by an up-draft medication nebulizer might have been used at the start and that these treatments might have been increased to every hour directly before the patient's transfer to the ICU. Similarly and appropriately, the therapist's initial suggestion of a Venturi mask to prevent the patient's CO_2 retention from worsening would have been appropriate. Frequent blood gas analyses are requested. The therapist notes that no acute infiltrates are noted on the chest X-ray film and suspects that the patient's hypoxemia may be chronic, given his elevated hematocrit. The therapist correctly obtains a sputum sample for culture and contacts the attending physician regarding the need for possible intubation.

Discussion with the physician in this case revealed that prior experience with this patient suggested that vigorous noninvasive respiratory care was enough to keep him from having to go on the ventilator. The therapist and physician agreed that they would observe the patient for a few more hours before making that decision. As it turned out, the patient continued to deteriorate and slipped into frank respiratory failure, ultimately requiring intubation.

The consulting therapist's role here is critical in that the monitors that he sets must be repeated frequently enough to allow for evaluation of the patient, essentially on a minute-to-minute basis.

Finally, repeating the chest X-ray examination after intubation (to check placement of the endotracheal tube, determine that a pneumothorax or acute pulmonary infiltrate has not developed, and establish a baseline film with the lungs well expanded from deep, respirator-delivered breaths) is a standard practice.

Case 2: Emphysema

SOAP 1

S "I'm so short of breath!"

O Obvious respiratory distress; vital signs: BP 155/110, HR 95, RR 25, and T 38.3° C (101° F). Malnourished (66 kg [146 lb], 180 cm [6 ft] tall); use of accessory muscles of inspiration, pursed-lip breathing; increased anteroposterior chest diameter. Depressed hemidiaphragms and generally diminished breath sounds; expiration prolonged; crackles in right lower lobe; CXR: apical scarring, large bulla in right middle lobe, pulmonary hyperexpansion, right lower lobe infiltrate consistent with pneumonia; cough: weak and productive of small amount of yellow sputum; ABGs (on 1.5 L/min O_2 by nasal cannula): pH 7.59, $Paco_2$ 40, HCO_3^- 37, Pao_2 38

A • Bronchitic exacerbation of COPD (history, general appearance, ABGs, CXR)
   • Increased work of breathing (increased respiratory rate, blood pressure, and heart rate)
   • Alveolar infiltrate in right lower lobe; presumed lobar pneumonia (CXR, fever)
   • Excessive bronchial secretions and poor ability to mobilize them (yellow sputum and weak cough)
   • Acute alveolar hyperventilation superimposed on chronic ventilatory failure with severe hypoxemia (ABGs and history)
   • Impending ventilatory failure
   • Possible malnutrition

P Upregulate Oxygen Therapy Protocol (e.g., O_2 per nasal cannula at 2.5 lpm) and Bronchopulmonary Hygiene Therapy Protocol (e.g., C&DB q 2 h with supervision; CPT with PD to right lower lobe qid; sputum culture). Begin trial of Aerosolized Medication Protocol (e.g., med. neb. treatments with albuterol 0.5 cc in 2.0 cc NS q 2 h 36, then q 4 h). Have ventilator on standby. Monitor closely (every hour, vital signs, pulse oximetry, ABGs).

SOAP 2

S "My chest feels tighter, and I'm more short of breath."

O Vital signs: BP 160/115, HR 97, RR 15 and shallow. T 37.8° C (100° F). Possibly getting fatigued (e.g., no use of accessory muscles of inspiration); diminished breath sounds; reduced air entry a possible reason for no crackles in right lower lobe; ABGs: pH 7.28, $Paco_2$ 82, HCO_3^- 36, Pao_2 41; Spo_2 68%

A • Continued increase in respiratory distress and fatigue (blood pressure, heart rate, shallow respiratory rate, no use of accessory muscles)
   • Right lower lobe infiltrate (dull percussion notes and admission CXR)
   • Excessive bronchial secretions (thick, yellow sputum)
   • Acute ventilatory failure superimposed on chronic ventilatory failure with severe hypoxemia ($Paco_2$ higher and pH lower than patient's normal baseline; general patient fatigue)

P Page physician stat. Recommend intubation and transfer to ICU. Recommend support via Mechanical Ventilation Protocol (e.g., Fio_2 1.00, V_T 900 cc, SIMV 12, PEEP 0). After intubation, perform deep tracheal suction for Gram stain and culture of secretions. Check ABGs 30 minutes after intubation. Continue Aerosolized Medication Protocol as earlier. Add mucolytic (e.g., acetylcysteine 2 cc of 20% solution q 6 h). Continue Bronchopulmonary Hygiene Therapy Protocol as earlier. Monitor closely and evaluate per ICU standing orders. Plan to review nutrition consult.

DISCUSSION

Emphysema is a slowly progressive destructive process involving lung parenchyma. In the case of panacinar (panlobular) emphysema, the loss of pulmonary function may be as much as 60 to 100 cc of forced expiratory volume in 1 second (FEV_1) per year. More rapid declines in pulmonary function are accompanied by conditions known to exacerbate chronic obstructive pulmonary disease (e.g., acute bronchitis, pneumonia and pneumothorax). In this case the patient's fever, history of a flulike syndrome, crackles in the right lower lobe, and a right lower lobe infiltrate on the chest X-ray all point to acute pneumonia as the reason for his deterioration. A correct response in this case was the rapid acquisition of a Gram stain and culture of the sputum. In addition, the patient was coughing up large amounts of thick, yellow sputum in the second assessment. Thus not only did the patient demonstrate many clinical manifestations associated with **Distal Airway and**

Alveolar Weakening (see Figure 9-11), but also the patient's condition was compromised by **Alveolar Consolidation** (see Figure 9-8) and **Excessive Bronchial Secretions** (see Figure 9-11).

A "red herring" in this case is the patient's earlier reported failure to improve after aerosolized medication therapy. Any exacerbation of COPD deserves an in-hospital trial of aggressive bronchial hygiene and aerosolized medication therapy because reversible bronchospasm may be one of the *only* components of the deterioration that does respond. Accordingly, putting the patient on an up-draft nebulizer treatment with bronchodilator, encouraging deep breathing and coughing, and using mucolytics and systemic hydration are indicated in this case, even though they were of little use in the past.

A good call for the treating team is to recognize the patient's malnutrition, quantitatively assess it, and bring early professional attention to the condition while he is in the hospital for this pneumonic exacerbation. Improved nutrition may improve respiratory muscle weakness and decreased cellular immunity.

That the patient suddenly (at the time of the second assessment, SOAP 2) slips into acute respiratory failure with significant CO_2 retention is not surprising. In some such patients, this event occurs more than 50% of the time, despite otherwise judicious use of oxygen and entirely appropriate respiratory care.

The patient previously requested that no heroic measures be taken on his behalf, but the attending physician was able to convince the patient to accept a period of mechanical ventilation when his clinical condition deteriorated despite the initial aggressive therapy prescribed. The organism responsible for this exacerbation (pneumococcus) was subsequently identified, and the patient gradually improved as antibiotic therapy and ventilator support were continued for a 10-day hospital stay. The patient was discharged on dietary supplementation and a program of multiple small feedings.

Attention must be drawn to the decreased adventitious breath sounds in the right lower lobe at the second assessment. The reader who correctly assumed that these sounds were due to decreased air entry in an airless, possibly obstructed right lower lobe should be congratulated! The fact that the crackles go away within 6 hours of admission does not suggest that the patient is improving. Indeed, it suggests just the opposite, as demonstrated by the patient's deteriorating arterial blood gas values.

Case 3: Asthma

SOAP 1

S "I feel horrible, and my chest is tight."

O Pursed-lip breathing; cyanotic appearance; use of accessory muscles of inspiration; frequent, strong cough productive of moderate amount of thick, white mucus; vital signs: BP 110/85, HR 190, RR 28, afebrile; bilateral diminished breath sounds, wheezing, and rhonchi. PEFR 150 lpm; CXR: air trapping and depressed diaphragm; Spo_2 (2 L/min O_2 by nasal cannula) 77%; ABGs: pH 7.45, $Paco_2$ 28, HCO_3^- 19, Pao_2 40

A • Status asthmaticus (general history and clinical data)
   • Increased work of breathing (HR, RR, and use of accessory muscles)
   • Bronchospasm (wheezing and PEFR)
   • Excessive bronchial secretions but effective cough (sputum production)
   • Acute alveolar hyperventilation and metabolic acidosis with severe hypoxemia (lactic acid probably causing pH and HCO3 − to be lower than expected for an acute decrease in Paco2 level)
   • Possible impending ventilatory failure

P Up-regulate Oxygen Therapy Protocol (e.g., 4 lpm nasal cannula or HAFOE at F_{IO_2} 40%). Begin aggressive Aerosolized Medication Protocol (e.g., albuterol aerosol per medication nebulizer). Initiate Bronchopulmonary Hygiene Therapy Protocol (e.g., C&DB q 2 h, bland aerosol therapy if tolerated, and prn suctioning). Maintain ventilator/intubation equipment on standby. Continue to monitor (e.g., vital signs, breath sounds, pulse oximetry, ABGs, and PEFR). Continue or increase frequency (6 puffs q 8 h) of beclomethasone inhaler as prescribed for home use.

SOAP 2

S "I'm wheezing too much, and I can't go to sleep."

O Pursed-lip breathing; cyanotic appearance; use of accessory muscles of inspiration; frequent, strong cough; moderate amount of thick, white mucus; PEFR 175 lpm; vital signs: BP 105/82, HR 180, RR 24; prolonged expiration; bilateral diminished breath sounds, wheezing, and rhonchi; Spo_2 95%; ABGs: pH 7.48, $Paco_2$ 34, HCO_3^- 24, Pao_2 73

A • Continued increased work of breathing (vital signs, use of accessory muscles, ABGs)
  • Bronchospasm (wheezing and PEFR)
  • Thick bronchial secretions (sputum production)
  • Acute alveolar hyperventilation with mild hypoxemia improving (metabolic acidosis corrected)
  • Impending ventilatory failure still a possibility
P Continue Oxygen Therapy, Bronchopulmonary Hygiene Therapy, and Aerosolized Medication Protocols. Continue beclomethasone inhaler as prescribed for home use. Maintain ventilator on standby. Continue to monitor and reevaluate closely.

SOAP 3

S "I feel like there is a weight on my chest."
O Use of accessory muscles; pursed-lip breathing; skin: damp, cool, and cyanotic; no cough or sputum; PEFR 145 lpm; vital signs: BP 160/100, HR 185, RR 13; diminished breath sounds bilaterally; no wheezing or rhonchi; Spo_2 79%; ABGs: pH 7.27, $Paco_2$ 57, HCO_3^- 24, Pao_2 51
A • Patient becoming fatigued (no wheezing, vital signs, ABGs)
  • Worsening bronchospasm ("silent chest," with decreased wheezing and decreased sputum production)
  • Acute ventilatory failure with moderate hypoxemia (ABGs)
P Contact physician stat regarding ventilatory failure. Consider intubation and mechanical ventilation. Until then, up-regulate Oxygen Therapy Protocol (e.g., nonrebreathing mask @ Fio_2 1.0). Continue Aerosolized Medication and Bronchopulmonary Hygiene Protocols. Continue beclomethasone inhaler as prescribed for home use. Monitor continuously. Request chest X-ray after intubation.

DISCUSSION

The historical point that the patient not only has asthma but also has had it severely enough recently to require hospitalizations and ventilator support is important and should alert the respiratory care practitioner that this patient is more than the run-of-the-mill asthmatic. That the patient's mother has stopped smoking, made environmental changes at home, and been conscientious enough to have the child on a home-recording program of peak expiratory flow rates (PEFRs) and that the child has been desensitized are all factors that speak to a compliant and intelligent patient and family.

The clinical manifestations presented in this case are all associated with **Bronchospasm** (see Fig. 9-10) and **Excessive Bronchial Secretions** (see Figure 9-11). The pursed-lip breathing, cyanosis, prolonged expirations, use of accessory muscles of respiration, frequent cough, thick and white mucus, increased heart rate and blood pressure, and the severity of the child's hypoxemia (despite alveolar hyperventilation on admission) are all good severity indicators and suggest that vigorous therapy is necessary. Many respiratory specialists feel that sputum and blood eosinophilia are good markers for allergic exacerbations of asthma. A circulating eosinophil count or Wright's stain for sputum eosinophilia, or both, might have been in order.

Note in SOAP 1 that the pH and HCO_3^- levels are lower than expected for a particular $Paco_2$ level, most likely because of the lactic acid caused by the severe hypoxemia. The lactic acid offsets the increased pH and HCO_3^- levels that should develop immediately in response to an acutely decreased $Paco_2$ level—according to the $Paco_2/HCO_3^-/pH$ nomogram. (A $Paco_2$ of 28 should move the pH to a level greater than 7.52.) The patient's arterial blood gas values (ABGs: pH 7.45, $Paco_2$ 28, HCO_3^- 19, and Pao_2 40) are often interpreted incorrectly as chronic alveolar hyperventilation with hypoxemia.

In this case, two primary indicators confirm that the patient has acute alveolar hyperventilation with hypoxemia and not chronic alveolar hyperventilation:

1. The patient's age and history of acute asthmatic episodes
2. The severe hypoxemia is enough to cause slight anaerobic metabolism

Because of the increased work of breathing (vital signs) and acute alveolar hyperventilation, the possibility of impending ventilatory failure is real.

At this point, however, the child is not retaining carbon dioxide, so increasing the nasal oxygen therapy to 4 L/min or, alternatively, using a Venturi mask is reasonable. The child needs frequent bronchodilator and inhaled steroid therapy, which should have been started. The semicritical nature of her illness and impending ventilatory failure should have been reported to the physician immediately after the first assessment. Intravenous corticosteroid medications are used almost always in this setting. Increasingly, *continuous* nebulized bronchodilator therapy is used in children such as this.

The time of the **second assessment** (SOAP 2) is more than 2 hours into aggressive therapy. The patient is improving slightly. The physical findings have changed little, and she still demonstrates mild hypoxemia. Assuming that the patient's oxygen therapy was increased correctly after the first assessment, a key point to note is that hypoxemia is present *despite oxygen therapy*. Further increase in the oxygen therapy would be safe. Use of a nonrebreathing oxygen mask would be appropriate. Hydration of the patient (and her secretions) would be helpful, probably via the parenteral route. Close monitoring of vital signs, pulse oximetry, breath sounds, PEFR determinations, and judicious use of arterial or capillary sample blood gas analyses should continue.

By the time of the **final assessment** (SOAP 3), the patient's status asthmaticus clearly has worsened to the point of acute ventilatory failure. Significant carbon dioxide retention and persistent severe hypoxemia are present. The silent chest does not represent improved bronchoconstriction. Rather, it suggests that a marked diminution of gas flow has occurred so that breath sounds are no longer generated. Confirmation comes from the fact that the patient can no longer cough up secretions. Presumably, they too are being expectorated with difficulty, given the obstructed airway. A chest X-ray to rule out bilateral pneumothorax as a cause of the bilaterally diminished breath sounds is a good idea.

The therapist at this point should not leave the patient and should be prepared to bag and mask or (if allowed in the individual institution) to go ahead with emergency intubation. The patient's hypertension and tachycardia suggest that further administration of bronchodilator aerosol alone is contraindicated, unless or until the patient has a mechanically open airway.

Case 4: Pneumonia

SOAP 1

S Patient states that he is very short of breath and has had a nonproductive cough for the last 4 days.

O Vital signs: BP 165/90, HR 120, RR 33, T 39.5° C (103° F). Cough: frequent, strong, hacking, productive of small amount of white and yellow sputum; skin: pale and damp; over right lower lobe, increased tactile and vocal fremitus, dull percussion note, bronchial breath sounds; SpO_2 87%; ABGs (on 2 L/min O_2 nasal cannula): pH 7.56, $PaCO_2$ 24, HCO_3^- 22, PaO_2 56; CXR: right lower lung infiltrate, air bronchograms, and alveolar consolidation; WBC 21,000/mm^3

A • Respiratory distress (vital signs, ABGs)
  • Right lower lobe pneumonia: consolidation (fever, fremitus, percussion notes, bronchial breath sounds, elevated WBC and CXR)
  • Bronchial secretions: infection likely (white and yellow sputum)
  • Good ability to mobilize bronchial secretions (strong cough)
  • Acute alveolar hyperventilation with mild hypoxemia (ABGs)

P Initiate Oxygen Therapy Protocol (e.g., increasing from 2 to 4 lpm per nasal cannula). Bronchopulmonary Hygiene Therapy Protocol (e.g., C&DB 2x /shift). Obtain sputum for Gram stain and culture; induce if necessary. Begin trial period of Hyperinflation Therapy Protocol (e.g., incentive spirometry 2x/shift). Monitor and reevaluate.

SOAP 2

S "I feel worse than when I came in."

O Vital signs: BP 140/70, HR 125, RR 35 and shallow, T 38.9° C (102° F); strong, barking cough; producing small amount of blood-streaked sputum; cyanosis; findings over right lower and middle lung lobes and left lower lobe: increased tactile and vocal fremitus, dull percussion notes, bronchial breath sounds, and crackles; SpO_2 86%; ABGs: pH 7.55, $PaCO_2$ 26, HCO_3^- 24, PaO_2 53

A • Continued respiratory distress (vital signs, ABGs)
  • Alveolar consolidation or atelectasis likely in right lower and middle lobes and left lower lobe; condition possibly worsening (percussion notes and breath sounds, crackles)
  • Bronchial secretions: small amount (sputum production)
  • Acute alveolar hyperventilation with moderate hypoxemia; essentially unchanged (ABGs)

P Update physician on patient's respiratory status. Continue Bronchopulmonary Hygiene Therapy Protocol. Continue trial period of Hyperinflation Therapy Protocol. Up-regulate Oxygen Therapy Protocol (e.g., simple oxygen mask or partial rebreathing oxygen mask @ F_{IO_2} 0.50). Ensure that patient is sitting up when taking oral medications, food, and liquids. Continue to monitor and reevaluate.

SOAP 3

S "I'm breathing easier."

O Vital signs: BP 135/85, HR 90, RR 19, T 37.3° C (99° F); cough: strong and nonproductive; CXR: resolving pneumonia, consolidation or atelectasis in lower and middle right and lower left lobes; increased tactile and vocal fremitus, dull percussion notes, and bronchial breath sounds; Spo_2 97%; ABGs on a 3 L/min O_2 nasal cannula: pH 7.44, $Paco_2$ 35, HCO_3^- 24, Pao_2 163

A • Consolidation or atelectasis in right lower and middle and left lower lobes—resolving (CXR, chest assessment data)
  • Normal acid-base status with overly corrected hypoxemia (ABGs)

P Down-regulate Hyperinflation Therapy Protocol (e.g., reducing incentive spirometry to 1x/shift with supervision, plus patient instruction). Continue to encourage C&DB. Down-regulate oxygen therapy per protocol (e.g., 3 lpm nasal cannula). Check final results of sputum culture. Reevaluate next shift.

DISCUSSION

This patient has a typical case of pneumonia, with cough, fever, increased blood pressure, heart rate and respiratory rate, dull percussion note, bronchial breath sounds, chest X-ray infiltrates, and acute alveolar hyperventilation with hypoxemia (see **Alveolar Consolidation**, Figure 9-8). Initially, the respiratory therapist's attention should be directed to identifying the causative agent by inducing a sputum specimen for culture and to oxygenating the patient, in this case with a low-flow oxygen cannula.

Unfortunately no effective, specific respiratory care treatment modality for alveolar consolidation exists. Hyperinflation therapy may be beneficial, especially when applied to partially consolidated alveoli. Just like any treatment modality, however, the effectiveness of the hyperinflation therapy must be assessed through the collection of objective data (e.g., arterial blood gases, chest X-ray, or vital signs). In addition, the response to oxygen therapy often is poor because the patient almost certainly has a right-to-left intrapulmonary shunt across the pneumonic segment. Some ventilated and perfused alveoli might be able to pick up some of the deficit (or so it is hoped), but a degree of oxygen refractoriness should be expected when alveolar consolidation is present.

This patient is so hypoxemic, despite alveolar hyperventilation, that close monitoring obviously is necessary. Asking questions about the patient's alcoholism and pneumonia vaccine status is worthwhile and shows that the therapist is thinking beyond the immediate acute episode during his evaluation and treatment of the patient.

The **second assessment** (SOAP 2) reflects the fact that patients with pneumonia often feel worse when they actually are improving. The production of sputum often is seen as a worrisome event when in fact it may herald the breaking up of the pneumonic infiltrate. Because the patient is still producing some sputum, bronchial hygiene therapy should be continued. The patient's Pao_2 really has not improved significantly, and a trial of a higher concentration of oxygen by Venturi or nonrebreathing oxygen mask may be helpful at this point. Improved oxygenation would help allay the patient's anxiety, as well as that of the physician and treating therapist.

The **third assessment** (SOAP 3) shows that the patient clearly is improving. Down-regulation of the oxygen therapy toward room air is all that remains for the therapist to do. Ordinarily, hyperinflation therapy would be reduced or discontinued in preparation for an early discharge. The reader should recognize that the average length of stay for patients with pneumonia in an American hospital today is approximately 4 days. Such patients may leave the hospital with a resolving, but not completely cleared, pneumonic process (and X-ray). Improvement in the patient's clinical status and resolution of fever, dyspnea, and signs of toxicity, however, can and should be expected in this short period unless complications such as bacteremia, abscess, or empyema arise. Attention to the event that precipitated the admission is worthwhile, and review of the situation and recollection that this patient is a problem drinker would be appropriate before discharge, when attempts to interdict this problem might be most helpful.

Case 5: Pulmonary Edema

SOAP 1

S "I don't think I'm having a serious problem."

O Vital signs: BP 100/50, HR 145 and irregular, RR 22, T normal; Spo_2 70%; anxiety and cough: small amount of frothy, pink secretions; bilateral, dull percussion notes over the lower lung areas; bilateral inspiratory crackles and expiratory wheezes over the lower lobes; ABGs (2 L/min O_2 by nasal cannula): pH 7.56, $Paco_2$ 28, HCO_3^- 20, Pao_2 51; CXR: dense, fluffy opacities in lower lungs; left cardiac enlargement

A • Respiratory distress (vital signs, ABGs)
  • Hypotension (blood pressure)
  • Acute pulmonary edema (crackles, distended neck veins, CXR)
  • Acute alveolar hyperventilation with moderate hypoxemia (ABGs)
  • Small airway secretions, alveolar flooding, interstitial edema or any combination of these (crackles)
  • Bronchospasm?? (wheezing most likely caused by airway secretions)

P Initiate Oxygen Therapy Protocol (e.g., increasing oxygenation to 50% Venturi mask). Hyperinflation Therapy Protocol (e.g., 5 cm H_2O CPAP mask qid for 15-30 min, or Bipap therapy at IPAP 6 cm H_2O, EPAP 4 cm H_2O; or if not tolerated, IPPB treatments for 15-30 min x 3). Begin Bronchopulmonary Hygiene Therapy Protocol (e.g., suctioning orally prn). Begin trial period of Aerosolized Medication Protocol (albuterol 0.25 cc in 2 cc normal saline qid). Monitor (e.g., vital signs, pulse oximetry, ABGs, cardiac enzymes and troponin levels) and reevaluate.

SOAP 2

S "I still don't feel great."

O Vital signs: BP 160/90, HR 105 and regular, RR 20, T 37.1° C (98.8° F); slight improvement in cyanosis; distended neck veins persistent; urine output: 650 ml last 2 hours; frequent, nonproductive cough; bilateral inspiratory crackles and expiratory wheezes over lower lobes; Spo_2 84%; ABGs: pH 7.54, $Paco_2$ 25, HCO_3^- 18, Pao_2 51

A • Continued respiratory distress (vital signs, ABGs)
  • Improved systemic hypotension (BP)
  • Persistent acute pulmonary edema (physical findings, CXR)
  • Worsening acute alveolar hyperventilation with moderate hypoxemia—more severe now than at admission (ABGs)
  • Small airway secretions (crackles)
  • Bronchospasm?? (wheezing most likely caused by airway secretions)

P Up-regulate Oxygen Therapy Protocol (e.g., increasing Fio_2 to 0.60). Up-regulate Hyperinflation Therapy Protocol (e.g., 10 cm H_2O CPAP mask qid for 15-30 min, or continuation of IPPB for 15 min). Continue Bronchopulmonary Hygiene Therapy Protocol (e.g., suction orally prn). Continue trial period of Aerosolized Medication Protocol as earlier. Continue to monitor closely (e.g., vital signs, pulse oximetry, ABGs).

SOAP 3

S "I'm breathing better."

O Vital signs: BP 140/115, HR 95 and regular, RR 16, T 37.3° C (99.1° F); no cyanosis; urine output: 850 ml over past 2 hours; neck veins no longer distended; cough: strong, nonproductive; bilateral crackles over lower lobes; Spo_2 97%; ABGs: pH 7.44, $Paco_2$ 36, HCO_3^- 24, Pao_2 190

A • Pulmonary edema (history and physical findings)
  • Condition appearing to improve
  • Small airway secretions (crackles)
  • Normal ventilatory/acid-base status with overly corrected hypoxemia (ABGs)

P Down-regulate Oxygen Therapy Protocol (e.g., 2 lpm per nasal cannula). Discontinue Hyperinflation Therapy Protocol (however, continuation of incentive spirometry tid still appropriate). Discontinue Bronchopulmonary Hygiene Therapy and Aerosolized Medication Protocols. Continue to monitor and evaluate (e.g., vital signs, Spo_2, ABGs in AM).

DISCUSSION

The patient's known cardiac history; cough productive of foamy, pink-tinged sputum; neck vein distention; peripheral edema; and rapid atrial fibrillation are virtually pathognomonic of acute pulmonary edema. The therapist should be aware that the following conditions may precipitate pulmonary edema in a given patient:

1. Acute myocardial infarction
2. Hypertension
3. Valvular heart disease
4. Rapid ventricular rate with inadequate filling time of atria and ventricles
5. Exogenous fluid overload

In this case, the patient demonstrated clinical manifestations associated with the following two specific anatomic alterations of the lungs: **Increased Alveolar-Capillary Membrane Thickness** (e.g., dense, fluffy opacities in lower lungs and low Pao_2; see Figure 9-9) and to a milder extent **Excessive Bronchial Secretions** (e.g., frothy, pink secretions and crackles; see Figure 9-11).

The treatment of this condition involves oxygen therapy, maintenance of alveolar volume with positive end-expiratory pressure (PEEP) or continuous positive airway pressure (CPAP) therapy, and bronchial hygiene therapy directed at mechanical removal of secretions from the airway. In the past, ethanol has been added to the inspirate to "reduce surface tension of the bubbles in the secretions," but this technique is falling from favor. Although trial periods may be appropriate, bronchodilator therapy typically is not required because smooth muscle bronchospasm usually does not occur in this condition.

In the **first assessment** (SOAP 1), the therapist may well have mentioned an interest in cardiac enzymes because treatment of the patient in whom acute myocardial infarction has caused pulmonary edema is somewhat different than that of patients with the conditions mentioned previously.

After the **second assessment** (SOAP 2), the patient clearly is not doing well, his Pao_2 is still low, and now the question of a coincident metabolic acidosis arises. This question is not uncommon in patients with cardiac disease who may be hypotensive. The blood gas observed in this case is more worrisome because the Pao_2 is low despite alveolar hyperventilation. If the patient were not tolerating mask CPAP, intubation for administration of PEEP therapy would be indicated at this point. If the patient were not already in the intensive care unit (ICU), transfer there would be indicated.

After the **third assessment** (SOAP 3), this case highlights the rapid therapeutic response that can occur in most patients with pulmonary edema. Even patients whose acute myocardial infarction was caused by pulmonary edema generally improve rapidly with therapy, such as is outlined in this case. The cardiac inotropic and chronotropic agents and the intravenous diuretic therapy started in the emergency room 9 hours or so earlier have by this time exerted their maximal effect. If monitoring of pulse oximetry and blood gases in the next 24 hours continues to provide reassuring results, the therapist can probably sign off this case and the patient can go on his planned trip to Alaska.

Case 6: Flail Chest

SOAP 1

S N/A (patient unconscious)

O Vital signs: BP 165/92, HR 120, RR 26 and shallow, T 36.2° C (97.2° F). Paradoxical movement of the anterior chest wall; skin: pale and cyanotic; diminished breath sounds bilaterally; CXR: multiple double rib fractures of the right and left anterior and lateral ribs, between ribs 4 and 9; sternum fractured in three places; atelectasis bilaterally; ABGs (Fio_2 0.8 by nonrebreathing mask): pH 7.17, $Paco_2$ 82, HCO_3^- 27, Pao_2 37; Spo_2 53%

A • Flail chest (paradoxical chest movement, CXR)
  • Atelectasis bilaterally (CXR)
  • Acute ventilatory failure with severe hypoxemia (ABGs)
  • Lactic acidosis most likely present—pH and HCO_3^- lower than expected for $Paco_2$ level
  • Acute alcohol intoxication with near-fatal blood alcohol level

P Initiate Mechanical Ventilation Protocol—stat. Also begin Hyperinflation Protocol and Oxygen Therapy Protocol. Monitor and reevaluate (e.g., in 1 hour).

SOAP 2

S N/A

O Cyanotic and pale appearance; distended neck veins; vital signs: BP 100/65, HR 145, RR 12 (controlled), T unchanged; auscultation: right lung, absent breath sounds and left lung, diminished breath sounds, rhonchi, and crackles; CXR: left lung, partially aerated and patches of atelectasis; right lung, completely atelectatic; hemodynamic indices: increased CVP, RAP, $\overline{PA}$, RVSWI, and PVR and decreased PCWP, CO, SV, SVI, CI, LVSWI, and SVR; oxygenation indices: increased $\dot{Q}s/\dot{Q}\tau$, $C(a-\overline{v})o_2$, and O_2ER and decreased Do_2 and $S\overline{v}o_2$; ABGs: pH 7.25, $Paco_2$ 65, HCO_3^- 25, Pao_2 54; Spo_2 80%

A • Atelectasis: patches throughout left lung; right lung airless (CXR)
  • Increased pulmonary vascular resistance and decreased cardiac output (distended neck veins, hemodynamic indices)
  • Acute ventilatory failure with moderate hypoxemia (ABGs)
  • Poor oxygenation status (oxygenation indices)

P Contact physician regarding patient's hemodynamic and oxygenation status; consider therapeutic bronchoscopy to treat atelectasis. Up-regulate Mechanical Ventilation Protocol to decrease $Paco_2$ (e.g., increasing rate or volume). Up-regulate Hyperinflation Therapy Protocol (e.g., increasing PEEP). Up-regulate Oxygenation Therapy Protocol (if not already at an Fio_2 of 1.0). Monitor and reevaluate (e.g., in 30 to 60 minutes).

SOAP 3

S N/A

O Cyanotic skin and distended neck veins; vital signs: BP 80/32, HR 190, RR 14 (controlled), T 38.9° C (102° F); right lung: no breath sounds; left lung: rhonchi and crackles; large amounts of yellow sputum; ECG: premature ventricular contractions; CXR: left lung partially aerated with patches of atelectasis (worsening) and right lung airless; early signs of ARDS; hemodynamics: worsening; ABGs: pH 7.22, $Paco_2$ 71, HCO_3^- 24, Pao_2 34; oxygenation status: worsening; Spo_2 61%

A • Atelectasis: patches throughout left lung (worsening); right lung completely atelectatic (CXR)
  • Early stages of ARDS (CXR)
  • Excessive bronchial secretions (sputum, rhonchi)
  • Infection likely (yellow sputum)
  • Increased pulmonary vascular resistance and decreased cardiac output: worsening (distended neck veins, hemodynamic indices)
  • Acute ventilatory failure with severe hypoxemia (ABGs)
  • Poor oxygenation status: worsening (oxygenation indices)

P Contact physician regarding patient's hemodynamic and oxygenation status; consider bronchoscopy. Up-regulate mechanical ventilation (if possible) per protocol to decrease $Paco_2$ (e.g., increasing in rate or volume). Up-regulate Hyperinflation Therapy Protocol. Continue Oxygen Therapy Protocol, and Bronchopulmonary Hygiene Therapy (e.g., in-line 2 cc 20% acetylcysteine with 0.5 cc albuterol). Obtain sputum culture. Monitor and reevaluate frequently.

DISCUSSION

This patient demonstrates the sequelae of an abnormally functioning diaphragm. The uneven ventilation that resulted from his multiple chest fractures gave him an unstable (flail) chest, causing atelectasis to develop. Several clinical manifestations associated with **Atelectasis** (see Figure 9-7) soon were evident in this case. For example, the patient's decreased lung compliance was manifested in his tachycardia and tachypnea, whereas his hypoxemia reflected the efforts seen with classic pulmonary shunting. His condition was extremely severe, as demonstrated by his first arterial blood gas values—pH 7.17, $Paco_2$ 82, HCO_3^- 27, and Pao_2 37.

In the **first assessment** (SOAP 1), the treating therapist correctly recognizes the patient's acute ventilatory failure, intubates him, and places him on mechanical ventilation per protocol. The patient's hypoxemia is treated by an increase in the inspired oxygen concentration, and an attempt should be made to stabilize the chest still further and treat his early **Atelectasis** with positive end-expiratory pressure (PEEP; see Figure 9-7). Many cases treated in this manner achieve "stability" of the chest wall much sooner than one would expect— that is, within a few days. This case, however, is an exception.

The **second assessment** (SOAP 2) shows that the patient is developing signs of pulmonary hypertension with increased pulmonary vascular resistance and a low cardiac output. The right lung has become completely atelectatic despite ventilatory care. A recommendation for therapeutic bronchoscopy is certainly timely. More PEEP could be added to the ventilator settings, and higher tidal volumes might well be used in such a patient. His respiratory acidosis certainly must be treated more aggressively with a change in ventilator settings (e.g., by increasing the rate or tidal volume). Mechanical dead space must be kept to a minimum in such patients.

The **third scenario** demonstrates that the patient has begun to slip into acute respiratory distress syndrome (ARDS) and that the atelectasis noted earlier is still a problem. His blood gases have worsened despite ventilator management, and the outlook has become increasingly grim. Repeat bronchoscopic examinations often are necessary in this situation, and an appropriate suggestion by the treating therapist would be to repeat the procedure. If the sputum is thick, mucolytic agents may be added. Prompt culture of the sputum is an excellent idea because the organisms may have changed during the patient's hospital stay.

Despite the aggressive care this patient received, he died 24 hours later.

Case 7: Pneumothorax

SOAP 1

S "I've been coughing so much and so hard, my chest hurts."

O Thin, but well-nourished appearance; use of accessory muscles of respiration; cyanosis, digital clubbing, pursed-lip breathing, and barrel chest; cough: frequent, strong, and productive—large amounts of thick, yellow-green sputum; vital signs: BP 145/85, HR 94, RR 20, T 37.9° C (100.3° F); hyperresonant percussion notes bilaterally; diminished breath sounds and rhonchi bilaterally; expiration prolonged; diminished heart sounds ; PFT (6 months previously): moderate-to-severe obstructive pulmonary disease; CXR: translucent, flattened hemidiaphragms and narrow heart; 10% pneumothorax on the left; ABGs (room air): pH 7.53, $Paco_2$ 48, HCO_3^- 38, Pao_2 57 (baseline: pH 7.42, $Paco_2$ 69, HCO_3^- 41, Pao_2 74).

A • Exacerbation of chronic bronchitis and emphysema (history, CXR)
  • Respiratory distress (vital signs, ABGs)
  • 10% Left pneumothorax: (CXR)
  • Excessive bronchial secretions (sputum, rhonchi)
  • Infection likely (yellow-green sputum)
  • Acute alveolar hyperventilation superimposed on chronic ventilatory failure (ABGs, history)

P Initiate Oxygen Therapy Protocol (e.g., HAFOE at F_{IO_2} of 0.28). Administer Aerosolized Medication Protocol (e.g., med. nebs. with 0.5 cc albuterol, in 2.0 cc 10% acetylcysteine). Begin Bronchopulmonary Hygiene Therapy Protocol (e.g., PD while awake and sputum Gram stain and culture). Monitor and reevaluate each shift.

SOAP 2

S "I feel horrible."

O Cyanosis, use of accessory muscles of respiration, and pursed-lip breathing; cough: frequent and weak; patient bracing himself when he coughs; small amount of yellow-green sputum; left anterior chest: hyper-inflated and fixed; vital signs: BP 95/55, HR 125, RR 28 and shallow; hyperresonant notes bilaterally; right lung: diminished breath sounds and rhonchi; left lung: no breath sounds; diminished heart sounds over right lung field; CXR: large, left-sided pneumothorax with mediastinal shift rightward; ABGs on 5 L/min nasal cannula: pH 7.24, $Paco_2$ 103, HCO_3^- 43, Pao_2 37; Spo_2 62%

A • Large, left-sided tension pneumothorax (CXR)
  • Treatment with tube thoracotomy
  • Respiratory distress (general appearance, vital signs, ABGs)
  • Left lung: collapsed or atelectatic or both (CXR)
  • Right lung: patches of atelectasis (CXR)
  • Excessive bronchial secretions (sputum, rhonchi)
  • Acute ventilatory failure superimposed on chronic ventilatory failure with severe hypoxemia (ABGs)

P Contact physician to consider transfer to ICU. Up-regulate Oxygen Therapy Protocol (e.g., FIO_2 at 0.6). Continue Bronchopulmonary Hygiene Therapy Protocol (e.g., continuing at present intensity; no physical therapy). Stay at patient's bedside. Do not begin mechanical ventilation per physician at present time (patient/physician directive). Hyperinflation Therapy Protocol (e.g., low CPAP mask trial). Stay at patient's bedside. Monitor and reevaluate (e.g., in 30 minutes).

SOAP 3

S "I'm feeling better."

O CXR: left lung reexpansion about 75%; right lung: no patches of atelectasis; cyanosis no longer present; pursed-lip breathing and use of accessory muscles of respiration; right lung: rhonchi and diminished breath sounds; left lung: diminished breath sounds; vital signs: BP 145/85, HR 105, RR 22, T 38° C (100.5° F); hyperresonant notes bilaterally; ABGs: pH 7.35, $Paco_2$ 85, HCO_3^- 41, Pao_2 64; Spo_2 90%

A • Left-sided pneumothorax and atelectasis: improving (CXR)
   • Excessive bronchial secretions (rhonchi, earlier SOAPs)
   • Chronic ventilatory failure with severe hypoxemia (ABGs)
   • ABGs not at patient's baseline level yet

P Continue present level of Hyperinflation Therapy Protocol (e.g., CPAP mask). Continue present level of Oxygen Therapy Protocol. Continue present level of Bronchopulmonary Hygiene Therapy Protocol. Monitor and reevaluate (e.g., in 4 to 6 hours).

DISCUSSION

The causes of pneumothorax include trauma to the chest wall, malignancy, infection of the pleural space or lung, rupture of subpleural bullae, and air leakage from tuberculous foci. The condition also may be without known cause (idiopathic) and pneumothoraces may be caused iatrogenically by needle tears of the pleura incurred during percutaneous needle lung biopsy or during aspiration of air or fluid from the pleural space.

This case demonstrates a pneumothorax caused by infection in a patient known to have chronic obstructive pulmonary disease (COPD). A rupture of a subpleural bulla or leakage of air from a parenchymal lung bulla may have accounted for his problem. The patient had pneumonia 4 years previously. If the pneumonia was due to a necrotizing organism, it could have weakened the visceral pleura, allowing air leakage. However, 4 years seems a bit long for that condition to be showing up at the current admission.

In the **first assessment** (SOAP 1), the therapist's attention to the patient's worsening pulmonary function is appropriate. Increasing his oxygenation by use of a Venturi oxygen mask would be acceptable, as would a trial of low-flow nasal cannula oxygen. The readers who recognized the small pneumothorax and noted its specific boundaries for bronchial hygiene therapy are certainly worthy of praise. The readers who saw the need to obtain an early sputum culture in the interest of promptly treating the infection also deserve commendation.

Three hours later, despite appropriate action, the patient is clearly worsening. Indeed, a stat has been called. The patient's chest X-ray film demonstrates a left tension pneumothorax, and the therapist at this point must ensure that a tube thoracostomy setup is available for the physician. Bilateral **Atelectasis** is present, reflected in the crackles, chest radiograph, cyanosis, and low Pao_2 (see Figure 9-7). The respiratory care practitioner's (RCP's) assessment would come after the chest tube has been placed and is functioning well, and he or she would so record that fact in the assessment. The RCP should note that the compressive atelectasis noted earlier has improved and help honor the patient's and physician's requests to avoid use of a ventilator if at all possible. However, the patient's CO_2 probably is high enough (103 mm Hg) to preclude this action. A trial of a respiratory stimulant, such as doxapram (Dopram), might be used in this setting. The therapist may try to increase the end-expiratory pressure to treat the atelectasis, but the reader should know that such therapy is fraught with the possibility of air trapping in patients with obstructive pulmonary disease.

Case 8: Acute Respiratory Distress Syndrome

RESPONSE 1

SOAP 1

S "I cannot move very well, and I am becoming very short of breath."

O Vital signs: BP 125/78, HR 93, RR 21, T normal. Skin: pale; no cough; nonproductive voluntary cough; tenderness over anterior chest; bilateral lung fields: dull percussion notes, bronchial breath sounds; Spo_2 95%; ABGs (3 L/min O_2 by nasal cannula): pH 7.51, $Paco_2$ 29, HCO_3^- = 22, Pao_2 68, CXR: bilateral "ground-glass" infiltrates worsening

A • Increased work of breathing (vital signs, ABGs)
  • Increased lung infiltrates: possible atelectasis or consolidation? Possible ARDS? Fat emboli? (CXR, chest assessment findings)
  • Acute alveolar hyperventilation with mild hypoxemia (ABGs)

P Hyperinflation Therapy Protocol (e.g., incentive spirometry with therapist qh until 2200; then q 2 h). Oxygen Therapy Protocol (e.g., HAFOE mask at Fio_2 0.4). Monitor and reevaluate (e.g., in 30 to 60 minutes with ABG).

SOAP 2

S "I'm feeling worse."

O Vital signs: RR 30, BP 165/95, HR 110, T 38.8° C (101.8° F); tender anterior chest; bronchial breath sounds and crackles bilaterally; Spo_2 75%; ABGs on Fio_2 = 0.80: pH 7.56, $Paco_2$ 24, HCO_3^- 218, Pao_2 35

A • Continued increased work of breathing (vital signs, ABGs)
  • Worsening of atelectasis or pneumonia (chest assessment, bronchial breath sounds and crackles)
  • Acute alveolar hyperventilation with moderate hypoxemia (ABGs)
  • Impending acute ventilatory failure (ABGs)

P Contact physician regarding impending ventilatory failure. Up-regulate Oxygen Therapy Protocol (e.g., partial rebreathing mask). Up-regulate Hyperinflation Therapy Protocol (e.g., changing incentive spirometry to IPPB or trial of nasal CPAP at 10 cm H_2O). Monitor and reevaluate (e.g., 1 hour).

SOAP 3

S N/A (patient unresponsive)

O Vital signs: RR 18, BP 170/97, HR 150, T 37.8° C (100° F). Skin: cyanotic; bronchial breath sounds and crackles bilaterally; Spo_2 69%; ABGs on Fio_2 = 1.0: pH 7.31, $Paco_2$ 48, HCO_3^- 22, Pao_2 31; CXR: increased infiltrates bilaterally

A • Worsening of interstitial lung process: ARDS or atelectasis versus pneumonia (chest assessment, CXR)
  • Acute ventilatory failure with moderate hypoxemia (ABGs)

P Contact physician regarding acute ventilatory failure stat. Prepare for immediate intubation and mechanical ventilation. Continue Hyperinflation Therapy with PEEP per Mechanical Ventilation Protocol. Continue Oxygen Therapy Protocol. Monitor and reevaluate closely.

DISCUSSION

Multiple trauma (including chest wall trauma) in a patient should in itself constitute notification to the therapist that respiratory expertise will be required. In this patient, who is hypotensive and has fractured teeth along with multiple bone fractures, three diagnoses should immediately come to mind: (1) the patient's potential for developing acute respiratory distress syndrome (ARDS), (2) the possibility that dental fragments were aspirated, causing obstructive pneumonia or atelectasis, and (3) fat emboli, which could complicate an already serious situation. A diagnosis of possible pulmonary contusion also would be in order, given the history of chest trauma, the short interval between the injury and the abnormal chest X-ray, and the fact that the X-ray abnormalities seemed out of proportion to the ABGs as measured. The patient's tachypnea, dyspnea, tachycardia, and hypoxemia all reflect the effects of the pathophysiologic abnormalities seen with **Atelectasis** (see Figure 9-7) and/or **Increased Alveolar-Capillary Thickening**—diffusion blockade (see Figure 9-9).

At the time of the **first evaluation** (SOAP 1), the development of progressive hypoxemia, "ground-glass" infiltrates in the chest film, and increasing dyspnea approximately 24 hours after multiple trauma are almost pathognomonic of ARDS. Examination and assessment have determined that despite his frontal chest injury, the patient does not have a flail chest. The probability that the patient will require intubation and mechanical ventilation with positive end-expiratory pressure (PEEP) or inverse ratio ventilation (IRV) is high.

A trial of hyperinflation therapy (e.g., with mask continuous positive airway pressure [CPAP]) is indicated in this setting but often is not successful because of patient intolerance. Preparation should be made for intubation and mechanical ventilation in case the pulmonary function decreases any further. Initially, the patient should be placed on mask oxygen therapy to improve oxygenation and supply him with a known F_{IO_2} so that the alveolar-arterial oxygen gradient can be calculated (with the assumption that the patient likely will be refractory, to some degree, to oxygen therapy). Hyperinflation therapy with incentive spirometry or intermittent positive-pressure breathing (IPPB) is indicated but may not be well tolerated because of chest pain. Prompt (30 to 60 minutes) reevaluation with repeat arterial blood gas (ABG) measurement is indicated.

At the time of the **second evaluation** (SOAP 2), 3 days after surgery, the patient has not improved—indeed, he is feeling worse. He is cyanotic and tachypneic, and his ABG values show profound deterioration, with a Pa_{O_2} of 35 mm Hg and a Pa_{CO_2} of 24 mm Hg. An attempt may be made at this point to increase his hyperinflation therapy with a positive expiratory pressure (PEP) mask or CPAP, but it will probably be futile. If the patient is not on an F_{IO_2} of 1.0, he should be. Review of the chest film is mandatory because a complicating problem such as a pneumothorax could theoretically have occurred or a large pleural effusion could have developed. If the reader believes that the patient should be intubated at this point, the concern is justified.

The **last evaluation** (SOAP 3) occurs 30 minutes after the second one. The patient is unresponsive. His auscultatory findings have not changed, but his blood gases have deteriorated still further. If protocol allows, the patient should be intubated immediately. If not, the attending physician should be called to request intubation and the immediate start of mechanical ventilation and PEEP.

With this aggressive therapy, the patient gradually improved. He remained on a mechanical ventilator for 14 days and then spent an additional 1 month recovering in the hospital. During this recovery, another pulmonary complication in the form of an acute pulmonary embolus developed. He recovered and eventually was discharged to his home on supplemental oxygen; he was subsequently lost to follow-up care.

Recent studies have suggested that lung function never completely returns to normal after a significant bout of ARDS. These effects, however, may be minimal. For example, exercise may produce mild oxygen desaturation as an effect of lung tissue remodeling.

Case 9: Idiopathic (Infant) Respiratory Distress Syndrome

SOAP 1

S N/A

O Mild respiratory distress: intercostal retractions, nasal flaring, and cyanosis; vital signs: BP 50/20, HR 180, RR 74, T 37.1° C (98.8° F). Grunting breath sounds and crackles bilaterally; CXR: mild haziness in lung bases; ABGs (F_{IO_2} 0.40): pH 7.52, Pa_{CO_2} 29, HCO_3^- 21, Pa_{O_2} 49

A • Impending infant respiratory distress syndrome (history, CXR)
   • Atelectasis, consolidation, and hyaline membrane formation likely (history, CXR)
   • Acute alveolar hyperventilation with moderate-to-severe hypoxemia (ABGs)

P Hyperinflation Therapy Protocol (e.g., nasal CPAP at 5 cm H_2O). Oxygen Therapy Protocol (e.g., F_{IO_2} at 0.30 via nasal CPAP). Monitor (e.g., vital signs, breath sounds, and acute changes in color and muscle tone) and evaluate closely. Place infant ventilator on standby.

SOAP 2

S N/A

O Vital signs: RR 30 (ventilator), BP 60/40, HR 184; harsh, bronchial breath sounds and fine crackles bilaterally; CXR: dense, "ground-glass" appearance in both lungs; ABGs (F_{IO_2} 0.60): pH 7.28, Pa_{CO_2} 53, HCO_3^- 19, Pa_{O_2} 57

A • Infant respiratory distress syndrome (history, CXR)
   • Worsening of atelectasis, consolidation, and hyaline membrane formation likely (history, CXR)
   • Acute ventilatory failure with severe hypoxemia (ABGs)

P Continue Hyperinflation Therapy per Mechanical Ventilation Protocol. Up-regulate Oxygen Therapy Protocol per Mechanical Ventilation Protocol. Constantly monitor ventilator settings to correct acute ventilatory failure (e.g., increasing rate and tidal volume). Monitor and reevaluate closely.

SOAP 3

S N/A

O Vital signs: BP 74/50, HR 120, spontaneous RR 42, T normal; normal vesicular breath sounds; CXR: normal; ABGs: pH 7.42, $Paco_2$ 37, HCO_3^- 24, Pao_2 162

A • Appearance that atelectasis, consolidation, and hyaline membrane no longer present (history, CXR)
   • Normal ventilatory status with overoxygenation (ABGs)

P Down-regulate Hyperinflation Therapy Protocol. Down-regulate Oxygen Therapy Protocol. Monitor and reevaluate.

DISCUSSION

Infant respiratory distress syndrome (IRDS) is one of the most common complications of prematurity. It can be prevented with aggressive respiratory care. IRDS often is referred to as *hyaline membrane disease* because of the formation of a hyaline membrane inside the alveoli. The problem also is complicated by inadequate surfactant production. The low levels of surfactant in the presence of immature lung tissue produce **Atelectasis** (see Figure 9-7). Hypoxia and pulmonary hypertension develop, which keeps the ductus arteriosus patent and thus allows continuation of fetal circulation after birth. The low Apgar scores on delivery also indicate impending respiratory distress. At this point, hypercapnia and respiratory acidosis occur, which ultimately may prove fatal.

IRDS often is due to lack of prenatal care for the mother. In this case, the premature delivery could have been stopped medically with tocolytic drugs, such as terbutaline. That the mother smoked throughout the pregnancy decreased the level of oxygen available to the infant, possibly resulting in the infant's being small for gestational age. The mother's youth in this case also suggests the possibility of a high incidence of complications with the birth.

Initially, the low Apgar score indicates that the infant needs constant monitoring. Although cyanosis and crackles are normal signs immediately after delivery, the nasal flaring and intercostal retractions are not. These signs, along with the grunting respirations, indicate impending respiratory failure. The blood pressure is normal, but the infant shows signs of tachypnea and tachycardia, which indicate increased work of breathing. The infant will require an immediate intravenous infusion because dehydration and humidification will be additional problems. The infant also should be placed immediately in an open-bed radiant warmer to ensure a neutral thermal environment.

At the **16-hour assessment** (SOAP 2), the infant is placed on mechanical ventilation because of the clinical findings. However, nasal continuous positive airway pressure (CPAP) could have been tried before intubation and placement on the ventilator. Nasal CPAP does not require the passing of a tube through the vocal cords but still aids in the distribution of surfactant into the distal alveoli.

The **last assessment** (SOAP 3) shows that the treatment has worked and that the infant continues to improve. The vital signs are all within the normal range; the ABGs indicate that the Fio_2 can continue to be decreased; and the infant can be weaned successfully from mechanical ventilation. The only concern (at this point) is the high Pao_2, because a value less than 100 mm Hg is required to prevent the development of retinopathy of prematurity.

The use of surfactant and the positive end-expiratory pressure (PEEP) or CPAP pressures for aerosol distribution successfully reversed the infant's condition. The short time needed to reverse the IRDS precludes any permanent damage to the lungs, which might have occurred if the infant had remained on the ventilator and developed bronchopulmonary dysplasia.

Case 10: Postoperative Atelectasis

SOAP 1

S "My gut really hurts, and I can't seem to get any air."

O Respiratory distress; cyanosis; vital signs: BP 185/90, HR 130, RR 35, T normal; tachypnea; frequent spontaneous, weak cough with yellow sputum production; LLL: diminished breath sounds; RLL: bronchial breath sounds and dull percussion notes; incentive spirometry (IS): 40% of preoperative value; Spo_2 (2 L/min O_2 by nasal cannula) 77%; ABGs: pH 7.57, $Paco_2$ 23, HCO_3^- 21, Pao_2 43; poor cooperation with IS

A • Labored breathing (general appearance, vital signs, ABGs)
  • Excessive yellow sputum accumulation (sputum)
  • Possible infection
  • Weak cough effort (observation)
  • Possible atelectasis or consolidation or both in RLL (dull percussion, bronchial breath sound, IS values)
  • Acute alveolar hyperventilation with moderate-to-severe hypoxemia (ABGs)
  • Poor patient cooperation with IS

P Oxygen Therapy Protocol (e.g., O_2 via HAFOE mask with Fio_2 0.60). Bronchopulmonary Hygiene Therapy Protocol (e.g., CPT and nasotracheal suction q 4 h and prn; sputum for culture). Hyperinflation Therapy Protocol (e.g., CPAP face mask at 10 cm H_2O 35 minutes q 2 h while awake). Aerosolized Medication Protocol (e.g., med. nebs. with 0.5 cc albuterol in 2 cc 20% acetylcysteine q 4 h). Monitor and reevaluate (e.g., checking ABGs in 30 minutes).

SOAP 2

S No response to questions

O Respiratory distress: cyanotic, cool, and damp skin; vital signs: BP 188/100, HR 135, RR 36, T 38.1° C (100.6° F). Right middle and both lower lung lobes: dull percussion notes, bronchial breath sounds, and crackles; CXR: RML, RLL, and LLL atelectasis and air bronchograms; Spo_2 72%; ABGs: pH 7.55, $Paco_2$ 29, HCO_3^- 22, Pao_2 46

A • Continued labored breathing (general appearance, vital signs, ABGs)
  • Sputum accumulation still excessive (cough and recent history)
  • Weak cough effort (observation)
  • RML, RLL, and LLL atelectasis (CXR, dull percussion, bronchial breath sounds)
  • Acute alveolar hyperventilation with moderate-to-severe hypoxemia (ABGs)
  • Impending ventilatory failure

P Call doctor stat and request transfer to ICU. Up-regulate Oxygen Therapy Protocol (e.g., increasing Fio_2 to 0.80). Up-regulate Bronchopulmonary Hygiene Therapy Protocol (e.g., increasing CPT to q 2 h). Up-regulate Hyperinflation Therapy Protocol (e.g., increasing CPAP mask to 15 cm H_2O). Up-regulate Aerosolized Medication Therapy Protocol (e.g., increasing med. nebs. to q 2 h). Continue to monitor and evaluate closely.

SOAP 3

S "I think I'm dying."

O Obvious respiratory distress; skin cyanotic, cool, and damp; no right-sided chest excursion; trachea deviated to the right; vital signs: BP 192/90, HR 142, RR 20, T 37.3° C (99.1° F); RML and RLL: bronchial breath sounds, crackles, and dull percussion notes; LLL: dull percussion notes and no breath sounds; SpO_2 62%; ABGs: pH 7.26, $Paco_2$ 53, HCO_3^- 22, Pao_2 37

A • Continued increased work of breathing (general appearance, vital signs)
  • Excessive sputum accumulation still likely (recent history)
  • RML and RLL atelectasis (dull percussion, bronchial breath sounds, CXR)
  • Possible LLL atelectasis (dull percussion note, CXR)
  • Likely caused by mucus plugging (no breath sounds)
  • Acute ventilatory failure with severe hypoxemia (ABGs)

P Contact physician stat. Recommend intubation and mechanical ventilation accompanied by the following: Oxygen Therapy Protocol, Bronchial Hygiene Therapy Protocol, Hyperinflation Therapy Protocol, and Aerosolized Medication Therapy Protocol.

DISCUSSION

By the time of the **first assessment** (SOAP 1), this overweight, tobacco-abusing woman with a chronic productive cough before surgery has developed postoperative atelectasis as a result of pain, splinting of the chest, or postoperative analgesia. The physical findings are classic for major **Atelectasis,** initially involving the right lung and associated with severe right-to-left shunt physiology (see Figure 9-7).

In the first portion of this case, the diagnosis and treatment of postoperative atelectasis with incentive spirometry (IS; and failing that, intermittent positive-pressure breathing [IPPB]) is fairly straightforward. The patient's severe hypoxemia, which persists despite alveolar hyperventilation, deserves careful monitoring. Giving this patient a much higher concentration of oxygen (e.g., 50%) by a Venturi oxygen mask probably is safe. However, careful attention must be paid to oximetry and blood gas analyses. If the patient did not wake up and become more cooperative at this point, the blood gases are severe enough to prompt consideration of intubation, mechanical ventilation, and therapeutic bronchoscopy at this time.

If the respiratory therapist has prepared the SOAP note carefully, a heavy preoperative cigarette smoking history should be noted. The alert reader would have started bronchial hygiene therapy per protocol. The mild diastolic hypertension, which has persisted despite analgesia, is worrisome and needs to be monitored carefully.

At the time of the **second assessment** (SOAP 2), the patient would not or could not cooperate with deep breathing and coughing and had categorically refused chest physical therapy. The blood pressure is even higher; the heart rate is rapid; and the patient has a fever as well. That the patient is now unresponsive raises the question of sedation overdose and possible CO_2 retention, but the blood gases clearly rule out the latter.

On the basis of the physical findings and the chest X-ray film, the therapist appropriately assesses the cause as right middle and lower lobe and possible left lower lobe atelectasis. Oxygen therapy is pushed correctly, with an increase in the F_{IO_2} by mask therapy. However, because of the right-to-left shunt physiology involved, this procedure may not be successful. Bronchopulmonary hygiene and aerosolized medication therapy per protocols are indicated as well, with vigorous bronchodilation, mucolysis, and consideration of therapeutic bronchoscopy. The patient's arterial blood gases are abnormal enough to make intubation and mechanical ventilation options at this point. Sputum from deep nasotracheal suctioning or bronchoscopy should be cultured promptly because the patient's fever likely represents pulmonary infection.

Certainly at the **final assessment** (SOAP 3), the patient must be mechanically ventilated; she has acute ventilatory failure and profound hypoxemia. Her bilateral atelectasis is still present and has not been improved by the treatments outlined previously. By the time of the final assessment, the patient has gone beyond the usual medical boundaries. The treating therapist's desire to contact the physician immediately and prepare for mechanical ventilation is entirely appropriate. Hyperinflation therapy with positive end-expiratory pressure (PEEP) as part of the mechanical ventilation order also would be appropriate because atelectasis clearly is the chief villain. Therapeutic bronchoscopy is part of the Bronchopulmonary Hygiene Protocol (see Protocol 9-2, page 138).

Despite vigorous therapy as outlined in this case, the patient did poorly. After 5 days, she was able to be weaned gradually from ventilator support; after 2 weeks, she was able to return home. Postoperative infection and retained secretions characterized her postoperative course. As of her last follow-up visit, she continued to smoke, against medical advice. Return demonstrations of IS and appropriate metered dose inhaler (MDI) use *were* never satisfactory in the course of her hospitalization.

Glossary

abscess Localized collection of pus that results from disintegration or displacement of tissue in any part of the body.

acetylcholine A neurotransmitter substance widely distributed in body tissue with a primary function of mediating synaptic activity of the nervous system.

acidemia Decreased pH or an increased hydrogen ion concentration of the blood.

acidosis Pathologic condition resulting from accumulation of acid or loss of base from the body.

acinus Smallest division of a gland, a group of secretory cells surrounding a cavity; the functional part of an organ. (The respiratory acinus includes terminal [respiratory] bronchioles, alveolar ducts, alveoli, and all other structures therein.)

acute Sharp, severe; of rapid onset and characterized by severe symptoms and a short course; not chronic.

adhesion Fibrous band that holds together parts that are normally separated.

adrenergic Term applied to nerve fibers that, when stimulated, release epinephrine at their endings. Includes nearly all sympathetic postganglionic fibers except those innervating sweat glands.

adrenocorticotropic hormone (ACTH) A hormone secreted by the anterior pituitary. It is regulated by the corticotropin-releasing factor (CRF) from the hypothalamus and is essential to growth, development, and continued function of the adrenal cortex.

aerosol Gaseous suspension of fine solid or liquid particles.

afebrile Without fever.

afferent Carrying impulses toward a center.

afferent nerves Nerves that transmit impulses from the peripheral to the central nervous system.

air trapping Trapping of alveolar gas during exhalation.

albumin One of a group of simple proteins widely distributed in plant and animal tissues. It is found in the blood as serum albumin, in milk as lactalbumin, and in the white of an egg as ovalbumin.

alkalemia Increased pH or decreased hydrogen ion concentration of the blood.

allele One of two or more different genes containing specific inheritable characteristics that occupy corresponding positions on paired chromosomes.

allergen Any substance that causes manifestations of allergy. It may or may not be a protein.

allergy Acquired hypersensitivity to a substance (allergen) that normally does not cause a reaction. An allergic reaction is essentially an antibody-antigen reaction, but in some cases the antibody cannot be demonstrated. The reaction is caused by the release of histamine or histamine-like substances from injured cells.

α_1-antitrypsin Inhibitor of trypsin that may be deficient in persons with emphysema.

α-receptor Site in the autonomic nerve pathways where excitatory responses occur when adrenergic agents such as norepinephrine and epinephrine are released.

anaerobic Metabolic pathway that does not require oxygen; such processes usually produce lactic acid.

anaphylaxis Allergic hypersensitivity reaction of the body to a foreign protein or drug.

anemia Condition in which there is a reduction in the number of circulating red blood cells per cubic millimeter, the amount of hemoglobin per 100 ml, or the volume of packed red cells per 100 ml of blood.

aneurysm Localized dilation of a blood vessel, usually an artery.

angiogram Serial roentgenograms of a blood vessel taken in rapid sequence after injection of a radiopaque substance into the vessel.

angiography Roentgenography of blood vessels after injection of a radiopaque substance.

anoxia Absence of oxygen.

anterolateral In front and to one side.

antibody Protein substance that develops in response to and interacts with an antigen. The antigen-antibody reaction forms the basis of immunity. Antibodies are produced by plasma cells in lymphoid tissue. Antibodies may be present because of previous infection, vaccination, or transfer from the mother to the fetus in utero or may occur without known antigenic stimulus, usually as a result of unknown, accidental exposure.

antigen Substance that induces the formation of antibodies that interact specifically with it. An antigen may be introduced into the body or may be formed within the body.

aortic valve Valve between the left ventricle and the ascending aorta that prevents regurgitation of blood into the left ventricle.

aperture Opening or orifice.

apex Top, end, or tip of a structure.

apnea Complete absence of spontaneous ventilation.

aponeurosis Flat, fibrous sheet of connective tissue that attaches muscle to bone or other tissues. May sometimes serve as a fascia.

arrhythmia Irregularity or loss of rhythm.

arteriole Minute artery that, at its distal end, leads into a capillary.

arthralgia Any pain that affects a joint.

arthropod Any member of a large group of animals that possess a hard external skeleton and jointed legs and other appendages. Many arthropods are of medical importance (e.g., mites, ticks).

asepsis The absence of germs; sterile.

asphyxia Condition caused by an insufficient uptake of oxygen.

aspiration Inhalation of pharyngeal contents into the pulmonary tree.

asymmetric Unequal correspondence in shape, size, and relative position of parts on opposite sides of the midline.

asystole Absence of contractions of the heart.

atelectasis Collapsed or airless lung. May be caused by obstruction of the airways by foreign bodies, mucus plugs, or excessive secretions or by compression from without, as by tumors, aneurysms, or enlarged lymph nodes.

atmospheric pressure Pressure of air on the earth at mean sea level. Approximately 14.7 pounds to the square inch (760 mm Hg).

atopic Of or pertaining to a hereditary tendency to develop immediate allergic reactions because of the presence of an antibody in the skin and sometimes the bloodstream.

atrial fibrillation Irregular and rapid randomized contractions of the atria working independently of the ventricles.

atrial flutter Extremely rapid (200 to 400/min) contractions of the atrium. In pure flutter a regular rhythm is maintained; in impure flutter the rhythm is irregular.

atrophy A wasting or decrease in size of an organ or a tissue.

atropine An alkaloid obtained from belladonna. It is a parasympatholytic agent.

autosomal recessive trait Pattern of inheritance in which the transmission of a recessive gene results in a carrier state if the person is heterozygous for the trait and in an affected state if the person is homozygous for the trait. Males and females are affected with equal frequency.

bacillus Any rod-shaped bacterium.

bacteria Unicellular ovoid or rod-shaped organisms existing in free-living or parasitic forms. They display a wide range of biochemical and pathogenic properties.

Bedsonia Former genus name for *Chlamydia*, now used as a common term denoting species of *Chlamydia* (e.g., bedsonias, *Bedsonia* organisms, bedsonial agents).

benign Noncancerous and therefore not an immediate threat, even though treatment eventually may be required for health or cosmetic reasons.

β-receptor Site in autonomic nerve pathways wherein inhibitory responses occur when adrenergic agents such as norepinephrine and epinephrine are released.

bicarbonate Any salt containing the HCO_3^- anion.

bifurcation A separation into two branches; the point of forking.

biopsy Excision of a small piece of living tissue for microscopic examination; usually performed to establish a diagnosis.

bleb Blister or bulla. Blebs may vary in size from that of a bean to that of a goose egg and may contain serous, seropurulent, or bloody fluid.

blood-brain barrier Membrane between circulating blood and the brain that prevents certain substances from reaching brain tissue and cerebrospinal fluid.

bradykinin Kinin composed of a chain of nine amino acids liberated by the action of trypsin or of certain snake venoms on a globulin of blood plasma.

bronchoconstriction Constriction of the bronchial tubes.

bronchodilation Dilation of a bronchus.

bronchograms Film of the airways after a radiopaque substance has been injected into them.

bronchoscopy A visual examination of the tracheobronchial tree with the bronchoscope.

bronchospasm Involuntary sudden movement or convulsive contraction of the muscular layer of the bronchus.

bulla Blister, cavity, or vesicle filled with air or fluid; a bleb.

cachexia General ill health and malnutrition marked by weakness and emaciation, usually associated with serious disease (e.g., tuberculosis, cancer).

calcification Process in which organic tissue becomes hardened by the deposition of calcium salts in tissue.

cannulation Placement of a tube or sheath enclosing a trocar to allow the escape of fluid after the trocar is withdrawn from the body.

capillary stasis Stagnation of the normal flow of fluids or blood in capillaries.

carbon dioxide (CO₂) Colorless, odorless, incombustible gas formed during respiration and combustion; normally constitutes only 0.03% of the atmosphere. Concentrations above 5% in inspired air stimulate respiration. CO₂ retention occurs in end-stage pulmonary disease.

carbon monoxide (CO) A product of incomplete combustion of fossil fuels. Also found in tobacco smoke, and highly toxic at high levels. Also used in pulmonary function testing to detect diffusion abnormalities.

carcinoma Malignant tumor that occurs in epithelial tissue. These neoplasms tend to infiltrate and give rise to metastases.

cardiogenic Originating in the heart.

cardiotonic drugs Drugs that increase the tonicity (contraction strength) of the heart.

carotid sinus baroreceptors Sensory nerve endings located in the carotid sinus. Changes in pressure stimulate the nerve endings.

cartilage Dense, firm, compact connective tissue capable of withstanding considerable pressure and tension; located in all true joints, the outer ear, bronchi, and movable sections of the ribs.

catecholamines Biologically active amines that behave as epinephrine and norepinephrine. Catecholamines have marked effects on the nervous and cardiovascular systems, metabolic rate, temperature, and smooth muscle.

cavitation The formation of cavities or hollow spaces within the body such as those formed in the lung by tuberculosis.

central venous pressure (CVP) Pressure within the superior vena cava. The pressure under which the blood is returned to the right atrium.

cerebrospinal fluid (CSF) Liquid cushion protecting the brain and spinal cord from shock.

chemoreceptor Sense organ or sensory nerve ending that is stimulated by and reacts to chemical stimuli and that is located outside the central nervous system. Chemoreceptors are found in the large arteries of the thorax and neck (carotid and aortic bodies), the taste buds, and the olfactory cells of the nose.

chemotactic Attraction and repulsion of living protoplasm to a chemical stimulus.

Chlamydia Genus of viruslike microorganisms that cause disease in humans and birds. Some *Chlamydia* infections of birds can be transmitted to humans (e.g., ornithosis, parrot disease). The organisms resemble bacteria but are of similar size to viruses and are obligate parasites.

chronic Denoting a process that shows little change and slow progression and is of long duration.

chronotropic Agent that increases heart rate.

cilia Small hairlike projections on the surface of epithelial cells. In the bronchi, they propel mucus and foreign particles in a whiplike movement toward the throat.

clinical manifestations Symptoms or signs demonstrated by a patient; may be subjective or objective.

coagulation Process of clotting. Coagulation requires the presence of several substances, the most important of which are prothrombin, thrombin, thromboplastin, calcium in ionic form, and fibrinogen.

coalesce To fuse, run, or grow together.

coccobacillus Short, thick bacterial rod in the shape of an oval or slightly elongated coccus.

coccus Bacterium with a spherical shape.

collagen Fibrous insoluble protein found in connective tissue, including skin, bone, ligaments, and cartilage. Collagen represents about 30% of the total body protein.

colloid Type of solution; a gluelike substance such as protein or starch whose particles (molecules or aggregates of molecules), when dispersed in a solvent to the greatest degree, remain uniformly distributed and fail to form a true solution.

compromise A blending of the qualities of two different things; an unfavorable change.

congenital Existing at and usually before birth; referring to conditions that are present at birth, regardless of their cause.

congestion Excessive amount of blood, tissue, or fluid in an organ or in tissue.

consolidation The process of becoming solid; a mass that has solidified.

contusion Injury in which the skin is not broken; a bruise. Symptoms are pain, swelling, and discoloration.

convex Having a rounded, somewhat elevated surface resembling a segment of the external surface of a sphere.

cor pulmonale Hypertrophy or failure of the right ventricle resulting from disorders of the lungs, pulmonary vessels, or chest wall.

corticosteroids Any of a number of hormonal steroid substances obtained from the cortex of the adrenal gland.

costophrenic angle The junction of the rib cage and the diaphragm.

cuirass A chest covering; breastplate, as in cuirass ventilator.

cyclic adenosine monophosphate (cAMP) Cyclic nucleotide participating in the activities of many hormones, including catecholamines, adrenocorticotropin, and vasopressin. It is synthesized from adenosine triphosphate and is stimulated by the enzyme adenylate cyclase.

cyst Closed pouch or sac with a definite wall that contains fluid, semifluid, or solid material.

cytoplasm Protoplasm of a cell exclusive of the nucleus.

demarcate To set or mark boundaries or limits.

demyelination The destruction or removal of the myelin sheath from a nerve or nerve fiber.

density Mass of a substance per unit of volume, the relative weight of a substance compared with a reference standard.

deoxyribonucleic acid (DNA) Type of nucleic acid containing deoxyribose as the sugar component and found principally in the nuclei of animal and vegetable cells, usually loosely bound to protein (hence termed *deoxyribonucleoprotein*).

depolarize To reduce to a nonpolarized condition. To reduce the amount of electrical charge between oppositely charged particles.

desensitization Prevention of anaphylaxis.

diabetes mellitus Chronic disease of pancreatic origin that is characterized by insulin deficiency or functional abnormality and a subsequent inability to process carbohydrates. This condition results in excess sugar in the blood and urine; excessive thirst, hunger, urination, weakness, and emaciation; and imperfect combustion of fats. If untreated, diabetes mellitus leads to acidosis, coma, and death.

diagnostic Pertaining to the use of scientific methods to establish the cause and nature of disease.

diastole Period in the heart cycle during which the muscle fibers lengthen, the heart dilates, and the cavities fill with blood.

dilation Expansion of an organ, orifice, or vessel.

dimorphic fungus A condition in which the organism has two distinct types of fungus.

dimorphism The quality of existing in two distinct forms.

disseminate Scatter or distribute over a considerable area; when applied to disease organisms, scattered throughout an organ or the body.

distal Farthest from the center, from a medial line, or from the trunk.

driving pressure Pressure difference between two areas.

ductus arteriosus Vessel between the pulmonary artery and the aorta. It bypasses the lungs in the fetus.

dynamometer An instrument for measuring the force of muscular contractions. For example, a squeeze dynamometer is one by which the grip of the hand is measured.

dysplasia Abnormal development of tissues or cells.

dyspnea Air hunger resulting in labored or difficult breathing, sometimes accompanied by pain. Symptoms include audible labored breathing, distressed anxious expression, dilated nostrils, protrusion of the abdomen with an expanded chest, and gasping.

edema A local or generalized condition in which the body tissues contain an excessive amount of fluid.

efferent Away from a central organ or section. Efferent nerves conduct impulses from the brain or spinal cord to the periphery.

efferent nerves Nerves that carry impulses having the following effects: motor, causing contraction of the muscles; secretory, causing glands to secrete; and inhibitory, causing some organs to become quiescent.

effusion Seeping or serous, purulent, or bloody fluid into a cavity, the result of such a seeping.

elastase Enzyme that dissolves elastin.

electrocardiogram (ECG) Record of the electrical activity of the heart.

electrodiagnostic Use of electric and electronic devices for diagnostic purposes.

electroencephalogram (EEG) Record of the electrical activity of the brain.

electrolyte Substance that, in solution, conducts an electrical current and is decomposed by the passage of an electrical current. Acids, bases, and salts are electrolytes.

electromyogram A graphic record of the contraction of a muscle as a result of electrical stimulation.

electrophoresis Movement of charged colloidal particles through the medium in which they are dispersed as a result of changes in electrical potential.

embolus Mass of undissolved matter present in blood or lymphatic vessels to which it has been brought by the blood or lymph current. Emboli may be solid, liquid, or gaseous.

empyema Pus in a body cavity, especially in the pleural cavity; usually the result of a primary infection in the lungs.

encapsulated Enclosed in a fibrous or membranous sheath.

encephalitis Inflammation of the brain.

endemic A disease that occurs continuously in a particular population but has low mortality, such as measles.

endocarditis Inflammation of the endocardium. It may involve only the membrane covering the valves, or it may involve the general lining of the chambers of the heart.

endothelium The layer of epithelial cells that lines the cavities of the heart, blood and lymph vessels, and the serous cavities of the body; it originates from the mesoderm.

enuresis Involuntary discharge of urine, usually referring to involuntary discharge of urine during sleep at night or bed-wetting beyond the age when bladder control should have been achieved.

enzyme Complex protein capable of inducing chemical changes in other substances without being changed itself. Enzymes speed chemical reactions.

eosinophil Cell or cellular structure that stains readily with the acid stain eosin. Specifically refers to a granular leukocyte.

epidemiology Scientific discipline concerned with defining and explaining the interrelationships of factors that determine disease frequency and distribution.

epinephrine Hormone secreted by the adrenal medulla in response to splanchnic stimulation.

epithelium Covering of the internal and external organs of the body, including the lining of vessels. It consists of cells bound together by connective material and varies in the number of layers and the kinds of cells.

erythema multiforme A hypersensitivity syndrome characterized by polymorphous eruptions of the skin and mucous membranes.

erythropoiesis Formation of red blood cells.

etiology Cause of disease.

exocrine gland Gland whose secretion reaches an epithelial surface either directly or through a duct.

expectoration To clear out the chest and lungs by coughing up and spitting out matter.

extravascular Outside a vessel.

exudate Accumulation of a fluid in a cavity; matter that penetrates through vessel walls into adjoining tissue.

fascia Fibrous membrane covering, supporting, and separating muscles.

febrile Pertaining to a fever.

fibrin Whitish, filamentous protein formed by the action of prothrombin on fibrinogen. The conversion of fibrinogen into fibrin is the basis for blood clotting. Fibrin is deposited as fine interlacing filaments in which are entangled red and white blood cells and platelets, the whole forming a coagulum or clot.

fibrinolytic Pertaining to the splitting of fibrin.

fibroelastic Composed of fibrous and elastic tissue.

fibrosis Formation of scar tissue in the connective tissue framework of the lungs.

fissure Cleft or groove on the surface of an organ, often marking the division of the organ into parts, as the lobes of the lung.

fistula Abnormal passage or communication, usually between two internal organs or leading from an internal organ to the surface of the body; designated according to the organs or parts with which it communicates.

flaccid paralysis Paralysis in which there is loss of muscle tone, loss or reduction of tendon reflexes, and atrophy and degeneration of muscles.

flare Flush or spreading area of redness that surrounds a line made by drawing a pointed instrument across the skin. It is the second reaction in the triple response of skin to injury and is caused by dilation of the arterioles.

fluorescent antibody microscopy Microscopic examination of antibodies tagged with fluorescent material for the diagnosis of infections.

foramen ovale Opening between the atria of the heart in the fetus. This opening normally closes shortly after birth.

fossa Hollow or depression, especially on the surface of the end of a bone.

galactosemia Presence of galactose in the blood.

gastric juice (or gastric secretions) Fluid produced by the gastric glands of the stomach. It contains pepsin, hydrochloric acid, mucin, small quantities of inorganic salts, and the intrinsic antianemic principle. Gastric juice is strongly acid, having a pH of 0.9 to 1.5.

genus In natural history classification, the division between the family or tribe and the species; a group of species alike in the broad features of their organization but different in detail.

globulin One of a group of simple proteins insoluble in pure water but soluble in neutral solutions of salts of strong acids; the fraction of the blood serum with which antibodies are associated.

glossopharyngeal nerve Ninth cranial nerve. Function: special sensory (taste), visceral sensory, and motor. Distribution: pharynx, ear, meninges, posterior third of the tongue, and parotid gland.

glycolysis Breakdown of sugar by enzymes in the body. This occurs without oxygen.

glycoprotein Any of a class of conjugated proteins consisting of a compound of protein with a carbohydrate group.

hematocrit Volume of erythrocytes packed by centrifugation in a given volume of blood. Hematocrit is expressed as a percentage of the total blood volume that consists of erythrocytes or as the volume in cubic centimeters of erythrocytes packed by centrifugation of the blood.

hematopoietic Pertaining to the production and development of blood cells.

hemoptysis Expectoration of blood.

hemorrhage Abnormal internal or external discharge of blood; may be venous, arterial, or capillary.

heparin Polysaccharide that has been isolated from the liver, lung, and other tissues. It is produced by the mast cells of the liver and by basophil leukocytes. It inhibits coagulation by preventing conversion of prothrombin to thrombin and blocking the liberation of thromboplastin from blood platelets.

hepatosplenomegaly Enlargement of both the liver and spleen.

heterozygote Individual with different alleles for a given characteristic.

hilus Root of the lungs at the level of the fourth and fifth dorsal vertebrae.

histamine Substance normally present in the body; it exerts a pharmacologic action when released from injured cells. The red flush of a burn is caused by the local production of histamine. It is produced from the amino acid histidine.

Homans' sign Pain in the calf with dorsiflexion of the foot, indicating thrombophlebitis or thrombosis.

homozygote Individual developing from gametes with similar alleles and thus possessing like pairs of genes for a given hereditary characteristic.

hormone Substance originating in an organ or gland that is conveyed through the blood to another part of the body where, by chemical action, it stimulates increased functional activity and increased secretion.

humoral Pertaining to body fluids or substances contained in them.

hydrostatic Pertaining to the pressure of liquids in equilibrium and to the pressure exerted on liquids by other forces.

hydrous Containing water, usually chemically combined.

hypercarbia, hypercapnea Excess carbon dioxide in the blood; indicated by an elevated $Paco_2$.

hypercoagulation Greater than normal clotting.

hyperinflation Distention of a part by air, gas, or liquid.

hyperplasia Excessive proliferation of normal cells in the normal tissue arrangement of an organ.

hyperpnea Increased depth (volume) of breathing with or without an increased frequency.

hypersecretion Secretion from glands or cells.

hypersensitivity Abnormal sensitivity to a stimulus of any kind.

hypertension Higher than normal blood pressure; greater than normal tension or tonus.

hypertrophy Increase in size of an organ or structure that does not involve tumor formation.

hyperventilation Increased rate and depth of breathing.

hypoperfusion Deficiency of blood coursing through the vessels of the circulatory system.

hypoproteinemia Decrease in the amount of protein in the blood.

hypoventilation Reduced rate and depth of breathing.

hypoxemia Below-normal oxygen content in blood.

hypoxia Tissue oxygen deficiency.

iatrogenic Any adverse mental or physical condition induced in a patient by the effects of treatment by a physician or by the patient himself.

idiopathic Disease or condition without a recognizable cause.

ileocecal valve Valve between the ileum of the small intestine and the cecum of the large intestine. It consists of two flaps that project into the lumen of the large intestine just above the vermiform appendix.

immunoglobulin One of a family of closely related but not identical proteins that are capable of acting as antibodies. Five major types of immunoglobulins are normally present in the human adult: IgG, IgA, IgM, IgD, and IgE.

immunoglobin E (IgE) An α-globulin produced by cells of the lining of the respiratory and intestinal tract. IgE is important in forming reagin antibodies.

immunologic mechanism Reaction of the body to substances that are foreign or are interpreted as foreign.

immunotherapy Production or enhancement of immunity.

incubation period Development of an infection in a person from the time of entry into an organism up to the time of the first appearance of signs or symptoms.

infarction Necrosis of tissue after cessation of blood supply.

inferior vena cava (IVC) Venous trunk draining the lower extremities, the pelvis, and the abdominal viscera.

inflammation Localized heat, redness, swelling, and pain as a result of irritation, injury, or infection.

inotropic (positive) Increasing myocardial contractility.

insertion Manner or place of attachment of a muscle to the bone.

intercostal retraction Retraction of the chest. Visible sinking-in of the soft tissues of the chest between and around the cartilaginous and bony ribs.

interstitial Placed or lying between; pertaining to interstices or spaces within an organ or tissue.

intrapleural pressure Pressure within the pleural cavity.

iodine Nonmetallic element belonging to the halogen group.

ion Atom, group of atoms, or molecule that has acquired a net electrical charge by gaining or losing electrons.

ischemia Deficiency of blood supply caused by obstruction of the circulation to a part.

isotope One of a series of chemical elements that have nearly identical chemical properties but differ in their atomic weights and electrical charges. Many isotopes are radioactive.

Kerley's lines Thickening of the interlobular septa as seen in chest roentgenography; may be caused by cellular infiltration or edema associated with pulmonary venous hypertension.

kinetic Pertaining to or consisting of motion.

Kulchitsky cell A cell containing serotonin-secreting granules that stain readily with silver and chromium; also known as an *argentaffin cell*.

lactic acid Acid formed in muscles during activity by the breakdown of sugar without oxygen.

latency State of being concealed, hidden, inactive, or inapparent.

lesion A wound, injury, or pathologic change in body tissue.

lethargy The state or quality of being indifferent, apathetic, or sluggish; stupor.

leukocytes White blood corpuscles, including cells both with and without granules within their cytoplasm.

leukopenia An abnormal decrease in the number of white blood cells to fewer than 5000 cells/mm³.

ligamentum nuchae Upward continuation of the supraspinous ligament, extending from the seventh cervical vertebra to the occipital bone.

linea alba White line of connective tissue in the middle of the abdomen from sternum to pubis.

lipid Any of numerous fats generally insoluble in water that constitute one of the principal structural materials of cells.

longitudinal Parallel to the long axis of the body or part.

lubricant Agent, usually a liquid oil, that reduces friction between parts that brush against each other as they move. Joints are lubricated by synovial fluid.

lumen Inner open space of a tubular organ such as a blood vessel or intestine.

lymphangitis carcinomatosa The condition of having widespread dissemination of carcinoma in lymphatic channels or vessels.

lymphatic vessels Thin-walled vessels conveying lymph from the tissues. Similar to veins, they possess valves ensuring one-way flow and eventually empty into the venous system at the junction of the internal jugular and subclavian veins.

lymph node Rounded body consisting of accumulations of lymphatic tissue. Found at intervals in the course of lymphatic vessels.

macrophage Cell whose major function is phagocytosis of foreign matter.

malaise A vague feeling of body weakness, fatigue, or discomfort that often marks the onset of disease.

malleolus The protuberance on both sides of the ankle joint, the lower extremity of the fibula being known as the *lateral malleolus* and the lower end of the tibia as the *medial malleolus*.

mast cell Connective tissue cells that contain heparin and histamine in their granules; important in cellular defense mechanisms, including blood coagulation; needed during injury or infection.

mechanoreceptor Receptor that receives mechanical stimuli, such as pressure from sound or touch.

meconium ileus Obstruction of the small intestine in the newborn by impaction of thick, dry, tenacious meconium, usually at or near the ileocecal valve. The condition results from a deficiency in pancreatic enzymes and is the earliest manifestation of cystic fibrosis.

meningitis Any infection or inflammation of the membrane covering the brain and spinal cord.

mesothelioma A rare, malignant tumor of the mesothelium of the pleura or peritoneum; associated with early exposure to asbestos.

metabolism Sum of all physical and chemical changes that take place within an organism; all energy and material transformations that occur within living cells.

metaplasia Conversion of one kind of tissue into a form that is not normal for that tissue.

methylxanthine Methylated xanthine. A nitrogenous extraction contained in muscle tissue, liver, spleen, pancreas, other organs, and urine; formed during the metabolism of nucleoproteins. The three methylated xanthines are caffeine, theophylline, and theobromine.

microvilli Minute cylindrical processes on the free surface of a cell, especially cells of the proximal convoluted renal tubule and the intestinal epithelium; they increase the surface area of the cell.

mitosis A type of cell division of somatic cells in which each daughter cell contains the same number of chromosomes as the parent cell.

mitral valve Bicuspid valve between the left atrium and the left ventricle.

mononucleosis Presence of an abnormally high number of mononuclear leukocytes in the blood.

motile Having the power to move spontaneously.

mucociliary clearing action In the large airways, a continuous blanket of mucus covering the tracheobronchial tree epithelium is mobilized by the forward motion of cilia. The ciliary action causes the mucus blanket to be mobilized in a continuous motion toward the hilus of the lung, eventually moving to the larynx, where the mucus is moved into the pharynx and swallowed or expectorated.

mucous Pertaining to or resembling mucus; also glands secreting mucus.

mucus The free slime of the mucous membranes. It is composed of secretions of the glands along with various inorganic salts, desquamated cells, and leukocytes.

myelin Insulating material covering the axons of many neurons; increases the velocity of the nerve impulse along the axon.

myeloma Tumor originating in cells of the hematopoietic portion of bone marrow.

myeloproliferative disorders A group of conditions characterized by proliferation of myeloid tissue, including agnogenic myelofibrosis, myeloid metaplasia, polycythemia vera, and chronic myelogenous leukemia.

myocardial infarction Development of an area(s) of cellular death in the myocardium, the result of myocardial ischemia following occlusion of a coronary artery.

myocarditis Inflammation of the myocardium.

myocardium Middle layer of the walls of the heart, composed of cardiac muscle.

myopathy An abnormal condition of skeletal muscle characterized by muscle weakness, wasting, and histologic changes within muscle tissue.

necrosis Death of areas of tissue.

neoplasm New and abnormal formation of tissue, such as a tumor or growth. It serves no useful function but grows at the expense of the healthy organism.

nephritis Inflammation of the kidney. The glomeruli, tubules, and interstitial tissue may be affected.

neuroendocrine Pertaining to the nervous and endocrine systems as an integrated functioning mechanism.

neuromuscular junction The area of contact between the ends of a large myelinated nerve fiber and a fiber of skeletal muscle.

nitrogen oxides Automotive air pollutant. Depending on concentration, these gases cause respiratory irritation, bronchitis, and pneumonitis. Concentrations greater than 100 ppm usually cause pulmonary edema and result in death.

nocturnal Pertaining to or occurring in the night.

nodule A small aggregation of cells; a small node.

nomogram Graph consisting of three lines or curves (usually parallel) graduated for different variables in such a way that a straight line cutting the three lines gives the related values of the three variables.

norepinephrine Hormone produced by the adrenal medulla, similar in chemical and pharmacologic properties to epinephrine.

normal flora Naturally occurring bacteria found in specific bodily areas. Normal flora has no detrimental effect.

occlude To close, obstruct, or join together.

olfactory Pertaining to the sense of smell.

oncotic pressure Osmotic pressure resulting from the presence of colloids in a solution.

opacity Opaque spot or area; the condition of being opaque.

opaque Impervious to light rays or, by extension, to roentgen rays or other electromagnetic vibrations; neither transparent nor translucent.

orbicularis oculi The muscular body of the eyelid; it is composed of the palpebral, orbital, and lacrimal parts.

orifice Mouth, entrance, or outlet to any aperture.

origin The more fixed attachment (usually proximal or central) part of a muscle.

orthopnea Respiratory complaint of discomfort in any but an erect sitting or standing position.

osmotic pressure Pressure that develops when two unequally osmolar solutions are separated by a semipermeable membrane.

osteoporosis Increased brittleness of bone seen most often in elderly persons.

oxygen content Total oxygen in blood.

ozone Formed by the action of sunlight on oxygen in which three atoms form the molecule O_3. It is an irritant to the respiratory tract.

palatine arches Vault-shaped muscular structures forming the soft palate between the mouth and the nasopharynx.

pancreas Fish-shaped, grayish pink gland that stretches transversely across the posterior abdominal wall in the epigastric region of the body. It secretes various substances, such as digestive enzymes, insulin, and glucagon.

pancreatic juice Clear alkaline pancreatic secretion that contains at least three different enzymes (trypsin, amylopsin, and lipase). It is poured into the duodenum, where, mixed with bile and intestinal juices, it furthers the digestion of food.

paracentesis A procedure in which fluid is withdrawn from the abdominal cavity.

paradoxical Occurring at variance with the normal rule.

paramyxovirus Subgroup of viruses including parainfluenza, measles, mumps, German measles, and respiratory syncytial viruses.

parasite Any organism that grows, feeds, and is sheltered on or in a different organism while contributing nothing to the survival of the host.

parenchyma Essential parts of an organ that are concerned with its function.

paroxysmal Concerning the sudden, periodic attack or recurrence of symptoms of a disease.

particulate Made up of particles.

patent ductus Open, narrow, tubular channel.

pathogen Any agent causing disease, especially a microorganism.

pendelluft Shunting of air from one lung to another.

perforation Hole made through a substance or part.

peribronchial Located around the bronchi.

peripheral airways Small bronchi on the outer portion of the lung where most gas transfer takes place.

peritoneal dialysis Removal of toxic substances from the body by perfusing specific warm sterile chemical solutions through the peritoneal cavity.

perivascular Located around a vessel, especially a blood vessel.

permeability The quality of being permeable.

permeable Capable of allowing the passage of fluids or substances in solution.

pH Symbol for the logarithm of the reciprocal of the hydrogen ion concentration.

phagocytosis Envelopment and digestion of bacteria or other foreign bodies by cells.

phalanges Bones of the fingers or toes.

phenotype Physical makeup of an individual Some phenotypes, such as the blood groups, are completely determined by heredity, whereas others, such as stature, are readily altered by environmental agents.

phenylketonuria Abnormal presence of phenylketone in the urine.

phlegmasia alba dolens Acute edema, especially of the leg, from lymphatic or venous obstruction, usually a thrombosis.

phosgene Carbonyl chloride ($COCl_2$), a poisonous gas causing nausea and suffocation.

phosphodiesterase Enzyme that catalyzes the breakdown of the second messenger cyclic adenosine monophosphate to adenosine monophosphate.

plaque A flat, often raised patch on the skin mucous surface or any other organ of the body. A patch of atherosclerosis. Also called dental plaque, a usually thin film on the teeth.

pleomorphic Multiform; occurring in more than one form.

pleurisy Inflammation of the pleura.

pleuritis Inflammation of the pleura.

polyarteritis nodosa Necrosis and inflammation of small and medium-sized arteries and subsequent involvement of tissue supplied by these arteries.

polycythemia Excess of red blood cells.

polymorphonuclear leukocyte Subclass of white blood cells, including neutrophils, eosinophils, and basophils.

polyneuritis Inflammation of two or more nerves at once.

polyneuropathy Term applied to any disorder of peripheral nerves, but particularly used to describe those of a noninflammatory nature.

polyradiculitis Inflammation of nerve roots, especially those of spinal nerves as found in Guillain-Barré syndrome.

polyradiculoneuropathy Guillain-Barré syndrome.

postpartum Occurring after childbirth.

postural drainage Drainage of secretions from the bronchi or a cavity in the lung by positioning the patient so that gravity will allow drainage of the particular lobe or lobes of the lung involved.

pressure The quotient obtained by dividing a force by the area of the surface on which it acts.

primigravida A woman pregnant for the first time.

prognostic Related to prediction of the outcome of a disease.

proliferation Increasing or spreading at a rapid rate; the process or results of rapid reproduction.

prophylactic Any agent or regimen that contributes to the prevention of infection and disease.

propranolol Beta-adrenergic blocker drug used in treating cardiac arrhythmias, particularly supraventricular tachycardia.

prostaglandin F One of a group of fatty acid derivatives present in many tissues, including the prostate gland, menstrual fluid, brain, lung, kidney, thymus, seminal fluid, and pancreas. Prostaglandin F is believed to cause bronchoconstriction and vasoconstriction.

prostration A condition of extreme exhaustion.

proteolytic An enzyme producing proteolysis.

protocol(s) A standard way of performing work. Usually consists of algorithms involving diagnostic and therapeutic components (e.g., Mechanical Ventilation protocol) (see page 143).

proximal Nearest the point of attachment, center of the body, or point of reference.

pulmonary Concerning or involving the lungs.

pulmonary blood vessels Vessels that transport blood from the heart to the lungs and then back to the heart.

pulmonary circulation Passage of blood from the heart to the lungs and back again for gas exchange. The blood flows from the right ventricle to the lungs, where it is oxygenated and carbon dioxide is removed. The blood then flows back to the left atrium.

pulsus paradoxus An exaggeration of the normal variation in the pulse volume with respiration. The pulse becomes weaker with inspiration and stronger with expiration. Pulsus paradoxus is characteristic of constrictive pericarditis and pericardial effusion. The changes are independent of changes in pulse rate.

purulent Containing or forming pus.

radiopaque Impenetrable to X-radiation or other forms of radiation.

recumbent Lying down or leaning backward.

refractory Resistant to ordinary treatment; obstinate, stubborn.

remission Lessening of severity or abatement of symptoms; the period during which symptoms abate.

reticular formation Located in the brain stem, it acts as a filter from sense organs to the conscious brain. It analyzes incoming information for importance and influences alertness, waking, sleeping, and some reflexes.

ribonucleic acid (RNA) Nucleic acid occurring in the nucleus and cytoplasm of cells that is involved in the synthesis of proteins. The RNA molecule is a single strand made up of nucleotides.

roentgenogram Film produced by roentgenography. An X-ray.

roentgenography Process of obtaining X-rays by the use of roentgen rays.

scintillation camera Camera used to photograph the emissions that come from radioactive substances injected into the body.

semilunar valves Valves separating the left ventricle and aorta and right ventricle and pulmonary artery. The aortic and pulmonary valves.

semipermeable Permitting diffusion or flow of some liquids or particles but preventing the transmission of others, usually used in reference to a membrane.

septicemia Systemic disease caused by pathogenic organisms or toxins in the blood; may be a late development of any purulent infection.

septum Wall dividing two cavities.

serotonin Chemical present in platelets, gastrointestinal mucosa, mast cells, and carcinoid tumors; a potent vasoconstrictor.

serum (1) Clear, watery fluid, especially that moistening surfaces of serous membranes; (2) fluid exuded in inflammation of any of those membranes; (3) the fluid portion of the blood obtained after removal of the fibrin clot and blood cells; (4) sometimes used as a synonym for *antiserum.*

sibilant Hissing or whistling; applied to sounds heard in a certain crackle (or rhonchus).

sign Any objective evidence or manifestation of an illness or disordered function of the body. Signs are more or less definitive, obvious, and, apart from the patient's impressions, in contrast to symptoms, which are subjective.

silicate Salt of silicic acid.

sinus tachycardia Uncomplicated tachycardia when sinus cardiac rhythm is faster than 100 beats per minute.

smooth muscle Muscle tissue that lacks cross-striations on its fibers; involuntary in action and found principally in visceral organs.

somatic nerve Nerve that innervates somatic structures (i.e., those constituting the body wall and extremities).

spasm Involuntary sudden movement or convulsive muscular contraction. Spasms may be clonic or tonic.

sphygmomanometer Instrument for determining arterial blood pressure indirectly.

sputum Substance expelled by coughing or clearing the throat. It may contain cellular debris, mucus, blood, pus, caseous material, and microorganisms.

stasis Stagnation of the normal flow of fluids, as of the blood, urine, or intestinal mechanism.

status asthmaticus Persistent and intractable asthma.

streptokinase Enzyme produced by certain strains of streptococci, capable of converting plasminogen to plasmin.

stroke volume Amount of blood ejected by the ventricle at each beat.

subarachnoid space Space occupied by cerebrospinal fluid beneath the arachnoid membrane surrounding the brain and spinal cord.

subcutaneous Beneath the skin.

sulfur dioxide Common industrial air pollutant; causes bronchospasm and cell destruction.

superficial Confined to the surface.

superior vena cava Venous trunk draining blood from the head, neck, upper extremities, and chest. It begins by union of the two brachiocephalic veins, passes directly downward, and empties into the right atrium of the heart.

surface tension Condition at the surface of a liquid in contact with a gas or another liquid. It is the result of the mutual attraction of molecules to produce a cohesive state, which causes liquids to assume a shape presenting the smallest surface area to the surrounding medium. It accounts for the spherical shape assumed by fluids such as drops of oil or water.

surfactant Phospholipid substance important in controlling the surface tension of the air-liquid emulsion in the lungs; an agent that lowers the surface tension.

symmetric Equal correspondence in shape, size, and relative position of parts on opposite sides of the body.

sympathomimetic Producing effects resembling those resulting from stimulation of the sympathetic nervous system, such as the effects following the injection of epinephrine.

symptom Any perceptible change in the body or its functions that indicates disease or the phases of a disease. Symptoms may be classified as objective, subjective, cardinal, and sometimes constitutional. However, another classification considers all symptoms as being subjective, with objective indications being called *signs.*

syncope Transient loss of consciousness resulting from inadequate blood flow to the brain.

syncytial Group of cells in which the protoplasm of one cell is continuous with that of adjoining cells.

systemic Pertaining to the whole body rather than to one of its parts.

systemic reaction Whole-body response to a stimulus.

systole Part of the heart cycle in which the heart is in contraction.

systolic pressure Maximum blood pressure; occurs during contraction of the ventricle.

tachycardia Abnormal rapidity of heart action, usually defined as a heart rate greater than 100 beats per minute.

tachypnea A rapid breathing rate.

technetium 99m Radioisotope of technetium that emits α-rays; used in determining blood flow to certain organs by use of a scanning technique. It has a half-life of 6 hours.

tenacious Adhering to; adhesive; retentive.

tension of gas Gas pressure measured in millimeters of mercury (mm Hg).

thoracentesis Puncture of the chest wall for removal of fluid.

thrombocytopenia Abnormal decrease in the number of blood platelets.

thromboembolism Blood clot caused by an embolus obstructing a vessel.

thrombophlebitis Inflammation of a vein in conjunction with the formation of a thrombus; usually occurs in an extremity, most frequently a leg.

thrombus Blood clot that obstructs a blood vessel or a cavity of the heart.

thymectomy Surgical removal of the thymus gland.

thymus Ductless gland situated in the anterior mediastinal cavity that reaches maximum development during early childhood and then undergoes involution. It usually has two longitudinal lobes. An endocrine gland, the thymus is now thought to be a lymphoid body. It is a site of lymphopoiesis and plays a role in immunologic competence.

titer A measurement of the concentration of a substance in a solution.

tone That state of a body or any of its organs or parts in which the functions are healthy and normal. In a more restricted sense, the resistance of muscles to passive elongation or stretch; normal tension or responsiveness to stimuli.

toxemia The condition resulting from the spread of bacterial products via the bloodstream; toxemic condition resulting from metabolic disturbances.

toxin Poisonous substance of animal or plant origin.

trachea Largest airway; a fibroelastic tube found at the level of the sixth cervical vertebra to the fifth thoracic vertebra; carries air to and from the lungs. At the carina it divides into two bronchi, one leading to each lung. The trachea is lined with mucous membrane, and its inner surface is lined with ciliated epithelium.

tracheobronchial clearance Mechanisms by which the airways are cleared of foreign substances; the act of clearing the airways by mucociliary action, coughing, or macrophages.

tracheostomy Operation entailing cutting into the trachea through the neck, usually for insertion of a tube to overcome upper airway obstruction.

tracheotomy Incision of the skin, muscles, and trachea.

transfusion Injection of blood or a blood component into the bloodstream; transfer of the blood of one person into the blood vessels of another.

translucent Transmitting light, but diffusing it so that objects beyond are not clearly distinguishable.

transmission Transference of disease or infection.

transpulmonary pressure The pressure difference between the mouth and intrapleural pressure.

transverse Describing the state of something that is lying across or at right angles to something else; lying at right angles to the long axis of the body.

trauma Physical injury or wound caused by external forces.

tricuspid valve Right atrioventricular valve separating the right atrium from the right ventricle.

trypsin Proteolytic enzyme of the pancreas.

tuberculosis Infectious disease caused by the tubercle bacillus *Mycobacterium tuberculosis* and characterized by inflammatory infiltrations, formation of tubercles, caseation, necrosis, abscesses, fibrosis, and calcification. It most commonly affects the respiratory system.

ulcerate To produce or become affected with an open sore or lesion of the skin.

underventilation Reduced rate and depth of breathing.

uremia Toxic condition associated with renal insufficiency that is produced by retention in the blood of nitrogenous substances normally excreted by the kidney.

urokinase Enzyme obtained from human urine and used for dissolving intravascular clots. It is administered intravenously.

vaccinia A contagious disease of cattle that is produced in humans by inoculation with cowpox virus to confer immunity against smallpox.

vagus Pneumogastric or tenth cranial nerve. It is a mixed nerve, having motor and sensory functions and a wider distribution than any of the other cranial nerves.

varicella Chickenpox.

vasoconstriction Constriction of the blood vessels.

venous stasis Stagnation of the normal flow of blood caused by venous congestion.

ventilation Mechanical movement of air into and out of the lungs in a cyclic fashion. The activity is autonomic and voluntary and has two components—an inward flow of air, called *inhalation* or *inspiration*, and an outward flow, called *exhalation* or *expiration*.

ventricle Either of the two lower chambers of the heart. The right ventricle forces blood into the pulmonary artery, the left into the aorta.

vernix Protective fatty deposit covering the fetus.

visceral pleura Pleura that invests the lungs and enters into and lines the interlobar fissures.

viscosity Stickiness or gumminess; resistance offered by a fluid to change of form or relative position of its particles caused by the attraction of molecules to one another.

viscous Sticky; gummy; gelatinous.

viscus Any internal organ enclosed within a cavity such as the thorax or abdomen.

volume percent (vol%) The number of cubic centimeters (milliliters) of a substance contained in 100 cc (or ml) of another substance.

wheal More or less round and evanescent elevation of the skin, white in the center, with a red periphery. It is accompanied by itching and is seen in urticaria, insect bites, anaphylaxis, and angioneurotic edema.

xenon 133 Radioactive isotope of xenon used in photoscanning studies of the lung.

Index